ORAL MICROBIOLOGY

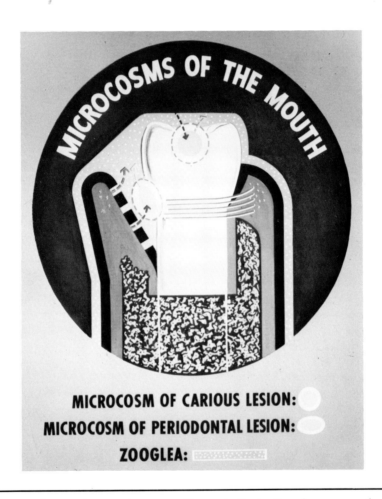

This schematic drawing depicts microcosms adherent to the tooth surface, one on the occlusal, and one in the periodontal pocket. The arrows indicate the route by which nutrients reach the microcosm, and the openings indicate the semipermeable nature of tissues and microcosm. The zooglea represents the sticky, tenacious, gelatinous coagulum that coats the teeth and mucous membranes; the zooglea also serves as an enveloping, semipermeable barrier within which the microcosm thrives. In addition to the colonized masses shown on the tooth surfaces, microcosms are found on the tongue, the mucous membranes, and the tonsils. (From Arnim, S. S.: J. Tenn. Dent. Assoc. **39**:1, 1959.)

ORAL MICROBIOLOGY

EDITED BY

William A. Nolte, B.S., M.S., Ph.D.

Professor and Chairman, Department of Microbiology,
The University of Texas at Houston Dental Branch,
Houston, Texas

With 270 illustrations

SECOND EDITION

The C. V. Mosby Company   SAINT LOUIS   1973

Contributors

HARRY BLECHMAN, B.S., D.D.S., M.A.

Dean, Professor, Department of Endodontics, New York University
College of Dentistry, New York, New York

PAUL R. COURANT, B.S., D.M.D.

Former Associate Professor of Periodontology, Boston University
School of Graduate Dentistry, Boston, Massachusetts

HEINER HOFFMAN, B.S., M.S., Ph.D., D.M.D.

Professor, Department of Microbiology, New York University
College of Dentistry, New York, New York

ISRAEL KLEINBERG, D.D.S., Ph.D.

Professor and Head, Biochemistry and Oral Biology (Graduate),
Faculty of Dentistry, The University of Manitoba,
Winnipeg, Manitoba, Canada

WILLIAM A. NOLTE, B.S., M.S., Ph.D.

Professor and Chairman, Department of Microbiology, The University
of Texas at Houston Dental Branch, Houston, Texas

SAMUEL ROSEN, B.A., M.S., Ph.D.

Professor of Dentistry, The Ohio State University College of
Dentistry, Columbus, Ohio

The price of teaching

It was his firm conviction that the teacher had failed in his intentions
if at the end of his discourse he was not mentally exhilarated and
physically exhausted.

Said of Noah Morris,
*late Professor of Therapeutics,
University of Glasgow*

Preface

The successful prevention and treatment of infectious diseases of man are related directly to knowledge of the microbial world. Most conditions that require dental treatment are directly or indirectly related to the metabolic activities and interrelationships of the indigenous oral microflora. Infectious diseases involving the teeth and supporting structures, such as dental caries, periodontal disease, and gingivitis, are of primary interest to the dental practitioner. Knowledge of the effect of these diseases on extraoral tissues and the recognition of oral manifestations of systemic diseases are his concern also, as a member of the health team. Therefore, knowledge of the fundamental principles of microbiology involving the characteristics of the infecting agent and the response of the host to infection is necessary in a course in microbiology for dental students.

This second edition has been brought up to date with current information that is considered to be essential and should be of interest to the dental student. This book follows the same sequence of chapter arrangement as the first edition. It considers the indigenous oral microflora in the role of the nonpathogen as well as the pathogen. It also considers important infectious diseases about which the dental student should be knowledgeable. This book has been written primarily as a text for the dental student. Details of technique have been excluded, since this basic information should be obtained from a general text or other selective sources. For the practicing dentist, this book may serve as a reference for basic as well as recent information on dental infectious diseases.

The chapters written by the late Dr. Henry Bartels have been rewritten and stress, with increased emphasis, the relationship between the cause, treatment, and prevention of dental disease of microbial origin.

This book represents the efforts of a number of contributors and those who assisted them. Appreciation is expressed by Dr. Heiner Hoffman to Mr. Gino Merlino and Dr. Sami Schaefler of the New York University College of Dentistry, and to his wife Claire for her steadfast encouragement; by Dr. Israel Kleinberg to Mrs. E. Okrainec and Dr. D. Summerfield of The University of Manitoba; by Dr. Sam Rosen to Miss Pamela Davis and Mr. Ralph Ulbrich of The Ohio State University College of Dentistry.

As editor, I wish to express my appreciation to Mrs. Judy Womack, Mrs. Sylvia Lacy, Miss Fern Fetters, and Mr. Reagan Brady of The University of Texas at Houston Dental Branch. Also, thanks is extended to each contributor for the special effort that made possible this second edition.

William A. Nolte

Contents

PART THREE   Control of microorganisms

ORAL MICROBIOLOGY

PART ONE / THE ORAL MICROFLORA AND THE HOST

1 / Oral ecology

MICROBIAL RELATIONSHIPS

Study of the relationships of microorganisms with one another and with their environment is called ecology. All forms of life are influenced in some way by the environment in which they live. Oral ecology, therefore, is a study of the interrelationships of members of the oral microflora and the influence of the oral environment on this microflora. Environmental factors appear to have a selective action on microbial populations. The environment seems to favor those microorganisms that possess the same or similar chemical, physical, and biologic properties. Of the environmental factors, nutrition appears to play an important role controlling the types and numbers of microbial populations in a community. The nutritional interrelationships of mixed microbial populations can be understood more completely when the nutritional requirements of individual types of the population are known.

An ecologic study is an investigation of the relationships of ecosystems, which are composed of abiotic factors, the habitat, and the biotic community, the microbial forms living in the habitat. The kind of nutrients in a microbial ecosystem is one of the most important factors that determines and controls the type of community that develops. Microbial communities vary in complexity. For example, if but one kind of food is available and its utilization by a specific organism results in degradative products that do not serve as food for other microorganisms, a simple community of this specific organism develops. Foods of animal and plant origin are chemically complex and favor the development and support of mixed microbial communities. Since man consumes these foods, mixed microbial populations inhabit the oral cavity and digestive tract.

A study of oral microbial ecosystems requires consideration of both quantitative and qualitative relationships between microorganisms. The effect of environment over a long period of time will be the selection of microorganisms best suited to survive in the oral cavity. Microbial associations nearly always exist even though different types may occupy separate niches differing perhaps in only one influential environmental factor. Those microorganisms that grow best in the absence of oxygen or at low oxygen tension in a mixed community live in those niches in which oxygen is reduced or eliminated.

The association between different kinds of microorganisms may be beneficial to both, may be beneficial to only one member, or may be detrimental to one or more members of the community. These complex interrelationships between microorganisms have been referred to as symbiosis, commensalism, antibiosis, and synergism. "Symbiosis" means the mutual beneficial relationships between two types of microorganisms; an example is anaerobes growing with aerobes. The aerobic microorganisms utilize atmospheric oxygen and create a low oxidation-reduction potential favorable for the growth of the anaerobes. In the oral cavity the accumulations of bacterial growth about the teeth, especially at the gingival margin and in the sulcus, where serum exudates flow, create an environment favorable for anaerobic microbial communities. For example, the spirochete *Treponema microdentium* is dependent on other organisms and the gingival sulcus anaerobic environment for survival.[22] The next microbial relationship is termed "commensalism," an association in which one species benefits while the other species is unaffected. A relationship between oral microorganisms showing commensalism may be demonstrated between *Bacteroides melaninogenicus* growing as a satellite colony within a *Staphylococcus aureus* colony on a blood plate. The *melaninogenicus* microorganisms require a vitamin K-like substance which is provided by the growing staphylococci. Rosebury[27] introduced the term "amphibiosis" for commensalism, since the indigenous flora can be beneficial or can cause disease. The indigenous microflora does not appear to be essential for life, because animals can be raised free of bacteria. The indigenous microflora does, nevertheless, contribute significantly to our overall nutrition, especially that microflora of the intestines which synthesizes large amounts of the B vitamins (riboflavin, thiamine, nicotinic acid, pantothenic acid) and vitamin K. Vitamins synthesized by organisms in the mouth and those contained within the microbial cells are swallowed. It is possible also that the oral flora may be of nutritional significance to man.[17] "Antibiosis" is a relationship of antagonism. An example is the inhibitory effect on proteolytic microbial types by accumulated acids that result from carbohydrate breakdown

by lactobacilli. Certain bacteria have been shown to produce substances called *bacteriocins*. The formative bacterial strains are active against some strains of the same or closely related species only. Certain indigenous oral streptococci produce bacteriocins that are antagonistic for *Streptococcus pyogenes* and some enterococcus strains, but not against unrelated bacteria. It has been suggested that bacteriocins may influence the intraspecies' stability in mixed microfloras.[18] The final relationship is termed "synergism," a relationship in which several organisms produce a reaction that neither can produce when growing alone. Vincent's infection of the oral cavity is often given as an example. There is a direct association here between the clinical picture of Vincent's infection and the tremendous increase in numbers of fusiform bacilli and spirochetes, as shown in smears of material made from infected mucosa.

In the relationship between the microorganism and the host, the former is known as the parasite. A parasitic microorganism is one capable of living and multiplying in or on the host body. When the proper condition presents itself, such as traumatic injury to tissue cells, the parasite may set up infection. When this happens the parasitic microorganism is frequently referred to as an opportunist.

The intrinsic sources of nutrient for microorganisms in the oral cavity are the materials from around the teeth, the exudates, epithelial cells undergoing degradation, and to some degree the salivary components. Whole saliva has been found to contain eighteen free amino acids, including aspartic acid, glutamic acid, threonine, serine, glycine, alanine, phenylalanine, leucine, isoleucine, proline, cystine, valine, methionine, tyrosine, tryptophan, histidine, lysine and arginine. Other intrinsic nutrients are hyaluronic acid and chondroitin sulfate, the principle carbohydrates of dentin. Cariogenic streptococci can use these compounds as carbon sources in their metabolism.[34] In addition, the food that we eat for our own nourishment serves as nutrient for oral microorganisms, from an extrinsic source. These two sources furnish the nutritional requirements necessary for the synthesis of protoplasm and for cell multiplication of the oral microbiota. Krasse[21] considers the intrinsic source the more important of the nutritional needs in stabilizing the oral flora.

For microorganisms to increase in size and multiply, certain types of nutritional and physiochemical environmental factors are required. The nutritional requirements for growth of parasitic microorganisms are: (1) compounds required as an energy source (carbohydrates); (2) compounds required for building new protoplasm (sources of carbon and nitrogen); (3) organic compounds required as growth factors; and (4) inorganic ions required as enzyme activators. Growth factors are organic compounds that are needed by the organism but which it cannot synthesize; therefore, these compounds must be supplied as nutrients. For example, the B vitamins and certain amino acids are required by lactobacilli, inositol is required by yeast, and a factor referred to as "K" is required for the growth of *Bacteroides melaninogenicus*. In addition to nutrients, the physiochemical requirements are favorable temperature, pH, carbon dioxide, oxygen tension, and moisture.

The process by which microorganisms obtain energy from substances from the environment is known as chemosynthesis. Microorganisms able to grow on organic substances are classified as heterotrophs or organotrophs. Heterotrophic types can be cultivated on artificial organic media in the laboratory. The microorganisms that constitute the normal oral microflora belong to the heterotrophic type. Other types of microorganisms, the viruses classified as hypotrophs, require living cells for their growth. These microorganisms lack the necessary enzyme systems needed to re-produce, and, therefore, they parasitize directly the enzyme systems of the host; they grow within the host's cells. A third type of microorganism, the autotrophs or lithotrophs, lives on inorganic substances. These microorganisms have complete enzyme systems and are able to manufacture from inorganic substances all the components required for their growth. Examples of this latter group are the sulphur and iron bacteria.

METHODS OF STUDYING THE ORAL MICROFLORA

The microflora of the oral cavity consists of bacteria, yeast, certain fungi, PPLO (pleuropneumonia-like organisms) forms, viruses, and protozoa. Each of these microbial forms has characteristic morphologic and physiologic properties that are controlled genetically.

The science of microbiology was born with the discovery of the simple microscope by Anton Van Leeuwenhoek around 1683 and his reporting the existence of small forms of life that could not be seen with the naked eye. Although Van Leeuwenhoek was the first to observe microorganisms in saliva and in material about the teeth, little advance in knowledge concerning microbial inhabitants of the oral cavity was made until about 1890 after the germ theory of disease was established and culture and staining techniques had developed. The first great worker in the field of dental microbiology who had a lasting influence in encouraging scientific investigations was W. D. Miller.

Today there are various types of microscopes: the brightfield, the darkfield, and phase contrast. These microscopes have a maximum magnification of 1,000× and are used to view and study the microbial characteristics of bacteria, yeast, molds, protozoa, PPLO forms, and rickettsiae. The size of these microscopic forms is measured in microns (μ) or the present equivalent unit of measurement, micrometer (μm).

A micron or micrometer is 0.001 of a millimeter or about 1/25 400 of an inch.

Except for Chapter 5, this book will refer to the old units of measurement, of which some of the important ones compare with present units as follows:

Present	EQUIVALENTS		Old	
Unit	*Symbol*		*Unit*	*Symbol*
micrometer	μm.	10^{-3} mm.	micron	μ
nanometer	nm.	10^{-6} mm.	millimicron	mμ

Since the brightfield microscope cannot resolve clearly particles that are less than 0.2 μ in diameter, minute forms such as the viruses cannot be seen with this type of microscope. Viral forms require an instrument that has a much higher resolving power, the electron microscope. It has an initial magnification of 20,000× to 50,000× and this can be increased by photographic enlargement to 1,000,000×. The unit of measurement of virus particles is the millimicron (mμ), or nanometer (nm.), 0.000001 of a millimeter. The relative size of different types of microorganisms, many of which are indigenous to the oral cavity, is shown in Fig. 1-1.

Although oral microorganisms were among the first to be observed by man, interest in oral microbiology lagged. Perhaps one of the reasons is that oral disease was not considered dangerous since the pain associated with a toothache could be easily remedied by extraction of the tooth. When it became apparent that the oral microflora did influence systemic diseases of the body, an interest was aroused in the nature and kinds of oral microorganisms in both the healthy and the diseased mouth.

To study the microflora of the oral cavity, two basic techniques have been employed, the direct smear and the culture plate. The first technique involves the direct smear made with material removed from different localities of the oral cavity, stained, and observed under the microscope. From these smears one learns something about the various morphologic types of microorganisms and their selective locations. Determinations of the numbers as well as microbial types may be made by employing techniques known as the Breed and the hemacytometer methods.

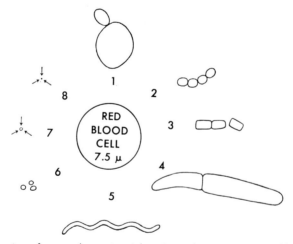

Fig. 1-1. Relative size of yeast, bacteria, rickettsiae, pleuropneumonia-like organisms, and viruses as compared with the red blood cell: **1,** *Candida albicans,* 2 to 3 μ by 4 to 6 μ; **2,** *Streptococcus salivarius,* 0.8 to 1.0 μ; **3,** *Lactobacillus casei,* 0.7 to 1.5 μ; **4,** *Leptotrichia buccalis,* 1 to 1.5 μ by 5 to 15 μ; **5,** *Borrelia vincentii,* 0.3 μ by 8 to 12 μ; **6,** *Rickettsia prowazekii,* 0.3 μ by 0.3 to 0.5 μ; **7,** pleuropneumonia-like organisms, 0.15 μ; **8,** serum hepatitis virus, 0.025 μ or 25 mμ.

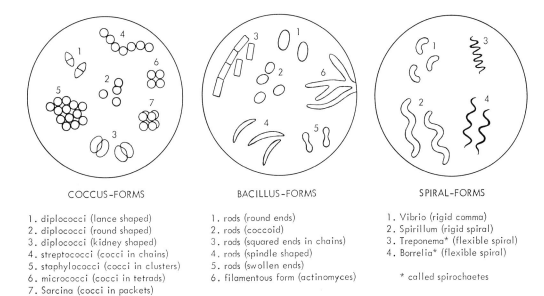

COCCUS-FORMS

1. diplococci (lance shaped)
2. diplococci (round shaped)
3. diplococci (kidney shaped)
4. streptococci (cocci in chains)
5. staphylococci (cocci in clusters)
6. micrococci (cocci in tetrads)
7. Sarcina (cocci in packets)

BACILLUS-FORMS

1. rods (round ends)
2. rods (coccoid)
3. rods (squared ends in chains)
4. rods (spindle shaped)
5. rods (swollen ends)
6. filamentous form (actinomyces)

SPIRAL-FORMS

1. Vibrio (rigid comma)
2. Spirillum (rigid spiral)
3. Treponema* (flexible spiral)
4. Borrelia* (flexible spiral)

* called spirochaetes

Fig. 1-2. Morphologic types of bacteria.

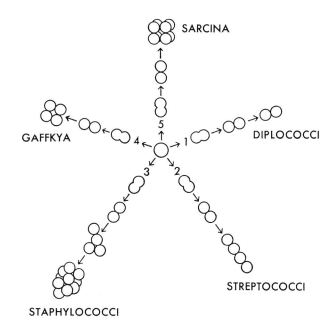

Fig. 1-3. Arrangements of cocci. Arrangement depends upon plane of division and attachment of cells after division. **1,** Diplococci occur generally in pairs; cell division is in one plane. **2,** Streptococci occur generally in chains; cell division is in one plane. **3,** Staphylococci occur in grapelike clusters; cell division is in three planes. **4,** *Gaffkya* organisms occur in groups of four; cell division is in two planes. **5,** Sarcinae occur in packets of eight; cell division is in three planes.

From the direct smears various forms such as cocci, bacilli, and spiral types can be distinguished (Fig. 1-2). Differences in the shapes of cocci (such as round, coffee-bean shaped or lenticular) and variations in the cellular arrangement (such as single, pairs, irregular masses, chains of cells and packets of four or eight) furnish additional information. Fig. 1-3 shows some of the different arrangements of cocci. When it comes to the bacilli or rod forms, one can distinguish their relative sizes as to diameter and length, whether they are pointed at one end or both, and whether they remain attached and form chains or occur singly or in pairs. Spiral forms are either rigid or flexible. The vibrio are short, single or united, and curved, and the spirilla are helicoidal or many-curved forms. Both of these are rigid. The flexible spiral forms constitute a group of organisms known as the spirochetes. In observing spirochetes darkfield microscopy is preferred to the use of fixed stained smears. In the former, spirochetes are observed in suspension and their coiled shape and movement can be studied, whereas in the direct smear the coiled shape of spirochetes is distorted.

Although the direct smear technique does furnish certain information regarding the basic morphologic types that inhabit the oral cavity, it does not furnish information as to species, such as fusobacteria, *Vibrio*, and *Selenomonas* as well as some cocci and short rod forms. Some streptococci may assume coccobacillus forms and some rods may appear coccoid in form. It is known that *Nocardia* and *Actinomyces* under certain culture conditions assume coccoid forms. It is possible that in the oral cavity these organisms may also assume such variations in shape. Therefore, a direct smear count as to types of microorganisms has limitations. The direct smear technique is used to determine the total number of microorganisms, both living and dead, re-

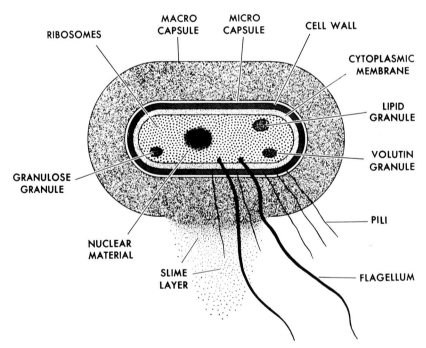

Fig. 1-4. Diagrammatic concept of a composite bacterial cell. Not all bacteria possess all of these structures, nor can certain ones of these structures be demonstrated in all bacteria of the same species.

moved from specific areas of the oral cavity.

By using selective staining techniques in preparing a fixed smear, one can learn something about the morphologic characteristics or anatomy of the bacterial cell. Gram's method is a differential staining technique and, when applied, shows that bacteria can be fairly well separated into two groups; one group gram-positive, which stains violet, and the other group gram-negative, which stains red. This difference in gram staining bears a relationship with certain chemical differences in the cell wall of bacteria.

Another differential staining technique determines the acid-fast property of certain microorganisms such as members of the genera *Mycobacterium* and *Nocardia*. This differential staining technique also aids in the separation of microorganisms based upon certain specific chemical differences.

Some of the more important structures of the bacterial cell and characteristics of these structures are presented in Fig. 1-4.

Capsule or slime layer
Macrocapsule

1. The macrocapsule is an extracellular slime, highly viscous, that adheres firmly to the cell wall of certain bacterial species.
2. True slime differs from capsular material in that it is more soluble, is easily lost from the cell, and does not assume the shape of the cell by which it is produced.
3. The capsule assumes the shape of the cell but is not an essential part of the bacterial cell. It probably originates as a secretion from the cell wall.
4. The presence of the capsule is genetically controlled and is determined by the environment under which the bacterium is growing. The presence of carbohydrates, serum, and ascitic fluid favors formation of capsular material by certain microorganisms. The anthrax bacillus forms a capsule when growing in the animal host. *Aerobacter aerogenes* forms its capsule in carbohydrate media when growth is slowing down. *Streptococcus salivarius* forms a heavy capsule in media containing 5% sucrose.
5. Capsule-forming cells develop colonies which have a glistening appearance and are mucoid. When touched with an inoculating needle, they prove to be of a stringy texture.
6. Smears made from mucoid colonies require a special staining technique, since capsular material is soluble in water and may be dissolved from the cell during preparation. The suspending medium can be serum or milk, and the smear may be stained by any of several methods, among them Anthony's and Frazer's methods.
7. Capsules appear to protect the cell from drying and from harmful environmental factors. Certain pathogenic microorganisms (pneumococcus, Friedländer's bacillus, influenza bacillus, anthrax bacillus, the plague bacillus, and others) form capsules that appear to protect the bacterial cell from phagocytosis.
8. Capsules are antigenic. Those that are chemically different from each other also are antigenically different. Pneumococci are separated into more than seventy different types based upon the chemical difference of their capsular material, which material reacts only with its specific antiserum. When an unknown capsulated pneumococcus is brought into contact with a specific antiserum, the capsule about the cell appears to swell if the unknown pneumococcus has the same type of polysaccharide material as was used in preparing the antiserum. The swelling of the capsular material, known as the quellung reaction, is used in diagnosis.

9. The chemical compositions of capsular materials differ in that some are polysaccharide, some are polypeptide, and others are complexes of these. Capsular material is continuous and appears to help hold the cells together after division leading to chain formation has occurred. Hyaluronic acid, a mucopolysaccharide, is one of the components of capsular material of certain streptococci. When such a streptococcus produces the enzyme hyaluronidase, it dissolves its own capsular material; the organism no longer appears in long chains, but rather it appears in pairs and in short chains of two and four cells.

Microcapsule

1. The microcapsule is a very thin layer close to the outer part of the cell wall and is formed by gram-negative bacteria.
2. The microcapsule is a lipopolysaccharide protein complex material and is antigenic.
3. Known as a somatic antigen or endotoxin, the microcapsule is thought to be responsible for the generalized physiopathologic changes associated with enteric infections.

Flagella

1. Flagella are delicate structures between 12 and 15 mμ in diameter and several times the length of the cell. Each flagellum consists of two or three fibrils twisted helically around each other to form a single unit.
2. Flagella originate from a granule within the cytoplasmic membrane.
3. Flagella are antigenic and are composed largely of protein (98%), with traces of carbohydrate and fat.
4. The formation of flagella is genetically controlled, but environmental factors influence their presence. They are generally found in young cultures growing slightly below the optimum temperature.
5. Flagella are difficult to stain but can be demonstrated by methods such as Leifson's in which the stain is precipitated or built up on the flagella.
6. Various arrangements and numbers of flagella are characteristic of different species and aid in classification. There are two main arrangements: (1) location of a single flagellum or a tuft of flagella at one or both ends (polar) of the bacterial cell; and (2) arrangement of many flagella about the entire bacterial cell.
7. Flagella are associated with motility, and some microorganisms can move at rates of between 25 and 200 μ per second.

Pili

1. Pili, extremely small structures about one-half the thickness of a flagellum or less, are between 100 and 300 mμ long. These structures surround the cell and vary in number between one hundred and two hundred per cell.
2. They are protein in nature and can be seen only with the electron microscope.
3. They are associated with gram-negative cells and are found on both motile and nonmotile bacteria. Their presence is not associated with motility.
4. They appear to function as organs of attachment and may agglutinate red blood cells.
5. Pili probably originate in the cytoplasmic membrane.
6. One or two pili appear to be special in that they are hollow and form a bridge in conjugation through which DNA is transferred from male to female cells.

Cell wall

1. The cell wall maintains the rigidity of the cell. It is several layers thick and

has some degree of ductility. The shape maintained by the cell appears to be associated with muramic acid.

2. The cell wall protects the vital part, the cytoplasmic membrane and its contents.

3. The wall can be demonstrated with the electron microscope. In old cultures in which the wall is partially broken down, the ghostlike structures seen are remnants of the cell wall. Plasmolyzing experiments cause the cell contents to shrink from the cell wall, allowing this rigid structure to be seen. The cell wall has a low affinity for dye but can be stained intensely with a mordant such as tannic acid (Webb's technique).

4. Of a porosity between 1 and 2 mμ, the cell wall possesses selective permeability.

5. The cell wall is between 10 and 25 mμ thick. Gram-positive bacteria possess thicker cell walls than do gram-negative bacteria.

6. The cell wall represents approximately 20% dry weight of the bacterial cell. Chemically it is composed of complexes of protein, lipids, and polysaccharides and is antigenic. Gram-negative cell walls are more complex than are the walls of gram-positive cells; gram-positive cells contain 0% to 2% lipids and 35% to 60% polysaccharides, while gram-negative cells contain 10% to 20% lipids and 15% to 20% polysaccharides. Lysozyme can hydrolize the cell wall of certain bacteria. When this occurs the living portion, the cytoplasm and its contents, is set free and becomes a spheric structure called the protoplast.

Cytoplasmic membrane

1. The outermost structure of the living portion of the cell, the cytoplasmic membrane, is encased within the cell wall.

2. Special staining techniques and plasmolyzing experiments are able to show the membrane.

3. The cytoplasmic membrane possesses selective permeability and represents from 10% to 20% dry weight of the cell.

4. The membrane is between 5 and 10 mμ thick; chemically of high lipid content, it contains between 20% and 25% lipid material.

5. The passage of material into and out of the cell by means of some type of transport system is controlled by the cytoplasmic membrane.

6. The membrane has little strength or rigidity and is forced against the inside of the cell wall by a hydrostatic pressure of about 20 atmospheres.

7. Invaginations of the cytoplasmic membrane form intracellular structures known as mesosomes, which appear to be sites of cytochrome enzymic activity.

Cytoplasm

Cytoplasm is the active, living material of the cell. In young cells it appears homogeneous and stains uniformly, whereas in old cells it is granular and stains unevenly. It contains ribosomes, various granules, nuclear material, and other structures.

Ribosomes

Ribosomes are ribonucleic acid–complexed protein particles, about 200 A in diameter. These particles stain very intensely with basic dyes and are distributed throughout the cytoplasm. Each cell may contain from 10,000 to 50,000 or more such particles. They appear to possess enzymic activity that synthesizes protein material.

Granules

Granules are deposits of reserved food but are not permanent structures of the cell since they disappear during periods of starvation. The types of granules that are commonly seen in microorganisms associated with the microflora of man are (1) metachromatic granules, also called volutin, that appear to contain metaphosphate, (2) fat or lipid granules, and (3) glycogen and starch granules. All of these bodies can be demonstrated with special staining techniques.

Chromatin material

Intracellular bodies of chromatin material have been shown to contain DNA when stained according to the Feulgen method. The DNA does not appear to be bound by a definite membrane as do nuclei characteristic of higher animals and plants. These bodies are difficult to demonstrate by staining since the entire bacterial cell stains uniformly with basic dyes because of its acid nature. The RNA–complexed protein particles, distributed throughout the cytoplasm of the bacterial cell, mask the DNA material because they, too, stain with basic dyes. In the demonstration of the presence of DNA (nuclear) material within a bacterial cell, the RNA protein particles are hydrolyzed either with ribonuclease or by treatment with one normal hydrochloric acid heated to 60° C. for 5 to 15 minutes. After this treatment the cell is stained with a basic dye such as Schiff's reagent used in Feulgen's test. The stained bodies are chromatin (DNA). If, after the hydrolysis treatment to destroy the RNA particles, the bacteria are exposed to deoxyribonuclease, the DNA material cannot be demonstrated in bacteria.

Experiments have demonstrated that during the growth of a bacterial culture, if small samples are removed at various intervals, hydrolyzed to destroy the RNA material, and then stained by the Feulgen method, the DNA material can be observed to divide as the cell divides. This would indicate that the DNA material contains the genetic characteristics of the bacterial cell.

Endospores

1. Of the bacteria that form endospores, members of the genera *Bacillus* and *Clostridium* are the most important.

2. The endospore may be considered a resistant phase in the life cycle of members of these genera. The spore resists chemicals, boiling water, and drying and does not take up stains by ordinary methods.

3. One spore forms within one vegetative cell undergoing sporulation. Therefore, it is not considered a method of multiplication. The spore may be located centrally, terminally, or subterminally. It may be the same size as the vegetative cell in which it forms, or may have a great diameter causing the cell to swell. Spores are either spheric or elliptical and differ in size.

4. The spore contains the living part of the cell from which it forms: the core containing chromatinic material, proteins, lipids, carbohydrates enzymes, minerals, and less water and a greater calcium content than the vegetative cell. The spore contains the compound dipicolinic acid, which is absent from vegetative cells and appears to be associated with heat resistance. Spores demonstrate low metabolic activity. The core is surrounded by a cortex and spore coat. Under favorable environmental conditions of moisture, nutrients, temperature, and oxygen tension, the spore germinates into an activity-multiplying vegetative cellular form.

To determine the living or viable microbial cells from oral material, the second basic technique, the culture plate, is employed. Material may be obtained from the oral cavity by using a sterile cotton swab, by scraping with a dental instrument or scalpel, or by securing a salivary sample, either stimulated or unstimulated. For the former salivary sample, the person may chew a piece of paraffin to stimulate his saliva. The samples may be streaked directly onto enriched culture media or they may be inoculated onto selective media. These streaked plates allow qualitative evaluation of the types of organisms present in the sample. Quantitative evaluation can be obtained by weighing the sample, making suitable dilutions, and then plating specific amounts of the dilutions on either enriched or selective media. Enriched media such as brain heart infusion agar and trypticase soy agar alone or fortified with serum or blood are frequently used to give the total number of cultivable microorganisms, whereas selective media such as Niven's medium, Rogosa's lactate medium, Rogosa's S L agar, Omata-Disraely agar, and Nickerson's medium give the numbers of specific microorganisms such as *Streptococcus salivarius*, *Veillonella*, lactobacilli, fusiform bacilli, and yeast for the respective media. On selective media the numbers of viable cells of specific organisms can be estimated.

The total count of microbial cells observed by the direct smear varies considerably from the total viable count obtained by culturing. The direct microscopic smear always gives higher counts. The ratio of the smear count to the cultivable count has been estimated as 40 to 1 or higher. In other words, the cultivation technique grows approximately only one microorganism out of forty. This does not necessarily mean that the remaining microorganisms are dead. It is known that selective media will not grow all of the specific microbial types for which they are selective. Selective media do have inhibitory effects even for some of the viable microorganisms they favor. Comparison of the number of fusiform bacilli in a direct smear made from a person having Vincent's gingivitis with the number of colonies of this organism developed on a selective medium shows that only a very small number of the bacilli are able to grow. The cells seen in the smear give evidence of normal morphologic traits and

stain uniformly, important characteristics of viable cells. It appears that many of the viable cells of the fusiform bacilli are not able to grow on the selective medium.

Enriched media will support the growth of larger numbers of specific microorganisms than will selective media, but these media cannot be used successfully in quantitative selective determinations. For example in gingival debris material, fastidious organisms such as the fusiform bacilli are not able to establish themselves early on enriched media; and in competition with other less fastidious organisms, they are either overgrown or inhibited. Selective media are of value in comparative studies for specific microorganisms of the oral cavity in health and in disease.

In order to determine the numbers of cultivable microorganisms, two sets of culture plates should be inoculated. One set should be incubated under aerobic conditions and the second set under anaerobic conditions. It is thought that when exposed to air anaerobic bacteria produce small amounts of hydrogen peroxide. Since strict anaerobes lack the enzyme catalase, this peroxide accumulates in the media to toxic concentrations and inhibits growth. Aerobic organisms possessing the enzyme catalase are able to degrade hydrogen peroxide as it is formed and thus prevent toxic concentration buildup. Another explanation is that atmospheric oxygen is not necessarily toxic for anaerobic organisms if the medium in which they are inoculated has an eH sufficiently low. The eH of the medium should be at least as low as −0.2 volts. The majority of microorganisms cultivated from the oral cavity are neither strict aerobes nor strict anaerobes. These organisms grow in either the presence or the absence of oxygen and are called facultative anaerobes. Strict anaerobic microorganisms do make up an important part of the oral microflora.

There are some microbial forms that are seen in the direct smear but have not been cultivated in the laboratory. For example, the organisms *Leptothrix racemosa* and *L. falciformis* have not been successfully cultivated on laboratory culture media. These two are considered complex microorganisms. There are also those organisms, the viruses and the PPLO forms, which will not grow on routine culture media and, therefore, are not easily detected. Spirochetes are difficult organisms to grow; their presence and numbers are generally determined in hanging-drop preparations made from dilutions of the test material and are observed under darkfield microscopy. Spirochetes indigenous to the oral cavity belong to the genera *Borrelia* and *Treponema*.

MAN'S ACQUISITION OF ORAL MICROFLORA

The oral cavity is accessible to the introduction of many different types of microorganisms. The microorganisms in water, foods, and air and on the hands readily gain entrance to the oral cavity. It has been stated that nearly every microorganism that has been identified has been isolated at one time or another from the oral cavity. The oral microflora is large in number and variable in type.

The oral cavity might be considered an ideal microbial incubator. It possesses a temperature of around 35° to 36° C. and has an abundance of moisture, an excellent supply of various types of foods, and differences in oxygen tension. Many aerobic, facultative, and anaerobic types find conditions favorable for their growth.

In the oral cavity, the microfloras differ basically with differences in the oral anatomy. The microbial population that forms on the surfaces of the crown of teeth differs collectively from those microbial forms that inhabit the gingival pocket and these differ from those found on the tongue and mucous membrane of the cheek. The salivary microbial population represents those microbial forms that are freed from

all oral surfaces as the result of the washing effect of the saliva.

What constitutes the normal microflora? The terms normal and indigenous are synonymous. It is difficult in some instances to distinguish between the indigenous and the transient. The indigenous microfloras are generally considered those that are ubiquitously present in man. They constitute a high percentage of the microbial population at any site; whereas the transient microfloras constitute only a small percentage and are not always present in a given site. For example, viridans streptococci are indigenous to the oral cavity, whereas coliform are considered transients; staphylococci are indigenous to the skin, whereas beta streptococci are transients. A third category referred to as supplementary is applied to those microorganisms detected in a significant percentage of the population, but not present in all. The oral lactobacilli are an example.[17]

The present concept of normal is dependent upon the techniques employed in obtaining the sample material, the types of culture media used, the conditions of incubation, the biochemical test used in classifying the cultivable microorganisms, and the techniques of direct wet and stained preparations. Although these techniques have limitations, the findings obtained describe the oral flora of the majority of subjects, young and old, living under specific environmental conditions.

Studies of the indigenous oral flora of man should begin with the first appearance of microorganisms in the oral cavity. This means that analysis of the oral flora should begin with the newborn. At birth, the mouth of the baby may be sterile or may be contaminated with several types of microorganisms including staphylococci, streptococci, coliform bacilli, and gram-positive rods. The source of these bacteria is the environment of which the child is gradually exposed during and after birth. The child comes in contact first with the microflora of the mother's vagina and then with the local environment of the outside world. The early oral microflora after birth is mainly aerobic and facultatively anaerobic. *Streptococcus salivarius* early establishes itself in the oral cavity of infants. In a study, it was isolated from most infants the day after birth and represented less than 1% of the total numbers of cultivated bacteria.[4] *S. sanguis* has been demonstrated in the mouths of infants only after the eruption of teeth, whereas *S. mutans* was not isolated during the first year.[9] The anaerobe *Veillonella alcalescens* has occasionally been isolated from infants less than two days old and regularly from infants after one week. The anaerobic fusiform bacilli have been cultivated from the mouth of infants younger than two months and from nearly all babies before the eruption of the first incisors. Fusiform bacilli appear to increase in number during the fourth and eighth months, and *Peptostreptococcus anaerobus* is reported to make its appearance in infants older than five months. The dominant flora of the oral cavity of the child before the eruption of teeth is mainly facultative in nature; with the eruption of teeth there is an increase in anaerobic forms.

According to a study of oral samples from newborn and one-year-old infants, *Streptococcus* was the only microorganism continuously cultured in quantities. Streptococci were reported to represent 98% of the cultivable microorganisms in initial samples, but declined to 70% at the end of the first year. Other microorganisms that were constantly present during the first year were staphylococci, *Veillonella*, and *Neisseria*. *Actinomyces*, lactobacilli, *Nocardia*, and fusiform bacilli were isolated from approximately one half of the infants, whereas species of *Bacteroides*, *Corynebacterium*, *Candida*, *Leptotrichia*, and coliform types were isolated from less than half. The dominant species of streptococci isolated from one half of the newborn was *Streptococcus salivarius*.

The quantitative and qualitative relationships of oral microorganisms change with the appearance of the dentition, the loss of the dentition, the use of artificial dentures, the type of diet, the subject's oral hygienic practices, and the degree of health or disease.

With the eruption of teeth there is an increase in anaerobic forms, the *Leptotrichia*, spirochetes, fusiform bacilli, spiral forms, and *Vibrio*. With partial loss of teeth, this microflora persists only where the teeth remain. The presence of fusiform bacilli and spirochetes appears to be associated with the natural dentition. Complete loss of the dentition causes a reversion of the microflora to a predominantly anaerobic facultative type. Anaerobic forms generally reappear with the wearing of dentures. In the neglected or diseased mouth, the bacterial types are mainly anaerobic and proteolytic, whereas in the well-kept mouth the dominant flora is mainly aerobic, facultative, and acidogenic.

The number of microorganisms that can be removed from the oral cavity by mouth rinsing varies throughout the day. Fig. 1-5 shows the variations in numbers of microorganisms that may be removed from the oral cavity by mouth rinsing. It is observed that bacterial counts are highest in the morning upon arising. As a result of eating breakfast, brushing the teeth, and rinsing the mouth, these numbers decrease. A gradual increase is noted before the noonday meal; after the meal a decrease occurs. A pattern of an increase followed by a decrease is seen after the evening meal. Counts taken the following morning are the highest and reflect the long, overnight incubation period.

There is considerable variation in the numbers of microorganisms cultured or determined by direct counts from oral samples. No doubt, the variations are the

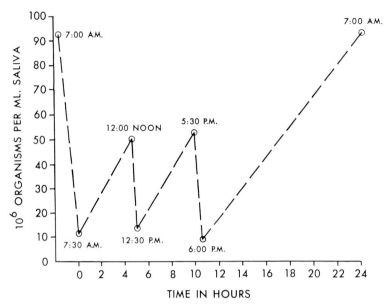

Fig. 1-5. Daily fluctuation in numbers of oral bacteria removed by saline rinse, based on viable aerobic plate count.

result of many factors: the differences in technique employed in obtaining samples, the types of culture media used, the conditions under which the culture plates are incubated, and the age and the general health of the subjects.

Culture analysis of unstimulated adult saliva has been reported to have a total aerobic microbial count of approximately 40 million per milliliter sample, with a range of from 5 to 114 million; and a total anaerobic count of 110 million per milliliter sample, with a range of from 10 to 384 million. The concentration of microorganisms cultured from gingival material is reported to average 15 billion aerobic count and 36 billion anaerobic count per gram, respectively. Microscopic counts from gingival material are reported to average 160 billion per gram of material. Bacterial analyses of gingival material from a group of normal and periodontally involved subjects show a mean microscopic count of 170 billion per gram, wet weight. The viable aerobic mean count was 16 billion, while the viable anaerobic

mean count was 40 billion. The high microscopic counts reported seem to indicate that the gingival material is composed almost entirely of bacteria. Comparison of the anaerobic viable count with the aerobic viable count indicates that most bacteria in the gingival crevice material are obligate anaerobes. Microscopic, aerobic, and anaerobic viable counts show that dental plaque also contains microorganisms in the billions. The mixed microbial communities that have established themselves on the tooth, in the gingival crevice, and in other areas of the mouth have been referred to collectively as microcosms.

At birth when the oral cavity is first contaminated with microorganisms, only those organisms that find conditions favorable for multiplication are able to establish themselves. The rate of multiplication, or the generation time, is defined as the time interval required for a single cell to divide and double itself. The theoretical doubling of cells for each generation is as shown in Table 1-1. The generation time for each type of microorganism differs. It

Table 1-1. Theoretic number of cells in a dividing bacterial population as related to the initial number and the number of generations

Generation	Number of cells after each generation
0	$200 \times 2^0 = 200^*$
1	$200 \times 2^1 = 400$
2	$200 \times 2^2 = 800$
3	$200 \times 2^3 = 1,600$
4	$200 \times 2^4 = 3,200$
5	$200 \times 2^5 = 6,400$
6	$200 \times 2^6 = 12,800$

*Initial number of cells.

also varies for the same microorganism under differences in incubation temperature, differences in culture media, and other environmental factors. *Lactobacillus acidophilus* when cultured in milk at 37° C. has a generation time of slightly less than 60 minutes; *Staphylococcus aureus* has a generation time of 30 minutes when growing in a broth medium. *Mycobacterium tuberculosis* inoculated into a synthetic medium requires approximately 14 hours or longer to reproduce itself, and the spirochete *Treponema pallidum* inoculated into rabbit testes has a generation time of between 30 and 33 hours.

The generation times for the different microorganisms growing in the oral cavity are not known. Total counts reported previously show that the oral cavity can support large numbers of different types of microorganisms. It has been demonstrated that microbial plaque, when removed from the tooth surface, regenerates in a matter of from 24 to 48 hours. The regeneration of plaque does vary with individual subjects, some requiring longer than 48 hours to develop. There appears an upper limit to which the microflora may increase in the oral cavity. This suggests that there are factors operating which control and limit the population of the oral microflora. One of these is the flushing action of saliva. It has been reported that from 1

to 2.5 gm. of bacterial cells are swallowed each day in saliva.[17] In addition, the mechanism of chewing, the action of the tongue, the lips, and the mucous membranes of the cheeks help to remove microorganisms from tooth surfaces. Currents and tissue fluids originating from the submucosal capillaries pass into the healthy gingival crevice and help remove organisms from this area. Desquamated exfoliated epithelial cells are shed, and with them microorganisms are removed and swallowed along with saliva.

Do microorganisms continually multiply in the oral cavity at a constant rate until they reach an X population density and then multiply at a slower rate? The growth of a pure culture of microorganisms in the test tube shows changes in numbers of viable cells with increased incubation time. Do microorganisms in the oral cavity follow a growth pattern somewhat similar to that demonstrated in the test tube? When a small inoculum of a microorganism (bacterium) is introduced into liquid medium and viable and total cell counts are determined at regular intervals, growth curves similar to those shown in Fig. 1-6 are obtained. The first part of the curve is referred to as a period of adjustment or lag phase and is shown on the graph by AB. The cells are adjusting themselves to the new environment, and a slight decrease in cell numbers occurs during the early part of this phase. Toward the latter part, often called physiologic youth, there is evidence of cell growth based on microscopic observations and chemical analyses of cultures. The size of the cells is larger here than in any of the other phases. They are not dividing, but they have increased in size; and the unit of metabolism per cell is reported to be greater than in any other part of the growth curve.

Following this increase in size, the cells begin to divide and multiply at a geometric rate. This phase shown on the graph

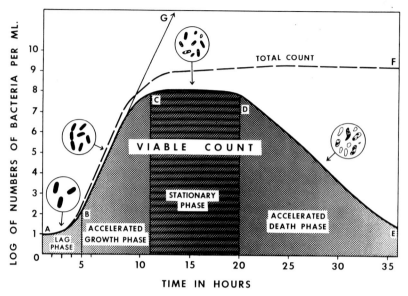

Fig. 1-6. Diagram of bacteria culture growth cycle showing: viable count curve, *AE*; total count curve, *AF*; continuous growth count, *AG*.

by BC is called the accelerated or logarithmic increase growth phase. The rate of multiplication is referred to as the generation time. Assuming that the generation time of an organism in a test tube culture is every 30 minutes, the number of cells can be determined from the following formula, $b = B \times 2^n$, in which B refers to the number of cells inoculated in the medium at the beginning of the experiment; b refers to the number of bacterial cells at the end of a given time period; and n refers to the number of generations. The generation time can be determined by dividing the number of generations into the time period which has lapsed between b and B, the formula being expressed as $G = \dfrac{t \text{ (time period)}}{n \text{ (number of generations)}}$. The generation time given for most organisms is determined during the early part of the accelerated growth phase. During the later part of this phase, microorganisms are not multiplying rapidly; in fact, some of the cells are dying. The deceleration of growth is caused by the accumulation of toxic products, the depletion in available food,

and overcrowding that results from rapid cell multiplication.

The third phase of growth, the stationary phase, is seen in the levelling off of the curve, CD on the graph. Here the numbers of viable cells are equalled by the numbers of cells that are dying. This balance reflects the effect of an increased accumulation of toxic products, a continued depletion of food, and continued overcrowding.

The last phase of growth is the accelerated death phase, DE. Here there is a constant decrease in the number of viable cells until finally the culture theoretically becomes sterile.

During the accelerated growth phase, microorganisms are considered to have their normal morphologic traits: they stain uniformly and demonstrate their true gram reaction. During the stationary phase, the microbial cells begin to show uneven staining and some may appear unstained and ghostlike, indicating they are dead. In the last phase, accelerated death, ghost cells become more predominant, and viable cells develop abnormal or involuted

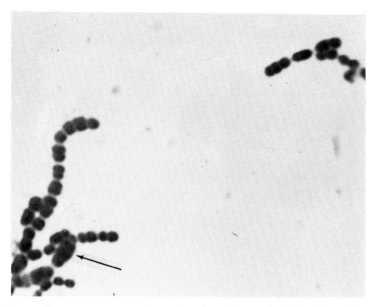

Fig. 1-7. Smear of a streptococcus culture showing abnormal cellular forms (arrow).

forms, the result of unfavorable environmental conditions (Fig. 1-7).

If microscopic and viable counts are made on a culture at the same time and both are plotted on the same graph, a second curve, AF, is formed. The microscopic or total count considers all organisms; therefore, it represents both living and dead cells. This curve demonstrates clearly why microscopic counts of the oral microflora are always many times greater than the viable counts.

AG on the graph shows that it is theoretically possible to extend the accelerated growth phase indefinitely. This can be achieved if fresh medium is added to the culture during this phase and toxic substances are neutralized or diluted. If an organism is a rapid acid former, the presence of some neutralizers, such as marble chips, will reduce the toxic effects of acid metabolic end products. The addition of nutrients also reduces metabolic toxic products by dilution. Growth of an organism under artificial conditons in the laboratory may be maintained at an accelerated pace for an indefinite period of time. Laboratory systems referred to as continuous culture have been developed to maintain organisms in the accelerated growth phase.

Conditions in the mouth seem to favor a modified continuous culture system. The intrinsic nutrients from the mucous membrane and gingival sulcus keep the microorganisms supplied more or less constantly with food; the extrinsic nutrients that we consume add to the intrinsic supply. The end products of microbial metabolism, toxic and nontoxic, are diluted and partially removed by the flow of saliva and also by the foods we eat.

It would appear that in the oral cavity conditions would vary in their effect on microbial growth. The microflora is complex, and each member's activity is controlled by its own genetic code; therefore, there would be differences in generation time, in the nutrient requirement, and in relationships with regard to antagonism, symbiosis, and synergism. The pattern of growth of individual types is no doubt dependent to some extent upon the pattern of growth of associated types and reflects the outcome of the ecosystem. We know that dental plaque regenerates on cleaned tooth surface within 24 to 48 hours. It may be during the period of regeneration that those organisms which are better established and whose nutrient requirements are not fastidious are able to multiply rapidly. It is during this period that these microorganisms may actually be in the accelerated growth phase. When they have increased to a certain population, competition between the different types may result in a retardation of growth and determine the decline into the stationary phase. From what is known about test tube cultures and what has been learned about oral organisms and the oral environment, one may theorize that microorganisms in the oral cavity probably represent two phases of the growth curve—at times, the accelerated phase and at times, the stationary phase. It is possible that they go into a beginning phase of decline; but it is doubtful that members of the indigenous oral microflora ever approach the final death phase and disappear from the oral environment in the normal subject (Fig. 1-8).

The morphologic characteristics of cocci in microbial accumulations on tooth surfaces (dental plaque) are reported to be similar to those of streptococci growing in the absence of amino acids. The bacterial cells show a thick cell wall, an increase in intracellular glycogen, a decrease in the volume of DNA, and little or no increase in numbers. It is reported that the growth rate of dextran-forming oral streptococci is slow. The extracellular dextran is thought to slow down growth by acting as a barrier in the diffusion of nutrients. It would also be expected to retard outward diffusion of metabolic products. The effect on growth was not observed when these streptococci were grown in a glucose medium or when dextranase was added to a sucrose medium. At slower

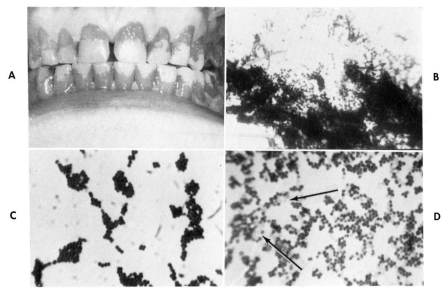

Fig. 1-8. Comparison of a stained smear of dental plaque, **B,** removed from teeth, **A,** with a staphylococcus 24 hour culture, **C,** and a staphylococcus culture 72 hours old, **D. B** and **C** show even staining and no abnormal morphologic forms. **D** shows ghostlike cells as well as unevenly stained cells (arrows). The ghost cells are characteristic of old cultures. Ghost-like forms are not observed in **B.**

growth rates, greater cell masses are produced. These observations indicate the importance of diffusion and the influence of nutrients on cell growth of oral mixed microcosms.[12]

DENTAL PLAQUE MICROFLORA

Supragingival dental plaque is generally defined as the nonmineralized microbial accumulation that adheres tenaciously to tooth surface, restorations, and prosthetic appliances, shows structural organization with predominance of filamentous forms, is composed of an organic matrix derived from salivary glycoproteins and extracellular microbial products, and cannot be removed by rinsing or water spray.[16]

In contrast, materia alba is considered to be the outer portion of dental plaque composed of an unorganized structure of microbial growth and desquamated epithelial and white and red blood cells adhering loosely to the organized structural portion of plaque and easily removed by rinsing and water spray.[23]

Some authorities, however, do not differentiate between the unorganized and organized microbial accumulations and consider dental plaque to be composed of the entire accumulating mass on tooth surface.[31]

Several ideas have been presented to explain the mechanism of microbial plaque formation. These are discussed in Chapter 8.

Quantitative and qualitative microbial determinations of plaque obtained from young subjects have been reported to have a mean total microscopic count of 250 billion organisms per gram, wet weight, an anaerobic mean viable count of 46 billion, and an aerobic mean viable count of 25 billion per gram, wet weight. Identification of the most cultivable microorganisms, based on shape, gram-staining reaction, and certain biochemical test reactions, shows the plaque to contain the following groups in these percentages:

Facultative streptococci	27
Facultative diphtheroids	23
Anaerobic diphtheroids	18
Peptostreptococci	13
Veillonella	6
Bacteroides	4
Fusobacteria	4
Neisseria	3
Vibrio	2

The identification technique missed organisms that comprise less than 1% or 2% of the plaque. None of the streptococci isolated were *Streptococcus salivarius*. Therefore, this microorganism does not predominate in dental plaque. *Bacteroides melaninogenicus* and lactobacilli were not detected and, therefore, if present, probably constituted less than 1% of plaque microorganisms. Based upon darkfield microscopic counts, spirochetes probably comprise less than 0.1% of dental plaque organisms.

The tooth appears to be the most favorable habitat for both *Streptococcus sanguis* and *S. mutans*.[7, 8] The tooth is covered with proteinaceous material (salivary mucoids–organic pellicle) containing amino acids and peptides that supply nutrients for growth. These zooglea-forming streptococci constitute the major streptococcal flora of the tooth and denture plaque. In the edentulous mouth, *S. sanguis* and *S. mutans* are reported not to be present in detectable numbers.[10]

S. mutans was first isolated from carious plaque in man by Clarke in 1924.[11] The organism was described as being small and pleomorphic, forming chained cocci in broth medium and coccobacilli on glucose agar, and producing artificial caries. *S. mutans* is normally found in the dense areas of plaque where ammonia and an anaerobic environment favor its growth. Its nutritional requirements are less fastidious than those of *S. sanguis*.[6]

The volume and cohesiveness of plaque is greatly influenced by a carbohydrate diet of sucrose. In the presence of sucrose, but not glucose, *S. mutans* forms extracellular dextran and levan; S. sanguis forms a dextran only, while S. salivarius forms a levan.[20] This latter streptococcal species is not considered important in plaque formations. When isolated from plaque, it is considered a contaminant from the saliva that washes the tongue, which is the normal environment for S. salivarius.[5]

de Stoppelaar and associates[13] reported the isolation from human dental plaque of a dextran-forming Streptococcus that was classified as resembling S. bovis.

Most cultivable bacteria from dental plaque possess the ability to form an intracellular iodine-staining polysaccharide. Streptococci, diphtheroids, fusiform bacilli, and Bacteroides have been shown to form large amounts of this polysaccharide; while others such as Veillonella, anaerobic streptococci, lactobacilli, and Vibrio sputorum form little or none. Plaque from caries-active subjects has been shown to contain as many as 60% iodine-staining polysaccharide microorganisms as compared to 13% from plaque obtained from noncarious subjects. Starved plaque has been shown to contain practically no extracellular polysaccharide and only a little intracellular polysaccharide. With an exposure to sucrose, intracellular polysaccharide forms first.[2]

Samples of developing dental plaque removed from the labial surfaces of upper and lower incisor teeth during a period of nine days and cultured showed that aerobic microbial types predominate during the early stages. Streptococci, Neisseria, and Nocardia were present in greatest numbers, with the streptococci predominating. At the ninth day's sampling, streptococci still predominated, followed by Actinomyces, Veillonella, Corynebacterium, and Fusobacterium; there was a decline in Neisseria and Nocardia (Fig. 1-9). This shift in microbial types suggests that the growth of anaerobes, such as Veillonella and Fusobacterium, was dependent upon the growth of aerobic and facultative types and that

with the increase in plaque thickness, conditions favorable for anaerobic growth were created.[25]

In studying the location of streptococci, Neisseria, and Veillonella and employing the indirect fluorescent antibody technique to frozen sections of plaque between 2 and 10 days old, Ritz[24] made the following observations: (1) Aerobic Neisseria were located peripherally in the outer layers of plaque and were more prominent in young plaque; (2) streptococci predominated, appeared to be more prevalent in younger than older plaque, and seemed to be randomly distributed throughout the plaque; (3) Veillonella, an anaerobe, was located in the deeper layers of plaque and was more prominent in old plaque than in young plaque. It was suggested that the aerobic forms, utilizing the oxygen, provide an environment in the deeper layers of plaque that favor the growth of anaerobic organisms.

A study of filamentous forms in plaque by use of fluorescent antibody technique showed that Actinomyces israelii, A. naeslundii, A. odontolyticus, Nocardia dentocariosus, and Odontomyces viscosus appeared as coccobacillary forms; whereas in culture they appeared as filamentous forms. Leptotrichia buccalis and Bacterionema matruchotii appeared as typical forms both culturally and when stained by the fluorescent technique in plaque.[29]

Human dental plaque was found to contain bacteriocin-forming streptococci. The findings of Kelstrup and Gibbons[19] suggest that these bacteriocins are not active in vivo and that streptococcal bacteriocins probably are not of ecologic importance in dental plaque.

Immature plaque, the first deposited on teeth after prophylaxis, appears to be composed of salivary mucoids and few microorganisms. The development of mature plaque shows that microorganisms grow out of surface defects and replace the mucoid material. Plaque that develops within 48

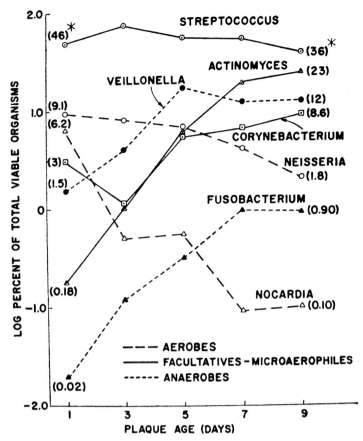

Fig. 1-9. Relative proportions of selected organisms in developing plaque. Numbers in parentheses indicate percent of given organisms in plaque at one and nine days. (Adapted from Ritz, H. L.: Microbial population shifts in developing human dental plaque, Arch. Oral Biol. **12:**1561, 1967.)

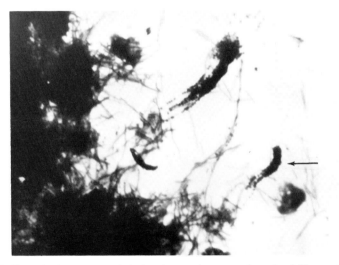

Fig. 1-10. Dental plaque material showing a dense meshwork of filaments, some rod and coccus forms, and a *Leptothrix racemosa* head at the point of the arrow.

hours is generally thicker in intraproximal areas and thinner on smooth tooth surfaces (Fig. 1-10).

GINGIVAL CREVICE MICROFLORA

The presence or absence of microorganisms in the normal gingival crevice has continued to be a broadly debated subject. The major technical difficulties have involved the avoidance of contamination from the gingiva at the necks of the teeth while one takes a sample from the crevice. Gingival crevice debris develops in an environment different from that of supragingival plaque in that it forms in an environment that might be considered free from saliva. The environmental nutrients such as gingival fluid, desquamated epithelial cells, and emigrated white blood cells create an environment favorable to strict anaerobic as well as facultative microbial microcosms. The crevice debris is reported to be a loosely attached unorganized aggregation of microorganisms that can be flushed away with a moderate spray of water.[16] Bacteria have been cultured twice as frequently from the mesial, distal, and palatal regions of the healthy gingival crevice of upper anterior teeth as from the buccal area. This difference may be explained by the relative ease of access of the buccal area to the cleansing effect of the toothbrush.

Studies of debris removed from the gingival crevice of normal subjects show a mean bacterial cell microscopic count of 130 billion per gram, wet weight. The mean total cultivable anaerobic bacterial count was 35.2 billion and the aerobic bacterial count, 19.7 billion per gram, wet weight. Mean counts for streptococci, fusiform bacilli, spirochetes, and *Bacteroides melaninogenicus* organisms show that the total count of streptococci represents 14 billion; facultative streptococci, 4.9 billion; *Bacteroides melaninogenicus,* 820 million; *Fusobacterium,* 12 million; and spirochetes, as determined by microscopic darkfield technique, 560 million per gram, wet weight (Fig. 1-11).

Investigations into the most numerous types of microorganisms that may be cultivated from gingival crevice debris obtained from children with deciduous dentition show gram-positive facultative cocci of the viridans group to be the most numerous of the coccus forms. Other cocci isolated

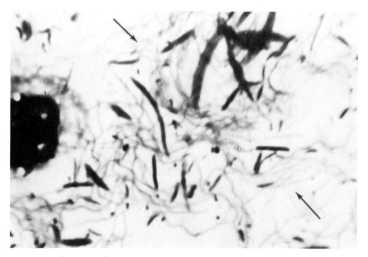

Fig. 1-11. Some morphologic forms seen in gingival crevice debris. Note the large number of spirochetal forms indicated by the arrows.

Oral ecology **25**

were identified as enterococci. Some of the gram-negative anaerobic cocci were identified as *Veillonella alcalescens,* and the gram-positive anaerobic cocci as peptostreptococci. Of the gram-negative anaerobic rods, a number were typical *Fusobacterium.* Several of the anaerobic gram-positive rods were considered lactobacilli. *Neisseria* were also found. *Bacteroides melaninogenicus* appears to be a late de-

veloper in the oral cavity of children. This organism may be isolated from the gingival margin in approximately 20% of children between the ages of 5 and 13 years. While it is rarely found in preschool children, it appears to increase during the period of mixed dentition, and by adolescence it is almost universally present.

Table 1-2 shows the groups of microorganisms cultivated from human gingival

Table 1-2. Relative proportions of groups of microorganisms found in the gingival crevice region*

Group	Approximate percentage of cultivable microbiota	Genera and/or species commonly found in this site
Gram-positive facultative cocci	28.8	Staphylococci Enterococci S. mutans S. sanguis "S. mitis"
Gram-positive anaerobic cocci	7.4	Peptostreptococcus
Gram-positive facultative rods	15.3	Corynebacterium Lactobacillus Nocardia O. viscosus B. matruchotii
Gram-positive anaerobic rods	20.2	A. bifidus A. israelii A. naeslundii A. odontolyticus P. acnes L. buccalis Corynebacterium
Gram-negative facultative cocci	0.4	Neisseria
Gram-negative anaerobic cocci	10.7	V. alcalescens V. parvula
Gram-negative facultative rods	1.2	
Gram-negative anaerobic rods	16.1	B. melaninogenicus B. oralis V. sputorum F. nucleatum S. sputigenum
Spiral organisms	1 to 3	T. denticola T. oralis T. macrodentium B. vincentii

*Adapted from Socransky, S. S.: Relationship of bacteria to the etiology of periodontal disease, J. Dent. Res. 49(suppl. 2):203, 1970.

crevice pooled debris from both normal subjects and subjects with periodontal disease. The same types of microorganisms appear to be present in both groups in relatively the same percentage. The one exception noted was the spirochetes, which showed approximately a threefold increase in the periodontal disease group. The same types of microorganisms appear in most adult subjects, although the proportions of organisms and species within groups appeared to vary from subject to subject and also from site to site within the same subject.[30]

TONGUE MICROFLORA

The predominant cultivable bacteria isolated from the human tongue fall within the following genera:

Faculative streptococci	38.3%
Veillonella	14.5%
Facultative diphtheroids	13.0%
Anaerobic diphtheroids	7.4%

Micrococci-staphylococci	6.5%
Bacteroides	5.3%
Peptostreptococcus-Peptococcus	4.2%
Neisseria	2.3%
Vibrio	2.1%
Fusobacterium	0.8%
Unidentifiable gram-negative rods	3.2%
Unidentifiable gram-negative cocci	2.6%

Of the total facultative streptococci isolated, *Streptococcus salivarius* was found to represent around 21%; other studies have shown concentrations of 55% and higher (Figs. 1-12 and 1-13). Of the bacteroides, *Bacteroides melaninogenicus* probably represents less than 1% of the isolates from the tongue. Spirochetes were not observed.

SALIVARY MICROFLORA

Dislodgement of microorganisms from colonizing aggregations in various locations of the oral cavity—the teeth, tongue, cheek, and pharyngeal mucous membrane—contributes to the microflora of the saliva.

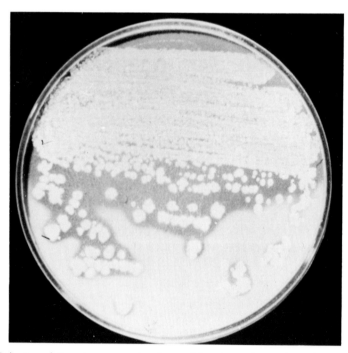

Fig. 1-12. Colonies of *Streptococcus salvarius* on Niven's medium. Note clearing of medium around colony resulting from acid production.

Much research involving oral organisms has been based upon the use of salivary samples as a substitute for dental plaque and gingival debris. Investigation of the possible source of salivary bacteria indicates that *Streptococcus salivarius* comprises 47% of the facultative streptococci present in saliva, 21% to 55% of the facultative streptococci on the tongue, and 10% of the facultative streptococci on the cheek. This organism was found to comprise less than 1% of the facultative streptococci of the plaque and gingival crevice. Dental plaque is not considered to be the source of *Streptococcus salivarius* found in saliva. Although *S. sanguis* is reported to be the dominant streptococci in early plaque from teeth, it constitutes only a minor portion of the flora of other sites in the oral cavity.[3] Therefore, dental plaque is not the major contributor to the salivary microflora. To ascertain whether gingival crevice material may be the source of salivary bacteria, analysis for *Bacteroides melaninogenicus* shows this organism to represent 5% or less of the total cultivable bacteria isolated from the gingival crevice. It represents less

than 1% of the isolates from plaque, cheek, and tongue, and also less than 1% of the isolates from saliva. These findings indicate that the gingival crevice is not the major source of salivary bacteria. Thus, the major source of salivary bacteria appears to be the tongue.

SPECIFIC GROUPS OF THE ORAL MICROFLORA

Lactobacilli reportedly form only a small minority of the plaque microflora. The ratio has been reported to be about one lactobacillus to 100,000 cocci. Lactobacilli have been found more frequently in plaque covering tooth surface with initial caries than in plaque that shows no evidence of caries activity. Prior to 1953, the gram-positive non–spore-forming rods isolated on tomato juice agar of pH 5 from dental plaque or saliva were called *Lactobacillus acidophilus* (Fig. 1-14). Since then it has been shown that of these gram-positive non–spore-forming rods *L. casei* is the predominant species isolated from the saliva of children with high lactobacilli counts, and not *L. acidophilus*. Research in which five hundred

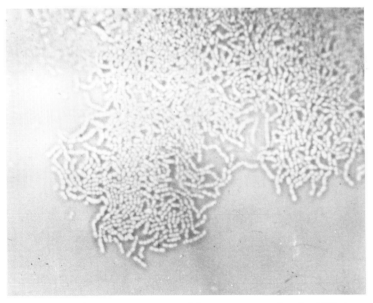

Fig. 1-13. Phase contrast view of *Streptococcus salivarius* (990x).

lactobacilli isolates were obtained from salivary samples from a large group of children indicated that of the homofermentative types *L. acidophilus* represented only 11% of the isolates; whereas *L. casei* made up the highest percentage—around 39%. *L. salivarius*, *L. plantarum*, and *L. arabinosus* constituted 2% or less; whereas of the heterofermentative types *L. fermenti* represented 30%; *L. buchneri*, 5%; *L. brevis*, 6%; and *L. cellobiosus*, 1% or less. Of the salivary bacteria, lactobacilli probably represent 0.1%.

The group of microorganisms identified as enterococci have been cultivated from slightly more than 21% of human salivary samples. Of the enterococci species identi-

fied, *Stretopcoccus fecalis* represented 82%; *S. liquefaciens*, 11%; and *S. zymogenes*, 6.6%. This group of organisms has not been found to be constantly present in all salivary samples each time tested. It has been isolated more consistently from subjects between the ages of 14 and 20 years, rather than in the younger and the older age groups. A correlation between lactobacilli and yeast counts indicated that when the enterococci count is high, the lactobacilli count is also high, while the yeast count is low. Enterococci have been isolated from the gingiva in 24%, and from the tonsils and pharyngeal area in about 18.5%, of subjects examined.

In a study comparing the occurrence of

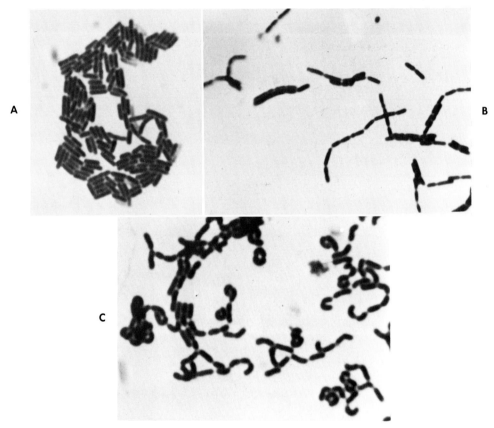

Fig. 1-14. Some variations in morphology and arrangement of lactobacilli isolated on LBS agar. **A,** Bacilli, occurring singly and in pairs showing palisade arrangement. **B,** Bacilli, occurring singly and in pairs and chains. **C,** Plump bacilli, curved and rod forms, occurring singly and in pairs (1,100×).

hemolytic stretococci on the gingiva, throat, and tonsils, they were present in 6.0%, 11.6%, and 43%, respectively, of normal adult subjects. The percentage of positive throat cultures is in agreement with other reports for normal individuals. The throat and tonsil areas may be considered the normal habitat for hemolytic streptococci (Fig. 1-15).

Although yeasts have frequently been isolated from the oral cavity, there is some difference of opinion as to whether they are a part of the normal microflora. It has been reported that the mouths of 54% of infants

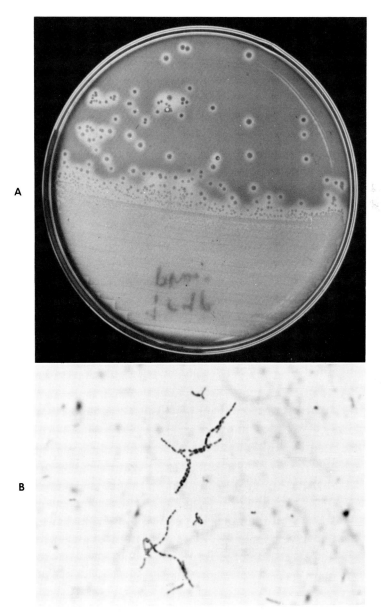

Fig. 1-15. A, Beta streptococci colonies showing clear hemolysis on blood agar streaked plate. **B,** Stained smear of a beta streptococcus colony.

between the ages of two and six weeks were positive for yeast, and between the ages of six weeks and one year 46.5% were positive. Young children between the ages of one and six years were found to be positive in 38.5%. Of a large group of healthy college students consisting of both men and women, yeasts were cultivated from salivary samples in 48.6%. The incidence of yeast was found to be somewhat higher in men than in women. Eighty-five percent of the subjects were positive for a period of a month, while 79% were positive for two months. Of the isolates, *Candida albicans* represented 93.8%, *Candida tropicalis*, 2.1%, and *Candida stellatoidea*, 1.4%. *Candida pseudotropicalis* and other, unidentifiable species represented less than 1%, whereas *Cryptococcus* species were found in 1% of the isolates. It was observed that the lower the salivary pH, the higher the percentage of yeast. Salivas of pH 5.0 yielded 100% isolates; pH 5.5, 83%; pH 6.0, 67%; pH 6.5, 52%; pH 7.0, 29%; and pH 7.5, 14%.

Another investigation of the presence of fungi in plaque material shows that positive cultures may vary between 20% and 58%. A higher frequency of positive cultures was found in females than in males, and the frequency was found to be higher in the summer than during the winter months. Approximately 70% of the positive findings were identified as *Candida albicans*.

A survey of the yeast population of a group of subjects between 20 and 30 years of age yielded yeast in 45% of the specimens. Of these, 75.8% were positive for *Candida* species: 60% were identified as *C. albicans*, 6.8% as *C. krusei*, 3.9% as *C. tropicalis*, 2.2% as *C. parapsilosis*, 0.8% as *C. guilliermondi, and* 2.2% as unidentified species of *Candida. Cryptococcus* was found in 10.9% of the specimens and *Saccharomyces* in 3.9%. The remaining 1.5% were unidentifiable yeast. The results of these investigations suggest that *C. albicans* is possibly a normal inhabitant of the oral cavity of man (Figs. 1-16 and 1-17).

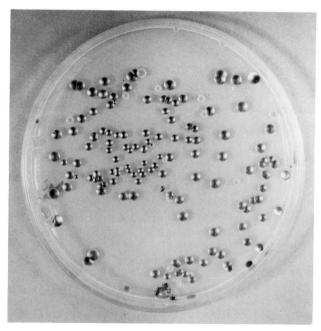

Fig. 1-16. Nickerson's agar plate inoculated with saliva from denture wearer. The dark (brown) colonies are *Candida albicans.*

Although filamentous microorganisms have not been cultured as predominating in high dilutions of dental plaque, smears made from plaque material show that these organisms make up the so-called fibrous bulk or meshwork of plaque. These microbial forms have characteristics of the *Actinomyces* group. Branching filaments identified as *Actinomyces israelii, A. naeslundii,* and *Bacterionema matruchotii,* formerly described as *Leptotrichia buccalis,* have been isolated from the oral cavity of healthy individuals. The fluorescent antibody technique has enabled identification of *B. matruchotii* as numerically the most frequent filamentous form observed in dental plaque specimens. *A. israelii* has been identified as the predominating organism in 40% to 50% of carious lesions and in 46.3% of plaques cultured from intact tooth surface. A filamentous form identified as *A. odontolyticus* has been isolated from carious dentin. There is confusion in the literature as to whether the actinomycetes isolated from the oral cavity are *A. israelii* or *A. bovis.* By the gel diffusion technique

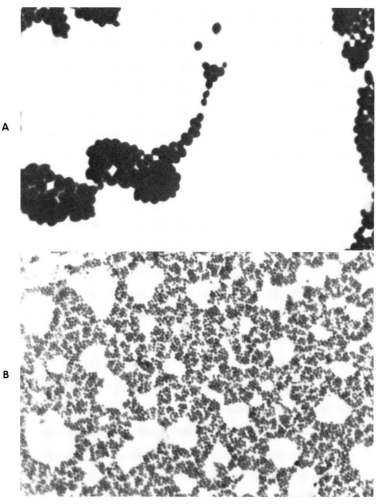

Fig. 1-17. Crystal violet-stained smear of a dark colony from Nickerson's medium. Typical oval yeast forms are seen in **A.** Compare size with *Staphylococcus aureus* shown in **B.**

employing the antibody reaction, it has been shown that *A. israelii* is antigenically distinct from *A. bovis. A. israelii* is the species normally present in the oral cavity of man; *A. bovis* is found in cattle. *A. naeslundii* shows cross-reactions with both *A. israelii* and *A. bovis.* Actinomycetes have an anaerobic respiration (Fig. 1-18).

The *Bacterionema matruchotii* differs morphologically from the *Actinomyces* in that certain filaments have an elongated terminal swelling. *Bacterionema* also has an aerobic type of respiration. This organism has been shown to have a complex growth cycle. When cultured for 36 hours on brain heart infusion agar, it forms flat colonies. Subcultures of these colonies to brain heart infusion broth develop bacillary variants resembling diphtheroids and streptococci. These morphologic forms are similar to those found for *Actinomyces*.[32] The genus *Nocardia* is closely related to the *Actinomyces* morphologically, but differs in that it is aerobic and that certain members have an acid-fast staining property.

Microorganisms resembling *Nocardia* have been reported isolated from carious teeth, from normal and inflamed gingival crevices, periodontal pocket debris, calculus, and oral lesions. The close relationship of this genus with other filamentous microorganisms isolated from the oral cavity makes its identification difficult. Strains isolated from various teeth have been named *Rothia dentocariosa* (*Nocardia dentocariosus*). Recent immunofluorescent staining using a prepared antinocardial rabbit serum suggests that *Nocardia* may play an important role in the initiation and development of plaque.

Although coliform bacteria have been listed as members of the oral flora, there is little evidence that they are permanent members. Salivary samples obtained from more than three hundred dental students show coliform organisms to be present in 32% of the samples. Of these coliform bacteria, 55% were identified as *Aerobacter aerogenes*, 34% as intermediate forms, and 3% as typical *Escherichia coli*. These mi-

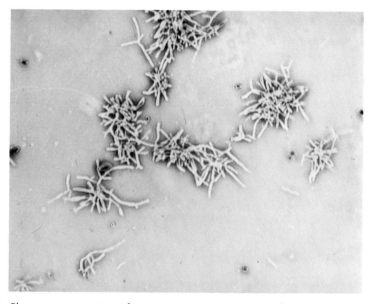

Fig. 1-18. Phase contrast view of an actinomycete prepared from a colony isolated on anaerobic blood plate inoculated with dental plaque. Note branching Y and V forms (950x).

croorganisms were found to be present in salivary samples sporadically and should not be considered permanent members of the oral flora. Serial dilutions of salivary samples from a number of positive subjects indicate that coliform organisms are present in low numbers.

Another group of microorganisms that are missed when culturing oral material unless specific culture media and culture conditions are provided is that of the pleuropneumonia-like organisms (PPLO). PPLO forms have been isolated from both male and female subjects. One study reported this organism in saliva of 45% to 46% of a group of male and female subjects. The finding of PPLO in relatively large numbers of oral cavities suggests a possible association of its presence with penicillin therapy, since in vitro studies with penicillin have demonstrated that some microorganisms dissociate into forms similar to PPLO. In vitro tests using *Proteus, Bacteroides,* streptococci, staphylococci, and others have shown that in the presence of certain concentrations of penicillin these organisms fail to synthesize the cell wall and assume morphologic forms quite characteristic of the known PPLO forms.

Also, lysozyme, an enzyme found in saliva and in various body fluids, results in the disintegration of the cell wall of certain bacteria, thus leaving the cytoplasmic membrane enveloping the living cell. The term protoplast is used to refer to the living cell devoid of its cell wall; whereas the term spheroplast refers to a living cell with some of the cell wall remaining. Usually when the influencing agent, such as penicillin, is removed, the form devoid of cell wall (L form) regenerates the cell wall and reverts to its original form. When reversion does not take place, the L form becomes stabilized and is then referred to as a PPLO by some investigators. These forms are filterable, are highly pleomorphic, and stain gram-negative. They develop very small colonies about 0.1 to 0.5 mm. in diameter; they require enriched media containing ascites or serum in approximately 50% and have characteristics similar to the pleuropneumonia organisms (PPO) originally isolated from cattle.

In a study to determine the possible relationship of oral PPLO forms and oral hygiene, a large group of young male naval recruits of an average age of 18 years were chosen as subjects. Saliva and gingival debris material were obtained and cultured for PPLO forms. Eighty-three percent of the subjects demonstrated PPLO oral forms. The results in this study indicated that there was no correlation between the presence of these forms and gingival disease, the amount of calculus, or the oral hygiene; there was a high rate of oral PPLO isolates in persons lacking caries activity and having low carious experience. Conversely, a low recovery rate of PPLO appeared to be associated with both high caries activity and high caries experience.

In another investigation, PPLO-like isolates identified as *Mycoplasma salivarium* were cultured from the gingiva of approximately 80% of subjects having natural dentition and none from edentulous subjects. PPLO forms are considered to be normal members of the anaerobic flora of the human mouth and are found mainly in the gingival sulcus. It is possible that the edentulous mouth does not supply the factors essential for the growth of this microbial form, factors such as oxygen tension, nutrition, and perhaps also a bacterial flora necessary for a symbiotic relationship.

Mycoplasma salivarium has been cultured from 86.7% of subjects with periodontal disease as compared to 31.8% of subjects with healthy sulci. Concentrations of this organism less than 10^4 per gram were not detected based on the sensitivity of the sampling technique. Therefore, the cause-and-effect relationship of *Mycoplasma salivarium* and periodontal disease cannot be concluded. The study does confirm other reports that this organism is found mainly in the sulcus and appears to be associated with the complex sulcus flora that causes gingivitis.[14]

It has been mentioned that environmental conditions do have some effect on the oral microflora. Low Arctic temperatures, $-14.7°$ F. to $-23°$ F., have been shown to lower the intraoral temperatures, because of mouth breathing, and to result in a significant decrease in lactobacilli counts. Studies of the environmental conditions of submarine living show that salivary lactobacilli, *Streptococcus salivarius,* and *Veillonella* do not change; therefore, submarine conditions would not be expected to increase the incidence of dental caries. In a recent study of the bacterial flora of saliva from a group of native Kalahari Bushmen, it was shown that the caries incidence was low and that the subjects showed pronounced attrition of the teeth. The fibrous nature of their food and the flattened occlusal surfaces of their teeth act in self-cleansing the teeth. Caries was noted to increase among middle-aged and old Bushmen in whom attrition had resulted in the wearing of the tooth beyond

the contact and allowed areas for food accumulations and stagnation. The Bushmen were found to have a high percentage of aerobic bacilli in their saliva. The bacilli are normally considered transient, but in the case of the Bushmen they appear to make up a normal part of the oral flora. These organisms are highly proteolytic; it is possible that their catabolic products may explain, in part, the low caries incidence among these people.

The organism *Micrococcus lactilyticus (Veillonella alcalescens)* has been consistently isolated from dental plaque and saliva of clinically normal subjects. It is present in the millions and constitutes a significant member of the indigenous anaerobic flora of human saliva. Since it utilizes lactate, an end product of acidogenic metabolism, the pH increases and this may have a deterring effect on dental caries.

A recent study has suggested that *Pseudomonas aeruginosa* be considered a member of the indigenous oral microflora for certain individuals. It was found in approximately 6.6% of salivas and was usually isolated from the same subjects over a period of a year. Two other species, *Ps.*

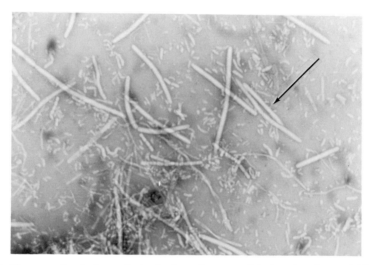

Fig. 1-19. Phase contrast view of gingival crevice material showing *Leptotrichia buccalis* (arrow). Note small size of other microbial forms by comparison.

putida and *Ps. fluorescens,* were found in 1.7% and 0.6%, respectively, and were considered transient. Other microorganisms that have been reported as members of the oral cavity are *Selenomonas sputigena, Leptotrichia buccalis, Leptothrix racemosa,* and *Leptothrix falciformis. Selenomonas sputigena* is a motile anaerobic spiral form that has been isolated from periodontal pockets.

Leptotrichia buccalis is one of the largest microorganisms found in the oral cavity. It requires anaerobiosis for initial isolation, but will grow on subcultural under microaerophilic or reduced oxygen tension atmospheres. The organism is a filament varying from 3 to 40 μ long and 1 μ wide. It is generally tapered at one end and rounded at the other. Young cells of *Leptothrix* stain gram-positive, whereas cells eight hours old or more generally stain gram-negative. These organisms are found in dental plaque material and also in gingival crevice debris (Fig. 1-19). The complex microorganism *L. racemosa,* shown in Fig. 1-20, is identified on the basis of morphologic characteristics. This organism is observed in areas about the teeth which are protected from the toothbrush and from the abrasive effect of cheek and tongue movements. The so-called fruiting head is characteristic in that there appears to be an orderly arrangement of teardrop-shaped to round bodies along the free end of the main stalk. Making direct smears of plaque material often results in the breaking off of these bodies. When a direct microscopic count of plaque is made, these free bodies are indistinguishable from cocci and are possibly counted as cocci. A series of photographs in Fig. 1-21 shows changes for the *racemosa* head when observed under slide culture. The complex microorganism *Leptothrix falciformis,* referred to as the "test-tube-brush" organism, is shown in Fig. 1-22. This organism is identified on morphologic bases only and is found in deep periodontal pockets.

Clostridia are not considered normal inhabitants of the oral cavity. Oral disease caused by these microorganisms has seldom been reported in dental publications. However, in a recent study, van Reenen and Coogan[35] reported the isolation of clostridia from the normal gingival crevice as well as periodontal pockets and carious teeth.

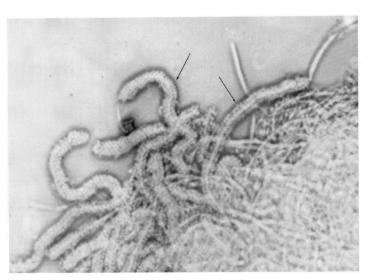

Fig. 1-20. Phase contrast view of a clump of *Leptothrix racemosa.* Note the orderly arrangement of the small bodies attached to the free ends of filaments shown by arrows.

Although certain members of the true fungi have been reported by a few workers as members of indigenous oral flora, there is little evidence to support their findings. The lack of adequate culture controls indicates these fungi to be contaminants.

Entamoeba gingivalis and *Trichomonas tenax* are examples of protozoa that have been isolated from oral specimens. These organisms are present in the clean and healthy mouth, and increase in the diseased mouth (Fig. 1-23). *E. gingivalis* is present in 75% or more of people older than 40 years. Published reports indicate that from a group of subjects who were considered to have clean and healthy mouths, 26% harbored *E. gingivalis*, 11.2% harbored *T. tenax*, and 6.4% harbored both of these protozoa. *E. gingivalis* was isolated from 100% of the patients with advanced periodontal disease, *T. tenax* from 80% of the patients.

The relation to infection of the oral cavity of these two oral protozoa is reported to be directly proportional to the amount of calculus present on teeth, the degree of coating on the tongue, and the progression of periodontal disease.[36]

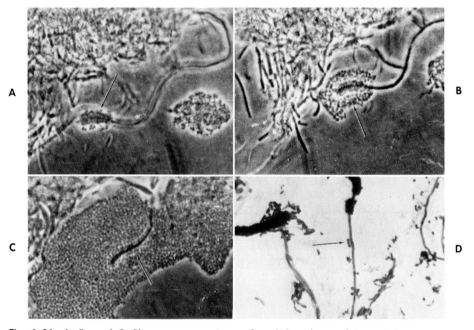

Fig. 1-21. A, B, and **C,** Phase contrast views of a slide culture of *Leptothrix racemosa.* **A** shows a filament with a small *L. racemosa* head free from a clump of dental plaque. **B** and **C** show that the coccoidal bodies attached to the head have increased in number during incubation. It was observed that these bodies first would swell, and then bud daughter bodies which would be set free in the surrounding medium. The freed bodies were then observed to divide by binary fission. No filaments developed from these bodies. With age the coccoidal bodies became ghostlike and the parent filament broke up into segments resembling large, rod shaped bacteria. Note the orderly arrangement of the bodies which appear attached to the central filaments in **B** and **C** (arrows). **D** is a stained preparation of a *racemosa* head. The head appears to have been partially freed of the coccoid bodies, the result of injury in preparing the smear; the freed bodies are seen throughout the smear. The arrow shows bodies which appear to be attached to the filament.

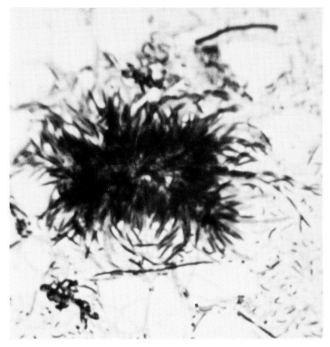

Fig. 1-22. Stained smear of the complex organism *Leptothrix falciformis.* This organism is found in deep periodontal pockets and has not been cultivated in the laboratory. Some authorities believe it represents the attachment of fusiform bacilli to some central body.

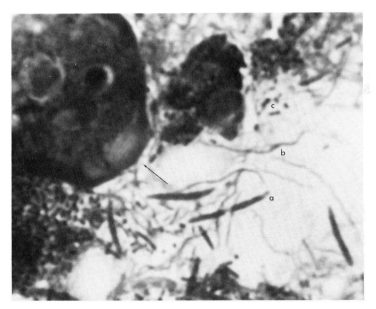

Fig. 1-23. Periodontal pocket material showing a large ameba at the end of the arrow. Note fusiform bacilli, *a,* spirochetes, *b,* and cocci, *c.*

Table 1-3. Some microbial factors that may influence virulence

Factor	Its action
Hyaluronidase (spreading factor)	Breaks down the intracellular substance, hyaluronic acid, and facilitates spread of infection through tissues Formed by many organisms including staphylococci, streptococci, pneumococci, diphtheroid bacilli, *Clostridium perfringens,* and other organisms
Coagulase	Causes clotting of human and rabbit plasma resulting in a fibrous covering about the microorganism or the lesion Protects the organism from phagocytosis Formed by many staphylococci, colon bacilli, *Pseudomonas, Serratia marcescens,* and other organisms
Kinase (fibrinolysin)	Causes the breakdown of blood clots and aids the organism in the spread of infection Streptokinase formed by many streptococci and staphylokinase formed by many staphylococci
Hemolysin	Causes lysis of red blood cells and other tissue cells Formed by many streptococci, staphylococci, and other organisms
Leukocidin	Destroys polymorphonuclear leukocytes Formed by many organisms, usually streptococci and staphylococci
Lecithinase	A lipolytic enzyme known as alpha toxin Combines with calcium, attacks phosolipids, and causes lyses of red blood cells and other tissue cells Formed by *Clostridium perfringens* and other *Clostridium* species
Neuraminidase or Sialidase	Causes loss of sialic acid from saliva resulting in precipitation of some of the glycoprotein components which may play a role in plaque formation on teeth. Formed by some oral streptococci, micrococci diphtheroids
Collagenase	An enzyme that hydrolyzes collagen Destroys collagen fibers Formed by many *Clostridium* and *Bacteroides* species
Chondrosulfatase	Hydrolyzes chondroitin sulfate, tissue-cementing polysaccharide Formed by some oral organisms
Exotoxin	Highly poisonous substance, generally protein Formed by many organisms including *Corynebacterium diphtheria* and *Clostridium tetani* Has a preference for certain tissues: nerve, heart, muscle, and kidney Blocks enzyme system Liberated by growing cells
Endotoxin	Poison of low potency Lipo-polysaccharide—protein complex Causes generalized physiologic change in host Formed by many gram-negative bacilli Appears to have no tissue selectivity Not easily separated from cell
Capsule Macro	A mucoid surface structure of the bacterial cell Generally polysaccharide or polypeptide in nature Formed by pneumococci, Friedländer's bacilli, and other organisms Protects cells from phagocytosis and other harmful agents
Micro	Closely associated with cell wall Is an endotoxin

Table 1-3. Some microbial factors that may influence virulence—cont'd

Factor	Its action
Diphosphorpyridine nucleotide	Associated with toxicity for leukocytes Formed by strains of *Streptococcus pyogenes*
Mucinase	A tissue-disintegrating enzyme formed by *Vibrio, Cholera, Shigella,* and *E. coli*
Necrotoxin	Formed by staphylococcus Kills tissue cell
Hypothermic factor	Lowers body temperature Formed by *Shigella dysenteriae*
Edema-producing factor	Formed by pneumococci Causes edema
Catalase	An enzyme that may be associated with pathogenicity of certain organisms *Mycobacterium tuberculosis* and *Pasteurella pestis*
Streptodornase (deoxyribonuclease)	Liquefies purulent exudates Formed by certain cocci

That certain viruses can be considered a part of the normal oral flora might be a debatable question. Generally, viruses are considered to be transient oral members, perhaps with the exception of herpesvirus hominis. This virus has been reported to be present in saliva of a very small percentage of asymptomatic individuals.

MICROBIAL FACTORS ASSOCIATED WITH PATHOGENICITY

The normal oral flora is made up of many types of microorganisms differing in nutritional and oxygen requirements. These microorganisms have established themselves in the oral cavity on the mucous membrane of the cheek, the gingiva, the tongue, in the gingival crevice, and on the teeth. Heavy accumulation of microbial growth about the teeth can be easily seen with the naked eye and can be partially removed by water spray. These accumulations are called materia alba. The adhering cellular mass is called bacteria or dental plaque. The various types of microorganisms of this natural flora live a facultative parasitic existence; these microorganisms

have established a normal relationship with one another and live in a more or less biologic equilibrium within the host.

Many members of this indigenous oral flora possess some pathogenizing properties and can cause infection and disease of the oral cavity as well as of other tissues of the body. Dental caries, periodontal disease, gingival inflammation, and subacute bacterial endocarditis are examples of infections associated with the indigenous oral microflora. Microorganisms that cause or are associated with disease are said to be pathogenic, and the degree of pathogenicity is referred to as virulence. There are many factors or attributes that microorganisms possess which enable them to produce infection and disease; these are called virulence factors. Certain virulence factors might be produced in vitro that are not in vivo, and vice versa.[28] The ability of a microorganism to produce disease is associated with its invasiveness or its toxicity or both. Listed in Table 1-3 are microbial factors that may be associated with diseases in man and animals.

Many of these factors are formed by

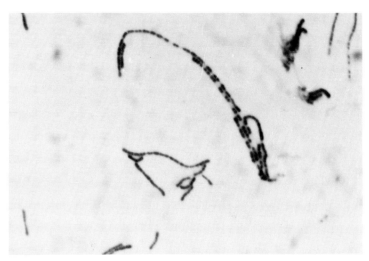

Fig. 1-24. Frazer capsule stain of guinea pig exudate showing the organism *(Diplococcus pneumoniae)* stained dark (red) surrounded by the capsule material (blue). (Courtesy Dr. D. H. Going, Houston, Tex.)

indigenous microorganisms isolated from gingival debris material and from other areas of the oral cavity (Figs. 1-24 and 1-25). Staphylococci and certain strains of *Streptococcus mitis* and *S. salivarium* isolated from the oral cavity have been demonstrated to form hyaluronic acid and beta glucuronidase, and microaerophilic diphtheroids have been shown to form chondrosulfatase. Certain strains of *Bacteroides melaninogenicus* have been shown to produce an enzyme that will hydrolyze collagen (Fig. 1-26). This microorganism also forms in the saliva high concentrations of ammonia, which is known to have lytic effect on epithelium of the mucous membrane. *Clostridium welchii* has been isolated from carious teeth and has been shown to disintegrate the organic matrix of decalcified dentin but does not affect carious or infected dentin.[15] Axenic *Trichomonas tenax* possesses the ability to depolymerize hyaluronic acid, a characteristic generally associated with certain members of the oral bacterial flora. This finding suggests a possible closer relation of this organism to periodontal disease.[33]

The endotoxins from gram-negative oral microorganisms of plaque are reported to cause rupture of polymorphonuclear leukocytes. This results in the release of the lysozomes of the leukocytes which break up and free acid phosphatase, esterases, and other enzymes that affect host gingival tissue and thus play an important part in periodontal disease. The quantity of bacterial endotoxin and the clinical degree of inflammation show a direct correlation.[1]

Microbial metabolites may also be considered factors associated with the pathogenicity of oral disease. Acids formed from carbohydrates by acidogenic-aciduric bacteria can result in decalcification of enamel and the beginning of the carious process. The periodontal pocket microflora consists of large numbers of anaerobic types—spirochetes, fusiform bacilli, *Vibrio*, *Veillonella*, and *Bacteroides*. These microorganisms possess the enzyme system to form hydrogen sulfide, a highly poisonous metabolite reportedly formed in deep periodontal pockets. Periodontal fluid contains nutrients for anaerobic bacteria and could furnish the substrate for hydrogen sulfide. This toxic gas could play a role in the pathologic changes observed in periodontal disease.[26]

Certain oral microorganisms possess mucolytic enzymes and are able to hydrolyze

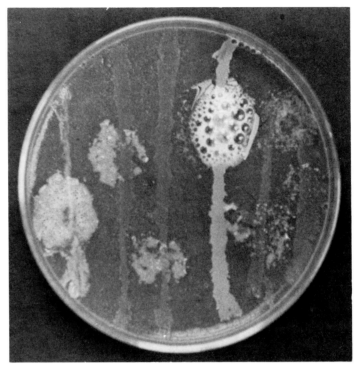

Fig. 1-25. Catalase production by *Micrococcus lysodeikticus.* Several drops of hydrogen peroxide placed on streaked growth show an effervescent effect for positive reaction.

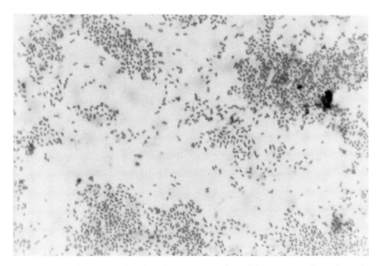

Fig. 1-26. Gram-stained smear of a black colony isolated from periodontal pocket material on laked blood menadione agar; identified as *Bacteroides melaninogenicus.* (Courtesy Dr. D. H. Going, Houston, Tex.)

salivary mucins with the release of sialic acid. This activity appears to have a relationship with plaque formation.

The more common oral diseases that concern the dentist appear to progress slowly, although many members of the oral microbiota possess pathogenizing properties. This observation suggests that the indigenous microflora consists of types of relatively low virulence.

CITED REFERENCES

1. Baboolal, R., Powell, R. N., and Prophet, A. S.: Hydrolytic enzymes in developing gingival plaque, J. Periodont. **41**:87, 1970.
2. Berman, K. S., and Gibbons, R. J.: Iodophilic polysaccharide synthesis by human and rodent oral bacteria, Arch. Oral Biol. **11**:533, 1966.
3. Carlsson, J.: Dental plaque as a source of salivary streptococci, Odont. Rev. **18**:173, 1967.
4. Carlsson, J.: The early establishment of *Streptococcus salivarius* in the mouth of infants, J. Dent. Res. **49**:415, 1970.
5. Carlsson, J.: Effect of diet on presence of *Streptococcus salivarius* in dental plaque and saliva, Odont. Rev. **16**:336, 1965.
6. Carlsson, J.: A medium for isolation of *Streptococcus mutans*, Arch. Oral Biol. **12**:1657, 1967.
7. Carlsson, J.: Presence of various types of non-haemolytic streptococci in dental plaque and in other sites of the oral cavity in man, Odont. Rev. **18**:55, 1967.
8. Carlsson, J.: Zooglea-forming streptococci resembling *Streptococcus sanguis* isolated from dental plaque in man, Odont. Rev. **16**:348, 1965.
9. Carlsson, J., Grahnen, H., Jonsson, G., and Wikner, S.: Establishment of *Streptococcus sanguis* in the mouth of infants, Arch. Oral Biol. **15**:1143, 1970.
10. Carlsson J., Soderholm, G., and Almfeldt, I.: Prevalence of *Streptococcus sanguis* and *Streptococcus mutans* in the mouth of persons wearing full-dentures, Arch. Oral Biol. **14**:243, 1969.
11. Clarke, J. K.: On the bacterial factor in the aetiology of dental caries, Brit. J. Exp. Path. **5**:141, 1924.
12. Critchley, P.: Effects of foods on bacterial metabolic processes, J. Dent. Res. **49**:1283, 1970.
13. de Stoppelaar, J. D., van Houte, J., and de Moor, G. E.: The presence of dextran-forming bacteria resembling *Streptococcus bovis*

and *Streptococcus sanguis* in human dental plaque, Arch. Oral Biol. **12**:1199, 1967.
14. Engel, L. D., and Kenny, G. E.: *Mycoplasma salivarium* in human gingival sulci, J. Periodont. Res. **5**:163, 1970.
15. Evans, D. G., and Prophet, A. S.: Examination of strains of *Clostridium welchii* isolated from teeth, Brit. Dent. J. **91**:199, 1951.
16. Genco, R. J., Evans, R. T., and Ellison, S. A.: Dental research in microbiology with emphasis on periodontal disease, J. Amer. Dent. Assoc. **78**:1016, 1969.
17. Gibbons R. J.: Significance of the bacterial flora indigenous to man, American Institute of Oral Biology, Twenty-sixth Annual Meeting, 1969, p. 27.
18. Kelstrup, J., and Gibbons, R. J.: Bacteriocins from human and rodent streptococci, Arch. Oral Biol. **14**:251, 1969.
19. Kelstrup, J., and Gibbons, R. J.: Investigations of *in vivo* bacteriocin activity, International Association for Dental Research, Abstract 175, Forty-seventh General Meeting, 1969, p. 84.
20. Krasse, B.: Caries etiology: Summary, International Symposium on Oral Disease, Alabama J. Dent. **5**:267, 1968.
21. Krasse, B.: The effect of nutrition on saliva and oral flora. In Blix, G. (ed): Symposia of the Swedish Nutrition Foundation 111, Nutrition and Caries Prevention, 1964, p. 21.
22. Loesche, W. L.: Importance of nutrition in gingival crevice microbial etiology, Periodontics **6**:245, 1968.
23. Mandel, I. D.: Dental plaque: Nature, formation and effects, J. Periodont. **37**:357, 1966.
24. Ritz, H. L.: Fluorescent antibody straining of *Neisseria*, streptococci, and *Veillonella* in frozen sections of human dental plaque, Arch. Oral Biol. **14**:1073, 1969.
25. Ritz, H. L.: Microbial population shifts in developing human dental plaque, Arch. Oral Biol. **12**:1561, 1967.
26. Rizzo, A. A.: The possible role of hydrogen sulfide in human periodontal disease. 1. Hydrogen sulfide production in periodontal pockets, Periodontics **5**:233, 1967.
27. Rosebury, T.: Microorganisms indigenous to man, New York, 1969, McGraw-Hill Book Company, p. 3.
28. Smith, H.: Biochemical challenge of microbial pathogenicity, Bact. Rev. **32**:164, 1968.
29. Snyder, M. L., Bullock, W. W., and Parker, R. B.: Morphology of gram positive filamentous bacteria identified in dental plaque by fluorescent antibody technique, Arch. Oral Biol. **12**:1269, 1967.

30. Socransky, S. S.: Relationship of bacteria to the etiology of periodontal disease, J. Dent. Res. 49(Suppl. 2):203, 1970.

31. Stephan, R. M.: The dental plaque in relation to the etiology of caries, Int. Dent. J. 4:180, 1953.

32. Streckfuss, J. L., and Smith, W. N.: Isolation of bacillary and streptococcal variants from *Bacterionema matruchotii,* J. Bact. **104:**1399, 1970.

33. Summersett, J. F., and Collins, W. T.: Degradation of hyaluronic acid by the oral protozoan *Trichomonas tenax,* International Association for Dental Research, Abstract 400, Forty-seventh General Meeting, 1969, p. 397.

34. Toto, P. D., Santangelo, M. V., and Madonia, J. V.: Use of hyaluronic acid and chondroitin sulfate by bacterial isolates from carious dentin, J. Dent. Res. 47:1056, 1968.

35. van Reenen, J. F., and Coogan M. M.: *Clostridia* isolated from human mouths, Arch. Oral Biol. **15:**845, 1970.

36. Wantland, W. W., and Lauer, D.: Correlation of some oral hygiene variables with age, sex and the incidence or oral protozoa, J. Dent. Res. **49:**293, 1970.

REFERENCES AND ADDITIONAL READINGS

Adams, R. J., and Stanmeyer, W. R.: Effects of prolonged Antarctic isolation on oral and intestinal bacteria, Oral Surg. 13:117, 1960.

Arnim, S. S.: Microcosms of the human mouth, J. Tenn. Dent. Assoc. 39:3, 1959.

Bailit, H. L., Baldwin, D. C., and Hunt, E. E.: The increasing prevalence of gingival *Bacteroides melaninogenicus* with age in children, Arch. Oral Biol. 9:435, 1964.

Bartels, H. A., and Blechman, H.: Limitations of mold establishment in oral cavity, J. Dent. Res. 43:136, 1964.

Bartels, H. A., and Blechman, H.: Survey of the yeast population in saliva and on evaluation of some procedures for identification of *Candida albicans,* J. Dent. Res. 41:1386, 1962.

Battistone, G. C., and Burnett, G. W.: The free amino acid composition of human saliva, Arch. Oral Biol. 3:161, 1961.

DeAraujo, W. C., and MacDonald, J. B.: The gingival crevice microbiota in five preschool children, Arch. Oral Biol. 9:227, 1964.

DeAraujo, W. C., and MacDonald, J. B.: The gingival crevice microbiota of preschool children, J. Periodont. **35:**285, 1964.

Dienes, L., and Madoff, S.: Differences between oral and genital strains of human pleuropneumonia-like organisms, Proc. Soc. Exp. Biol. Med. **82:**36, 1953.

Egelberg, J., and Cowley, G.: The bacterial state of different regions within the clinically healthy gingival crevice, Acta Odont. Scand. **21:**289, 1963.

Ennever, J. J.: The occurrence of *Micrococcus lactilyticus* in the dento-bacterial plaque, J. Dent. Res. 30:423, 1951.

Gergely, L., and Uri, J.: The mycotic flora of the healthy mouth, Arch. Oral Biol. 3:125, 1961.

Gibbons, R. J., Socransky, S. S., DeAraujo, W. C., and VanHoute, J.: Studies of the predominant cultivable microbiota of dental plaque, Arch. Oral Biol. 9:365, 1964.

Gibbons, R. J., Kapsimalis, B., and Socransky, S. S.: The source of salivary bacteria, Arch. Oral Biol. 9:101, 1964.

Gibson, J.: Nutritional aspects of microbial ecology. In Microbial ecology, Seventh Symposium of the Society of General Microbiology, New York, 1957, Cambridge University Press, p. 22.

Gordon, D. F., Jr., and Gibbons, R. J.: Studies of the predominant cultivable microorganisms from the human tongue, Arch. Oral Biol. 11:627, 1966.

Howell, A., Jr., Stephan, R. M., and Paul F.: Prevalance of *Actinomyces israelii, A. naeslundii, Bacterionema matruchotii,* and *Candida albicans* in selected areas of the oral cavity and saliva, J. Dent. Res. 41:1050, 1962.

Hurst, V.: Bacterial flora of the mouth, J. Periodont. 27:87, 1956.

Jablon, J. M., and Zinner, D. D.: Indigenous character of human oral strains of cariogenic streptococci, Bact. Proc. **20:**66, 1967 (Abstract M35).

Kelstrup, J.: The incidence of *Bacteroides melaninogenicus* in human gingival sulci, and its prevalance in the oral cavity at different ages, Periodontics 4:14, 1966.

Krasse, B.: The proportional distribution of *Streptococcus salivarius* and other streptococci in various parts of the mouth, Odont. Rev. **5:**203, 1954.

Lindhe, J., and Mansson, U.: The bacteriology of the gingival crevices of erupting human incisors, J. Periodont. Res. 1:14, 1966.

McCarthy, C., Snyder, M. L., and Parker, R. B.: The indigenous oral flora of man. I. The newborn to the 1-year-old infant, Arch. Oral Biol. **10:**61, 1965.

McDougal, W. A.: Studies on the dental plaque. II. The histology of the developing interproximal plaque, Aust. Dent. J. 8:398, 1963.

Mandel, I. D.: Dental plaque: Nature, formation and effects, J. Periodont. 37:357, 1966.

Massler, M., and MacDonald, J. B.: The occurrence of beta hemolytic streptococci on the gingiva of normal young adults, J. Dent. Res. **29**:43, 1950.

Mazzarella, M.: Effect of prolonged submarine patrol on oral microbiota, The program of abstracts and papers, The International Association for Dental Research, Forty-fifth General Meeting, 1967 (Abstract #234). Published by J. Dent. Res., p. 95.

Mazzarella, M. A., and Shklair, I. L.: Clinical significance of pleuropneumonia-like organisms in the oral cavity, Great Lakes, Illinois, 1960, Dental Research Facility, U. S. Naval Training Center, 1-9.

Morton, H. F., Smith, P. F., and Williams, N. B.: Isolation of pleuropneumonia-like organisms from human saliva: A newly detected member of the oral flora, J. Dent. Res. **30**:415, 1951.

Razin, S., Michmann, J., and Shimshoni, Z.: The occurrence of mycoplasma (pleuropneumonia-like organisms, PPLO) in the oral cavity of dentulous and edentulous subjects, J. Dent. Res. **43**:402, 1964.

Richardson, R. L., and Jones, M.: A bacteriologic census of human saliva, J. Dent. Res. **37**:697, 1958.

Ritz, H. L.: Localization of *Nocardia* in dental plaque by immunofluorescence (28533), Proc. Soc. Exp. Biol. Med. **43**:925, 1963.

Ritz, H. L.: Microbial populations in developing dental plaque, The program of abstracts and papers, The International Association for Dental Research, Forty-fifth General Meeting, 1967 (Abstract #202). Published by J. Dent. Res., p. 86.

Roth, G. D., and Thurn, A. N.: Continued study of oral nocardia, J. Dent. Res. **41**:1279, 1962.

Snyder, M. L., Bullock, W. W., and Parker, R. B.: Morphology of gram-positive filamentous bacteria identified in dental plaque by fluorescent antibody technique, Arch. Oral Biol. **12**:1269, 1967.

Socransky, S. S., Gibbons, R. J., Dale, A. C., Bortinick, L., Rosenthal, E., and MacDonald, J. B.: The microbiota of the gingival crevice area of man. I. Total microscopic and viable counts and counts of specific organisms, Arch. Oral Biol. **8**:275, 1963.

Sutter, V. L., Hurst, V., and Landucci, A. O. J.: Pseudomonads in human saliva, J. Dent. Res. **45**:1800, 1966.

Tilden, E. B., and Svec, M.: Further studies of a differential culture technique for estimation of acidogenic bacteria in saliva, J. Dent. Res. **31**:9, 1952.

van Reenen, J. F.: Dentition, jaws and palate of the Kalahari Bushman: Part III, J. Dent. Assoc. S. Afr. **19**:67, 1964.

Wantland, W. W., and Wantland, E. M.: Incidence, ecology and reproduction of oral protozoa, J. Dent. Res. **39**:865, 1960.

Williams, N. B., Forbes, M. A., Blau, E., and Eickenberg, C. F.: A study of the simultaneous occurrence of enterococci, lactobacilli and yeast in saliva from human beings, J. Dent. Res. **29**:563, 1950.

Winkler, K. C.: The mechanism of the dental plaque, Int. Dent. J. **8**:561, 1958.

Young, G., Resca, H. G., and Sullivan, M. T.: The yeasts of the normal mouth and their relation to salivary acidity, J. Dent. Res. **30**:426, 1951.

2 / Defense mechanisms of the mouth

INTRODUCTION

Throughout his life man harbors within and on his body a great variety of microorganisms that are potentially pathogenic. The relationship between the healthy host and his indigenous oral microflora represents a balanced biologic system that permits the survival of both. The inherent oral flora establishes and maintains itself without causing any observable harmful change in the host.

The microflora of the oral cavity can be separated into the resident and transient floras. The resident floras represent those microorganisms constantly demonstrated by culture, staining, and immunologic techniques to be in specific areas of the oral cavity; these floras are influenced to some extent by the diet of man and by his geographic location. The transient microfloras, on the other hand, represent those microorganisms isolated sporadically from the oral cavity; they appear unable to survive for any length of time with the resident floras. In the study of oral diseases of man, knowledge of the normal and transient microfloras is essential in determining which organisms cause or are associated with different clinically recognized oral diseases.

The pathogenic traits of the normal microflora do not manifest themselves until something occurs which upsets the balance in the host-parasite relationship; the parasite gains control and causes changes that result in disease. Members of the normal oral flora appear unable to cause disease unless introduced into unprotected or different areas of the body through injury or through some systemic change that favors the parasite. There is evidence that calculus formation about teeth serves as an irritant to the surrounding gingival tissue. Calculus is responsible for much of the inflammation that is associated with the quantitative increase in microorganisms noted in periodontal disease. Much evidence suggests that dental calculus, in vivo, is the result of mineralization by plaque microorganisms.[4, 6]

Employing both cultural and fluorescent antibody staining techniques in studying the microflora of calculus, Slack and coworkers[12] demonstrated the presence of gram-positive filaments and diphtheroid forms: *Actinomyces israelii, A. naeslundii, A. odontolyticus, A. viscosus, Arachina propionica, Rothia dentocariosa, Bacterionema matruchotii,* and *Corynebacterium acnes.*

The microbial flora of the gingival crevice possesses pathogenic properties in terms of its ability to attack oral host tissue. Many members of this mixed population elaborate enzymes and toxic substances that cause cell breakdown resulting in tissue necrosis. The gram-negative bacteria possess endotoxins that have been shown to elicit allergic reactions in laboratory animals.

45

Certain members of the oral bacteria possess enzymes that attack polysaccharides and proteins of the host cells. From salivary samples, *Streptococcus* organisms of Lancefield groups A and K, isolates of *Staphylococcus aureus*, and *Streptococcus mitis* have been shown to produce the enzyme hyaluronidase. This enzyme facilitates the spread of infection through tissues. It has been observed that upper-respiratory tract infections, dental caries, and periodontal disease cause a marked increase in salivary hyaluronidase titers, the increase in hyaluronidase in saliva appearing to be of microbial origin. Certain gingival bacteria form an enzyme that contributes to the breakdown of collagen fibers, and histologic study of gingival tissues shows disorganization of these fibers. This change is seen in periodontitis. Quantitative change in the oral microbiota seems to be one of the dominant characteristics evident when tissue resistance is lowered, as in subjects with malnutrition or debilitation.

Members of the oral flora are adaptable parasites able to survive in the host without obvious damage to host tissue. Their low virulence is indicated by the inability of most members to colonize in previously uninhabited areas elsewhere in the body. When forced into the bloodstream, as occurs during the extraction of teeth, these microorganisms are removed within a matter of from 10 to 30 minutes by the host's phagocytic cells (Fig. 2-1). On the other hand, when forced into the bloodstream and given opportunity to colonize on weakened tissues, as on the heart valves in a rheumatic subject, viridans streptococci in particular may set up vegetative growths on the inactive or the healed alveolar heart lesion and effect the condition, subacute bacterial endocarditis. Many conditions, local or systemic, lowering tissue resistance of the host illustrate the pathogenic potentialities of the indigenous oral flora.

It has been demonstrated that the bacteriologic difference between the normal and the diseased mouth is essentially quantitative. The same organisms appear to be present both in the normal and in the diseased condition; but in the latter, the microbial population has greatly increased in numbers. A periodontally involved mouth

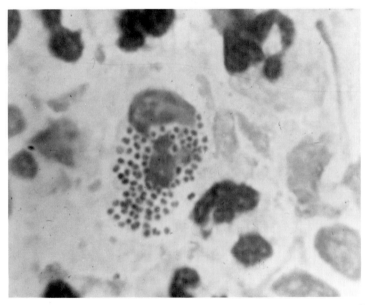

Fig. 2-1. Phagocytosis by a polymorphonuclear leukocyte cell showing intracellular cocci.

may contain from five to ten times or more bacterial debris than that of a normal mouth. Thus it is obvious that the increase in numbers of organisms in disease results in a total increase in the amounts of potentially pathogenizing enzymes, toxins, and other substances of microbial origin.

To be enduring parasites, the microorganisms must learn to live with the host without inciting any overt inflammatory defense response of the host. This relationship represents what might be called a balanced, peaceful coexistence or a commensal existence. The indigenous microflora in the healthy mouth of man is an example of commensalism. Certain indigenous microbial types may afford protection to the host by preventing the colonization of other types, referred to as nonindigenous. The indigenous flora may stimulate the development of humoral and cellular resistance. By an increased stimulation of phagocytosis and antibody response on the part of the host, this resistance could aid in controlling those nonindigenous types that bear common antigens. Humoral antibodies in turn could possibly help in controlling the num-

bers and the spread of the indigenous microbes, especially those that inhabit the gingival crevice.

Frequent and accidental injury to the mucous membrane of the oral cavity generally does not result in serious infections. The many factors that appear to be associated with the defense mechanism of the mouth may be grouped under these three basic headings:

1. The first line of defense—those anatomic and physiologic barriers such as the mucous membrane, the epithelium, the flow of saliva, the anatomy and chemical composition of teeth, antagonistic substances of microbial origin, and others
2. The second line of defense—cellular, normal phagocytosis; cells involved: the leukocytes and the macrophages
3. The third line of defense—humoral immunity, the result of antibody formation

THE ORAL MUCOSA

The stratified squamous epithelium of the oral mucosa forms a continuous surface

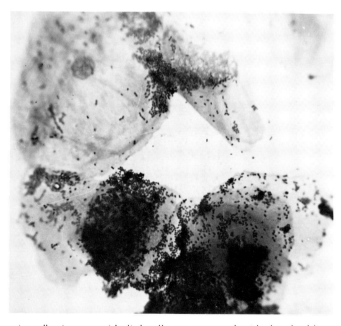

Fig. 2-2. Bacteria adhering to epithelial cells are removed with the shedding of these cells.

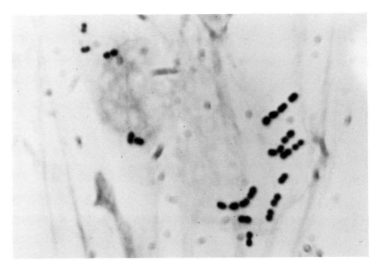

Fig. 2-3. Smear made with throat swab showing cocci adhering to mucuslike material.

that protects the underlying tissues of the oral cavity by functioning as a mechanical barrier. The protection afforded by the epithelium is dependent to a great extent upon its keratinization and its ability to desquamate or shed epithelial cells (Fig. 2-2).

It has been shown that the epithelium of the cheek possesses a minimal keratinization or lacks it completely, whereas complete keratinization is notable of the epithelium of the hard palate and the gingiva. The gingival pocket epithelium is not keratinized and is composed of a very few cell layers; therefore, it offers a rather weak barrier for oral defense. However, it does contribute to the self-cleansing tendency of the gingival pocket, since it is renewed considerably faster than the oral epithelium. Also, there is a continuous outward migration of epithelial cells, which is followed by their desquamation at the entrance of the pocket. The movement of these cells from the sulcus outward mechanically aids in removing microorganisms and other debris from this area. The close contact between the pocket epithelium and the tooth surface does minimize the penetration of microorganisms and other material into the sulcus or pocket area.

Microorganisms are held on and within a slimy or mucous coat that covers the oral cavity, including the teeth (Fig. 2-3). It is generally thought that the attachment of bacteria to oral epithelial cells is associated with the adherence of bacterial capsular material and mucoid carbohydrate of saliva that cover the epithelium. Experimentally, use of digestive enzymes and surface-active agents has been shown to be ineffective in removing microorganisms. It has been suggested that bacterial attachment to oral epithelial cells may be caused by a reaction involving antibody.[5] Immunoglobulins demonstrated in the human gingiva are thought to be a response to the bacterial antigens that inhabit the gingival sulcus. Antigenic substances are thought to pass through the epithelial barrier of the gingiva and stimulate immunoglobulin formation. Thus, the intact epithelium probably serves also as a humoral defense barrier.[13] There is some evidence that the healthy mucosa has an inhibitive effect on the nonindigenous microorganisms which enter the oral cavity, and also that it retards the proliferation and the invasion of members of the indigenous flora.

When carbon particles or microorganisms are placed in specific areas of the oral cavity, they move backward in the throat and are swallowed. This backward motion is caused by a sucking action set up by movement of the tongue, the cheeks, the lips, and the palate. Salivary flow is also a factor in the movement of these particles from the lingual and buccal mucosa areas especially. Carbon particles have been shown to be removed from the oral cavity within a period of 30 minutes, and nonindigenous microorganisms within several minutes to a few hours. The rapid clearance of streptomycin-resistant and streptomycin-dependent lactobacilli from the oral cavity can be attributed to tissue trapping, the flushing action of saliva, and the swallowing reflex. Movement of the lips and tongue during the mastication process keeps food particles on the occlusal surfaces of teeth, and the chewing process helps to clean these surfaces of microbial growth. Food particles and microbial clumps are directed toward the throat by saliva flow and movement of the tongue, and are swallowed with the masticated food bolus.

The epithelium and its mucous coat, coupled with the irrigating effect of saliva, the movement of the tongue, cheeks, and lips, and the effect of chewing, swallowing, expectorating, and coughing represent mechanisms that help to remove microorganisms and thereby control, within certain limits, the microbial populations of the oral cavity.

SALIVA

The lubricating property of saliva is due to its mucin content. Mucins contain carbohydrate and amino acids, and these may serve as possible nutrients for microorganisms. Salivary mucins have been found to coat bacteria and to protect the organism against phagocytosis.

Salivary flow rate

The effectiveness of the saliva's flow rate and cleansing action is influenced by the location of the salivary glands and their ducts. Numerous studies have been conducted to determine the flow rate of saliva within the oral cavity; but technical difficulties in obtaining true salivary samples have produced conflicting results. Some reports indicate a higher rate of salivary flow in caries-inactive than in caries-active subjects. It has been noted that rampant caries usually occurs in subjects with impaired salivary flow. The quantity of saliva secreted between meals is reported to be somewhat less than at mealtime.

The flow of saliva from the large salivary ducts demonstrates a protective mechanism in that it restrains the movement of microorganisms into the duct. The slowing down of salivary flow, noted to occur in the state of shock and dehydration, appears to favor infection of the parotid glands. Such concurrence has been observed in the severe dehydration of subjects following cholera and dysentery infections.

A recent study of a large group of subjects between the ages of 17 and 22 years showed statistically a higher parotid fluid flow rate in subjects with the lowest DMF score. The study provided evidence, though, that the carious status of individuals could not always be predicted, since there was considerable overlapping of flow rate values between the different DMF score groups.

In an attempt to correlate salivary flow rate with caries activity and caries inactivity, consideration of the buffering effect of saliva is most important. Saliva acts to neutralize and dilute acids formed by dental plaque from ingested carbohydrates. Saliva from caries-inactive subjects shows a greater buffering capacity or carbon dioxide combining power; it appears also to be more highly supersaturated with calcium and phosphate ions and has slightly more ammonium than saliva from caries-susceptible individuals. Fig. 2-4, *A* and *B*, shows the buffering effect of caries-active and caries-inactive salivary samples in the presence of dental plaque.

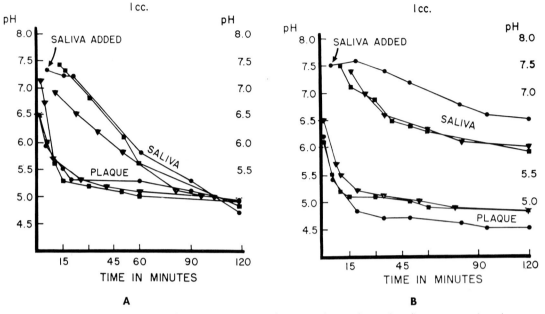

Fig. 2-4. Changes in pH of dental plaque and surrounding saliva. The plaque was placed in a cup glass electrode; sugar was added and saliva was placed in contact with the outer surface of the plaque. Changes in pH of the plaque in A and B show the characteristic drop. Comparison of pH change of saliva shows that saliva from caries active subjects, **A,** dropped rapidly, whereas saliva from caries inactive subjects, **B,** showed less change in pH and never reached a critical pH (5.2). The caries inactive saliva demonstrates greater buffering effect. (From Nolte, W. A., and Arnim, S. S.: J. Dent. Res. **35**(1):83-89, 1956.)

Salivary pH

Optimum pH for growth of most bacteria is between pH 6.5 and 7.5. In general, it may be stated that the minimum pH for the growth of these microorganisms is between pH 4.5 and 5.0, and the maximum between pH 8.0 and 8.5. Although the pH range for growth of the majority of microorganisms is quite wide, pH exerts some degree of selective action on survival and growth of certain species. In the oral cavity, a low pH around 4.0 to 5.5 favors the survival and growth of acidogenic, aciduric types such as lactobacilli, yeast, and some streptococci. Lactobacilli do not survive long in saliva as it changes to the alkaline side of neutrality. On the other hand, saliva of pH 5.0 or lower has a growth inhibitory effect for strong proteolytic types. Salivary samples from caries-resistant adults appear to have significantly higher pH levels than do samples from caries-active adults. No clear relation of this kind has been shown for the saliva of children.

Inhibitory factors in saliva

Saliva has been demonstrated to have a bactericidal and a lytic effect on many pathogenic and nonpathogenic microorganisms. Substances found in saliva that inhibit the growth of different bacterial species are called inhibins; those particular substances that inhibit the growth of the diphtheria bacillus have been called zidins. In vitro tests have shown that the diphthericidal activity of saliva results from the presence of hydrogen peroxide, produced by strains of oral alpha streptococci.

Much of the inhibitory activity of saliva appears to be associated with an antagonism among oral organisms themselves. Bacterial antibiosis probably plays a very important role in selecting and controlling the oral flora. Freshly stimulated saliva has been shown to inhibit beta hemolytic streptococci and to prevent the germination of *Clostridium tetani* spores.

The microbial balance of the oral flora can be changed with the use of antibiotics. Inhibition of many types of the indigenous flora with the tetracycline antibiotics leads to the rapid appearance of the yeast in the oral cavity. The use of penicillin troches changes the oral flora, and gram-negative coliform organisms soon appear. When use of the antibiotic is discontinued, the inhibited indigenous microflora reappears. The yeast and coliform types in turn decrease in number, apparently through the antagonism of the reappearing normal types.

In addition to inhibitory factors of microbial origin, there are several antimicrobial substances produced by the host and found in the saliva. The most important of these substances will be discussed.

Lysozymes

Fleming, in 1922, reported the presence of a substance in nasal secretions that caused the dissolution of the bacterium *Micrococcus lysodeikticus*; the substance was called lysozyme. This substance is widely distributed in the tissues of the body, in body fluids, including the saliva, in gingival tissue, and in the gingival crevice fluid as well as in leukocytes. It has not been shown to be present in pus, cerebrospinal fluid, or urine. Since this enzyme is widely distributed in the tissues and fluids of man, it is thought to play a very important role in man's native resistance to infection. It is active against strains of *Neisseria*, micrococci, *Sarcina*, *Klebsiella*, streptococci, staphylococci, and *Mycobacterium*.

Lysozyme is a mucopolysaccharide enzyme; it is protein in nature and has an iso-electric point at pH 10.5 to 11.0. The

activity of egg white lysozyme has been shown to be rendered nonlytic for the organism *Micrococcus lysodeikticus* by treatment at pH 7.0 with submaxillary mucoid. This mucoid-lysozyme complex can be reversed by sodium chloride. Uncentrifuged saliva is reported to have 50% more lysozyme activity than does centrifuged saliva. It is thought that salivary lysozyme complexes with mucin, is precipitated, and is removed by centrifugation. Variations in lysozyme activity of saliva may result in part from variations in the mucopolysaccharide content.

Laboratory tests have indicated that lysozyme appears to act on the mucoid-polysaccharide substance of the bacterial cell. Gram-positive bacteria contain a mucocomplex which maintains the structural integrity of the cell wall. Dissolution of this complex, acetyl-aminopolysaccharide, by lysozyme affects the protoplast, a result of a breakdown of the cell wall and the liberation of the cytoplasmic membrane with its content.

The effectiveness of lysozyme as a host resistance factor to infection is debatable. Higher concentrations of lysozyme have been found in the inflamed gingiva than in the normal gingiva; also, greater lysozyme activity has been found in gingival fluid from subjects with increased periodontal inflammatory changes. This increase in lysozyme activity of gingival fluid over that of serum or saliva is attributed to leukocytes which infiltrate the gingiva and migrate out to the pocket. It has been shown that injured granulocytes release an active enzyme that behaves much like lysozyme. Since the number of disintegrated leukocytes appears to be much higher in fluid from the inflamed gingival pocket than that from the clinically healthy gingival pocket, the increase in lysozyme activity in fluid from the inflamed pocket is possibly the result of disintegrated leukocytes. In addition to causing lyses of susceptible bacteria, lysozyme may inhibit growth without causing the cell to disintegrate.

A report has shown that several strains of the indigenous microflora appeared to be resistant to the action of lysozyme. Members of the indigenous microflora identified as *Bacteroides oralis, B. melaninogenicus,* anaerobic diphtheroids, facultative diphtheroids, fusiform bacilli, a species of lactobacilli, peptostreptococci, staphylococci, a streptococci identified as *mitis,* also one identified as *salivarius,* a spirochete *Treponema microdentium, Veillonella alcalescens,* and *Vibrio sputorum* were not lysed by this enzyme, nor were they inhibited from growing. In studies in which gingival crevice material was incubated with lysozyme, the bulk of the organisms found in this material were not lysed. These findings seem to indicate that lysozyme has little effect on the indigenous oral microflora.

Other antibacterial factors

Human saliva contains, in addition to lysozyme, other antibacterial agents. It has been demonstrated that saliva from immune mouths will not support the growth of *Lactobacillus acidophilus* and, when sugar is added, does not permit the formation of acid as rapidly as does saliva from caries-susceptible subjects. In vitro tests have shown that saliva possesses bactericidal action for various bacteria including the typhoid bacillus, the tuberculosis bacillus, the diphtheria bacillus, and colon bacilli.

It has been reported that the majority of aerobic bacteria found in human saliva form hydrogen peroxide in vitro. If hydrogen peroxide accumulates in certain areas of the oral cavity, it should inhibit anaerobic types.

Freshly stimulated whole saliva has been shown to prevent the growth of beta streptococci. The inhibitory substance is distinct from lysozyme and hydrogen peroxide; it is associated with the viable indigenous oral flora and appears to act as an antibiotic against the beta streptococci. It is possible also that this substance is some essential growth requirement and that its utilization by other members of the oral microflora makes it unavailable for the beta streptococci. Freshly stimulated whole saliva has also been demonstrated to inhibit *Clostridium tetani,* the inhibitory factor having the same properties as the substance that inhibits beta streptococci.

Numerous studies have reported the presence of a lactobacillus-bactericidin system in parotid and submaxillary saliva, but not in serum (Fig. 2-5). The activity of this bactericidin system has been shown to depend upon two components; one is identified as peroxidase and the other, thiocyanate. The system appears to be associated with the salivary glands themselves and is not of microbial origin. The inhibitory effect of this system is decreased by catalase and serum. It is absent from the saliva of premature new infants and is not found in the majority of newborns until after the first four days of life. Lactobacillus-bactericidin titers appear to show a systematic increase during the first decade of life, at which time they level off. The level of the antilactobacillus system in saliva appears to vary in the same individual from time to time. Some individuals' saliva shows a decrease in antilactobacillus activity during sieges of upper-respiratory tract infection. As health returns, the usual titer of activity reappears.

It has been shown that the albumin portion of serum has a depressant activity on the factor, this depressing effect apparently being associated with the reactive sulfhydryl groupings.[14]

It has been observed that all lactobacilli isolates are not always inhibited by salivary specimens. Isolates of *Lactobacillus acidophilus, L. casei, L. salivarius, L. plantarum, L. fermenti, L. buchneri, L. brevis,* and *L. cellobiosis* have been shown to demon-

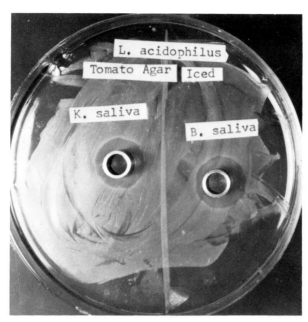

Fig. 2-5. Antilactobacillus factor. Tomato juice agar, lawn seeded with *Lactobacillus aci-dophilus*. Filtered saliva of individuals K and B was added to steel cylinders, and the Petri dish was placed in a refrigerator overnight to permit diffusion of the factor. The plate was then incubated for 24 hours. Zones of inhibition of growth are observable about each saliva specimen.

strate a wide range in sensitivity to the antilactobacillus system in salivary specimens. A variable that affects the demonstration of the factor is the kind of medium used in testing. Rogosa's medium was shown to give the best reproductive results, while brain heart infusion broth appeared to inactivate the factor.[2] The present findings agree with those of Matsumura and associates[8, 9] in that the factor is bacteriostatic rather than bactericidal.

Smoking reportedly increases the antibacterial activity of saliva for lactobacilli. The increase in activity is reported to be possibly associated with the increase in thiocyanate ion noted in smokers' saliva. The antilactobacillus activity was evident during the first few minutes of cigarette or pipe smoking.[3] The presence of this system in saliva is thought by some to help in the selection of the oral microbial population.

Another factor which differs from the antilactobacillus system has been found in saliva. This factor is present in the saliva of caries-immune subjects and absent in caries-susceptible. It appears to be associated with gamma globulins and requires complement for its activity. Cultures 72 hours old appeared to be more susceptible to its lytic effect than were cultures 24 to 48 hours old. This lytic factor appears to be antibody-like and shows more or less specific activity for gram-positive microorganisms.

Antibodies

General information. Antibodies are modified serum globulins formed by plasma and lymphoid cells of the reticuloendothelial system. These globulins, given the name immune globulin (Ig), constitute normally about 1% of the total protein of the serum.

From investigations during the past 10 years, immunoglobulins appear to have certain basic structure. The basic immunoglobulin (7S) has four polypeptide chains, two heavy chains with a molecular weight of about 50,000 each and two light chains of 25,000 mol. wt. each. The chains are held together by disulfide bonds. The entire molecule has 150,000 mol. wt. and possesses two binding sites. The specific determinants of the binding groups for antigen are associated with the heavy chains, whereas the common determinants of binding with antigens are associated with the light chain.

When immunoelectrophoretic technique is employed on serum, antibody globulins are found mainly in the gamma fraction and can be separated into three major distinct classes referred to as IgG, IgM, and IgA; and two minor classes, IgE and IgD. These antibodies have also been referred to as γG, γM, γA, γE, and γD.

Based upon chemical, physical, and immunologic properties, antibodies have been shown to possess certain characteristics. In the following paragraphs, the antibodies and some of their important characteristics are noted.

IgG is an immunoglobulin that has a sedimentation constant of 7S (Svedberg units) in the ultracentrifuge, about 150,000 mol. wt., has two combining sites and therefore a valence of two, fixes complement, passes placenta in human beings, and constitutes about 70% of the total immunoglobulin. It is the most important of the immunoglobulins, highly specific and active against toxins, bacteria, and virus. It appears to follow IgM in antibody response. It can be demonstrated in animals to produce passive cutaneous anaphylaxis.

IgM is known as a macroglobulin, 19S sedimentation constant and 900,000 mol. wt. It is composed of five 7S monomers and, theoretically, it should have ten binding sites. However, it appears to have a valence of only five, and therefore there is possibly a masking of the other binding sites. This is the first antibody formed. It does not pass the placenta nor does it show passive cutaneous anaphylaxis. It represents about 7% of the immunoglobulin and is found to a lesser extent in the extravascular fluids. It is found to predominate in infants and is synthesized in the fetus in utero. This antibody is highly bactericidal for gram-negative bacteria. It has been referred to as the "killer" antibody. IgM appears to be less specific in combing with antigen than IgG and it fixes complement.

IgA is an antibody that exists in two forms: 7S and 11S with 170,000 and 390,000 mol. wt., respectively. The IgA of the 7S type is found in serum. The IgA of the 11S type is composed of two 7S serum molecules and is linked by a nonglobulin secretory piece referred to as "T" piece. The T piece is synthesized in mucous membrane epithelial cells, whereas the IgA molecule is synthesized by plasma cells. This antibody is antibacterial and antiviral. Secretory IgA is found in saliva, tears, the gastrointestinal and genitourinary tracts, urine, and colostrum. It is found to be the second highest in concentration in man. It may represent the first line of antibody defense against bacteria and virus invasion via mucous membranes, for example, those of the oral cavity.

IgE is an 8S antibody, 200,000 mol. wt. It is known as the reaginic antibody mediating atopic and anaphylactic allergic reactions. IgE is present in low concentration in normal individuals, and it is found to increase in allergic individuals.

IgD is an antibody known as a 7S, 150,000 mol. wt. Its antibody activity has not been definitely established. It is present in concentrations in serum.

There is evidence that specific antibody formation is mainly dependent upon lymphocytes, which appear in the germinal centers of the thymus in the embryo after the second month. As the thymus develops, lymphocytes migrate and establish active germinal centers of lymphocytic tissues (nodes) in the spleen, tonsil, adenoid tissues, and throughout the body. When in contact with antigenic substances, the lymphocytes differentiate into antibody-producing plasma cells. The importance of the thymus in immunity is stressed by the fact that if it is removed early in life, the adult shows the absence of or a defective immunologic response. The most important cites of antibody production are the spleen and lymph nodes.

Antigens

Substances that stimulate antibody formation and react with the formed antibody are called antigens. Antigens are foreign to the host and are generally protein in nature. Some polysaccharide material has been shown to have antigenic properties. Lipoid substances, nonantigenic polysaccharides, and other chemicals can be coupled to protein. These substances are called haptens or partial antigens and, when combined with an antigenic protein, they influence the specificity of antibodies that are formed. Haptens do not stimulate antibody production but do combine with antibodies produced by the stimulation of the hapten-protein-complex antigen.

For a substance to be antigenic, the minimum molecular weight is about 5,000. In general, the greater the molecular weight, the greater the stimulation in antibody production. Most of the microbial antigens are protein hapten complexes. Specificity of antigens is determined by their chemical structure and the spacial relation of chemical radicals in the molecule. The antigenic portion that combines with the antibody is called "determinant group." Determinant groups vary in number from two to many, and they are known as valences of the antigen or its combining

power. Specificity may be changed by altering chemical groups of the antigenic molecule by treatment with formaldehyde by heat or other means.

Some antigens are found in widely distant species; these are known as heterophile antigens. An example is the Forssman antigen, present in the organs of the guinea pig, in the dog, sheep, human red blood cells, certain other animals, plants (corn), and certain strains of enteric and pneumococcal bacteria. Isoantigens are substances present in some members of the same species that are antigenic for other members of the species. The A, B, and Rh substances of the erythrocytes and histocompatability antigens of man are examples of isoantigens.

There are antigenic substances of the body such as the lens protein of the eye, thyroglobulin, and certain other substances that are normally isolated from antibody-forming cells. When these substances come in contact, possibly through injury, with lymphocytes, their antigenicity is recognized as foreign or "nonself" and specific antibody is formed against them. The reaction against one's own antigens is known as autoimmunity.

Microorganisms contain many different antigenic substances. The virulence of a specific microorganism is probably associated with only one or two of its antigens. Therefore, antibodies produced against these antigens should give protection to the host. In the case of beta streptococci, virulence appears to be associated with surface "M" protein of the cell; for the pneumococci, it is the different polysaccharide capsule material; for gram-negative bacteria, it is the endotoxin (polysaccharide-lipid-protein complex); and for the diphtheria bacillus, it is the exotoxin.

Several factors found in serum, collectively known as complement, are associated with certain immunologic reactions. Complement is concerned with lysis of bacteria, red blood cells in the presence of their specific antibody. It is involved in phagocytosis and also in a possible, non-specific resistance system involving a serum protein known as properdin.

The kinds of antibodies stimulated by antigenic substances have been given various names such as antitoxins, agglutinins, precipitins, lysins, opsonins, and neutralizing, complement-fixing, and blocking antibodies. These names are descriptive of the type of in vitro or in vivo reactions that occur between an antibody and its specific antigen.

1. Antitoxins are antibodies which neutralize or flocculate antigenic toxins or toxoids.
2. Agglutinins are antibodies which cause an aggregation or clumping of particulate antigen such as bacterial cells and red blood cells.
3. Precipitins are antibodies which complex with soluble antigens and form precipitates.
4. Lysins are antibodies which react and cause dissolution of cells in the presence of a component known as a complement.

Table 2-1. Some antigen-antibody reactions

Name of test	State of antigen	Name of antibody	Reaction
Animal protection	Soluble: toxin	Antitoxin	Neutralization of toxin by antitoxin occurs when mixed in proper proportions.
Agglutination	Particulate: suspension of intact bacterial cells, R.B.C., etc.	Agglutinin	There is clumping of cells by antibody.
Precipitation or flocculation	Soluble: extracts of cells and tissues, serum	Precipitin	A visible precipitate occurs with the union of antigen and antibody.
Cytolysis	Particle: bacterial cell	Cytolysins	Bacterial cells react with cytolysins in the presence of complement, and cells lyse.
Opsonic index	Bacterial cell	Opsonin	Bacterial cells react with the opsonin and are made more suspecptible to phagocytosis by leukocytes.
Hemagglutination inhibition	Virus	Antiviral antibodies	Virus coats type O human R.B.C. and causes them to agglutinate. In the presence of immune sera the antibodies combine with the virus and agglutination of R.B.C. is inhibited.
Complement fixation	A. Soluble (unknown system) PLUS B. R.B.C. (hemolytic system)	C-F antibody Hemolysin	Positive / No hemolysis / (Antigen + antibody react in the presence of complement) — Negative / Hemolysis / (R.B.C. + hemolysin react in the presence of complement)
Quellung reaction	Capsule about bacterial cell	Capsular antibody	Capsule appears to swell in presence of specific immune sera.
Fluorescent antibody	Virus or bacteria	Fluorescent labelled antibody	The union of fluorescent labelled antibody with antigen fluoresces under ultraviolet light.

5. Opsonins are antibodies which effect the particulate antigen and render the antigen more readily phagocytized by leukocytes.

6. Neutralizing antibodies, sometimes referred to as protective antibodies, render the antigenic microorganism, commonly a virus, noninfective.

7. Complement-fixing antibodies involve reaction in which a known system containing red blood cells and its specific hemolysins are employed in determining whether the complement has been fixed in the unknown or test (antigen + serum antibody) systems.

8. Blocking antibodies combine with antigen; their reaction is not demonstrated unless they can be shown to inhibit or prevent the reaction between a known antigen and its specific antibody.

Table 2-1 presents tests that indicate the physical manifestation of some antigen-antibody reactions.

Salivary antibodies. Reports show that antibodies against *Vibrio*, the spirochete of syphilis, and *Brucella* have been found in saliva. These antibodies, called "natural antibodies," may be found in saliva and serum of subjects who have had no evidence of previous infection. Antibodies are present in parotid fluid as well as in whole saliva. Natural antibodies which react with *Salmonella typhosa* and *Shigella dysenteriae* have been detected in parotid fluid. Antibody globulins of the γA (11S), some γG (7S), and to a lesser extent γM (19S) are found in saliva, while the bactericidal activity of parotid fluid appears to be associated with the γA fraction. Parotid fluid has been shown to contain IgA that readily agglutinates *Streptococcus sanguis*.[1] Some workers have suggested that the antibodies found in saliva are the result of gingival pocket fluid which contains serum protein. The pocket fluid could be one of the sources for the antibodies found in saliva. Antibodies have been found in parotid fluid collected free from serum contamination. The salivary gland itself may be capable of synthesizing immune globulin, or the antibodies found in parotid fluid may be the result of the passage of blood into the parotid gland and then to the fluid that is secreted. Experimental evidence suggests that both mechanisms are possibly involved.

Opsonizing antibodies to *Lactobacillus acidophilus*, streptococci, and *Sarcina lutea* have been detected in unstimulated saliva. A phagocytic index of from 20% to 60% was shown for caries-free saliva and from 0% to 10% for caries-active saliva. The passive transfer of antibodies to saliva occurs when immune serum is administered. Antibodies stimulated by the injection of the typhoid vaccine do find their way to the saliva; the saliva of typhoid fever patients has been reported to show both H and O agglutinins. Respective salivary and serum samples from subjects have shown detectable antibody titers by the hemagglutination or agglutination tests for *Staphylococcus aureus*, *Staphylococcus albus*, *Streptococcus pyogenes*, *Streptococcus salivarius*, *Streptococcus mitis*, *Streptococcus faecalis*, *Diplococcus pneumoniae*, *Bacillus subtilis*, *Corynebacterium hoffmanii*, *Clostridium perfringens*, *Actinomyces israelii*, *Neisseria catarrhalis*, and *Escherichia coli*. Antibody titers for these organisms were always lower in saliva than in respective serum. Some salivary samples were negative when the respective serum samples were positive. These antibodies were detected in saliva samples only when they were present in the respective serum sample; therefore, these salivary antibodies probably came from the plasma.

This finding suggests that members of the indigenous flora are capable of inducing antibodies in man and that these antibodies may help to determine and regulate the quantitative relationship among the oral microfloras. Submaxillary saliva was shown to have an elevated concentration of IgA and albumin in caries-resistant subjects.[15]

Lehner and co-workers[7] demonstrated that the sera from subjects with a high DMF score had a significantly higher antibody titer for two cariogenic streptococci than sera from subjects with a low DMF index. Noncariogenic bacteria did not reflect a difference in antibody titers for these subjects. Therefore, examination of the antibody titers in man against bacteria that are cariogenic in animals might aid in establishing a relationship of these bacteria to human caries.

Parallel studies employing the immunofluorescent technique have shown the presence of antibodies to *Candida albicans* in serum and saliva of subjects with candidiasis, carriers of candida, and control subjects. The highest titers were found in patients having candidiasis, and the titers were higher in the serum than in the saliva.

The fungus *Cryptococcus neoformans* is frequently associated with infections in man. It is considered to be an opportunist, and infection is thought to be related to variations in host resistance. Anticryptococcal substances have been detected in serum and saliva of normal subjects. The fungus inhibitor in the saliva is different from the serum inhibitor. Both are possibly associated with man's natural resistance to cryptococcosis.

Salivary corpuscles

It is well known that the leukocyte count of blood, of cerebrospinal fluid, of urine, and of other fluids furnishes valuable clinical information. The presence of leukocytes or corpuscles in saliva has recently received considerable notice. Subjects with clinically healthy gingiva have few salivary leukocytes. As gingivitis develops, the number of leukocytes increases. The number of leukocytes varies from person to person and for a given person during the day; it appears to be the lowest in the morning, increases during the day, and decreases at night.[10]

In diseases of the oral cavity, attention has been directed to the number and kinds of microorganisms in saliva rather than to the salivary corpuscle count of saliva. It has been reported that the leukocyte count ranges from 110,000 to 1,364,000 per milliliter of saliva for dentulous subjects with clinically healthy mouths; 770,000 to 11,896,000 per milliliter of saliva from subjects with inflamed and carious mouths; and 1,000 to 143,000 per milliliter of saliva from edentulous subjects with healthy mouths. There is a marked fluctuation in the leukocyte count of saliva as compared with that of blood.

The source of the oral leukocyte is of considerable interest. Leukocytes have not been found in glands or in the ducts of saliva. The entire mucous membrane is a source of the salivary corpuscles, the highest numbers coming from the gingiva. It is reported that leukocytes make up an average of 47% of the somatic cell scrapings from the gingival sulcus and 1.6% of the total somatic cells from other areas of the mouth. The mechanical stimulation of chewing and brushing and the metabolic activity of microorganisms induce leukocytes to migrate from capillaries to the connective tissues and then to the gingiva.

Very few lymphocytes have been found in saliva or in smears from the sulcus. These cells are found in the epithelium of the gingiva, and they probably play a major role in local humoral defense. The polymorphonuclear leukocytes represent the overwhelming majority of white blood cells found in saliva and in smears from the oral cavity. Salivary leukocytes that come from the oral mucous membrane are thought to come either directly through the epithelium or from small, specific glands.

Once the oral leukocyte reaches the free tissue surface, its survival and activity are dependent upon the presence of the mucous coat. Mucus from the salivary glands protects the viability of the leukocytes. It has been observed that leukocytes break up when they come into contact with the serous part of saliva.

Leukocytes have been found in the soft plaque material removed from teeth. When these leukocytes come into contact with saliva, they ball and become inactive. When plaque is placed in an isotonic solution, such as Ringer's, the leukocytes show vigorous phagocytic activity. Leukocytes from caries-resistant subjects phagocytize cariogenic streptococci to a greater degree than those from caries-active subjects. Concentrated parotid saliva from both caries-resistant and caries-active subjects was shown to enhance phagocytosis of cariogenic streptococci in in vitro tests. The presence of specific antibody has been given as the possible explanation for the immunity of the caries-free group.[11]

It is suggested that the intact viable leukocyte is actually a main line of defense in the oral cavity and that it may help also to control the microbial population.

GINGIVAL FLUID
Flow

The removal of india ink particles inserted into a healthy gingival pocket indicates that the flow of fluid from the pocket probably proceeds outward at a much faster rate than saliva can penetrate inward. Microorganisms are hindered from entering the gingival sulcus by the intact crevicular epithelium, by the flow of gingival fluid into the oral cavity, and by the continuous shedding of epithelial cells which line the sulcus. The movement of gingival fluid and epithelial cells that line the crevice outward into the oral cavity prevents the entrance of, and encourages the removal of, extraneous matter from the gingival crevice, thus contributing to defense against gingival disease. The flow of gingival fluid outward also furnishes an intrinsic nutrient supply, which influences favorably the development of plaque on teeth at the gingival margin (Fig. 2-6).

Antimicrobial factors

Gingival fluid contains antibacterial factors in addition to lysozyme. Globulins having the property of antibodies are present in this fluid. The gingival fluid seeps out of the sulcus into the oral cavity and in so doing adds antibodies to saliva. The amount of fluid that flows from the gingival pocket under experimental conditions has been shown to increase with the severity of gingival inflammation. Studies have indicated that the fluid flow begins before

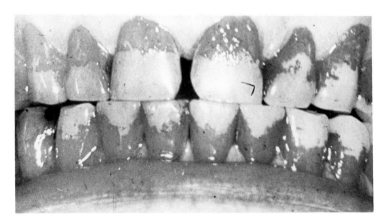

Fig. 2-6. Heavy plaque accumulations at the gingival margin necks of teeth as shown with a disclosing stain. (Courtesy Dr. S. S. Arnim, Houston, Tex.)

pathologic changes in tissue can be observed at a clinical level and that it persists in many instances after clinical inflammation has subsided. The gingival fluid is an inflammatory exudate, and its absence or presence may represent a definite clinical criterion in distinguishing the normal from the inflamed gingiva.

By the use of fluorescin it has been possible to demonstrate the passage of blood from the tissues of the sulcus into the crevicular environment. It has been shown that more fluorescin passes into the inflamed gingival pocket than into the healthy sulci. This may be taken to indicate that there is an increase in the amount of plasma present as the result of increased capillary permeability of the sulcus tissue in inflammation. The flow of tissue fluid into gingival pockets can be increased by vigorous chewing, by pressing on the gingiva, and also by toothbrushing. The amount of gingival fluid in the crevice reflects the degree of inflammation.

A comparison of the proteins of the gingival pocket fluid with those of the serum and saliva, using immunoelectrophoretic techniques, has shown that the gingival pocket fluid contains γG, γA, and γM globulins, albumins, and fibrinogen. These proteins were present in concentrations comparable to those in the plasma. Unconcentrated saliva was shown to contain γG and γA globulins and albumins in concentrations much lower than those in the serum; γM globulin was not detected in this study. The ratio of γG to γA globulins was found to be approximately 1 to 1 in saliva; whereas that in serum and gingival fluid was 8 to 1.

The presence of antibodies in the gingival pocket fluid represents a defense mechanism of this gingival area. The presence of a fibrinolytic enzyme system in this fluid is equally important in that it helps remove fibrin formed as a result of the inflammatory response. The development of fibrin clots could reduce the flow of

fluid from inside of the pocket outward and thus hinder a defense mechanism which retards the ingress of microorganisms to the sulcus area.

Gingival fluid is rich in nutrients and it will support the growth of many different types of bacteria. Any restriction of the outflow of this nutrient would create a culture environment within the sulcus; rapid colonization of microorganisms within the sulcus would result. Polymorphonuclear leukocytes have been found in this fluid, and it has been observed that phagocytosis takes place in the gingival sulcus.

The fluorescent antibody technique has shown that specific antibodies are present within the gingival tissue adjacent to the sulcus. It has been observed that there is a difference in the intensity of fluorescent staining in different areas of gingival tissue, indicating that tissue globulins are probably present in varying amounts. The increase in the number of plasma cells and in the globulins in the inflamed gingiva suggests that a protective mechanism is directed against bacteria found in the crevice. The presence of plasma cells and antibodies within this tissue, coupled with the failure to find microorganisms, may be taken to indicate a successful defense mechanism against bacterial invasion.

The presence of antibodies in the sulcus is the result of diffusion of these antibodies from the surrounding tissues containing plasma cells. The antibodies may control the bacterial population within the sulcus or may react with soluble microbial antigens which have diffused into the surrounding tissues. Plasma cells are sources of antibody production, and their presence indicates this activity within gingival tissue. The reaction observed between various microorganisms of the gingival sulcus, identified microscopically as gram-negative and gram-positive bacilli, cocci, coliforms, and others, suggests that a spectrum of antibodies is produced within gingival tissue. The finding of plasma cells in normal gingival tissue suggests that antibodies against oral microorganisms are always present and that they maintain a relatively constant defense in the tissues.

There are those who have reported that the clinically normal human gingiva does not show any flow of fluid. Not finding fluid in the clinically normal crevice reflects, first, a difference in criteria used to determine what is clinically normal and,

second, a difference in the sensitivity and variations of technique employed in sampling the gingival crevice.

OTHER DEFENSE MECHANISMS

The enamel of the tooth increases in hardness with progressive age and protects the internal structures from invasion of microorganisms. Enamel is nonvital and, once it is damaged, does not repair itself.

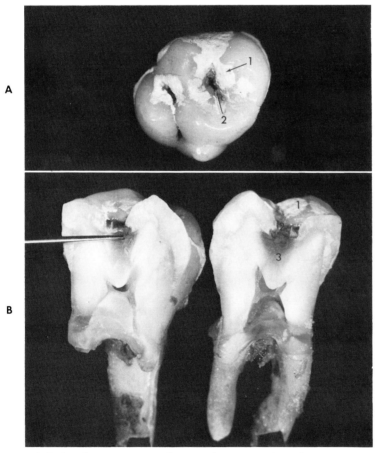

Fig. 2-7. **A,** Calculus formation is evident on the crown, *1,* with active caries within the central fossa, *2.* **B,** Split tooth shows soft carious lesion. The formation of calculus, *1,* and decay, *2,* occurs simultaneously but in different areas, indicating the flexibility of the microbial masses associated with these processes. When cariogenic foods collect within the cavity and are held for long periods of time, the tooth demineralizes. Organisms on the tooth surface are not exposed to cariogenic foods for long periods; therefore, their chief nutrient differs from those in the cavity, with the end result that mineralization occurs. Evidence of sclerosis of dentinal tubules between the carious lesion and the pulp is seen, *3.* (Courtesy Dr. S. S. Arnim, Houston, Tex.)

It is one of the hardest substances of the body; it is hardest on the occlusal and incisal surfaces. Although it is resistant to diseases that affect the soft tissues, it is susceptible to acids produced by certain types of microorganisms. It is when the pH is reduced to around 5.2 and lower that acids decalcify the inorganic structures; but not all microorganisms produce acids in sufficient quantity to bring about decalcification (Fig. 2-7). Dental plaque through its buffering capacity exerts some protection against acid foods and microbial acids.

Under the enamel is the dentin, which possesses restoratory powers. The protective action of dentin against bacterial invasion is its forming sclerotic dentin within the tubules and its laying down secondary dentin over the pulp end of the tubules. These two mechanisms form a barrier against bacterial invasion of the pulp.

If the pulp is invaded, a typical inflammatory response is shown by the infiltration of polymorphonuclear leukocytes, small lymphocytes, and macrophages. A wall of connective tissues is produced by fibroblasts in an attempt to prevent the spread of these microorganisms. If invasion is carried to the periapical tissues, an abscess may form which protects and localizes the microorganisms in this area. A chronic infection is likely to involve the development of a granuloma. This structure affords a barrier and helps to prevent further spread of microorganisms into periodontal tissues. The flow of blood or serum as the result of injury to oral tissues washes away microorganisms and other foreign material from the environment and thus acts in defense of the host.

The gingival papillae fill the interproximal space between the teeth and in such manner assist in preventing the stasis of food about the teeth. Calculus formation on the crowns of teeth may actually exert a protective action.

Thus the mouth exhibits many effective defense mechanisms that tend to prevent infection and maintain a condition of oral health.

CITED REFERENCES

1. Balekjian, A. Y., Tow, H. D., and Hoerman, K. C.: In vitro agglutination of oral microorganisms by parotid fluid, International Association for Dental Research, forty-ninth General Session, Abstracts, 1971, p. 101.
2. Bartels, H. A., Blechman, H., and Hammer, H.: Factors which influence the assay of the antilactobacillus agent in saliva, J. Dent. Res. 48:22, 1969.
3. Courant, P.: The effect of smoking on the antilactobacillus system in saliva, Odont. Rev. 18:251, 1967.
4. Dawes, C.: The nature of dental plaque, films, and calcareous deposits, Ann. N. Y. Acad. Sci. 153:147, 1968.
5. Hoffman, H., and Valdina, J.: Mechanism of bacterial attachment to oral epithelial cells, Int. Acad. Cytol. 12:37, 1968.
6. King, W. J., Eigen, E., and Fine, N.: Calculus production in vitro, Ann. N. Y. Acad. Sci. 153:147, 1968.
7. Lehner, T., Wilton, J. M. A., and Ward, R. G.: Serum antibodies in dental caries in man, Arch. Oral Biol. 15:481, 1970.
8. Matsumura, T., Morioka, T., Iwamoto, Y., Ueda, M., and Hamada, K.: Studies on the antibacterial factor in human saliva. V. Mode of action of the S. A. factor, J. Osaka Univ. Dent. Sch. 2:81, 1962.
9. Matsumura, T., Morioka, T., Onishi, T., and Iwamoto, Y.: Studies on antilactobacillary factor in human saliva. III. Relationship between active saliva and concentration of bacterial suspension, Dent. Bull. Osaka Univ. 1:31, 1961.
10. Rindom Schiott, C., and Loe, H.: The origin and variation in number of leukocytes in the human saliva, J. Periodont. 5:36, 1970.
11. Shklair, I. T., Rovelstad, G. H., and Lamberts, B. L.: A study of some factors influencing phagocytosis of cariogenic streptococci by caries-free and caries-active individuals, J. Dent. Res. 48:842, 1969.
12. Slack, J. M., Landfried, S., and Gerencser, M. A.: Identification of Actinomyces and related bacteria in dental calculus by the fluorescent antibody technique, J. Dent. Res. 50:78, 1971.
13. Toto, P. D., Gargiulo, A. W., and Kwan, H.: Immunoglobulins of intact epithelium, J. Dent. Res. 49:179, 1970.
14. Ueda, M., Morioka, T., Iwamoto, Y., Hamada,

K., and Matsumura, T.: Characterization of serum depressor on the human salivary anti-bacterial factor, Arch. Oral Biol. **11**:849, 1966.

15. Zengo, A. N., Mandel, I. D., and Goldman, R.: Salivary studies in caries resistant adults, International Association for Dental Research, forty-eighth General Session, Abstracts, 1970, p. 165.

REFERENCES AND ADDITIONAL READINGS

Abramoff, P., and La Via, M. F.: Biology of the immune response, New York, 1970, McGraw-Hill Book Company.

Alexander, J. W., and Good, R. A.: Immunobiology for surgeons, Philadelphia, 1970, W. B. Saunders Co.

Austin, L. B., and Zeldow, B. J.: Quantitative changes of a human salivary bactericidin for lactobacilli associated with age, Proc. Soc. Exp. Biol. Med. **7**:406, 1961.

Bartels, H. A., and Blechman, H.: The inhibitory action of stimulated whole saliva on the in vitro growth of *Clostridium tetani,* Oral Surg. **12**:1141, 1959.

Bartels, H. A., and Blechman, H.: The rapid clearance from the oral cavity of introduced streptomycin dependent and resistant strains of lactobacilli, J. Oral Med. **21**:111, 1966.

Bartels, H. A., Blechman, H., and Cavallaro, J.: The inhibitory action of saliva on the in vitro growth of beta hemolytic streptococci, J. Dent. Res. **37**:654, 1958.

Bartels, H. A., Blechman, H., and Pokowitz, W.: The in vitro activity of the antilactobacillus factor toward various species of lactobacilli, J. Dent. Res. **44**:829, 1965.

Brandtzaeg, P.: Immunochemical comparison of proteins in human gingival pocket fluid, serum and saliva, Arch. Oral Biol. **10**:795, 1965.

Calonius, P. E. B.: The leukocyte count in saliva, Oral Surg. **11**:43, 1958.

Cattoni, M.: Lymphocytes in the epithelium of the healthy gingiva, J. Dent. Res. **30**:627, 1951.

Collins, A. A., and Gavin, J. B.: An evaluation of the antimicrobial effect of the fluid exudate from the clinically healthy gingival crevice, J. Periodont. **32**:99, 1961 .

Cranstoun, G. B.: An evaluation of the natural defenses of the mouth, The McGill Dent. Rev. **14**:10, 1952.

Dodds, A. E.: Protective reactions against bacterial invasion with special reference to the tooth and surrounding structures, J. Dent. Assoc. S. Afr. **8**:304, 1953.

Dogon, I. L., and Amdur, B. H.: Further characterization of an antibacterial factor in human parotid secretions, active against *Lactobacillus casei,* Arch. Oral Biol. **10**:605, 1965.

Eichel, B., and Lisanti, V. F.: Leucocyte metabolism in human saliva, Arch. Oral Biol. **9**:299, 1964.

Evans, R. T., and Mergenhagen, S. E.: Occurrence of natural antibacterial antibody in human parotid, Proc. Soc. Exp. Biol. Med. **119**:815, 1965.

Gibbons, R. J., deStoppelaar, D., and Harden, L.: Lysozyme insensitivity of bacteria indigenous to the oral cavity of man, J. Dent. Res. **45**:877, 1966.

Gilbert, V. P.: An evaluation of the natural defenses of the mouth, J. Canad. Dent. Assoc. **17**:668, 1951.

Green, G. E.: Properties of a salivary bacteriolysin and comparison with serum beta lysin, J. Dent. Res. **45**:882, 1966.

Igel, H. J., and Bolande, R. P.: Humoral defense mechanisms in cryptococcosis: Substances in normal human serum, saliva, and cerebrospinal fluid affecting the growth of *Cryptococcus neoformans,* J. Infect. Dis. **116**:75, 1966.

Kamienski, M. A.: An evaluation of the natural defenses of the mouth, J. Canad. Dent. Assoc. **17**:616, 1951.

Klebanoff, S. J., and Luebke, R. G.: The antilactobacillus system of saliva—role of salivary peroxidase, Proc. Soc. Exp. Biol. Med. **118**:483, 1965.

Klinkhamer Tandarts, J. M.: Human oral leukocytes, Periodontics **1**:109, 1963.

Krasse, B., and Gustafson, B.: Buffer effect of saliva stimulated between and at meals, J. Amer. Dent. Assoc. **56**:50, 1958.

Kraus, F. W., and Konno, J.: Antibodies in saliva, Ann. N. Y. Acad. Sci. **106**:311, 1963.

Lehner, T.: Immunofluorescent investigation of *Candida albicans* antibodies in human saliva, Arch. Oral Biol. **10**:975, 1965.

Loe, H., and Holm-Pedersen, P.: Absence and presence of fluid from normal and inflamed gingiva, Periodontics **3**:171, 1965.

Mahler, I. R., and Lisanti, V. F.: Hyaluronidase producing microogranisms from human saliva, Oral Surg. **5**:1235, 1952.

Mason, D. K., Harden, R. M., Rowan, D., and Alexander, W. D.: Recording the pattern of salivary flow, J. Dent. Res. **45**:1458, 1966.

Nemes, J. L., and Wheatcroft, M. G.: Action of salivary lysozyme on *Micrococcus lysodeikticus,* Oral Surg. **5**:653, 1952.

Nolte, W. A., and Arnim, S. S.: In vitro changes in pH of dental plaque material and surrounding saliva, J. Dent. Res. **35**:83, 1956.

Nungester, W. J., Bosch, J. K., and Alonso, D.: Resistance lowering effect of human respiratory tract mucin, Proc. Soc. Exp. Biol. Med. **76:**777, 1951.

Raust, G.: A review of the literature on salivary mucins, J. West. Soc. Periodont. **10:**48, 1962.

Schneider, T. F., Toto, P. D., Gargiulo, A. W., and Pollock, R. J.: Specific bacterial antibodies in the inflamed human gingiva, Periodontics **4:** 53, 1966.

Shannon, I. L., and Terry, J. M.: Higher parotid fluid flow rate in subjects with resistance to caries, J. Dent. Med. **20:**128, 1965.

Sharawy, A. M., Sabharwal, K., Socransky, S. S., and Lobiene, R. R.: A quantitative study of plaque and calculus formation in normal and periodontally involved mouths, J. Periodont. **37:** 53, 1966.

Sharry, J. J., and Krasse, B.: Observations on the origin of salivary leucocytes, Acta Odont. Scand. **18:**347, 1960.

Simmons, N. S.: Studies on the defense mechanisms of the mucous membranes with particular reference to the oral cavity, Oral Surg. **5:**513, 1952.

Singer, A. J.: Salivary bacteria. II. The ureolytic activity of micrococci isolated from saliva, Oral Surg. **4:**1568, 1951.

Stewart, F. S.: Bacteriology and immunology for students of medicine, ed. 9, Baltimore, 1968, The Williams & Wilkins Co.

Weinberg, S.: The natural barriers to infection in the mouth, J. Canad. Dent. Assoc. **27:**213, 1961.

Weinstein, E., and Mandel, I. D.: The fluid of the gingival sulcus, Periodontics **2:**147, 1964.

Wright, D. E.: The source and disintegration rate of leucocytes in saliva from caries-free and caries active subjects, Brit. Dent. J. **106:**278, 1959.

Zeldow, B. J.: Studies on the antibacterial action of human saliva. I. A bactericidin for lactobacilli, J. Dent. Res. **38:**798, 1959.

Zeldow, B. J.: Studies on the antibacterial action of human saliva. III. Cofactor requirements of a lactobacillus bactericidin, J. Immun. **90:**12, 1963.

PART TWO / ORAL LESIONS INCITED BY MICROORGANISMS

3 / Bacterial infectious agents

Microbial lesions of the oral cavity are caused by organisms that may be divided into three major groups, according to their ecologic and pathogenic characteristics. Most of the lesions are caused by microorganisms that ordinarily occur in the mouth without causing overt symptoms or abnormal changes to indicate their presence. These are normal inhabitants that act as opportunists, gaining access to the oral tissues through dental caries extending into the pulp and the periodontal membrane or through minor trauma such as a scratch from toothbrush bristles. A second, or intermediary, group may be recognized consisting of pathogens, such as the pneumococcus or the diphtheria bacillus, which have managed to attain a carrier or persister state in the oral cavity or oropharynx of certain individuals. The third major group of microorganisms are frank pathogens, such as the tubercle bacillus or the spirochete of syphilis, which produce the initial lesion either elsewhere in the body or directly in the oral cavity, but do not specifically colonize in the oral cavity or oropharynx.

The complex structural features of the oral cavity in relation to the cranium and the neck, and the anatomic features of the oral cavity itself, have important aspects that act either as defense mechanisms or as pathways of infection that are discussed with the appropriate clinical infection.

RESIDENT OPPORTUNISTS
STAPHYLOCOCCI: STAPHYLOCOCCAL INFECTIONS

The staphylococci[71] are gram-positive spheric bacteria, nonmotile, nonsporulating, and aerobic. A number of species have been recognized, among which *Staphylococcus aureus* is the most pronounced pathogen. *S. aureus* strains, however, present such a large and continuous range of subtly varying characteristics that they are difficult to identify with precision in epidemiologic investigations unless bacteriophage typing is used. With phage typing, it is possible to identify, in some instances, a specific carrier who may be the source, for example, of an outbreak of surgical infections in a hospital.

Pathogenicity has been attributed to the ability of staphylococci to produce a number of extracellular factors, including several hemolysins, leukocidin, enterotoxin, coagulase, and hyaluronidase. The pathogenic strains, constituting *S. aureus*, are usually identified by their production of pigment, fermentation of mannitol, hemolysis of blood, and coagulation of plasma. They produce such pyogenic lesions as furuncles and osteomyelitis, as well as various other infections, including pneumonia and septicemia.

The pathologic picture of a staphylococcal infection is characteristically found in a localized abscess. The bacteria cause ne-

67

crosis of the tissue which is surrounded by a wall of fibrin resulting from coagulase activity. Inflammatory cells, including leukocytes, gather about the lesion. The center of the lesion liquefies, and the lesion then points to the surface to drain. As the liquefied center drains out, granulation tissue fills up the cavity. The staphylococci may spread from one site to another by way of the lymphatic or blood vessels to set up new abscesses.

Because of their ability to rapidly develop resistance to most antibiotics, these bacteria may present serious therapeutic problems. Staphylococci isolated from clinical cases should be tested in the laboratory for their range of antibiotic sensitivities to guide therapy. Agents of the erythromycin group or novobiocin have a tendency to cause a rapid development of resistance among the staphylococci so that these drugs, in particular, should not be used singly for treatment of chronic staphylococcal infections.

Ecology

The natural sites for body colonization by S. aureus include the oral cavity[213] and the skin, especially that within the anterior nares, which is the main reservoir for seeding other body surfaces or for contaminating the environment.[305] A person tends either to be a persistent carrier or to be persistently free of S. aureus in the nasal passages following exposure to the organism in the first days of life. Coagulase-positive S. aureus may also be found regularly in the oral cavity of man[146] along with several other less pathogenic staphylococcal species such as S. candidus, S. citreus, S. epidermidis, and S. salivarius.[101, 135, 276] The micrococci as a group, however, constitute but a small fraction of the total oral flora.

In the normal mouth, S. epidermidis occurs more frequently than S. aureus, while the reverse relationship occurs in mouths with open suppurative lesions such as periodontitis.[135] Diabetics tend to have a higher incidence of S. aureus in the mouth than do nondiabetics.[188] The normally small numbers of staphylococci in the oral cavity may be the result of the effects from other bacterial species present, although there is a lack of evidence to support this possibility.

Staphylococci have been implicated in a number of oral and dental lesions. Infected root canals often yield S. aureus; parotitis, facial cellulitis, and osteomyelitis of the jaws have also been found in many instances to result from staphylococcal infection.

Staphylococcal osteomyelitis of the jaws

S. aureus is the microorganism most frequently causative of osteomyelitis,[170] being found in at least 75% of the cases—the only other commonly found agents being the beta hemolytic streptococcus and the pneumococcus. There is very little information to explain the predominance of staphylococci. It has been observed that in longer surgical procedures for the removal of ectopic mandibular third molars S. aureus and Corynebacterium xerosis tend to occur more frequently in the blood of the sockets following the tooth removal than in the sockets of teeth that were quickly removed. Apparently there was greater opportunity for implantation from the flora of the fingers during the longer procedures. Experimental infection of laboratory animals, including the rabbit and guinea pig, has also yielded suggestive observations. Intravenous injection of virulent S. aureus leads to localized abscesses of the long bones, but infection of the jaws apparently does not occur.[282] However, it has been found[167] that an experimental model of chronic osteomyelitis in the maxilla or mandible can be obtained if a hole is drilled into the bone, a cotton pellet inserted into it, and then staphylococcal culture injected into the bone through the cotton. The site is then sutured, with the cotton pellet left in place. With a similar procedure, it has also been found that both alpha hemolytic and beta hemolytic streptococci give much the same histologic picture of localized infection even though highly invasive strains are used.[83] These results suggest that the jaws have relatively great resistance to infection and that osteomyelitis of the jaws, in the cases following extraction, may in part result from the implantation of staphylococci or other bacteria in the company of foreign bodies.

Clinically, the acute phase of osteomyelitis of the long bones, including the jaws, begins with constant, intense, pounding pain, high fever, chills, prostration, and sometimes vomiting.[125] The pain is felt in the neighborhood of the infection. The initial tissue changes consist of an acute exudative inflammation of the bone marrow, an increase in intra-osseous tension, local thrombosis, obliteration of the blood supply, necrosis of the bone, and toxic exudation. The entire maxilla or mandible may become necrotic in the most developed cases. In children and adolescents, osteomyelitis is often caused by hematogenous infection, especially following trauma. Osteomyelitis of the maxillae and mandible in the adult is rarely produced by the hematogenous route, but rather may follow dental extractions, fractures, the injection of local anesthetics, or from the direct extension of a facial skin lesion such as a furuncle or carbuncle.[26]

The single most important factor is associated with extraction of the teeth, for osteomyelitis of the jaws very rarely develops in the edentulous person.[211] Some cases of acute osteomyelitis apparently arise from a periapical or periodontal infection or from direct extension of a severe infection of the maxillary sinus.[144] This latter case is a rare occurrence apparently because there is no subperiosteal network of blood vessels to spread the infection. The more frequently occurring circumstance, that of osteomyelitis from dental infection, may go on to involvement of the maxillary antrum and facial bones. In fractured jaws, infection of the fracture line in either the maxillae or the mandible is extremely rare today since antibiotic therapy is usually started as soon as possible.[154] An even rarer occurrence following fracture is actinomycotic infection of the bone, which usually develops two months or longer after the injury (see the section on actinomycotic infections).

Osteomyelitis of the mandible in adults is six times more common than osteomyelitis of the maxillae.[273] This difference is related to the anatomic characteristics of the two regions.[169] The intra-oral maxillary infections, especially those connected with the dentition, have dependent drainage and less contamination from the saliva. The mandible, on the other hand, is constantly bathed by the saliva, and intra-oral drainage is not always adequate. Moreover, there is a poorer blood supply and a denser bone structure in the mandible.

That the frequent occurrence of periapical abscesses in either jaw does not result in osteomyelitis more frequently probably may be accounted for by certain additional anatomic characteristics of the tissues involved. Among these is the fact that the distance of the abscess from the red marrow is relatively much greater than its distance from the surface of the bone; in fact, there is very little red marrow in the jaw bones, and this small amount is separated from the alveolar process by a dense bony structure. In other words, an abscess usually breaks and discharges externally before it reaches the marrow. Only rarely does the pus spread through the cancellous spaces or spread under the periosteum, which results in a progressive avascular necrosis of the cortical plate of the bone.

The incidence and the severity of all acute osteomyelitis have decreased greatly since the introduction of antibiotic therapy, but effective chemotherapy still depends upon prompt initiation of treatment.[271] If it is delayed, the antibiotic has difficulty reaching the infecting bacteria because of the bone necrosis. This point is so important that it is advisable to begin the antibiotic therapy before results of laboratory studies are available. If the infecting organism is a staphylococcus, treatment is best initiated with a penicillinase-resistant penicillin, such as methicillin, until it is determined whether or not the infecting strain is resistant. This is the most desirable plan of therapy since about one third of staphylococcal infections acquired outside of hospitals are resistant to penicillin G, as are most of hospital-acquired staphylococcal infections.

If treatment is started too late or discontinued too soon or if an incorrect choice of antibiotic had been made, acute osteomyelitis may become chronic.[153] In this case, the single microbial agent usually initially involved in oral infections is in most cases joined by others such as *Streptococcus viridans* or gram-negative rods such as *Escherichia coli* or *Klebsiella pneumoniae.*

Chronic osteomyelitis usually is characterized by sequestered dead bone enclosed in a heavy involucrum. A sinus develops that may intermittently open and close for years. Dense scar tissue, harboring bacteria, surrounds the sinus tracts and acts as a membrane impervious to antibiotics. A broad-spectrum antibiotic is required for therapy, but a successful outcome also requires surgical intervention to remove the dead, infected bone and scar tissue and requires also the drainage of any abscesses present.[49]

Another clinical syndrome involving bone that may occur following tooth extraction is commonly called "dry socket," referring to a tooth socket following extraction in which the blood clot disintegrates, with the production of a foul odor, without pus, but with severe pain persisting for several days.[176] There is a widespread belief that bacteria cause this condition, but no definitive studies have yet appeared to demonstrate this.[36]

Infection of a maxillary tooth with roots lying in close relation to the antrum, such as the first or second molar, may lead to S. *aureus* infection of the antrum by way of the bone, and then, possibly cavernous sinus thrombosis and infection.[38] Even extraction of an infected mandibular tooth,[141] in certain cases, may lead to cavernous sinus thrombosis (see p. 72). On the other hand, a root canal infected with S. *aureus* may lead to staphylococcal subacute bacterial endocarditis if the patient has had heart damage.[70]

Parotitis

Bacterial parotitis is a nonspecific infection that may possibly be confused for the swelling that accompanies some cases of osteomyelitis of the mandible. A distinguishing clinical feature easily determined is the discharge of purulent exudate from Stensen's duct.

Acute suppurative parotitis is most commonly caused by S. *aureus*,[221] although hemolytic or nonhemolytic streptococci or *Diplococcus pneumoniae* may be among a large variety of microorganisms sometimes responsible.[198] The disease is usually caused by one bacterial species, but mixed infections do occur. The infection usually starts from the oral cavity, ascending Stensen's duct from an unhealthy condition brought about by poor oral hygiene, an ill-fitting denture,[8] or stomatitis.[269] Acute parotitis has been known to follow prophylactic treatment of the teeth, dental extraction, infection of the buccal mucous membrane, pericoronitis, or in association with acute osteomyelitis of the jaws.[250] Drying of the oral mucosa through decreased parotid salivary flow from drugs with an atropine-like action, including the phenothiazine derivatives used by psychiatric patients,[223] increases the liability toward developing parotitis. The postoperative period, when a patient may not be receiving fluids and food by mouth and when the salivary flow is diminished, is a period of particular risk. Occasionally parotitis may arise by a hematogenous or lymphogenous route or by direct extension from contiguous tissues.

Experimental work with animals tends to support the idea that ascending duct infection is the most probable route of infection. In one study,[22] when the Stensen's duct of each side in four dogs was infected with S. *aureus*, all but one of the parotid glands developed marked suppuration, while only two of nine dogs developed recognizable inflammation when an artery to the parotid was injected.

Under normal conditions, the parotid of man is protected from infection by the flushing effect of the free-flowing saliva, by certain antibacterial factors in the saliva such as lysozymes and antibodies, and by the corkscrew configuration of the parotid duct which hinders the backflow of excreted saliva contaminated by the oral microflora.[198]

Epulis (pyogenic granuloma)

Staphylococci in pure culture are commonly found in a granulomatous lesion often occurring on the gingiva, but which may also occur on the tongue,[181] referred to as epulis granulomatosa or pyogenic granuloma.[275] Epulis is a tumorous growth developing at the site of an injury that recurs promptly if it is clipped off, a characteristic that has led to its being mistaken for a malignant cancer. These tumors grow rapidly and consist of newly formed vascular tissue so fully permeated with blood vessels that it resembles a hemangioma. The growth is densely infiltrated with polymorphonuclear leukocytes. Treatment requires excision and cauterization with the electrocautery.[280]

Other staphylococcal infections of the mouth, face, and lips
Stomatitis

An ulcerative stomatitis of the oral cavity caused by staphylococci may arise in infants following mechanical injury to the mucosa.[143] Ulcerative stomatitis caused by coagulase-positive S. *aureus*, accompanied by severe pharyngitis, has been observed following oxytetracycline therapy.[140] A chronic disease of the oral mucosa, with miliary abscesses from which S. *aureus* has been isolated, is known as pyostomatitis vegetans.[172] The mucosa exhibits an inflammatory hyperplasia, thrown into folds, and is studded with miliary abscesses from pinpoint to pinhead in size. Rupture of the miliary abscesses is followed by the development of a fibrinopurulent exudate. The process may gradually spread to involve the entire oral cavity. It is not caused by the microorganisms cultured from the lesions, so they must be regarded purely as opportunists.

Botryomycosis

The clinical entity known as botryomycosis is a granulomatous inflammation of tissues, with draining sinuses, which contains funguslike granules within suppurative foci.[307] The granules are very much like the actinomycosis sulfur granules in their structure. It is usually caused by the staphylococcus although various other bacteria have been found in some cases. All these organisms seem to be characteristically possessed of low virulence, and the lesion is primarily a result of hypersensitivity to the bacteria involved. The tongue has been reported to be infected by such a process, involving staphylococci,[263] although the usual site is not the oral cavity.

Gingivitis

Clinically inflamed gingiva contains cellular components of staphylococci in approximately half of the cases that have been studied by direct fluorescent antibody techniques.[285]

Root canal infections

Staphylococcal infections of the root canal are not rare. Subacute bacterial endocarditis from a hemolytic S. *aureus* may occur following root canal therapy of a tooth with this organism infecting the root apex.[70]

Upper facial and lip infections

Staphylococcal infections of the upper lip, nose, upper facial skin, or the maxillary portion of the oral cavity are very dangerous because of the numerous venous anastomoses with the deeper veins, which establish communication with the cavernous sinus.[7] The distance to the cranial sinuses from the face is very short, and the venous system involved lacks the protective valves found in other parts of the body. Before the introduction of chemotherapeutic agents in 1937 for the treatment of cavernous sinus thrombosis, this condition was fatal in all cases. Even today, once the infection reaches the sinus, mortality may be as great as 80%, and the survivors usually have residual nerve damage. Antibiotic therapy, combined with judicious surgical drainage when indicated, has greatly decreased the incidence of such infections and offers the only hope once it does appear.

STREPTOCOCCI

The streptococci are a large group with widely varying characteristics that are capable of independent pathogenicity, causing a number of specific diseases, and of participating in mixed infections with many other microorganisms. They are therefore of considerable interest.

The streptococci are spheric or ovoid cells arranged in long or short chains, or in pairs. They are gram-positive, nonsporulating, usually nonmotile, and most species are aerobic and facultative. The genus *Streptococcus*, a member of the family Lactobacillaceae, has presented considerable difficulty in classification, prompting the development of various taxonomic schemes, elements of which are commonly used for convenience in what is admittedly still a rather confused situation.

The streptococci were divided into four groups by Sherman: the pyogenic, the viridans, the enterococcal, and the lactic groups. Another commonly used classification, developed by Brown on the basis of red blood cell lysis on blood agar plates, divides the streptococci into a beta hemolytic group (Fig. 3-1), a greening or alpha hemolytic group, and a group of streptococci referred to as gamma or indifferent

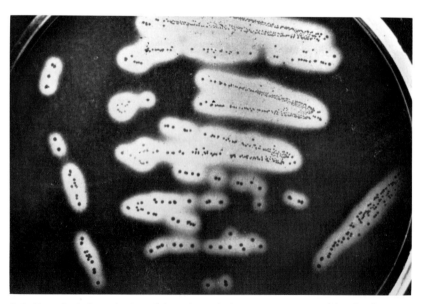

Fig. 3-1. Hemolysis by colonies of beta hemolytic streptococcus on blood infusion agar.

strains that have no hemolytic effect. Using precipitin techniques, Lancefield found that many of the hemolytic streptococci contain cell wall polysaccharide (C antigens) by which they can be differentiated into a number of serologic groups. Among these, group A contains the beta hemolytic streptococci pathogenic for man; group D contains the enterococci, which may or may not be hemolytic; groups F and G are commensals of the mouth and throat that have a low virulence; and groups H and K are commensals in the nose and throat, but without known pathogenicity. Many streptococci isolated from mucous membranes, however, have not been classified yet since the established Lancefield antigens do not occur in them.

In addition to the C carbohydrate, group A streptococcal cell walls also contain an M protein antigen that is closely associated with virulence. It is found principally in strains that produce matt or mucoid colonies. The M protein hinders ingestion by phagocytes.

Therapy for group A beta hemolytic streptococcal infections relies upon penicillin G since the entire group is uniformly sensitive to this antibiotic. Sensitivity tests in the laboratory are not needed for infections by these organisms. The alpha hemolytic streptococci and enterococci, on the other hand, vary so greatly in their antibiotic sensitivities that it is necessary to do laboratory studies to find the most effective agent against them.

Four principal groups of streptococci are of special interest to the oral microbiologist: the beta hemolytic streptococci, the alpha hemolytic streptococci, the enterococci, and the anaerobic streptococci.

Beta hemolytic streptococci

Group A beta hemolytic streptococci are the cause of such diseases as septic sore throat, scarlet fever, and rheumatic fever in human beings. Certain extracellular products elaborated by group A strepto-

cocci have been related to the pathogenesis of these diseases. Among these are: hyaluronidase, streptokinase, deoxyribonuclease, and hemolysins.

The occurrence of beta hemolytic streptococci in the oral cavity is of considerable interest for their possible role in the spread of infection. Although the throat and oral cavity are at best but several inches apart, it has been found that in one study of 500 medical and dental students, predominantly male, beta hemolytic streptococci were present in the throat alone in 61%, on the gingiva alone in 24%, and on both throat and gingiva in only 14% of the subjects. Only 12% of the 500 students were demonstrated to be carriers of the streptococci. The saliva of patients with positive throat cultures may or may not contain beta hemolytic streptococci. In general, the saliva of patients with upper-respiratory tract streptococcal infection whose tonsils have been removed contains fewer hemolytic streptococci than saliva from those patients who have retained their tonsils. During the first few days of an upper-respiratory tract infection, the saliva may contain as many as 1 million or more streptococci per milliliter. Beta hemolytic streptococci have been isolated from root canals of infected teeth in approximately 5% or less of the cases studied.

The currents of salivary fluid toward the esophagus and antibiosis by the oral microbiota may be factors in inhibiting their colonization in the mouth. These factors are discussed in Chapter 2.

Scarlet fever

Tonsillitis and pharyngitis, commonly called sore throat, are frequent infections caused by beta hemolytic streptococci, group A. Scarlet fever[306] also begins as a streptococcal throat infection with a high temperature, but in addition a widespread rash occurs on the skin, the result of an erythrogenic exotoxin produced by the streptococci. The appearance of erythrogenic toxin is dependent upon the streptococcal strain being lysogenic. Not all strains of group A streptococci are able to produce the toxin, but those that do are known as scarlatinal strains. In most instances, similar to the diphtheria bacillus and its exotoxin, the streptococci remain as inhabitants of the throat and tonsils but liberate the erythrogenic toxin, which is absorbed into the bloodstream.

Scarlet fever is a highly contagious disease having an incubation period of from several days to a week, following which there appear the sore throat and a fever ranging between 100° and 103° F. Within several days a rash appears on the trunk and later may appear on the face and limbs; the lips, nose, and chin are not involved. The rash fades after three or four days, and the skin desquamates around the middle of the second week. In some patients otitis media, mastoiditis, cervical lymphadenitis, or nephritis may follow.

An acute streptococcal pharyngitis may cause petechiae on the oral mucosa of the soft palate. In the case of scarlet fever, oral mucosal changes are similar to those in the skin, but they begin earlier and are more marked. At the height of the skin eruption the oral mucosa is uniformly congested. The hard palate mucosa exhibits a red, punctiform mottling. The tongue is at first furred. The fungiform papillae of the tongue become enlarged and swollen, and, since they are not capped by keratinized epithelium as are the more numerous neighboring filiform papillae, the fungiform papillae appear as reddened protuberances. This topography of the tongue simulates the appearance of a strawberry, hence the so-called strawberry tongue; as the lesions subside and the redness fades, the tongue is said to simulate more the appearance of a raspberry and is then referred to as a raspberry tongue. Eventually the tongue becomes normal both in color and in size of the papillae. In scarlet fever cases reported since the advent of

antibiotics, it has been found that only 16% develop these lingual signs of scarlet fever.[109]

Diagnosis presents some difficulties in certain cases since there may be confusion with measles, rubella, drug eruptions, or other disease states. In addition to culture of the pharynx for beta hemolytic streptococci, the Dick test and the Schultz-Charlton test may be useful. The Dick test consists of the intracutaneous injection of erythrogenic toxin; and a susceptible person will experience an area of redness within 24 hours at the site of injection. If an area of more than 1 cm. persists throughout the course of the infection, a diagnosis of scarlet fever is questionable; but if the positive result changes to negative early in the course of the disease, then the test result is highly suggestive of scarlet fever. The Schultz-Charlton test consists of the intradermal injection of scarlet fever antitoxin into an area where the rash is present. If the rash blanches at the site of injection within from 6 to 12 hours, the erythrogenic toxin was neutralized, and the test result is positive, indicating that scarlet fever is present.

Erysipelas

Erysipelas[65] is a disease recognized since ancient times. It is an acute inflammatory reaction developing upon the invasion of dermal lymphatic channels by group A hemolytic streptococci that probably come from the nose.[27] The face is the most common site for this infection, since it is involved in 90% of the cases, but there may be extension into the mucous membranes. Much less commonly, erysipelas may start in mucous membranes, chiefly those of the pharynx and fauces, but sometimes in the nose, eustachian tube, or middle ear.

The bacteria gain entry into the lymphatics of the skin or mucosa through an infection caused by another organism, an abrasion, fissure, wound, or surgical procedure. Since there is an incubation period of from three to seven days, the initial break in the surface structure may have healed by the time the typical lesion of erysipelas appears, giving the impression of spontaneous eruption.

Facial erysipelas begins abruptly with a short prodromal phase of malaise, pyrexia, and chills. The skin lesion appears around the mouth or nares as a bright red, tense, raised area with a distinct but irregular outline. The general condition of the patient then deteriorates, with the appearance of toxemia, pyrexia, insomnia, and restlessness. If the disease is not treated, the periphery of the lesion advances as a raised edge over the cheeks, where it is generally stopped at the lines where the skin is bound down to the underlying bone of the zygomatic arches, orbits, and nose, giving a so-called butterfly appearance. The acute stage resolves after from three to ten days, leaving a dry and desquamating skin. The infection occurs most frequently between December and May, as do other hemolytic streptococcal infections. Facial erysipelas, starting at the lip, has been known to follow shortly after dental extraction, but it is not known whether there is any causal relationship. Erysipelas of the face also may occur upon operative drainage through the skin of a streptococcal parotitis.[269] Facial cellulitis from an infected maxillary cuspid when seen first by a physician rather than a dentist may be mistaken for erysipelas, especially if an erysipeloid reaction has developed from the toxins produced by the dental infection.[237]

Before antiseptic and aseptic techniques were developed, erysipelas was a common and virulent disease that often reached epidemic proportions. Control was greatly advanced on the application of listerian principles, and today, with the antibiotics readily available, erysipelas rarely appears. These infections now are rarely fatal unless they occur in infants or in aged and debilitated adults.

Rheumatic fever

Rheumatic fever, mainly a childhood disease, usually starts with a sore throat and causes a temperature of from 100° to 102° F. The course is protracted, during which there is widespread involvement of fibrous tissues of the joints, heart, and other organs. The affected joints are hot, red, swollen, and painful. Arthritis is a consequence of the joint involvement, but there are more serious consequences for the heart valves. Skin eruptions are common during the course of the acute phase but do not last long. Subcutaneous nodules may also occur, usually over bony prominences.

Several lines of evidence implicate group A beta hemolytic streptococci in the development of rheumatic fever. First, the group A streptococci are the only bacteria causing human infection such as acute pharyngitis or otitis with an epidemiologic pattern that parallels the seasonal incidence and geographic distribution of rheumatic fever. Second, this group causes repeated infections at intervals throughout childhood; such repetition probably establishes the conditions for the first attack of rheumatic fever. Third, rheumatic fever can be prevented if the streptococci are attacked with vigorous antibiotic therapy early in the course of the infection. Fourth, a specific immune response to streptococcal antigens occurs almost uniformly in patients with acute rheumatic fever. The mechanism by which streptococcal infection leads to rheumatic fever is not clear, but it most probably involves autoimmune reactions.

Rheumatic fever leads to a number of important effects of special interest to the dentist. Since perhaps 1.5% of the dentist's patients may have had rheumatic fever,[277] there is a good possibility that the dentist will eventually encounter these conditions among his patients. The damage to their heart valves that often occurs requires antibiotic cover during dental procedures, including prophylaxis and extraction, as a precaution against a possible subacute bacterial endocarditis from the bacteremia that occurs.[247]

Part of the rheumatic disease complex includes inflammatory changes involving the joints and leading to arthritis. Rheumatoid arthritis produces widespread pathologic lesions. It is a generalized disease in which the joints are the principal site for destructive changes. Symptoms include muscle stiffness, joint stiffness, aching, pain, and swelling. As the process develops, there is generalized decalcification and destruction of the joint structures that may lead to ankylosis. The temporomandibular joint may become involved,[183] although it is rarely the first to be so; usually this involvement of that joint is associated with generalized rheumatoid arthritis.[19] The proportion of cases in which that joint suffers some disability is very great, perhaps 50%,[53] although few of these cases have persistent, residual joint symptoms.[59] In rare cases both sides of the mandible may become ankylosed.[54] In the case of juvenile rheumatoid arthritis affecting the temporomandibular joint, the result often is micrognathia if the process occurs early enough.[12]

Rheumatoid arthritis is diagnosed essentially on the basis of clinical findings, but positive results of serologic tests for the rheumatoid factor are useful for confirmation of the diagnosis and give information important for prognosis. In addition to the rheumatoid factor being present in the serum of patients with rheumatoid arthritis, the levels of IgG and IgM tend to be raised; there is also a rise in IgA levels.[292]

Greening streptococci

Most of the so-called viridans or alpha hemolytic streptococci do not belong to any of Lancefield's serologic groups. Serologic study of a large number of oral strains has shown that only 37% are members of Lancefield groups. Groups H and K, and to a lesser extent groups F and O, are the most common among these. Members of more than one group are often found in the same mouth.[77]

Because of the problem in specific identification, it has been difficult to implicate the greening streptococci in pathologic processes.[241] As a result of recent studies, however, five divisions can now be recognized among the viridanslike streptococci of man[52]: *Streptococcus salivarius, S. sanguis, S. mutans, S. milleri,* and *S. viridans. S. salivarius, S. mutans,* and *Diplococcus pneumoniae* are readily recognized and are homogeneous species. *S. milleri, S. sanguis,* and *S. viridans* do not form equally clearcut entities and should be regarded as aggregations of similar strains.

Oral infection by greening streptococci

The alpha hemolytic streptococci are the predominant streptococci in the oral cavity. The two species found most frequently are *S. mitis* and *S. salivarius,* which are readily differentiated by their colonial characteristics on mitis-salivarius medium. *S. mitis* grows as a small, bluish-black colony from 0.5 to 2 mm. in diameter, while *S. salivarius* grows as a larger colony, because of the abundant production of extracellular levan, which looks like a convex gumdrop in shape. Both of these species are often found, alone or most frequently together with other oral microbes, in abscesses, ulcerative stomatitis, root canals, periodontal pockets, calculus, and carious lesions. Their significance alone or in combination with other oral microbes in these various disease processes is still under study.

Alpha hemolytic streptococci have been obtained in pure culture in cases of acute ulcerative stomatitis that differ materially from the usual clinical forms containing a mixture of Vincent's microorganisms, including spirochetes, fusobacteria, and gram-positive cocci.[295] This streptococcal stomatitis clinically is very much like Vincent's infection, being characterized by widespread ulcerative lesions of the lips, buccal cavity, and pharynx; but, in addition, it has an associated mild purulent conjunctivitis. It differs clinically by the absence of the typical foul odor of Vincent's infection and by the fact that the patients are acutely ill and may even show an alarming prostration. The infection may arise as a primary condition resembling diphtheria, or it may be a complication of pneumonia. The pathogenesis of this infection has not been elucidated, although it is thought that it may involve nutritional deficiencies.

Greening streptococci have also been associated with a less severe form of stomatitis, hypertrophic in character, whose outstanding features are swelling, pain, and redness of the gums, palate, and throat.[309] The disease is acute in its onset and is accompanied by fever, salivation, and malaise. The gingival margin is bright red, rolled, and edematous, the papillae are pushed up between the teeth. There is no ulceration, erosion, vesiculation, or membrane formation.

A form of nonhemolytic streptococcal oropharyngitis has been described,[121] with membrane formation, which has a tendency to spread to the soft palate, the gingiva, and the gingivolabial folds. The disease is most easily mistaken for diphtheria and Vincent's angina, so that a bacteriologic examination is necessary to establish its identity. The infection results in a good deal of local discomfort and dysphagia, especially when the soft palate is involved, but it seems to be only mildly infectious.

In spite of these isolated and infrequent observations, it may well be found in the future that infection of the oral mucosa by greening streptococci is not a rare event for it is now known that the marginal gingiva of patients with grossly inflamed gingivae contains antigens of S. *mitis*, indicating possible invasion of the tissue by antigenic products of this hemolytic streptococcus.[308]

Alpha hemolytic streptococci, on entering the blood, may localize in the heart to cause subacute bacterial endocarditis, discussed in Chapter 11.

Recurrent aphthous stomatitis

This disease of the oral mucosa[89] is a recurrent necrotizing ulceration of undetermined origin. A strain of S. *sanguis* has been isolated from these oral ulcers, and the patients show an increased delayed type of skin reactivity to these organisms as compared to normal patients. It has been suggested, therefore, that recurrent aphthous stomatitis may represent a delayed type of hypersensitivity to S. *sanguis*.[102]

Pneumococcal pneumonia: *Diplococcus pneumoniae*, referred to by some as *Streptococcus pneumoniae*

The pneumococcus, the etiologic agent of pneumococcal pneumonia, is a small, lanceolate, gram-positive diplococci which often occurs in short chains resembling streptococci. It is nonmotile, nonsporulating, and typically encapsulated. The pneumococcus is difficult to separate from the viridans streptococci that are also found on the mucosa of the upper respiratory tract. This can be accomplished, however, with the bile solubility and inulin fermentation tests, results of both of which are positive for the pneumococcus and negative for the other greening streptococci. In addition, the pneumococcus is lethal for the laboratory mouse upon intraperitoneal inoculation and gives a specific capsule swelling reaction when mixed with type-specific capsular antiserum on a slide (quellung reaction).

The pneumococcal capsule is associated with virulence, apparently because it impedes phagocytosis. The capsular polysaccharide confers antigenic specificity that divides these organisms into approximately 80 types, of which types 1 to 32 account for about 95% of the cases of pneumococcal pneumonia. The reservoir for the agent of this infection is man himself, consisting of persons with active disease and asymptomatic carriers. In addition to pneumonia, the pneumococcus may cause infections of the middle ear, the sinuses, the mastoid, the meninges, or the heart valves.

Since the organisms are found to reside in the upper respiratory tract, including the oral cavity, they are chiefly spread through airborne dissemination of the saliva and the discharges of the respiratory tract.[301] The occurrence of the pneumococcus in the saliva is of considerable historic interest for the oral microbiologist since it was first isolated from this source almost simultaneously by two masters of early bacteriology in the latter part of the nineteenth century. In 1880 Pasteur attempted to isolate the agent of rabies from the saliva of a boy under treatment for this disease. He found instead an organism that proved to be highly pathogenic to rabbits that he designated as *microbe septicemique du salive*. About the same time Sternberg in the United States found the same organism in the saliva of healthy persons upon its subcutaneous inoculation into rabbits.[122] In subsequent years, however, repeated investigations have shown that the virulent types of pneumococci and those most frequently associated with primary acute pulmonary infections can be recovered only rarely from normal mouths.[82] Recent findings[199] suggest that the absence of the more pathogenic pneumococci from the oral cavity may be the result of excretion of antipneumococcal IgA antibody into the saliva.

The pneumococcus occasionally causes oral lesions. In infants ranging from a few days old to 16 months of age, primary infection of the mouth may occur upon exposure to persons with respiratory disease. The incubation period appears to be very short, perhaps only two or three days.[56] The lesions involve, in order of frequency, the buccal mucosa, palate, anterior pillars of the fauces, lower lip and under surface of the tongue, and the tonsils. The lesion initially resembles that of thrush, consisting of silvery flecks, pinpoint

in size, which are widely separated. There may be six or eight of these on a side, and they become pinhead ulcers. Secondary infection with staphylococci or *Candida* organisms commonly follows, and systemic reactions of fever, vomiting, and dehydration result. In well-advanced cases the infection results in a membrane on the mucosa which gradually thickens. The infection may be life-threatening without apparent lung changes.

Parotitis caused by the pneumococcus occurred in only four cases among 153 cases in the records of two St. Louis hospitals.[269] A much higher ratio was found among children in New Orleans. Of 21 cases studied there, eight yielded pneumococci upon cultivation of saliva from Stensen's duct. These included types 3, 16, 17, and 18. Pneumococcal parotitis is a much more acute type of parotitis than that caused by *Streptococcus* of the viridans group's. In these former cases, the parotid saliva is purulent, with a characteristic greenish tinge. Sialographic examination of the gland shows much greater gland destruction than in the viridans *Streptococcus* cases. Pneumococcal parotitis also has a tendency to become chronic with abscess formation within the gland.[240]

Treatment of pneumococcal infections rests upon any of a number of quite effective antibiotics. The penicillins especially are valuable, but it is nevertheless desirable to not delay treatment, especially for the very young infant and the elderly. In recent years, drug-resistant strains have been appearing, and resistance to tetracyclines, erythromycin, and lincomycin has been noted in some isolates from patients.

Enterococci

These gram-positive, nonmotile streptococci, among the group D streptococci of Lancefield, are a characteristic group that occur usually as diplococci, are unusually resistant to heat, almost always ferment mannitol, and very seldom ferment raffinose. They are able to grow in the presence of bile, and most strains produce no change on a blood agar plate. Isolation of enterococci in primary plates of clinical specimens is readily carried out on Pfizer Selective Enterococcus agar plates* (PSE medium), which relies upon bile and sodium chloride to suppress unwanted species of bacteria and permits identification of the enterococ-

*Pfizer Laboratories Division, Pfizer, Inc., New York, N. Y.

cal colonies by their hydrolysis of esculin, the products of which form black iron salts surrounding the enterococcal colonies (Fig. 3-2). The colonies are round, entire, convex, and small.[138] Among the species and varieties recognized are S. *faecalis,* S. *faecalis* var. *liquefaciens,* S. *faecalis* var. *zymogenes,* S. *bovis,* S. *faecium,* and S. *faecium* var. *durans.*[224]

Enterococci have been found in a large number of infections in man, including dental cellulitis, trismus, pharyngitis, otitis

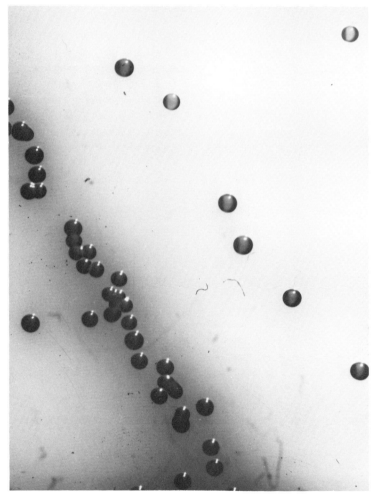

Fig. 3-2. Colonies of enterococci on Pfizer selective enterococcus agar medium. Enterococcal colonies are surrounded by black iron salts. (Courtesy of Dr. H. D. Isenberg, Long Island Jewish Medical Center, New Hyde Park, N. Y.)

media, mastoiditis, meningitis, peritonitis, septicemia, and endocarditis.[187] Since the enterococci are commonly found in the oral cavity,[279] it may well be that it is from this source that the bacteria come which cause these infections. The enterococci do not seem to be among the streptococci involved in dental caries,[107] however, but hyaluronidase-producing strains of enterococci have been isolated from scrapings of teeth in human beings with peridontal disease.[239] The enterococci are common in root canal infections,[208] constituting a problem in therapy since they may have a relatively high resistance to penicillin and thus are difficult to eliminate if this antibiotic is used for therapy.[74] In the presence of streptomycin, however, they become much more susceptible to penicillin.[120]

Peptostreptococci

The peptostreptococci,[281] very commonly referred to as anaerobic streptococci, are a group of gram-positive cocci imperfectly known because of the technical difficulties encountered in their study. Veillon in 1893 was the first to mention their occurrence in pathologic states, including Ludwig's angina. It was not until 1910 that attention was first called to their frequent involvement in puerperal sepsis.

These gram-positive cocci become almost all gram-negative after 24 hours' cultivation. The cells show no particular arrangement under the microscope, although some isolates may exhibit chaining. Continued cultivation very rarely leads to increased oxygen tolerance to the point of allowing aerobic growth. Eight species of anaerobic streptococci are recognized as producing putrefactive wound infection in the seventh edition of *Bergey's Manual of Determinative Bacteriology*,[30] while Prévot in the first American edition of his *Manual of Classification and Determination of Anaerobic Bacteria*[219] recognized nine anaerobic species, listed in the genus *Streptococcus*. Recent study has shown, however, that serologic relationships between *Peptostreptococcus* and *Streptococcus* are generally weak.

Among the more well-defined species of *Peptostreptococcus* are *P. anaerobius, P. putridus*, and *P. foetidus. P. putridus* appears to be the most common pathogen, being especially involved in puerperal infections. These species, according to Prévot, vary in their growth in glucose broth: *P. anaerobius* forms a flocculent sediment; *P. putridus* clouds the medium; and *P. foetidus* forms a stringy, clotted mass in broth. In their decomposition of native proteins foul gases are produced, one of which is hydrogen sulfide. All these species attack unheated proteins with the production of hydrogen sulfide, although coagulated proteins are rarely denatured.

The anaerobic streptococci are generally noninvasive endogenous parasites that inhabit the skin, respiratory and intestinal tracts, the vagina, and the oral cavity. They have been isolated not only from the normal flora but also from purulent and gangrenous processes,[298] which include lung abscesses, sinusitis, suppurative adenitis, gingivitis, and ulcerative stomatitis, as well as from dental caries, osteomyelitis of the mandible, deep submandibular abscesses, apical and alveolar abscesses,[84] and infected root canals.

In disease states, these bacteria are very frequently associated with other microorganisms,[126] especially with anaerobic bacilli, fusiform bacilli, and spirochetes, indicating a good possibility that the pathologic effects are not caused by the anaerobic streptococci alone. It has been suggested, however, that those strains that have no apparent independent pathogenicity may, in fact, play a significant role in the pathogenesis of an infectious lesion by lowering the local pH by fermentation of carbohydrates or organic acids so that the local defensive mechanisms cannot cope with other microorganisms that may also be present.

There are no extensive studies with laboratory animals on the pathogenicity of anaerobic streptococci. Only a few investigators have shown that pure cultures of the organism are capable of producing lesions in animals, the general experience being that they are practically nonvirulent for laboratory animals.[175]

In clinical cases, the possibility of an anaerobic streptococcal infection must be considered if the infection does not respond to use of the standard antibiotics or if the infection involves actinomyces.[66] The difficulties of treatment are well illustrated by a case of bacteremia that responded to a combination of penicillin and streptomycin after unsuccessful trials with penicillin alone, and tetracycline alone and with ampicillin, and cephalothin.[299]

LACTOBACILLI

Lactobacilli are microaerophilic to anaerobic gram-positive rods, nonsporulating, usually nonmotile, and with complex nutritional requirements. They fall into two groups on the basis of glucose fermentation: homofermentatives, which produce lactic acid predominantly, and heterofermentatives, which also produce other aliphatic acids, ethyl alcohol, and carbon dioxide. They typically occur in fermenting dairy and plant products and in the vagina, the alimentary tract, and the oral cavity of mammals and man. They may participate in the production of dental caries. Root canal cultures yield lactobacilli in approximately 12% of all positive cultures,[208] and these have been detected in postextraction bacteremias.[20] It is not surprising, therefore, that lactobacilli have been found in some cases of endocarditis.[24]

A number of animal studies have shown that the lactobacilli have the pathogenic capacity for producing serious disease. Animal inoculations have shown[238] that capsulated strains have a much greater capacity to produce skin lesions in rabbits than do nonencapsulated strains. The repeated intraperitoneal injection of large numbers of *Lactobacillus acidophilus* produces joint lesions in rabbits.[128] Encapsulated *Lactobacillus casei* var. *rhamnosus* has been found capable of killing mice upon intravenous injection.[260]

VEILLONELLA

The genus *Veillonella*[235] consists of small nonmotile, gram-negative, oxidase-negative, anaerobic cocci, which are included in the family Neisseriaceae. Two species are recognized: *Veillonella parvula* and *V. alcalescens*. These bacteria occur in the natural cavities of certain animals and man, being present in large numbers in the human mouth. Cultivation of clinical specimens for primary isolation has been greatly facilitated by the development of a simple yeast trypticase plating medium that is incubated in anaerobic jars.[236]

Veillonella organisms are characterized by a lack of carbohydrate fermentation, but they have marked activity upon lactic, succinic, and certain other organic acids.

Although carried normally without pathogenic effects, they have been isolated as part of a mixed flora from various suppurative processes such as periodontitis, pulmonary gangrene, tonsillitis, and appendicitis. The role played by *Veillonella* organisms in these mixed infections is unknown; but since they yield lipopolysaccharide extracts with the characteristics of endotoxins,[25] it seems possible that they may have a significant role in the development of these mixed infections. They also may perhaps participate in the development of plaque-mediated dental diseases such as caries and periodontitis since they are able to contribute actively to plaque development once the initial deposit has been made upon the teeth by other bacteria.

The antibiotic sensitivity spectrum of *Veillonella* organisms consists of a sensitivity toward penicillin, erythromycin, and bacitracin, and a resistance toward vancomycin, streptomycin, and neomycin.[85]

BACTEROIDACEAE

The family Bacteroidaceae contains a number of genera of gram-negative, strictly anaerobic bacilli with rounded or pointed ends, which do not form spores. In the seventh edition of *Bergey's Manual of Determinative Bacteriology*,[30] several dozen species are listed among the genera in this family, but it is questionable that they are all valid. On the basis of extensive experience a more recent evaluation has concluded that these bacteria may be separated into five major groups. Among these many organisms, when subjected to analysis by the methods of numerical taxonomy, it was found that members of the genera *Fusobacterium* and *Sphaerophorus* are so closely similar that they form a single phenome which also includes *Bacteroides melaninogenicus*. *Bacteroides* forms a phenome of its own that contains *B. fragilis* and *B. oralis*.[14]

As a group, the *Bacteroides* organisms appear to have but low pathogenicity, and only a few species among these bacteria have been considered to be pathogenic for man; in particular, *Sphaerophorus necrophorus*, *B. fragilis*,[179] and *B. melaninogenicus*.[266] This pathogenicity, however, requires special circumstances in which the bacteria may act as opportunists. Normally, these organisms inhabit the oropharynx, the gastrointestinal tract, and the female genital tract. In the bowel, they outnumber coliforms 100 to 1. The *Bacteroides* species occuring in the oral cavity have been detected in the saliva, in material obtained from the tongue surface, in the gingival sulcus and periodontal pocket, and in some instances in root canals. Among the species found in these oral sites are *B. melaninogenicus*, which is thought to play a role in periodontal disease, and *B. oralis*.

When the normal sites of colonization are injured or diseased, bacteroides may gain entrance into the tissue or may become systemically distributed by gaining entrance into the lymphatic or blood vessels. In these latter instances, secondary foci of infection may be established in neighboring or distant sites such as the lung, liver, brain, bone, or various joints.[34] There is also reason to suspect that there may be transmission of the organisms from patient to patient within the hospital.[18] Characteristically, *Bacteroides* infections also contain many other types of bacteria. There is a high incidence, in particular, of anaerobic streptococci.[288] There has been reported an increasing number of bacteroides infections recently, increasing tenfold in one hospital within a period of 10 years.[182] This may be due to widespread use of antibiotics that suppress gram-positive bacteria, in part to greatly improved methods of anaerobic cultivation, and in part to a greater realization of the great frequency of such infections.

Sphaerophorus necrophorus in pus is a short, slender rod, gram-negative, non-sporulating, non–acid-fast, often showing a granular appearance on staining and closely resembling *Haemophilus influenzae*. Structure in culture is more variable than that in pus[5] and includes filaments to 50 or 100 μ, with fusiform or globular swellings. Anaerobic conditions and an enriched medium are required for laboratory growth. Primary cultivations from lesions usually show streptococci so closely associated that it is extremely difficult to obtain a pure culture. A wide variety of human infections occurs with this organism that includes pharyngitis, otitis media, mastoiditis, lung abscess, pneumonia, arthritis, osteomyelitis, liver abscess, peritonsillar and sublingual abscesses, empyema, pyemia, and septicemia. The portal of entry commonly is the throat or tonsils, or the genital tract in the case of women.[6] Therapy is effective with tetracycline or ampicillin. This bacterium is resistant to erythromycin.[81]

Bacteroides fragilis is a small bacillus of constant form that produces local infections, but only rarely does it produce a septicemia. It is the commonest bacteroides isolated from human purulent material, other than from the mouth or respiratory tract. Among the lesions from which it has been isolated are cerebral abscess, scrotal abscess, bartholinian abscess, tubo-ovarian abscess, and postappendectomy wound infection.

On blood agar cultivated anaerobically the organism forms small colonies after 48 hours' incubation. The organism is resistant to penicillin, streptomycin, neomycin, and polymyxin, but fully sensitive to tetracyclines, chloramphenicol, erythromycin,[92] and lincomycin.[136] The last two antibiotics appear to be the most useful for clinical use.

Bacteroides melaninogenicus at present is difficult to place within a clearly defined phenome, so that more thorough study is required.[152] This organism is described as a small coccobacillus that usually occurs singly, but occasionally, especially in old cultures, in pairs, or in chains of varying length. This species is a strict anaerobe and is difficult to culture. Its growth is promoted by from 5% to 10% CO_2 in its atmosphere. Optimal growth requires hemin and some form of vitamin K such as menadione.[97] Fortuitous contaminants in the inoculum may supply these needs. Growth is slow, especially on primary culture. After five days' incubation (Fig. 3-3), surface colonies on blood agar plates show a blackening which accounts for the species name. It has been found, however, contrary to the original opinion, that the black color is not melanin, but rather hematin.[251] Various isolates from different sources show heterogeneity in both their biochemical and immunologic characteristics.[55]

This species constantly inhabits healthy mucous membranes but takes a prominent part in various pathologic processes.[41] It is a member of the gingival crevice and salivary flora in the adult. In the infant mouth, it may occur in a few cases before the teeth erupt,[133] but it only becomes al-

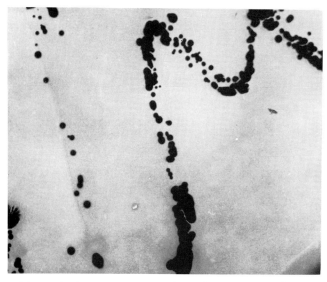

Fig. 3-3. *Bacteroides melaninogenicus.* Anaerobic cultivation at 37° C. was incubated 5 days on 5% human blood added to Difco blood infusion agar base. Colonies are convex and deep black in color, and vary in size from 0.5 mm. to 2 mm. Colonies may be either smooth or rough.

most universally present upon the creation of gingival sulci upon tooth eruption. The organism is found more frequently in deep than shallow gingival sulci, although no correlation is found between its occurrence and inflammation of the sulci.[151] *B. melaninogenicus* has been reported to be a component of various mixed anaerobic infections such as pulmonary abscesses, appendicitis, puerperal fever, nephritis, surgical infections. It has also been isolated from the oral cavity of hamsters,[147] guinea pigs, dogs, cattle, sheep, and swine. It is often associated with *Actinomyces*, and it is difficult to isolate from them in the laboratory.[48] *B. melaninogenicus* is very highly sensitive to penicillin, almost as sensitive to erythromycin, and relatively much more resistant to streptomycin.[92]

Bacteroides oralis is a gram-negative, nonmotile rod with rounded ends. Surface colonies on blood agar are round, smooth, gray to white in color, nonhemolytic, and small. It is strictly anaerobic and has been isolated from the gingival crevice area of man.

Fusobacterium

The genus *Fusobacterium* is distinguished from the others in the family Bacteroidaceae by the cells characteristically having either one or both ends pointed. These gram-negative bacteria are anaerobic, some strains are motile, and all are highly fastidious in their growth requirements upon primary isolation. It has been found to be more difficult to isolate and maintain than any other of the gram-negative nonsporulating anaerobic bacilli.[92] A number of species have been described, but among these only *Fusobacterium polymorphum* and *F. nucleatum* have been thoroughly studied. Fusobacteria are normal members of the oral microbiota and ordinarily exhibit low pathogenicity. Under some circumstances they may participate in mixed infections with spirochetes and streptococci in the mouth, such as

acute necrotizing ulcerative gingivitis or in similar mixed infections of other mucosal surfaces, especially of the genitalia. In other cases they may participate in the production of abscesses in various organs such as the lungs or brain. Infections by fusobacteria alone occur much more rarely.

MIXED MICROORGANISMS
Infections of floor of mouth and neck

Most soft-tissue infections of the mouth are caused by the heterogenous mixture of microorganisms occurring in the oropharynx or the oral cavity, which can participate in varying proportions in these processes.[108] These infections in the oral cavity or the neck are largely determined by the anatomic relations of the structures involved. Since the inception of the antibiotic era, deep neck infections originating from a dental source have become relatively more frequent, and the salivary glands in the floor of the mouth have also become a more frequent portal of entry for such infections. In the pre-antibiotic era the predominating microorganism of deep neck infections appeared to be either hemolytic or nonhemolytic streptococcus, occurring in more than 40% of the cases, with the staphylococcus as the second most frequently occurring bacterium; diphtheroides, bacteroides, *E. coli*, spirochetes, spirilla, and pneumococci were also found to be present, although not all in the same case. It appears, however, that since antimicrobial agents have come into common use the staphylococcus has become the predominating microorganism.

Ludwig's angina

Among the most serious clinical forms of the mixed infections is Ludwig's angina (Fig. 3-4), a cellulitis of the floor of the mouth in which streptococci and staphylococci are the most common bacteria found in the infected area, but Vincent's organisms and other oral spirochetes may be either primary or secondary invaders.[106] In a few cases only a single bacterial species, for example, an enterococcus, has been found upon laboratory study of material from the lesion.[201] Ludwig's angina usually has its origin in a periapical infection of a carious lower molar tooth and develops either before or after extraction. The teeth most often involved are the second and third molars, with the first molar and the bicuspids less frequently responsible. Perforation through bone by an abscess of the third molar occurs on the lingual side because of the extreme thickness of the buccal wall of the alveolus. If perforation occurs superior to the attachment of the mylohyoid muscle, the infection progresses along the fascial planes to the sublingual space. Further extension through the mylohyoid muscle into the submandibular space occurs in uncontrolled infections.

The symptoms that develop with the extension of the infection are swelling with induration, pushing of the tongue upward toward the side opposite that of the infection, and difficulty in opening the mouth, in swallowing and breathing; pain and an increase in temperature are also noticeable. Respiratory obstruction from the developing cellulitis may result in death unless a tracheotomy is done promptly. If antibiotic therapy and surgical drainage when indicated are used early enough, the necessity for tracheotomy and the danger to life are very largely avoided. The present striking successes form a sharp contrast to the situation in 1836, the year in which Wilhelm Frederick von Ludwig reported the condition first, when the disease was almost invariably fatal.[145] Deep neck infections arising in soft tissues seem to yield to antibiotic therapy more readily and more rapidly than infections having their origin in the dental alveolus or the temporal bone.[17]

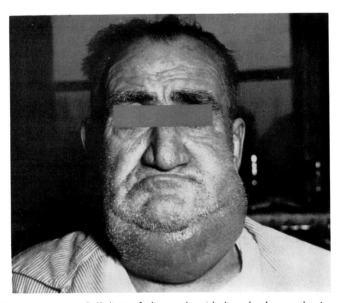

Fig. 3-4. Ludwig's angina. Cellulitis of the neck with lymphadenopathy is subsequent to an abscess of the floor of mouth. *Staphylococcus aureus*, anaerobic streptococcus, and a *Bacteroides* species were isolated from exudate. (Courtesy Dr. I. W. Scopp, Veterans Administration Hospital, New York, N. Y.)

Infections of the lungs
Aspiration pneumonia

Aspiration pneumonias varying through a wide range of severity may develop when predisposing factors occur such as dental sepsis, extraction of teeth, anesthesia, or chronic bronchitis with aspiration of sputum. It is most commonly seen in patients with poor oral hygiene and in states of deep unconsciousness when the gag reflex becomes depressed by trauma or barbiturate or alcohol intoxication.[23]

Lung abscess

A lung abscess is an area of necrosis localized in the pulmonary tissue, surrounded by an inflammatory reaction. Putrid lung abscess may develop upon inhalation of contaminated material from the mouth or pharynx and consequent infection of the lung parenchyma with a mixed microbial flora, dominated by anaerobes. No single organism can be considered to be the causative factor since staphylococci, anaerobic streptococci, diphtheroids, pneumococci, *Klebsiella* organisms, fusobacteria, spirochetes, and spirilla are found in different proportions from one case to another.[37] The fusospirochetal organisms, however, appear to account for a very large proportion of the cases.[264]

Severe gingivodental disease with advanced oral sepsis is the single most commonly associated disease in cases of lung abscess.[252] Surgical procedures in the mouth or pharynx, such as dental extractions or tonsillectomy, and depression of the natural protective reflexes of the pharynx and larynx from the anesthetic are additional factors associated with the development of lung abscess. Alcholism or the inhalation of infected material during sleep may also lead to lung abscess. Early diagnosis and prompt treatment are of great importance.

Treatment includes use of antibiotics and postural drainage; surgical drainage in a few cases may be necessary.[252] Pre-extraction scaling and periodontal treatment are among the measures instituted that are highly effective in reducing the incidence of this infection.[210]

ENTEROBACTERIACEAE

The family Enterobacteriaceae consists of gram-negative, nonsporulating, rod-shaped bacteria that grow well on artificial media. Some species have no flagella, while others are flagellated peritrichously. Nitrates are reduced to nitrites, glucose is fermented with the formation of acid or of acid and gas. Result of the indophenol oxidase test is negative. The antigenic composition is complex, with interrelationships among the different genera. Saprophytes as well as animal and human pathogens are among the different genera.

The enteric bacteria are usually considered to be only transiently present in the human oral cavity, but the oral structures nevertheless have been known to become infected with them, although other sites of the body are much more frequently involved. There have been an increasing number of gram-negative infections in recent years, and especially in hospitals, where they have supplanted the staphylococci in importance.[178] This situation may result from the widespread use of antibiotics and the subsequent suppression of gram-positive bacteria; but hospital transfer of the bacteria through direct contact, contaminated solutions, instrumentation, operation, and catheters also is significant.[171]

In some cases an infection may involve gram-positive cocci in addition to the enterics, requiring a mixture of antibiotics for therapy. Osteomyelitis of the mandible, for example, by a mixed flora with *Enterobacter aerogenes* as the predominant organism, and with alpha hemolytic streptococci and *E. coli* also present, has been reported.[186] Among the other clinical conditions of the oral structures involving enterics, there has been reported[244] post-extraction cellulitis of the floor of the mouth and neck caused by *Salmonella choleraesuis* and an infection of a maxillary epithelial cyst caused by *Salmonella typhimurium*.[158]

These infections of the oral cavity appear to be diagnosed correctly only after failure to respond to treatment with the most commonly useful antibiotics for gram-positive oral infections, such as penicillin.[186]

Klebsiella

The genus *Klebsiella* consists of non-motile, gram-negative, nonsporulating, aerobic bacilli which form large and regular capsules. Surface colonies are large and very mucoid, a consequence of the prominent capsules. These organisms frequent many carbohydrates. The capsules, consisting of polysaccharides, are of varied antigenicity, thus allowing the differentiation of several capsular types.

Most prominent among the *Klebsiella* is *K. pneumoniae* (Friedländer's bacillus), an organism that occurs in the respiratory tract of a small number of normal persons and may produce a dangerous pneumonia with high mortality in untreated cases. About 1% of the bacterial pneumonias are caused by *K. pneumoniae*.

In the oral cavity, *K. pneumoniae* has been known to cause a chronic osteomyelitis of the mandible[2] and a membrane-forming stomatitis in infants.[78] The stomatitis may be accompanied by a diarrhea from the same organism.[270] An unidentified species of *Klebsiella* has also been isolated from a suppurative infection of the parotid space.[186] A small proportion of root canal cultures yield *Klebsiella* species.[88] These isolates were found to be resistant to erythromycin, penicillin, and oleandomycin, but sensitive to neomycin, nitrofurantoin, streptomycin, and kanamycin. Other studies indicate that Friedländer's bacillus is also sensitive to the sulfonamides, tetracycline, and chloramphenicol.

Cephalothin and polymyxin B are effective against many strains.

Another *Klebsiella* species of interest to the oral microbiologists is *K. rhinoscleromatis*. This organism has been isolated from rhinoscleroma, a destructive but chronic granuloma of the nose and pharynx that may involve the upper lip, cheeks, soft and hard palates, and the superior alveolar process. It is uncertain what the role of *K. rhinoscleromatis* is in this disease since it cannot evoke the disease in laboratory animals and since the bacterium is also found in healthy persons.[197]

Donovania granulomatis

This gram-negative organism, the agent of granuloma inguinale, is a plump bacillus that is nonsporulating but does have prominent polar granules. It can be cultivated in the yolk sac of the developing chicken embryo and in rich media such as beef heart infusion. The organism, therefore, has highly fastidious growth requirements.

Its growth is characteristically mucoid, bearing in this respect a resemblance to *K. pneumoniae*, to which it is closely related antigenically. In smears from lesions or in biopsy material, *D. granulomatis* is found to be capsulated also and is found both free and within polymorphonuclear leukocytes or large mononuclear cells.

The disease caused by this organism is a slowly progressing granulomatous ulceration, destructive of tissue, which usually occurs in the genital region, but it is not entirely certain that it is a true venereal disease, that is, contracted primarily by sexual contact. The incubation period is from one to four weeks, following which there often develops a swelling in the groin that goes on to rupture.

The original report describing granuloma inguinale was from India by Donovan and was based upon a patient with a buccal lesion. This was an unusual circumstance for, as it became evident in the course of time, extragenital lesions are found in but 6% of all cases and are usually secondary to genital granulomas. The extragenital sites commonly involved are skin, subcutaneous tissues, and the mucous membranes around the oropharynx and eyes.[47]

Of special interest for the dentist are the lesions that may occur on the face, at the corners of the mouth, on the lips, buccal mucosa, tonsils, uvula, hard palate, gingiva, or in the neck as cervical abscesses.[80] In the case of buccal lesions, if the oral infection has been long standing, scar formation and subsequent contraction of cheek tissue may result in extreme limitations of mouth opening and abolition of lateral excursions of the mandible. Involvement of the uvula or faucial pillars may lead to their destruction.[258] These facial and oral lesions apparently develop by self-inoculation through the fingers from the primary inguinal lesion. Metastasis or abnormal sexual practices are other possibilities that have been considered for some cases. Secondary infections involving especially the fusobacteria and spirochetes, and resulting in foul-smelling, painful, and progressive ulcers, often complicate the disease.[104]

Epidemiologic studies indicate that in the United States the infection occurs primarily among blacks but does also occur among whites. It has been found in the Americas, the Far East, and Africa, being more common than had once been thought. At least 10,000 cases are known to have occurred in the United States.

Diagnosis is made from the case history, the clinical picture of the lesions, and demonstration of the organism in the fresh tissue smear. The technique for this latter procedure requires tissue obtained by a punch biopsy forceps or by scraping the lesion. The tissue is macerated on glass slides, stained with Giemsa solution, and studied in the microscope for the presence of Donovan bodies.

Treatment with the antibiotics chloramphenicol, the tetracyclines, or dihydrostreptomycin has been highly effective.

Proteus

The genus *Proteus* consists of gram-negative, motile, aerobic bacilli, only a few species of which infect man. *Proteus* species are distinctive because of their rapid spread over the surface of agar culture medium, referred to as "swarming," and because of their rapid liquefaction of gelatin. Lactose is not fermented. *Proteus vulgaris* normally inhabits the intestinal tract of man but may produce disease in various parts of the body. These infections tend to present special problems in therapy because of their marked resistance to most of the antibiotics. Kanamycin and nitrofurantoin are the most effective agents currently available for treatment for proteus infections.

Proteus vulgaris has been described as the sole agent found in a few reported cases of submandibular abscess[155] and as a rarely occurring organism in infected root canals[261] or bacterial parotitis.[240]

Pseudomonas

The bacilli belonging to the first genus of the family Pseudomonadaceae constitute the genus *Pseudomonas*. These rod-shaped, gram-negative forms are primarily water and soil parasites and are of low pathogenicity for man, with the exception of *Pseudomonas aeruginosa*, which is particularly a problem with debilitated patients. Most species of the genus are motile with one monotrichous flagellum. The bacteria grow in large round colonies, with a tendency toward spreading and with a range of variations in form. Fermentation of some sugars is weak, and lactose is never fermented. A characteristic property is the ability to form water-soluble pigments that may be separated into two groups. One of these is pyocyanin, a deep blue phenazine derivative that is not fluorescent. It is easily extracted by chloroform from crude cultures. The pigments of the other group show a bright fluorescence in daylight and ultraviolet light, but they cannot be extracted from the water phase in cultures.

Oral relationships of *P. aeruginosa* are significant. The organism has been found to colonize the gingiva[193] and occurs in the saliva of a small proportion of Americans as an established member of the microbiota.[257] It has a much higher incidence in the oral cavity of African tribesmen living in primitive circumstances.[50] *P. aeruginosa* has also been isolated from a small percentage of infected root canals.[88] Its presence in some nonvital intact teeth following trauma to the teeth is thought to be probably an anachoretic effect.

Ordinarily, *P. aeruginosa* has but very limited ability to invade the body unless the body defenses are not fully developed, as in the infant, or when these defenses have been weakened as in debilitated adults. Under suitable conditions *P. aeruginosa* may be the cause of a great variety of suppurative and other affections in man. Bacteremia, septicemia, endocarditis, pyelonephritis, bacteriuria, pneumonia, peritonitis, osteomyelitis, and skin infections are among the lesions known to occur. Oral infections with *P. aeruginosa* may occur after oral surgical procedures.[100] *Pseudomonas* bacteremia also may occur after oral surgery.[99] Reports have been published of mandibular infection following the surgical extraction of impacted molars and of infection in the mandibular molar region of a patient undergoing simultaneous endodontic and periodontal therapy in that same region.[100] Drainage and tetracycline therapy were effective in clearing these cases.

Neonatal suppurative parotitis caused by *P. aeruginosa* has been but rarely observed,[162] although such cases usually develop following invasion of the tissues upon a septicemia. In the adult, acute suppurative parotitis from a mixed infection involving staphylococcus and pseudomonas has been observed.[113]

Chronic osteomyelitis, with sequestrum formation, of the maxilla in an adult, associated with a pseudomonas infection, has also been reported.[228] This rare infection occurred following the start of endodontic treatment and then extraction of the maxillary right lateral incisor tooth. Resistance to tetracyclines by the pseudomonad isolated from the lesion required the use of streptomycin for therapy. The polymyxin group or gentamicin have also been useful therapeutic agents, but, unfortunately, it is not always possible to find a satisfactory antibiotic for pseudomonas infections if the toxic effects of the useful drugs prohibit their use in a particular case.[58]

The use of a high-humidity environment for newborn infants with respiratory problems has resulted in a number of pseudomonas infections that have frequently been fatal. Among such cases has been reported an infection of the lips which progressed to a noma involving the cheeks and nose.[123] Death quickly followed in this instance in spite of oxytetracycline and polymyxin therapy. Autopsy showed scattered abscesses on the pleural surfaces of the lungs.

For the past ten years there appears to have occurred a steadily rising rate of pseudomonad infection in hospitals, especially among patients in debilitated condition with severe underlying disease.[156] Certain sites such as the urinary tract and burned skin are especially liable to infection in such patients. Intensive studies in hospitals have shown that *P. aeruginosa* apparently colonizes in the gastrointestinal tract and that autoinfection may occur commonly from the feces by way of the patient's hands. *Pseudomonas* organisms colonize hospital equipment soon after use by an infected person. Such equipment often is too large or too intricate to be sterilized easily after use, and this may become a new source of infection.[178]

SMALL GRAM-NEGATIVE RODS
Brucella

The brucellae[61] constitute a genus of closely related, small, aerobic, gram-negative rods, nonmotile and nonsporulating, which are capable of causing various but similar acute and chronic diseases of domestic animals and man. Each species has a preferred host, but all are able to infect other animals and man. *Brucella abortus* has its reservoir in cattle, *B. suis* in swine, and *B. melitensis* in sheep and goats.[268]

Most infections in man are subclinical, or brief or low-grade illnesses that escape diagnosis. In acute brucellosis, there is a generalized spread through the body by way of the blood, with a wide variety of nonspecific symptoms occurring throughout the body. The first localization is, in most cases, the lymph glands or lymphoid tissue such as the tonsils. A number of cases have been observed[61] of oral infections involving the mucosa, and with a consequent stomatitis. One such reported case[218] resulted from ingestion of large quantities of raw milk. The patient had red and edematous gingivae, small ulcers scattered about the oral mucosa, and grayish patches that somewhat resembled those of thrush. The anterior cervical and submental lymph nodes were enlarged, firm, and tender. Although the patient was acutely ill, his condition responded rapidly to treatment with immune blood serum.

In cases of long-lasting chronic infections, the organisms are no longer in the blood, having localized in the tissues and particularly in the reticuloendothelial system. The organisms have been recovered from local lesions in practically every tissue of the body and are found predominantly intracellularly. Granulomas commonly develop at the sites of localization that consist primarily of collections of epithelioid cells and lymphocytes. These localized lesions may persist for years, producing chronic or recurrent ill health.[173] Dental sepsis, especially periapical abscesses, play

a role in increasing the severity of the disease. Patients with osteoarthritis have a coexisting periodontitis or dental abscess. In one case,[203] *B. abortus* was isolated from the follicular cyst of an impacted maxillary third molar, extraction of which led to prompt disappearance of an iritis. Another instance of chronic infection was localized in the parotid gland.[148] The infection was cleared only upon intensive systemic treatment with oxytetracycline combined with operative drainage of the brucella abscess in the parotid. In a significant number of cases brucellosis has been initially diagnosed incorrectly as stomatitis, dental caries, mumps, actinomycosis, tonsillitis, or infectious mononucleosis.[61]

Salivary antibodies against brucella have been demonstrated in human cases of brucellosis by agglutination and complement-fixation techniques.[300]

Haemophilus

The genus *Haemophilus* consists of small gram-negative, nonmotile, nonsporulating, aerobic rods that must be supplied with hemoglobin porphyrins for the synthesis of cytochrome, cytochrome oxidase, peroxidase, and catalase, and with di- and triphosphopyridine nucleotides. The species of special interest to the oral microbiologist is *H. influenzae*.

Varied infections

H. influenzae is carried in the nasopharynx and the oropharynx and also can be isolated from the saliva.[220] Its pathogenicity, especially among the young, makes it one of the important bacterial species producing serious clinical infections in children.[253] Among these are pharyngitis, epiglottitis, sinusitis, otitis media, meningitis, pericarditis, osteomyelitis, subcutaneous abscesses, and appendicitis. *H influenzae* may have a role as a secondary invader during outbreaks of pandemic influenza, although it is regarded as an uncommon pathogen in the adult.[150]

Infants and young children between the ages of six months and two years may develop cellulitis from *H. influenzae* type b.[79] Typically, the lesion is localized on the face, especially a cheek, and is accompanied by fever, upper-respiratory tract infection, and swelling of the involved area. In a few cases there may be otitis media or teething at the onset of the cellulitis. The buccal mucosa may be pale and slightly edematous on the involved side, and the tonsils enlarged and injected.[103] There is a bluish-purple discoloration present in the area of the cellulitis only during the first few days of the infection. The temperature is markedly elevated. Nose and throat cultures, as well as blood cultures, usually yield the organism. The occurrence of these infections during such a sharply demarcated period in early life is illuminated by the observation that 80% of cases of *H. influenzae* type b meningitis occur between the ages of two months and three years.[87] Moreover, defibrinated blood from subjects less than two months and more than three years of age has considerable bactericidal effect on cultures of *H. influenzae* type b, while blood from children in the intervening age group lacks this ability. Early diagnosis is very important since treatment is most effective when given early. Chloramphenicol is the drug of choice for chemotherapy for clinical states that are life-threatening[253]; otherwise, ampicillin or a sulfonamide combined with erythromycin may be used.

Whooping cough

Bordetella pertussis, the agent causing pertussis (whooping cough), greatly resembles *H. influenzae* in its microscopic characteristics. Cultural characteristics also resemble those for the genus as a whole. On the basis of colonial growth, four phases may be distinguished, of which phase 1 is the most virulent. In this phase the organisms form smooth colonies consisting of encapsulated cells; phase 4 cells are without capsules and form rough colonies. Phases 2 and 3 are intermediate in their characteristics.

Whooping cough is an acute, highly contagious disease characterized by recurring attacks of spasmodic cough and is generally seen in young children. It has a long course with a slow convalescence. In full-blown cases the paroxysms of coughing result in hemorrhages from the mouth that may have their origin either in the pharynx or the bronchi. The frenum of the tongue may develop an erosion or deeper ulceration that may lead to its partial or total destruction. This lesion results from protrusion of the tongue during the coughing episodes and consequent friction against the sharp, newly erupted lower incisors.[124] On the other hand, however, pertussis may occur in a very mild form that lasts for only from 7 to 14 days and may not include the classic whooping cough.

Diagnosis depends, in the early phase of the disease, upon culturing the organism on a plate of Bordet-Gengou medium held close to the mouth for inoculation upon coughing. With fully developed symptoms of whooping cough, clinical observations of the patient readily allow recognition of the disease. Later in the course of the infection, the patient develops circulating antibodies that are also useful for diagnosis. For therapy, antibiotics early in the course of the illness may be useful,[140] but recourse is also made to the injection of hyperimmune globulin together with pertussis vaccine made from phase 1 culture. Prevention is routinely practiced today by the injection into the infant less than one year old of a vaccine consisting of killed phase 1 organisms, together with diphtheria and tetanus toxoids.

Oral involvements

Among the species of *Haemophilus* is *Bacteroides corrodens*, an organism that had been mistaken initially for a bacteroides.[139] This is a gram-negative, non-motile, small rod. It is oxidase-positive, and its growth is enhanced by 7.5% CO_2 in its atmosphere. It is facultative in its atmospheric requirements for oxygen and has a marked need for hemin. This species is fairly inactive in its biochemical reactions with carbohydrates. Surface colonies on blood agar plates give rise to tiny depressions in the agar surface within from 36 to 48 hours, a characteristic accounting for the species name. The colonies are round, smooth, gray-white, and as large as 2 mm. in diameter after five days' incubation at 37° C. Strains have been isolated from the gingival crevice, bacteremia, mandibular abscess, dental granuloma, buccal abscess, and the sputum.

Pasteurella

The *Pasteurella* organisms are gram-negative, nonmotile (at 37° C.), nitrate- and catalase-positive, aerobic, pleomorphic coccobacilli with bipolar staining. Of the several species in the genus *Pasteurella*, which comprises organisms producing hemorrhagic septicemia, plague, and pseudo-tuberculosis, only two have special interest for the oral microbiologist: *P. multocida* and *P. pneumotropica*.

P. multocida (synonym *P. septica*) is a widely distributed bacterium that has a virtually unlimited range of hosts.[29] It is carried in the mouths and appears in the saliva of apparently healthy wild and domestic animals, although under suitable circumstances it may act as an animal pathogen causing hemorrhagic septicemia, a highly contagious and usually fatal infection. *P. multocida* may enter the human body through the respiratory tract (in inhaled droplets from the sneeze of an animal) or through the wound from an animal scratch or bite. That infections with *P. multocida* are not more common is surprising since animal bites, especially by the dog or cat, are a common medical problem. The number of people, and particularly children, bitten each year is truly phenomenal. It is estimated that in the United States 660,000 people are bitten by dogs alone each year. Approximately one of seven victims of dog bite shows signs of infection.[39]

Most of the human infections caused by *P. multocida* fall within one of three clinical pictures: (1) chronic pulmonary infection, in which *P. multocida* may be a secondary invader; (2) a systemic form of infection with meningitis; and, most commonly, (3) local infection with adenitis almost always following the bite of an animal.[256] This last syndrome consists of extensive swelling and severe pain, starting from a few hours to several days or a week after an animal bite. There frequently develops a local abscess with or without involvement of underlying bone. The infection progresses to frank osteomyelitis of the bone especially after a deeply penetrating wound.[4] Ulcer of the mouth due to *P. multocida* has been reported.[131] In some cases a mixed infection may develop containing additional bacteria such as alpha streptococcus, beta streptococcus, *E. coli*, or *Clostridium*. Circulating antibodies are not usually found during local infections, but in systemic infections there may be a vigorous antibody response.

Diagnosis is greatly facilitated if the possibility of a *P. multocida* infection is kept in mind in any cases of injury where animals have been involved. Cultural identification of the organism is indispensable for establishing the diagnosis, but careful bacteriologic study is necessary.[29]

Penicillin is an effective antibiotic in treatment, as are cephalothin, chloramphenicol, erythromycin, and the tetracyclines, but antibiotics alone may not eradicate an established infection.[29] Careful debridement of the bite wound is of great value in prevention or rapid control of an infection, especially in the case of facial wounds.[283]

P. pneumotropica, distinguished by its

ability to ferment maltose, has been found in a fatal case following a dog bite. The infection was highly virulent, killing the bitten 51-year-old man within 48 hours. The bacterium was isolated from both the patient's blood and the dog's mouth.[190]

Francisella

Formerly known as *Pasteurella tularensis,* *Francisella tularensis* is a small, gram-negative, aerobic, nonmotile coccobacillus on initial isolation, but becomes rodlike on continued cultivation. It requires special media containing cysteine or cystine for growth. The optimal incubation temperature is from 35° to 37° C.

Tularemia

Francisella tularensis is the etiologic agent of tularemia, an acute infectious disease man acquires in most cases from the handling of infected animals, from the eating of rare meat of infected animals, such as the rabbit or ground squirrel, or from the bite of a vertebrate or a tick. It has been estimated, however, that 90% of infections in the United States follow exposure to the tissues or secretions of rabbits. Transmission from one human being to another is unknown.

The incubation period for tularemia is usually from two to five days. Onset is abrupt, with chills, fever, and general malaise. The course of the illness is prolonged, but recovery without unfavorable sequelae usually occurs. Mortality before streptomycin became available was approximately 7%, but the chances of recovery have since been greatly improved. Six clinical types are recognized: the ulceroglandular, oculoglandular, glandular, pulmonary, cryptogenic (also referred to as the typhoidal), and the oropharyngeal.

The ulceroglandular form is the most common, constituting about 80% of reported cases. In this type of infection there is inflammation and subsequent ulceration at the site of inoculation, and regional adenopathy. Metastatic lesions may occur in various parts of the body. The bite or scratch of wild rabbits may sometimes result in this clinical type. More rarely, it has been known to occur with the bite of a domestic cat.[46]

The oculoglandular form of tularemia is the best known, although it rarely occurs. In this type the organism produces an inflammation of the mucous membrane of the eyes as a result, usually, of self-inoculation with the fingers. This is followed by lymphatic and systemic involvement.

The pulmonary form results from the inhalation of infectious droplets. It is most commonly seen among laboratory workers who have come into contact with infected laboratory animals. In this form of tularemia, an ulcerative stomatitis may develop involving the tongue, gingiva, and buccal mucosa.[212]

In the typhoidal form of tularemia, there is general systemic involvement, with fever and prostration, but without a local lesion. The oropharyngeal type is characterized by the development of buccal, gingival, and lingual lesions in some cases. In other instances, there may be marked swelling in the parotid region. Some cases have been observed in which the only manifestation of the tularemia was an acute tonsillitis. The tonsils are covered with an exudate or grayish-white membrane, which may sometimes involve the posterior pharyngeal wall, the anterior faucial pillars, the base of the tongue, the soft palate, uvula, and the nasal and buccal mucosae, resembling diphtheria at times. The cervical lymph nodes are enlarged, are usually tender, and may suppurate.[132]

Diagnosis depends upon taking a careful, accurate history and cultivating early the fluid from obvious local lesions. Although isolates have been obtained from the blood (during the first two weeks of the disease), these have been relatively rare in human cases, except in instances of untreated fulminating infection.

Treatment with streptomycin for at least eight days, or with the tetracyclines, gives good therapeutic results. Use of penicillin and sulfonamides is ineffective.[9]

CORYNEBACTERIUM
Diphtheria

Diphtheria is an acute infectious disease whose etiologic agent, *Corynebacterium diphtheriae,* was first reported by Klebs in 1883 in microscopic examination of pseudomembranous material removed from the tonsils. The bacterium was cultivated on coagulated beef serum by Löffler in 1884. The disease is primarily one of childhood, more than 60% of cases occurring in children less than ten years of age. The bacillus is not invasive but produces an exotoxin at the site where it has localized, generally the tonsils. The exotoxin enters the blood stream and causes a toxemia.

Morphology. The bacillus stains readily with the simple stains and is gram-positive, nonmotile, nonsporulating, and noncapsulated. This slender bacillus is pleomorphic and may be wedge or dumbbell shaped or slightly curved. Granules, generally present in the bacillus, are often found at the extremities and are then called polar bodies. These bodies stain more intensely with Löffler's alkaline methylene blue than does the rest of the bacillus and appear to be tinted red.

Cultivation. Growth is readily obtained upon beef heart infusion agar with from 5% to 10% horse serum enrichment. A small quantity of potassium tellurite added to the medium makes it both selective and differential. Commensal residents of the nose and throat are inhibited, and diphtheria bacilli that vary in their exotoxin potency may be differentiated into the gravis, intermedius, and mitis strains, depending on their colonial characteristics. The gravis strain yields colonies that are large with a raised center and dull gray; the intermedius colonies are small and grayish; the mitis-strain colonies are small and have black centers and gray peripheries. These characteristics, together with starch hydrolysis and blood hemolysis, are used especially for epidemiologic studies.

Cultivation on blood agar yields small, raised, grayish, granular colonies; hemolysis may or may not occur. The coagulated serum medium of Löffler is still used. It is prepared by adding one part of dextrose infusion broth to three parts of horse or bovine serum and then coagulating this mixture in slanted tubes at a low degree of heat in an inspissator.

Toxin. The most significant effects of the diphtheria bacillus in a diphtheritic infection are usually caused by the powerful exotoxin that it produces. It has been found that the toxigenic strains of *C. diphtheriae* are lysogenic and that some strains of nontoxigenic diphtheroids may become toxigenic by conversion to the lysogenic state.

The toxin causes primarily damage in the heart muscle, kidneys, liver, and peripheral nerves. Death is usually caused by heart failure in an acute infection. Intensive efforts have been made to determine the mechanism of action of the toxin, but this problem still remains unresolved.

Pathogenicity. Within from several days to a week after the bacillus has lodged in the upper respiratory tract, multiplication begins and a small amount of exotoxin is formed which causes necrosis of the neighboring epithelial cells. The diphtheria bacillus continues to multiply with an increase in toxin, and the necrotic area becomes deeper and extends laterally. An inflammatory reaction then occurs, with migration of leukocytes and diapedesis of red blood cells. A pseudomembrane forms consisting of necrotic epithelial cells, blood cells, and fibrin; it covers the tonsillar area and in some individuals extends over the pharynx and into the trachea. While these local injuries cannot be considered insignificant, the most severe damage is caused by the systemic distribution of the toxin through the bloodstream.

Immunization. Diphtheria alum toxoid combined with tetanus toxoid and pertussis vaccine (DTP) is injected intramuscularly into infants after the first month of life. Three doses are given, each at four-to six-week intervals, and a reenforcing dose is given one year after the third injection. Booster doses are required at intervals later in life.

If a child is exposed to diphtheria and it is not known whether he is immune, a Schick test should be given as well as treatment with penicillin for five days, the incubation period for diphtheria. In the Schick test, a small quantity of diphtheria toxin is injected intracutaneously; if no reaction occurs at the site of injection, the child is not susceptible to the toxin. An erythematous reaction indicates lack of immunity, and the child, therefore, should then receive a full schedule of toxoid for immunization in addition to the prophylactic penicillin.

Diagnosis. In addition to the clinical observations, laboratory determinations are necessary to firmly establish a diagnosis of diphtheria in a patient. Smears and swabs are taken of the suspected lesion for microscopic examination and cultivation. Smears are stained with Gram's and alkaline methylene blue methods. Swabs are streaked out on blood agar and tellurite plates and on a Löffler slant. Isolated colonies after two days' incubation at 37° C. are studied. Since pathogenicity relies principally upon toxin production, which may or may not be present in the particular strains found, the isolates are tested in animals by a virulence test. This may be either an intracutaneous injection of the culture into rabbits or a subcutaneous injection of the culture into guinea pigs. In the case of skin-tested rabbits, necrosis may develop at the site of injection, while in the case of the guinea pig given organisms subcutaneously, the test animal unprotected by antitoxin will die.

Treatment. Therapy for suspected active diphtheria requires the injection of antitoxin as soon as possible after completion of sensitivity test to the antiserum. Bacteriologic confirmation of the diagnosis should not be awaited before administering the antitoxin. Antibiotic, usually penicillin, is also administered. The antitoxin is necessary to counteract the diphtheria toxin, and the antibiotic aids in removal of the organism from the body.

Since the exotoxin of *C. diphtheriae* is rapidly fixed to nerve tissue cells and, once combined, cannot be neutralized by antitoxin, it is essential that the antitoxin be given as early as possible in the disease. Subcutaneous injections of antitoxin are absorbed less rapidly than those injected either intramuscularly or intravenously. In a severe case the latter two routes are both used. Early in mild cases, from 3,000 to 5,000 units may be adequate; but later in the disease, and depending on the severity of the symptoms, parenteral administration of from 30,000 to 100,000 units is used. Children who have not been previously immunized, who are free of symptoms, but who have been exposed to persons with diphtheria should receive a prophylactic dose of 10,000 units while the first dose of toxoid is given to start active immunization. The antitoxin protects the child for several weeks while active immunity is developing.

Oral lesions. Diphtheritic infections confined entirely to the oral cavity occur but rarely. Such lesions have been reported at the commissures of the mouth[229] and on the facial skin, especially if a crack or herpetic sore is present. Lesions have also been observed on the buccal and labial mucosa,[231] the tongue,[217] the soft palate,[73] and in the sockets of recently extracted teeth. The oral infections, however, usually develop only after some traumatic injury and usually are secondary to late severe faucial diphtheria. They are ulcerous and possess no definite characteristics that render them readily distinguishable from other infectious ulcerous lesions. Pharyngeal diphtheria results in a swelling of the soft palate that may be mistaken for a peritonsillar abscess.[210] In some cases, swelling of the neck and submaxillary region develops to the point of suggesting a diffuse cellulitis such as is seen in Ludwig's angina.[294]

In about 10% of diphtheria patients in temperate climates, paralytic phenomena appear that tend to be limited to the cranial nerves. As a rule, paralysis begins in and is limited to the uvula and the palatal muscles. Such cases are first recognized by the appearance of nasal speech and the regurgitation of fluid through the nose.[249] The facial muscles and tongue are rarely involved.

Carriers. Perhaps the most important factor in the perpetuation of certain infectious diseases, and especially diphtheria, is the presence of carriers of the infectious agent. In the case of diphtheria bacillus carriers, the bacilli may remain in the upper respiratory tract after all clinical signs have disappeared if some abnormal condition is present; and in some cases the carriers may harbor the bacilli without ever having been ill or having had active signs of the disease.[10] Under ordinary conditions, 1% or 2% of the population harbor virulent diphtheria bacilli. During epidemics, this rate is very much greater and rises to perhaps 15%.[117] In a certain number of carriers of *C. diphtheriae*, the bacillus can be found readily in the saliva obtained by having the subject spit into a tube,[163] but swabs of the nose, tonsils, or posterior wall of the pharynx are the most productive. In most cases the carrier harbors the bacilli in the tonsils. In a small number the bacilli are found only in the nose. Isolates must be checked for virulence in the laboratory before a confident judgment can be made of their significance. It is doubtful that diphtheria bacilli properly identified by biochemical and virulence tests have ever been reported from root canals.

The detection of bacilli at a superficial site sampled by a swab is misleading in regard to the actual site of parasitization. In fact, the bacteria are often deeply imbedded in the tissues, so that clearing a carrier requires systemic administration of antibiotic at a high enough level to secure a high tissue concentration. Penicillin or erythromycin has been used effectively for this purpose, but treatment requires ten days. A series of six negative cultures for a period of two weeks following treatment is needed to assure that the carrier has indeed been cleared. The failure to cure the carrier with this regime probably indicates some abnormality of the upper respiratory system that must be corrected before success can be obtained. Among the possible abnormalities that may require attention are those involving the tonsils or the teeth, such as caries, or perhaps gingivitis.[67]

The exact mechanism by which the body rids itself of diphtheria bacilli is not entirely clear. It was noted as early as 1909 that there is an apparent antagonism between the diphtheria bacillus and staphylococci in the throat for when the throats of diphtheria bacillus convalescent carriers become infected with staphylococci the bacilli disappear.[21] Subsequent experimental studies on artificial culture media with large numbers of *S. aureus* strains have shown that only a few are capable of inhibiting diphtheria bacilli. These principally consist of strains sensitive to a single phage (type 71) or of closely related strains.[209] A further group has been found that is not characterized by phage sensitivity. Moreover, the conditions apparently needed for the production of the antibiotic effect by the staphylococci are such as to make it very questionable that this effect can operate effectively in the tonsillar crypt, which is the most favorable site for diphtheria bacillus localization in carriers.

Other early observations suggested that there may be local production of specific immune protective globulins which are active against diphtheria toxin, and that diphtheria antitoxin is excreted in the saliva.[274] Recent investigations have shown that this indeed is the case and that these immune bodies consist principally of the IgA fraction.[202] They are found in both saliva and nasal fluid. Saliva has been shown to have an inhibitory effect upon *C. diphtheriae* that is caused by the viridans streptococci. Further study has indicated that the antibacterial action is from hydrogen peroxide formed by the streptococci.

Diphtheroids

Gram-positive, nonsporulating, nonmotile bacilli that resemble the diphtheria bacilli and may possess metachromatic granules are referred to as diphtheroids. They are part of a large and heterogeneous group, and some workers place them with the actinomycetes and other forms in the order Actinomycetales.[194] Most of these microorganisms have a similar type of cell wall structure and a common antigenic determinant, which seems to lie in the deeper layers of the cell wall. The diphtheroids are found in the mouth, throat, and nose, on the conjunctiva, and also on the skin and about the genitalia of apparently normal persons. In a number of cases of subacute bacterial endocarditis, diphtheroids have been isolated from blood cultures. Although some of these isolations may have been a result of contamination from the skin while the blood sample was being drawn, this is probably not true for all instances.[207]

A salivary incidence of 67% is found for oral diphtheroids. These are heterogeneous in their biologic characteristics, but most of them are saccharolytic. They have also been isolated from a large proportion of infected root canals.[57] At times, filamentous microorganisms of the oral cavity such as *Actinomyces israelii* and *Actinomyces naeslundii* may appear in the diphtheroid form, probably as the result of filament fragmentation.

Anaerobic diphtheroids have been isolated along with other microorganisms from various kinds of lesions, but their causative relationship to these lesions is not yet established. An anaerobic diphtheroid, *Corynebacterium acnes*, is considered to be possibly involved in the pathogenesis of acne.

CLOSTRIDIUM

The bacterial genus *Clostridium* consists of anaerobic or microaerophilic rods that produce endospores. The spores are usually wider than the rod, producing a swelling of the cell. These organisms are generally gram-positive. Many of the species in the genus are pathogenic for man, acting particularly by the production of powerful exotoxins or by their powerful proteolytic action upon devitalized tissue. Their natural habitat is the soil and the intestinal tract of animals and man.

Since the human oral cavity contains ecologic niches that harbor anaerobes and microaerophiles, there is a real possibility that clostridia also may establish themselves in this environment. Indeed, cultivations of both carious and sound extracted teeth have yielded *Clostridium welchii* type A in about 60% of the carious teeth and 10% of the sound teeth.[75] *C. welchii*, *C. tetani*, and other clostridial species have also been isolated from human saliva, although only infrequently.[110] The low incidence of these bacteria in the saliva appears to be the result of the presence of the mixed salivary flora which inhibits both their growth and their production of toxin. Clostridia have been isolated from periodontal pockets in from 9% to 10% of the pockets sampled, while 38% of normal gingival crevices contain clostridia.[290] The species isolated, in order of decreasing frequency, are *C. sporogenes*, *C. bifermentans*, *C. botulinum*, *C. oedematiens*, and *C. perfringens*.

There have been many attempts to identify the mechanisms that allow clostridia and the other anaerobes to colonize in the mouth. It is known that the oxidation-reduction potential of the medium in which the anaerobes are contained is of critical importance.[119] The limiting oxidation-reduction potential of growth of *Bacteroides vulgatus* and *Clostridium sporogenes* is eH+150 mv. at pH 6.6; at potentials more positive than this the organisms do not grow, while at more negative potentials they grow consistently.[111] Other species of clostridia, such as *C. welchii* and *C. histolyticum,* have different redox requirements, but these also are lower than those suitable for aerobes.

Free-flowing saliva has a high positive redox potential ranging between 240 mv. and 400 mv.,[68] which is considerably greater than that required for the anaerobes.[230] On the other hand, however, the potential of the saliva shifts toward the negative side with the elapse of time,[69] which suggests that saliva in stagnant areas such as the periodontal pocket and the dental interproximal space, where oxygen uptake may be retarded, has redox potentials low enough to permit anaerobic growth.[159]

Attempts have been made to identify the origin of the reducing capacity of saliva. Approximately 70% of the reducing characteristics is found in the sediment of centrifuged saliva, which consists of bacteria, desquamated epithelial cells, leukocytes, and some debris.[204] The reductase activity of saliva has been found to be correlated significantly with numbers of salivary anaerobes.[242] The formed elements of the saliva, therefore, appear to provide the principal source for lowering the redox potential. Other factors that may be acting to promote suitable growth conditions in the saliva for oral anaerobes include the lack of peroxides in the saliva, the presence of salivary catalase, and the depletion of oxygen by the aerobic flora.[160]

Tetanus

Tetanus was a clearly recognized disease centuries ago, and was very accurately described by Hippocrates. Its cause, however, was not uncovered until 1884 when Nicolaier published the results of his investigations, implicating *Clostridium tetani* (Fig. 3-5). Tetanus in the United States remains as a problem primarily among

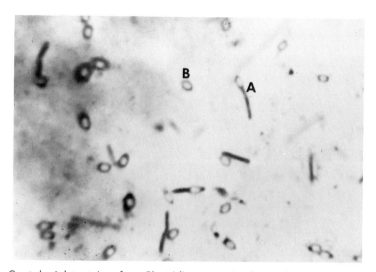

Fig. 3-5. Crystal violet stain of a *Clostridium tetani* culture showing unstained spores. Some spores are terminal to vegetative cells, *A,* while the vegetative portion of others has disintegrated, leaving the free spore, *B.*

infants less than one year of age and among drug addicts who use unsterilized needles, syringes, or contaminated drugs.[166] Otherwise it is a relatively rare disease, with fewer than 500 cases occurring annually. This is largely the result of the well-established use of prophylactic anti-toxin following injuries.[11]

In spite of the low normal oral incidence, the clostridia apparently are capable of initiating pathologic conditions from sites in the oral cavity. This seems to be the case especially for tetanus infection, which produces a toxin acting on the motor nerve cells. A carious tooth may be the portal of entry for the organism. There are several reports claiming that tetanus developed following extraction of teeth,[105, 255, 284] but most of these are open to question because of difficulties encountered in obtaining adequate bacteriologic supporting data. Tetanus has also been reported as occurring after a bite on the thumb by the family dog[129] and from a bite on the arm by a horse.[278]

In some cases, tetanus first comes to the attention of a dentist rather than a physician because of the involvement of oral structures, although the initial lesion may have had no relationship to dental problems. The following case[192] illustrates this point: A man, aged 55, had a lame jaw for which he went to the dentist; but while on his way to the dental office he underwent convulsions. Later he developed trismus and spasms of the neck and leg muscles. He had cut his thumb on a bottle 16 days before the onset of symptoms. Recovery followed the intravenous and intra-muscular injection of 340,000 units of anti-toxin.

Many conditions may cause confusion with tetanus so that a differential diagnosis may be difficult. Among the possible confusing diseases that may come to the attention of the dentist are osteomyelitis of the mandible, dislocated mandible, impacted lower third molar,[297] mumps,[265, 304]

and arthritis of the temporomandibular joint.[142]

The incubation period between initial infection with the tetanus bacillus and the active phase of the disease is usually from about one week to ten days. However, there may be a range of several days to several weeks, or even one year, before symptoms appear.[304] The symptoms of tetanus are classified as either: (1) prodromal, or those occurring before the frank development of the disease; or (2) classic, or those occurring with the disease in full progress and not necessarily preceded by the prodromal symptoms.

The prodromal symptoms of tetanus occur several days before the frank onset of the disease. They include such spastic muscle manifestations as a stiff jaw (trismus) and a stiff tongue which trembles and is drawn to one side when protruded; and pain and spasm in the muscles of the face, jaws, neck, and at deglutition. The trismus, caused by spasm of the masseter muscles, is the most dependable of the clinical signs,[265] occurring in 80% of the cases. The constancy of trismus as one of the initial symptoms, it has been suggested,[90] may result from the short length of the fifth cranial nerve and from an unusual susceptibility to the toxin. Measurement of the degree of opening of the jaw at the incisors is an index useful for determining whether the symptoms are getting more severe or are diminishing. Because of a lack of suspicion of the possibility of tetanus, it is estimated that perhaps as many as 2% of cases of this disease are initially treated by the extraction of a tooth or by palliative treatment for disease of the nose or throat. This is very unfortunate for it is during the early, prodromal, state that treatment should be instituted for the best chance of recovery.[234]

In view of the difficulties in establishing a definite diagnosis at the time a patient presents himself, it has been suggested[130] that any patient who has difficulty in opening the mouth which cannot be attributed to a local infection or other obvious cause should be considered for tetanus treatment.

The classic symptoms of tetanus are those of a full-blown, well-developed case and include the following characteristics: (1) Involvement of the jaws, which become firmly fixed; in these cases, the patient cannot talk and has difficulty in opening his mouth, hence the term "lockjaw." (2) The sardonic grin, or risus sardonicus, which results from a spasmodic contraction of the facial muscles that causes the forehead to become wrinkled, the eyes fixed, the facial muscles drawn back, and the teeth to be bared. Trismus or lockjaw and risus sardonicus usually appear early but in some cases may not occur until late in the course of the disease. (3) Dysphagia, or difficulty in swallowing, a clinical aspect which is caused by spasms of the muscles of deglutition. (4) Opisthotonos, in which the body is stiffened and bent backward because of spasms of whole groups of body muscles. (5) A slight rise in temperature, but with profuse sweating. (6) Difficulty in breathing, leading to death from asphyxia.[304]

Hospital patients under treatment for tetanus present problems for the dentist, involving maintenance of oral hygiene, for which gentle suction is used to clean the mouth. This procedure aids in preventing secondary aspiration pneumonia or sinusitis.[291] In some cases the spasm of the masseter muscles may become so great that the jaw is fractured. Use of tetanus antitoxin, which is a routine part of prophylactic therapy for puncture wounds, may result in masseter muscle spasm from a serum reaction which presents the difficulty of ruling out a tetanus possibly developing.[287] A serum reaction may also result in facial diplegia. In such cases the patient may not be able to use the muscles of facial expression, wrinkle his forehead, or close his eyes. The tongue protrudes in the midline, although there is no disturbance of sensation in the anterior two thirds of the tongue. There is polyneuritis in the rest of the body, and the cerebrospinal fluid albumin level rises without a concomitant rise in cell count.[196]

Gas gangrene

Gas gangrene results in extensive destruction of muscle and connective tissue by the activity of a number of clostridial species, including *C. perfringens*, *C. septicum*, and *C. novyi*. Fermentation of muscle sugar results in gas that in combination with various enzymes and toxins produced by the bacteria initiates a vicious circle of destruction. Infection of the hand by *C. perfringens* along with the other oral bacteria has been known to occur from laceration by the teeth during an argument. In spite of the great chances for soiling, gas gangrene is extremely rare following maxillofacial wounds, probably because of a large soft tissue mass and a very large blood supply. Treatment involves debridement of involved tissues and administration of polyvalent antitoxin and an antibiotic such as penicillin.

Botulism

Botulism is an intoxication caused by *C. botulinum*, an organism commonly found in the soil, which regularly contaminates human plant and animal food products. Inadequate precautions in processing and handling of certain foods will allow this organism to grow and produce one of the most powerful exotoxins known. The site of action is the nerve endings, where the toxin prevents the release of acetylcholine and consequently results in muscle paralysis. The question has been studied whether simple tasting of the food contaminated with botulinum toxin and prompt expulsion without swallowing any of it will result in significant absorption through the oral mucosa. Experimental studies with mice and monkeys indicate that in the monkey if absorption does in fact occur it must be about fifty times less effective than if the toxin is placed directly into the stomach. Polyvalent antitoxin should be administered as soon as possible when botulism is suspected.

BACILLUS

The bacterial genus *Bacillus* consists of strictly aerobic gram-positive rods that produce endospores. It contains but a single frankly pathogenic species, *Bacillus anthracis*. The bacillus of anthrax is one of the largest pathogenic bacteria. The rods' ends are characteristically square-cut or even depressed. Under suitable conditions long chains or filaments may develop. The spores have a very pronounced resistance to heat, desiccation, and various chemicals, so that in nature they may survive for decades.

Anthrax

Anthrax is characteristically a disease of domesticated animals that may be transmitted to man by way of their wool, hides, hair, or tissues. It is primarily an industrial disease in the United States, occurring among those who work with imported hair, bristles, or other animal products.[28] Infection is usually through the skin of exposed parts of the body, rarely from inhalation of infected material or from swallowing the vegetative cells or spores. From the superficial lesion, referred to as a malignant pustule if on the skin, the bacilli may possibly enter the bloodstream, causing a septicemia and death if not adequately treated. Antibiotics have been highly effective in therapy.

There are occasionally oral aspects to anthrax. Infection of the palate has been reported in the United States[31] that apparently was caused by a toothbrush with imported animal bristles. Recovery occurred only after a protracted course, with several false starts in therapy, because of the failure to establish the correct diagnosis promptly. The malignant pustule of the skin most commonly occurs upon the face, fingers, and hands. Its occurrence on the face usually results from inoculation by contaminated fingers. The histopathologic nature of an anthrax pustule of the lip has been described,[289] including features that resemble erysipelas. In the erysipelatous form of anthrax, there is extensive edema of the face or the mucous membranes of the conjunctiva or mouth. On the neck, a malignant pustule may be followed by extension of edema from the neck and face to the lips, into the mouth, throat, and larynx.

MYCOBACTERIUM

The genus *Mycobacterium* contains a number of species pathogenic for animals and man. Among these are *Mycobacterium tuberculosis*, the agent of human tuberculosis, *M. bovis*, the agent of bovine tuberculosis, *M. ulcerans*, an agent causing skin ulcers in man, *M. kansasii*, an atypical mycobacterium, and *M. leprae*, which causes human leprosy.

Tuberculosis

The causative agent of human tuberculosis, *M. tuberculosis*, is an acid-fast, slender rod. It is aerobic, nonmotile, and nonsporulating. Characteristic small granules are found within the cell. Growth occurs best at 37° C. Resistance to physical factors varies somewhat from the vegetative cells of other bacteria. Heat killing resemble that for other bacteria, but tubercle bacilli are relatively resistant to drying, chemical germicides, and other environmental factors, perhaps because of the presence of various lipids in the tubercle bacillus cell.

The high content of lipid materials in tubercle bacilli, as much as 40% of the dry weight, accounts for a number of the biologic characteristics of these microorganisms, including growth and staining. Growth on the surface of the usual solid media is generally dry and irregularly heaped, while in broth cultures a thick, wrinkled pellicle develops on the surface of the broth. The tubercle bacilli are difficult to stain and require special techniques. The most useful is the acid-fast stain, which is based upon carbolfuchsin staining solution. The retention of the fuchsin in spite of treatment with alcohol and dilute hydrochloric acid is associated with the presence of mycolic acid in the cell. Mycolic acid is found in a complex acid-fast material that also contains polysaccharides, a complex glyceride wax, and an unsaponifiable wax made up of higher alcohols, mycolic acid, and other constituents.

Primary isolation of tubercle bacilli is made from clinical specimens, such as tissues, exudates, excretions, or washings of the stomach, mouth, or other body cavity.

Three general types of media have been developed to meet the various special circumstances that may arise. The first type, of enriched solid medium, usually contains glycerol and egg and is used for primary isolation from clinical specimens. The second type is designed to yield dispersed growth of bacilli that have adapted to artificial cultivation. This is a fluid medium to which a wetting agent such as polysorbate 80 (Tween 80), an oleic acid ester, has been added. The third type of medium is chemically defined, simple in nature, and is used for investigational studies in the biology of the tubercle bacillus.

The soluble cell substances of tubercle bacilli grown in broth evoke a delayed hypersensitivity reaction in the skin of sensitized animals or man. The soluble material, referred to as tuberculin, is obtained from a concentrate of glycerol-broth culture filtrate. As first prepared by Koch it was concentrated by evaporation on a water bath, and it is referred to as O.T. (old tuberculin). If the protein antigen is obtained from culture in a synthetic glycerol-asparagin-citrate broth medium by precipitation with trichloroacetic acid, the preparation is referred to as P.P.D. (purified protein derivative). These tuberculin preparations are used principally for diagnostic purposes in man. Intradermal inoculation of tuberculin in graded doses will evoke a positive reaction if the person has been exposed to tubercle bacilli, either from infection or from vaccination. In young children, a positive reaction probably indicates infection, and in the adult a positive reaction is good reason for further study to make certain that an active tuberculosis is not present.

In spite of great advances in the therapy for and public health control of tuberculosis, this disease is still present in significant numbers. It attacks the lungs most frequently, but extrapulmonary disease is not uncommon. The kidneys and bones are the other organs most commonly affected, but additional sites may also become involved.

It is striking that secondary oral infections in patients with pulmonary tuberculosis are rare in spite of the large number of bacilli that may be expectorated.[62] Primary infections of the oral cavity, however, occur even more rarely than do secondary infections.[195] Infections, either primary or secondary, that particularly involve structures in or related to the oral cavity and that may attract the dentist's attention are conveniently divided into five groups: (1) tuberculosis cutis orificialis; (2) lupus vulgaris; (3) tubercular osteomyelitis; (4) salivary gland infections; and (5) pulmonary tuberculosis.

Tuberculosis of the mouth. Tuberculosis cutis orificialis most commonly occurs as an ulcer of the mucosa. Its intraoral localization in order of decreasing frequency is: tongue, cheeks, gingiva, floor of the mouth, and lips. The palate, uvula, tonsils, or faucial pillars are less frequently involved. Tubercular lesions of the tongue frequently have a history of mechanical irritation from the sharp edges of decayed and abraded teeth, broken silver amalgam fillings, gold inlays, crowns, or broken artificial teeth.[40]

The lesion starts as a small yellowish nodule that breaks down and ulcerates. The developed ulcer is a very painful sore, especially when the tongue is involved. Sour, salty, and spicy foods are irritating to the exposed nerve endings of the raw ulcer. The pain may be so severe as to interfere seriously with the patient's nutrition. These patients may give a history of repeated dental treatments for "Vincent's" ulcerations that did not effect relief.[51] Prognosis for patients with oral tuberculous ulcers is poor since these lesions almost always indicate an advanced case of pulmonary tuberculosis. Additional lesions commonly occur in the nares and on the mucocutaneous border of the anus.[267] In those rare instances when the oral lesion is a result of primary inoculation, prognosis is excellent since chemotherapy combined with simple surgical excision of the lesion, when indicated, usually means complete cure.[185]

Tuberculosis of the skin. Lupus vulgaris, or tuberculosis of the skin, is of dental interest because the face is the most commonly involved site. This is a slowly developing disease that almost always begins in childhood[177] and is characterized by periods of retrogression and exacerbation extending over many years. The lesions consist of reddish brown plaques of small, soft tubercles that progress by the formation of satellite nodules, which in turn coalesce to form groups of various sizes.[275] The infection may spread from the face into the oral cavity.[44] Lupus may also involve the nose and palate.[164] The skin is infected by the tubercle bacilli either from without, by inoculation, or from the blood vessels or lymphatics, or directly by contiguity from a tubercular lesion of lymph node, bone, or other tissue. Mouth-to-mouth respiration has been known to result in primary inoculation tuberculosis of the skin around the mouth when the emergency patient has tuberculosis.[114]

Tubercular osteomyelitis. Tubercular osteomyelitis may involve the facial bones, including the maxilla and the mandible, either secondary to pulmonary tuberculosis or as a primary infection.[86] Involvement of the bone often becomes evident following extraction of a tooth,[63,] [157] or it may occur upon fracture of the mandible.[86] These cases are characterized by a chronic course,[3] severe pain, the presence of sinuses, and sequestration of bone.[254] Of the infections involving the maxilla or the mandible, 60% occur in children less than 16 years of age. Cases are so rare that the level of clinical suspicion is low. In some instances it has been reported that initial therapy was based upon the assumption of a purely localized pyogenic infection due to some dental cause. Only upon failure to respond to such treatment was a more probing search made to establish a diagnosis.[296]

A tubercular granuloma may occur at the root apex of teeth, most probably as a result of tubercle bacilli entering the root canal of decayed teeth from sputum. This lesion is difficult to distinguish from ordinary periapical granulomas and indeed may be a superimposed infection of an originally nonspecific periapical granuloma. It is easily overlooked, and occasionally it heals after the same treatment is given as for the ordinary granuloma.[33]

Infection of salivary gland. Salivary gland infection by the tubercle bacillus may be either primary or secondary to a tubercular lesion elsewhere in the body, but in either case it is a rare occurrence. The submaxillary gland is more commonly involved rather than the parotid.

Pulmonary tuberculosis. Pulmonary tuberculosis, in the open form that is actively releasing viable tubercle bacilli, presents a serious risk to the dentist, dental hygienist, and dental technician since it releases into the mouth innumerable bacilli. These may be found contaminating the lips, gingiva, teeth, and oral mucous membrane, as well as the saliva.[1]

Epidemiologic aspects. Epidemiologic considerations are of importance to the dentist since the oral cavity is one of the principal routes by which the patient sheds tubercle bacilli into the environment from the lungs. It has been shown that such patients have living tubercle bacilli about the site of dental procedures, and the possibility therefore must be considered that the dentist may be at increased risk of acquiring tuberculosis and may also be a source for further spread of the infection.[233] Unfortunately, however, there is but little evidence available on these possibilities—not enough to give a clear picture.

The Registrar-General of Great Britain reported for 1931 that the proportion of deaths from respiratory tuberculosis among dental practitioners was 11.4%, or approximately twice that of physicians (5.2%), and that the rate for dentists was also greater than the overall mortality (8.5%) for people in all occupations in the same social class.[16]

In Australia, on the other hand, the risk of acquiring tuberculosis does not appear to be great since the actual known incidence of tuberculosis among Australian dentists is lower than that of the general population. It has been estimated that the Australian dentist, on the average, probably has three sittings a year with a patient who has undiagnosed tuberculosis.[310]

A study of tuberculosis in medical and dental students for the period from 1945 to 1950 at Guy's Hospital in London revealed greater morbidity for the dental students, although the difference was not statistically significant. Reports from Sweden and America, on the other hand, have indicated appreciably higher rates occur among the medical students.[16, 312]

The possibility of a dentist or dental technician acquiring tuberculosis from dental impression material after it has been removed from the mouth of a tubercular patient has received some attention. It has been found that the tubercle bacillus does remain on the impression material after removal from the mouth,[226] indicating a possible hazard for those working with these impressions. This is discussed in Chapter 12.

The distribution of tuberculosis in the population is not uniform so that the degree of exposure to possible infection for the dentist is closely related to the character of his clientele. In New York City, Puerto Ricans, blacks, and other nonwhites account for the largest part of the tuberculosis.[286] Urban areas characterized by poor socioeconomic conditions have much higher rates of tuberculosis than do areas with high incomes and low population densities. It is evident that hospitals for the tubercular present an increased risk for attending or staff dentists and that special precautions must be taken in administering dental treatment to patients in such institutions.[191]

Immunization with BCG vaccine, an attenuated strain of a bovine tubercle bacillus, is used for persons at special risk of incurring tuberculosis, particularly if they are tuberculin-negative. Such persons include members of tuberculous families, health personnel working with tubercular patients, and laboratory workers exposed to the organisms.

Diagnosis. Diagnosis of oral lesions requires a number of approaches. Biopsy is especially useful and should be carried out in the case of any persistent lesion that cannot be otherwise explained.[227] However, biopsy alone may not be enough to differentiate from syphilis, carcinoma, or traumatic ulcers, so that radiologic examination of the lungs, bacterial cultivation, serologic tests for syphilis, and the skin test with tuberculin may also be necessary. Result of the tuberculin skin test, in the case of orificial tuberculosis, is usually negative. Animal inoculations in some cases has proved to be useful[12] but is only rarely used because of the expense. The guinea pig and rabbit are the most useful laboratory animals. The guinea pig is highly susceptible to both human and bovine types of tubercle bacilli, whereas the rabbit is susceptible only to the bovine type.

Treatment. Since the initial choice of therapy often determines whether treatment will be a success or a failure, diagnosis must also result in the isolation of the organism in order to determine the antimicrobial sensitivities of the infecting strain.

Therapy consists of a combination of surgical excision of the diseased tissue, when indicated, with chemotherapy and in recent years has proved to be highly effective.[165] The current number of deaths from tuberculosis in the United States is about 6,000 yearly, a very significant reduction from the start of the century when tuberculosis was the leading cause of death. The reduction is largely a result of a number of factors, undefined in some part, which are not related to therapeutic techniques. The reduction in the most recent years, however, probably rests primarily on effective therapy. Several drugs have proved to be important, and new ones are still being evaluated. Among those that have established themselves are isoniazid (INH), streptomycin, and para-aminosalicylic acid (PAS).

INH, the most effective established drug presently used, is included in the therapy of every case. It diffuses rapidly and is quickly absorbed from the gastrointestinal tract. It is rarely the cause of untoward reactions when given in the usual doses.

Streptomycin is a strongly basic amine compound whose toxicity limits its use. It is conventionally given only during the first 6 to 12 weeks of treatment, and its use may be discontinued earlier if toxic symptoms begin to appear.

PAS is only weakly antitubercular. It is important because it is able to prevent or delay the development of resistance to INH

and to streptomycin and is always given in combination with these or other agents. This drug has an irritating effect upon the gastrointestinal tract so that its administration presents a problem.

Bovine tuberculosis

Mycobacterium bovis is distinguished from the other mycobacteria pathogenic for man by its greater virulence for cattle and its ability to easily infect laboratory rabbits, whereas *M. tuberculosis* has a much reduced virulence for rabbits. Human infections with *M. bovis* may occur with the ingestion of infected milk. Primary infection of man with bovine tubercle bacilli most commonly occurs in bone or joint but has been observed in the gingiva.[91]

The true incidence of bovine tuberculosis of the oral cavity, however, is not known since reported cases rarely include laboratory studies that were pursued to the point of differentiating the various species. Nevertheless, it appears from statistical studies in Denmark[180] that in the case of pulmonary tuberculosis, at any rate, the risk of developing the disease is much greater in those infected from human sources than in those infected from bovine sources. This, in all probability, is likely to be the case for oral tuberculosis as well. Tuberculin testing of dairy herds and slaughter of all positive reactors together with the required pasteurization of milk used for human consumption have markedly reduced the incidence of bovine tuberculosis in man in the United States.

Infections by atypical mycobacteria

There are certain types of mycobacteria other than the tubercle bacillus that occasionally cause disease in man. Referred to as atypical mycobacteria,[246] they have been arranged in four groups as follows: Group 1 (photochromogens), which has light-conditioned pigmentation, and Group 3 (nonphotochromogens, or Battey bacilli), which has no pigmentation, are the groups with the most important pathogens; Group 2 (scotochromogens) and Group 4 (rapid growers) are the least important among these pathogens.

Tuberculin testing of American medical and dental students has shown that a larger number of these students give a positive reaction for Battey bacilli than for the tubercle bacilli.[312] It has been found that atypical mycobacteria may infect the parotid gland or paraparotid lymphatic tissue.[311] Submaxillary and cervical lymph nodes have been known to become infected by nonphotochromogens (Group 3),[293] and it has been estimated that the atypical mycobacteria may be responsible for at least 70% of the cervical lymphadenitis occurring in children.[184] These submaxillary and cervical infections have presented problems in differential diagnosis, especially in differentiating from dental infection or mumps.[149]

The atypical mycobacteria are resistant to chemotherapeutic drugs in comparison to *M. tuberculosis,* a circumstance making surgical treatment the most effective approach for management of a patient's condition. If the facial nerve is too closely involved with the lesion, however, it nevertheless may be necessary to resort to drug therapy.[248]

Leprosy

The causative agent of leprosy is *M. leprae,*[259] an acid-fast bacillus also known as Hansen's bacillus, after its discoverer. Although the acid-fast bacilli are found in large numbers in the nasal mucous and in the lesions, yet there still remains doubt as to their pathogenicity. Animals are not susceptible to the injection of either the acid-fast bacilli or ground-up suspensions of lepromatous nodules containing many of the bacilli. Numerous attempts to transmit the disease to man by similar inoculations have also proven futile. Lepers have been known to live with their families for years without there being any evidence

that the disease is readily transmitted. It is also rare for physicians, nurses, nuns, or priests in daily contact with lepers to become diseased. It has been estimated that in 1970 there were about 11 million lepers in the world.[302] There are areas of the world (Uganda, South Sea Islands, Philippines) where leprosy is endemic. Whether these acid-fast bacilli are saprophytes living in the diseased tissue or are the causative agents requiring specific unknown factors absent in most normal individuals is still undetermined.

Transmission of the disease apparently is aided by a tropical climate, lack of an adequate diet, and possibly a hereditary predisposition. The period of incubation may be rather long in some infected persons; several years or a decade or more may elapse between the initial exposure and the occurrence of symptoms. Such periods of incubation are far longer than the incubation periods in tuberculosis and may indicate the *M. leprae* is of low virulence or that the host's body does not provide favorable biochemical factors for the growth of the leprosy bacillus.

The lesions of leprosy are of two types, nodular lepromatous and anesthetic. The nodular lepromatous type is characterized by masses of granulomatous tissue that proliferate and may coalesce to form nodular, tumorlike masses called leproma. These may occur in various parts and organs of the body; in the skin they lead to disfigurement and mutilation of tissues. Leproma may occur in the oral cavity, on the cheeks, soft palate, tongue, and lips and has been known to invade and perforate the palate. Lesions of the lips and face distort the facial appearance and may involve destruction of the nasal bones and cartilage.[189] Involvement of the nerves in the anesthetic type is a slower manifestation of leprosy and is accompanied by loss of sensation; the feet are readily traumatized by knocks against objects, and secondary infections occur. Attempts at healing result in bizarrely shaped feet.

Prevention of leprosy has been approached by the use of BCG vaccine. In Uganda, where one child of every ten contracts the disease, BCG vaccination has succeeded in reducing the incidence among children by 80%.

Treatment consists of the extended administration of long-acting sulfonamides and sulfones (especially diaminodiphenylsulfone, referred to as DDS). DDS is the most useful, but there is a serious danger of the lepra bacillus strain becoming absolutely resistant to it if the dosage is inadequate. These drugs, nevertheless, represent a very significant advance over the hopeless prognosis that once confronted the leprosy patient.[43]

ACTINOMYCETACEAE

Actinomycetaceae is a family of parasitic or pathogenic gram-positive, branching, filamentous microorganisms (Fig. 3-6) that have in the past been thought to occupy a taxonomic position between the true fungi and the bacteria. It appears today, however, that they are closer to the bacteria than the fungi in a number of significant respects, including cell wall composition and sensitivity to penicillin, and they seem especially close to the gram-positive bacteria.

The filaments of these organisms are less than 1 μ wide and have a pronounced tendency to fragment into coccoid and bacillary bodies that then may develop into filaments in their turn.

Three genera have been recognized, *Actinomyces*, *Nocardia*, and *Rothia*. The species found are nonproteolytic and nonhemolytic; they have an optimal temperature for growth of 37° C. Most of the identified species are capable of causing disease in various parts of the body in addition to the oral cavity.

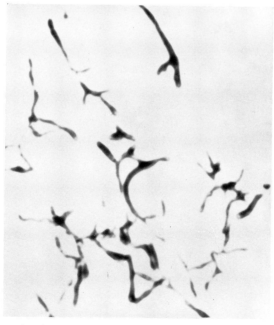

Fig. 3-6. Gram-stained colony smear showing gram-positive filamentous branching with swollen ends and bacillary forms (950 ×).

Actinomyces

Actinomyces is distinguished from the other genera by its anaerobic or micro-aerophilic growth and by its non–acid-fast staining. Considerable difficulty has been encountered in determining the species of *Actinomyces* because of serious problems in isolation, cultivation, and determination of differential characteristics. Taxonomy has relied primarily upon such classic characteristics as colony structure, sugar fermentations, and physiologic tests. How-ever, even in strains from morphologically and serologically identical original group-ings, there may occur differences in fer-mentative capacity. Nevertheless, at least six species have been differentiated: *Actino-myces bovis, A. israelii, A. naeslundii, A. odontolyticus, A. viscosus,* and *A. eriksonii.* The two appearing most commonly in lesions are *A. bovis,* in lumpy jaw of cattle, and *A. israelii,* in actinomycosis of man. The pathogenicity of the several other species occurring in the oral cavity of man is not established.[72, 95]

A. israelii is a gram-positive slow-grow-ing, anaerobic to microaerophilic organism forming small, white, coherent, "bread-crumb" or "cauliflower" colonies that grow at the bottom of tubes of fluid media. Mi-croscopically it is a nonsporulating, branch-ing, filamentous organism whose filaments seldom exceed 1 μ in width. Microcolonies on the surface of agar are filamentous, with no distinct central area, the so-called spider colony. Mature colonies on agar usually are irregular, rough, and heaped up, but smooth colonies may also be pro-duced. Atmospheric requirements are facul-tative, although growth is best under anaerobic conditions. Biochemical reac-tions are primarily saccharolytic rather than proteolytic, but the fermentation reactions are quite variable; nevertheless, they are useful for identification.[127] Two serologic types have been distinguished. Identifica-tion of this species requires knowledge of the total pattern of reactions, including serologic studies.[32]

A. naeslundii is a common inhabitant of the human oral cavity and resembles *A. israelii.* It is a facultative organism, grow-ing as well aerobically as under reduced oxygen tension. Most strains, however, grow best under microaerophilic or anaero-bic conditions in the presence of CO_2. The cells are gram-positive, consisting of diph-theroids and branched filaments that often show clubbed ends. Microcolonies on the surface of agar are highly filamentous and spiderlike. Mature colonies are usually fairly flat, but with smooth surfaces and entire edges. The organism is catalase-negative. In human lesions, *A. naeslundii* does not form granules readily, as does *A. israelii,* but it does develop freely in the tissues. *A. naeslundii* antigen has been found at least in one instance to react with the antisera prepared from one of three strains of *A. israelii,* indicating a closer rela-tionship to this species than that of *A. bovis* to *A. israelii.*[94]

A. bovis may be distinguished from *A. israelii* by its smooth colonial growth, in contrast to the rough, dry, grayish colonies of *A. israelii.* These latter colonies adhere tenaciously to the surface of the medium whereas the smooth colonies of *A. bovis* do not. It hydrolyzes starch rapidly and completely, in contrast to *A. israelii* and *A. naeslundii.*[215] Antisera prepared against strains of *A. bovis* and *A. israelii* do not cross-react with antigens of these two species.

A. eriksonii is distinguished by the fol-lowing characteristics[95]: (1) generally smooth colonies that are soft, entire-edged, and nonadherent; (2) inability to grow in the presence of oxygen, and stimulation by CO_2; (3) ability to hydrolyze starch and coagulate milk; (4) inability to reduce nitrates; and (5) marked ability to ferment sugars. This species is similar to the other *Actinomyces* in its general structure and form, catalase negativeness, and inability to liquefy gelatin. Its cell wall constitution places it firmly in the same group as the other *Actinomyces* species.

A. *viscosus*[96] is a filamentous, facultative, gram-positive organism requiring CO_2 for growth under all conditions of cultivation. The filaments segment to produce short diphtheroid cells. Mature colonies are smooth, strongly convex, cream to white in color, and dry to viscous in consistency. No spores or aerial mycelium are formed. It is catalase-positive and nonhemolytic and ferments sugars with the production of acid only.

Actinomycosis

Actinomycosis[161] is a chronic infectious disease affecting man, but also occurring in cattle, horses, and swine. It was one of the first diseases recognized as being of microbial origin. Bollinger in 1877 reported the presence of branching mycelia in the material discharged from a diseased mandible of a cow. He considered these to be the cause of the suppuration and the bony destruction. Harz studied this organism given him by Bollinger and named it *strahlenpilz* (ray fungus), or actinomyces, from its microscopic appearance. Israel in 1878 was the first to find the causative agent in human necropsy material, and in 1879 Ponfick first recognized infection during life. Although the usual species involved in human infections is *A. israelii*, *A. naeslundii* and *A. eriksonii* have also been occasionally implicated.

The clinical picture is a faithful reflection of the low pathogenicity of the microorganism, which is unable to penetrate intact mucosa, requiring a breach in the tissues to establish itself. About half of all human cases occur in the cervicofacial region. The disease here ordinarily follows several weeks or months after a tooth extraction[116] or some other surgical or accidental trauma to the oral cavity, such as a compound jaw fracture,[134] but it may also result from a partially erupted third molar, periodontal disease[45] (Fig. 3-7), or the infected root canal of a carious tooth.[98] The first signs of infection, several weeks after implantation of the organisms, consist of induration and relatively nontender swelling. Located especially at the angle of the jaw or in the vicinity of the parotid gland, the swelling is generally a dark reddish-purple; it eventually becomes fluctuant

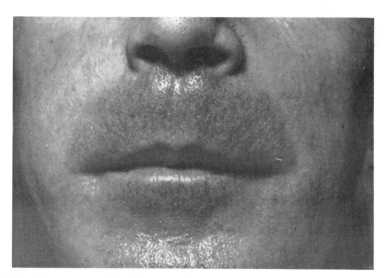

Fig. 3-7. Lip of patient swollen because of periodontal abscess about upper left lateral incisor. He experienced pain and a temperature of 102° F. Purulent exudate was removed from the abscess and an actinomyces was isolated.

and goes on to drain through sinuses opening upon the skin or, more rarely, upon the oral mucosa. From the initial site of infection the lesion extends directly to structures that lie in relation to the oral and pharyngeal cavities, including the tongue and other muscles, salivary glands, jaw bones, larynx, skin, mucosa, maxillary sinus, brain, and skull.

In actinomycosis of the bone, reactions to the infection take place at a very slow rate, with several months elapsing before any significant change is observed. The mandible is involved much more frequently than the maxilla. Lingual actinomycosis, much more prevalent in men than in women, may occur at any age and in any walk of life. Lingual infection results in slightly painful and nodular masses that become ulcerated. If the infection is not treated, it progresses to the point that the tongue and adjacent tissues become fixed and the tongue can no longer be protruded.

Involvement of the skin of the neck is characterized by ridgelike elevations or folds with sulci between, associated with the sinus openings. The fistulas often heal with much scarring, but new sinus tracts develop that will open upon a surface to also drain off the exudate from the lesions. Trismus from involvement of the muscles of mastication, pain, swelling, and limitation of jaw movement are also prominent symptoms. Of these, trismus is the most important sign before the formation of pus. In advanced cases the temporomandibular joint on the affected side may become almost or completely ankylosed. Although cervicofacial actinomycosis is usually localized, there is always the possibility of dangerous complications by spread of the infection from the initial lesion by continuity to other parts of the body, and especially to the spinal or cranial region. Actinomycotic meningitis may occur in this manner, but it is very rare.

Thoracic actinomycosis may result from extension of the cervicofacial form, but most commonly it appears to result from inhalation of infected material from the tonsil among those from 10 to 20 years of age, and from dental sepsis among those from 30 to 50 years of age. In rare cases, aspirated fragments of carious teeth have been reported as the cause of an actinomycotic lung abscess. The second most frequently occurring cause of thoracic lesions is extension from an abdominal focus into the thorax. Thoracic actinomycosis is a slowly developing disease that generally gives rise to multiple sinuses at an early stage; these may open upon the chest wall or may even extend to the heart.[15] Since there is a marked tendency for mixed infections with other oral bacteria in pulmonary abscesses (see p. 86), a diagnosis of pulmonary actinomycosis is tenable only when the actinomycetes are found within the tissue itself.[222] A mixed infection with tubercle bacilli may also occur in the lungs. Actinomycotic bronchopneumonia occurs occasionally as a complication of an existing pulmonary infection.

Approximately 30% of actinomycotic cases are in the abdomen, which is twice the frequency found for thoracic actinomycosis. In some instances abdominal actinomycosis may be secondary to thoracic infection. Usually it involves the ileocecal region, starting with an abscess of the appendix; it may then spread to the liver, spleen, urinary tract, or spinal column. The skin over the affected part may be reddish-brown and may be the site for ulcers. Rupture into the genitourinary tract may result in a purulent discharge into the urine or into the vagina. Most cases of genital tract actinomycosis are considered to be secondary to intestinal infection.[272]

Actinomycotic lacrimal canaliculitis and conjunctivitis have been reported.[214] Transmission by human bite has also been reported, but is a rare event. Generalized infection through the bloodstream is also not commonly observed, and is usually fatal. It occurs only in untreated cases and

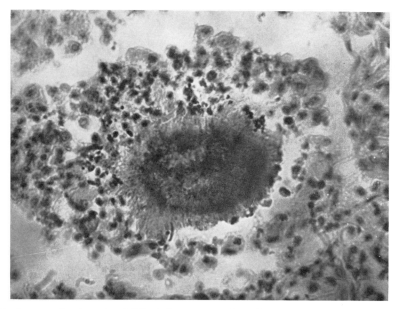

Fig. 3-8. Gram-stained section (450 ×) showing a nidus of actinomyces filaments surrounded by numerous polymorphonuclear leukocytes.

is characterized by secondary involvement of the skin, vertebra, liver, kidneys, and ureters.

The pathologic reaction of the tissues in actinomycosis is that of an infective granuloma, which develops without regard to tissue barriers. There is a progressive, slow, chronic invasion of blood vessels, fibrous connective tissue, and bone, with formation of granulation tissue, necrosis, and abscess. The lesion tends to point, and numerous fistulae may form, connecting the abscesses to the outside skin or intra-oral mucosa, which exude purulent material. Soft, bluish-red granulation surrounds the openings of the fistulae. Much scarring occurs as the lesions progress.[118]

Within the abscesses are microcolonies of the filamentous and branching microorganisms, the so-called sulfur granules. The granules when sectioned in tissue (Fig. 3-8) or crushed and gram-stained are seen to be made up of extremely fine, branching, gram-positive filaments. Their undisturbed structure, as seen in a tissue section, is much more complex. The center consists of intertwined mycelia, while at the periphery are radiating clubs composed of radial mycelia slightly thicker at the tip, surrounded by sheaths that take the acid rather than the basic dyes and also stain gram-negatively. These clubs vary in size, being up to 10 μ long and 5 μ wide; they are acid-fast.

Formation of the sulfur granules seems to require the tissue reactions associated with the chronic infection. Controversy exists as to the origin of the clubs in the sulfur granules. Some consider that they represent the swollen tips of the mycelia, or a capsule of a polysaccharide-protein complex,[216] while others claim that the sheaths surrounding the clubs are derived from a nonspecific reaction between the infective agent and the host, possibly related to hypersensitivity.[232]

The sulfur granule within the tissue is surrounded by a polymorphonuclear infiltration. Peripheral to this are collections of plasma cells, lymphocytes, and macrophages which in turn may be surrounded by a fibrous tissue capsule.

Why *Actinomyces* species that are a common member of the normal oral microbiota should become pathogenic has not been explained, although many investigations have attempted to clarify this question. Suspensions of pure culture injected intraperitoneally into mice or hamsters may cause abscesses on the peritoneal wall and in the intestinal lymph nodes, liver, spleen, and other viscera. In many instances, however, no lesions develop. It has been suggested that an allergic reaction may have a role in the development of the lesions, but other possibilities have also been considered. In particular, there are good reasons to suspect that mixed cultures of aerobes and anaerobes are necessary to provoke disease, acting synergistically. In numerous cases, especially of cervicofacial actinomycosis, the actinomycetes are found associated with streptococci, fusobacteria, *Bacteroides corrodens,* or *Actinobacillus actinomycetemcomitans.* In the opinion of some investigators, the presence of these other microorganisms is probably the reason the actinomycetes become pathogenic,[118] so that actinomycosis is in fact a nonspecific disease.[108]

Epidemiologic considerations. Epidemiologic aspects originally were considered to hinge upon the occurrence of free-living forms and upon the occurrence of lumpy jaw in cattle, but it is now well established that actinomycosis is caused by endogenous members of the oral microbiota that are worldwide in distribution. Within the mouth, actinomycetes, including *A. israelii* and *A. naeslundii,* have been isolated from the saliva, the gingival sulcus, the gingiva, dental plaque, dental calculus, carious teeth, the root canal of infected teeth, and tonsillar crypts.[57] Presumably, the microorganisms pass by contact, direct or indirect, from man to man as part of the normal oral flora. The time and manner, however, by which the actinomycetes become part of the oral flora is not known. Seasonal influences upon incidence are not apparent.

Males incur the disease much more often than females, the ratio in some series being perhaps as much as 3.5 cases for each case among females. Most cases occur after the age of 20 years, during the third and fourth decades of life, but the disease can start at any age. There is a fairly even distribution of actinomycosis between rural and urban populations. The frequency of the various types of actinomycosis appears to vary from one country to another. Thoracic infections, for example, have been reported from many different countries, but particularly from Europe and the United States. A high incidence occurs in Germany; in the United States, it is greater in southern California than in the other states. Twenty-one deaths from actinomycosis occurred in the United States in 1958. Mortality data, however, are greatly overshadowed by the number of infections actually occurring. Undoubtedly, the actual incidence is much greater than is indicated by the reported cases. In Great Britain, it has been estimated that dental centers serving a population of half a million people may expect to see approximately half a dozen cases of oral actinomycosis each year.

Diagnosis. Specific diagnosis of actinomycosis is often easy and simple clinically,[137] but it may present difficulties nevertheless. This is especially the case in the early stages when it may closely simulate various inflammatory conditions and tumor formations. It should always be kept in mind when one is confronted with chronic inflammatory processes of the oral cavity or the parts associated with it. Most desirably, the diagnosis should be made before chemotherapy is started since otherwise the difficulties of making an accurate diagnosis are increased.

The diagnosis is made from the history; the persistence of the swelling; a possible slight rise in the temperature, usually not more than one degree; histologic study of biopsy sections; microbiologic investigation of clinical specimens; and radiologic examination.[76]

Exudate collected from a draining sinus tract of the lesion is examined by ordinary vision for the presence of sulfur granules, which are almost invariably present. These granules, seen by the bare eye, on more precise examination do not always prove to be composed of actinomycetes, but their presence in the exudate is highly suggestive. Whitish or pale yellow in color, the actinomycotic granules in human lesions range in size from a fraction of a millimeter to about 2 mm. in diameter. They usually consist of a soft mycelial mass, whereas in cattle they become hard and calcified.

A search for actinomyces in gram-stained biopsy material is successful in only about 10% of cases, but biopsy nevertheless may demonstrate the characteristic changes of actinomycosis. A firm diagnosis should include evidence of this kind. For decisive diagnosis, however, cultivation is useful in addition to the study of tissue sections. For this purpose, sulfur granules from the exudate may be washed in sterile saline solution or broth medium to lessen possible contaminants from the mouth; the granules are then broken up so as to allow greater dispersion; and then they are inoculated into dextrose infusion broth or thioglycollate broth. For surface growth, the granules may be pressed into the medium of a 1% yeast brain heart infusion agar or blood brain heart infusion agar plate.

Surface growth on primary isolation requires strict anaerobic incubation at 37° C. for several days or perhaps for as much as a week in some instances. It is important to make repeated cultures and smears if the initial findings are negative, but great care must also be taken to avoid confusion with actinomycotic organisms normally present in the mouth which in fact may not be responsible for the clinical lesions in a particular case.

The only characteristic radiologic changes produced by actinomycosis, especially of the thorax, are the result of bone change. Periostitis of the ribs occurs in the presence of a pulmonary infection without empyema. Bone involvement with actinomycosis results in bone destruction simultaneously with new bone formation.

Animal inoculation of clinical specimens is not a satisfactory method for detecting actinomycetes since the inoculated animals do not consistently develop lesions that are useful for diagnosis.

Treatment. Treatment[245] presents some difficult problems because of the type of characteristic tissue reaction. The involved areas are usually quite extensive, markedly indurated, and relatively avascular in the region of the growing microorganisms.[112] This creates difficulties, first, in getting effective levels of the therapeutic agent within the lesion, and, second, in restoring the involved tissues to a normal functional state.

Before antibiotics became available, treatment was a prolonged and uncertain affair that included surgical drainage, irrigation of sinuses with potassium iodide, the injection of autogenous vaccine, and x-ray therapy. Pulmonary infections rarely were cured, generally causing death. Prognosis has greatly improved in recent years. Chemotherapy with sulfonamides and antibiotics, together with supportive treatment and surgical drainage, has proven very successful, although surgical procedures such as excision of diseased tissue may still be necessary to assure efficient diffusion of antibiotic into the lesion.

While *A. israelii* strains vary in their sensitivity to penicillin, most are inhibited if the dosage is great enough. Some clinicians use from 5 million to 8 million units intramuscularly daily for 14 days. Treatment should be continued until complete healing is seen and for a short time after. This may require that therapy be administered for several weeks, and in some cases several months, before the infection is overcome.

Penicillin has been shown to effect a cure rate of 90% for thoracic actinomycosis when given in combination with excisional surgery when possible. The newer semisynthetic penicillins remain to be evaluated clinically for their effectiveness in treating actinomycoses.[313] Other antibiotics, especially tetracycline, may be necessary if the infecting strain is resistant to penicillin or if the patient has a history of a prior allergic reaction to penicillin.[205]

Nocardia

The genus *Nocardia*[13] is distinguished from the other actinomycetes by its aerobic growth and partial or non–acid-fast staining. Among the several pathogenic species of *Nocardia* that have been described, only *Nocardia asteroides* is commonly found in nocardiosis occurring in the United States and Europe. *N. asteroides* grows well under aerobic conditions on ordinary media. It has a wide temperature range for growth, but does best from 20° to 37° C. Growth may be observed in broth within from one to three days, but as long as four or six weeks may be needed in some cases to obtain recognizable growth. The colonies are pigmented, and on aging they become wrinkled. Carbohydrates are not fermented. In tissues and exudates, fine granules are found which differ from those of *A. bovis* by the absence of clubs.

Nocardiosis

Nocardiosis is a localized or systemic disease that appears to be increasing in incidence. The clinical picture is varied, although it usually consists of an acute or chronic pulmonary involvement. There may, however, be chronic suppuration of the skin, subcutaneous tissues, or bone. In rare instances oral lesions have been noted, including gingival infection in one case,[225] and secondary infection of the oral mucosa in a generalized infection with osteomyelitis and abscesses in the adrenal, heart, and brain.[60] There is a clear association of nocardiosis with serious underlying diseases such as glomerulonephritis under cortisone treatment.[200] Therapy includes use of antimicrobial drugs and surgery when indicated. The sulfonamides have been useful agents for treatment.[303]

Rothia

The genus *Rothia* contains but a single species, now known as *Rothia dentocariosa*, but previously known as *Actinomyces dentocariosus*, *Nocardia dentocariosus*, and *Nocardia salivae*.[93] *R. dentocariosa* has a preference for aerobic growth, but its cell wall constituents differ from *Nocardia* in that diaminopimelic acid (DAP) is not present.[64] It is simple to distinguish in the laboratory from *Nocardia* species by the fact that it does not grow on Sabouraud dextrose agar whereas *Nocardia* species do. It is a gram-positive filamentous organism isolated from a variety of human tissue in various clinical states such as dental caries, chest abscess, throat abscess, and postoperative wounds.[35] In regard to pathogenicity, very little is known. Experimental studies have shown that intramuscular inoculation of mice results in abscess formation.[243]

CITED REFERENCES

1. Abbott, J. N., Briney, A. T., and Denaro, S. A.: Recovery of tubercle bacilli from mouth washings of tuberculous patients, J. Amer. Dent. Assoc. **50**:49, 1955.
2. Agranat, B. J.: Friedlander's osteomyelitis of the mandible: Report of case, J. Oral Surg. **27**:293, 1969.
3. Allan, I. McD.: Tuberculous osteomyelitis of the mandible: Report of a case, Brit. J. Plast. Surg. **9**:240, 1956.
4. Allott, E. N., Cruickshank, R., Cyrlas-Williams, R., Glass, V., Meyer, I. H., Straker, E. A., and Tee, G.: Infection of cat-bite and dog-bite wounds with *Pasteurella septica,* J. Path. Bact. **56**:411, 1944.
5. Alston, J. M.: Human infections with organisms resembling Bang's necrosis bacillus, Second International Congress on Microbiology, London, 1937, Report of Proceedings, p. 181.
6. Alston, J. M.: Necrobacillosis in Great Britain, Brit. Med. J. **2**:1524, 1955.
7. Ammenwerth, B. K., and Doherty, E. C.: Cavernous sinus thrombosis of dental origin treated with methicillin, J. Amer. Dent. Assoc. **71**:55, 1965.

8. Anderson, O. E.: Acute nonspecific infections of the parotid gland, Arch. Otolaryng. 47:649, 1948.
9. Anderson, R. A.: Oculoglandular tularemia: A case report, J. Iowa Med. Soc. 60:21, 1970.
10. Anderson, T.: Advances in the treatment of acute infectious diseases, Practitioner 193: 482, 1964.
11. Axnick, N. W., and Alexander, E. R.: Tetanus in the United States: A review of the problem, Amer. J. Public Health 47: 1493, 1957.
12. Bache, C.: Mandibular growth and dental occlusion in juvenile rheumatoid arthritis, Acta Rheum. Scand. 10:142, 1964.
13. Ballenger, C. N., and Goldring, D.: Nocardiosis in children, J. Pediat. 50:145, 1957.
14. Barnes, E. M., and Goldberg, H. S.: The relationships of bacteria within the family Bacteroidaceae as shown by numerical taxonomy, J. Gen. Microbiol. 51:313, 1968.
15. Bates, M., and Cruickshank, G.: Thoracic actinomycosis, Thorax 12:99, 1957.
16. Batty Shaw, A.: Tuberculosis in medical and dental students: A study at Guy's Hospital, Lancet 2:400, 1952.
17. Beck, A. L.: The influence of the chemotherapeutic and antibiotic drugs on the incidence and course of deep neck infections, Ann. Otol. 61:515, 1952.
18. Beigelman, P. M., and Rantz, L. A.: Clinical significance of Bacteroides, Arch. Intern. Med. 84:605, 1949.
19. Bellinger, D. H.: Arthritis of the temporomandibular joint: Diagnosis and management, J. Oral Surg. 10:47, 1952.
20. Bender, I. B., Seltzer, L., Meloff, G., and Pressman, R. S.: Conditions affecting sensitivity of techniques for detection of bacteremia, J. Dent. Res. 40:951, 1961.
21. Berger, U.: Ueber die pro- und antibiotische Beeinflussung des Corynebacterium diphtheriae durch pathogene Staphylokokken der Mundhöhle, Schweiz. Med. Wschr. 81:130, 1951.
22. Berndt, A. L., Buck, R., and Buxton, R. von L.: The pathogenesis of acute suppurative parotitis, Amer. J. Med. Sci. 182:639, 1931.
23. Besman, I. R., and Lyons, H. A.: Aspiration pneumonia, Dis. Chest 35:6, 1959.
24. Biocca, E., and Seppilli, A.: Human infections caused by lactobacilli, J. Infect. Dis. 81:112, 1947.
25. Bladen, H. A., Gewurz, H., and Mergenhagen, S. E.: Interactions of the complement system with the surface and endotoxic lipopolysaccharide of Veillonella alcalescens, J. Exp. Med. 125:767, 1967.
26. Blum, T.: Clinical experiences with osteomyelitis of the jaws, Arch. Clin. Oral Path. 1:156, 1937.
27. Boycott, J. A.: Seasonal variations in streptococcal infections, Lancet 1:706, 1966.
28. Brachman, P. S., and Fekety, F. R.: Industrial anthrax, Ann. New York Acad. Sci. 70: 574, 1958.
29. Branson, D., and Bunkfeldt, F., Jr.: Pasteurella multocida in animal bites of humans, Amer. J. Clin. Path. 48:552, 1967.
30. Breed, R. S., Murray, E. G. D., and Smith, N. R.: Bergey's manual of determinative bacteriology, ed. 7, Baltimore, 1957, The Williams & Wilkins Co.
31. Briggs, O. C.: Anthrax of the oral cavity, J. Oral Surg. 5:173, 1947.
32. Brock, D. W., and Georg, L. K.: Characterization of Actinomyces israelii serotypes 1 and 2, J. Bact. 97:589, 1969.
33. Brodsky, R. H., and Klatell, J. S.: Tuberculous periapical granulomata, J. Dent. Res. 22:345, 1943.
34. Brown, A. E., Williams, H. L., and Herrell, W. E.: Bacteroides septicemia: Report of a case with recovery, J. A. M. A. 116:402, 1941.
35. Brown, J. M., Georg, L. K., and Waters, L. C.: Laboratory identification of Rothia dentocariosa and its occurrence in human clinical materials, Appl. Microbiol. 17:150, 1969.
36. Brown, L. R., Merrill, S. S., and Allen, R. E.: Microbiologic study of intraoral wounds, J. Oral Surg. 28:89, 1970.
37. Brunn, H.: Lung abscess, J. A. M. A. 103: 1999, 1934.
38. Brunner, H.: Intracranial complications of ear, nose and throat infections, Chicago, 1946, Year Book Medical Publishers, Inc., p. 219.
39. Brunsdon, D. F. V., and Mallett, B. L.: Local infection with Pasteurella septica following a dog-bite, Brit. Med. J. 2:607, 1953.
40. Bryant, J. C.: Oral tuberculosis, Amer. Rev. Tuberc. 39:738, 1939.
41. Burdon, K. L.: Bacterium melaninogenicum from normal and pathologic tissues, J. Infect. Dis. 42:161, 1928.
42. Burket, L. W., Oral medicine, diagnosis and treatment, ed. 2, Philadelphia, 1952, J. B. Lippincott Co., p. 392.
43. Bushby, S. R. M.: The chemotherapy of leprosy, Pharmacol. Rev. 10:1, 1958.
44. Calmette, A.: Tubercle bacillus infection and tuberculosis in man and animals. Soper, W.

B., and Smith, G. H. (trans.), Baltimore, 1923, The Williams & Wilkins Co. p. 228.

45. Caron, G. A., and Sarkany, I.: Cervico-facial actinomycosis, Brit. J. Derm. **76:**421, 1964.

46. Chambers, W. E.: Human tularemia infection through bite of the domestic cat, Med. Bull. Veterans Admin. **19:**206, 1942.

47. Cherny, W. B. V., Jones, C. P., and Peete, C. H.: Disseminated granuloma inguinale and its relationship to granuloma of the cervix and pregnancy, Amer. J. Obstet. Gynec. **74:**597, 1957.

48. Chertkow, S.: Studies on *Bacteroides melaninogenicus,* J. Dent. Res. **47:**953, 1968.

49. Clawson, D. K., and Stevensom, J. K.: Treatment of chronic osteomyelitis, Surg. Gynec. Obstet. **120:**59, 1965.

50. Clement, A. J.: Field studies in the Southern Kalahari: August, 1951, J. Dent. Res. **32:**697, 1953.

51. Cole, H. N., and Driver, J. R.: Tuberculosis orificialis, Arch. Derm. Syph. **40:**327, 1939.

52. Colman, G.: The application of computers to classification of streptococci, J. Gen. Microbiol. **50:**149, 1968.

53. Comroe, B. J., Collins, L. H., and Crane, M. P.: Internal medicine in dental practice, London, 1954, Henry Kimpton, p. 400.

54. Cook, H. P.: Bilateral ankylosis of the temporomandibular joints following rheumatoid arthritis, Proc. Roy. Soc. Med. **51:**694, 1958.

55. Courant, P. R., and Gibbons, R. J.: Biochemical and immunological heterogeneity of *Bacteroides melaninogenicus,* Arch. Oral Biol. **12:**1605, 1967.

56. Crawford, J. A.: Pneumococcal stomatitis, Tri-State Med. J. **11:**2308, 1939.

57. Crawford, J. J., and Shankle, R. J.: Application of newer methods to study the importance of root canal and oral microbiota in endodontics, Oral Surg. **14:**1109, 1961.

58. Crowder, J. G., and White, A.: A serologic response in human *Pseudomonas* infection, J. Lab. Clin. Med. **75:**126, 1970.

59. Crum, R. J., and Loiselle, R. J.: Incidence of temporomandibular joint symptoms in male patients with rheumatoid arthritis, J. Amer. Dent. Assoc. **81:**129, 1970.

60. Cruz, P. T., and Clancy, C. F.: Nocardiosis: Nocardial osteomyelitis and septicemia, Amer. J. Path. **28:**607, 1952.

61. Dalrymple-Champneys, W.: Brucella infection and undulant fever in man, London, 1960, Oxford University Press, p. 82.

62. Darlington, C. C., and Salman, I.: Oral tuberculous lesions, Amer. Rev. Tuberc. **35:**147, 1937.

63. Davidson, J. B., Roberts, J. B., and Roberts, E. P.: Tuberculosis of the mouth, Ann. Dent. **2:**103, 1944.

64. Davis, G. H. G., and Freer, J. H.: Studies upon an oral aerobic actinomycete, J. Gen. Microbiol. **23:**163, 1960.

65. Dawson, M. H.: Erysipelas. In Cecil, R. L. (ed.) A textbook of medicine by American authors, Philadelphia, 1943, W. B. Saunders Co., p. 143.

66. Degnan, E. J., Hinds, E. C., and Sills, A. H., Jr.,: Role of anaerobic streptococci in oral surgery, J. Oral Surg. **18:**464, 1960.

67. Deuel, R. E., Jr., Putney, B., and Morabito, S. J.: A survey of tonsil and adenoid surgery, New York J. Med. **54:**1617, 1954.

68. Eisenbrandt, L. I.: Initial oxidation-reduction potentials of saliva, J. Dent. Res. **22:**293, 1943.

69. Eisenbrandt, L. I.: Studies on the oxidation-reduction potentials of saliva, J. Dent. Res. **24:**247, 1945.

70. Eisenbud, L.: Subacute bacterial endocarditis precipitated by nonsurgical dental procedures, Oral Surg. **15:**624, 1962.

71. Elek, S. D.: *Staphylococcus pyogenes* and its relation to disease, Edinburgh, 1959, E. & S. Livingstone.

72. Emmons, C. W., Binford, C. H., and Utz, J. P.: Medical mycology, Philadelphia, 1963, Lea & Febiger, p. 55.

73. Emory, L.: Prosthetic restoration of soft palate lost as a result of diphtheria, J. Amer. Dent. Assoc. **41:**75, 1950.

74. Engström, B.: The significance of enterococci in root canal treatment, Odont. Rev. **15:**87, 1964.

75. Evans, D. G., and Prophet, A. S.: Examination of strains of *Clostridium welchii* isolated from teeth, Brit. Dent. J. **91:**199, 1951.

76. Everts, E. C.: Cervicofacial actinomycosis, Arch. Otolaryng. **92:**468, 1970.

77. Farmer, E. D.: Streptococci of the mouth and their relationship to subacute bacterial endocarditis, Proc. Roy. Soc. Med. **46:**201, 1953.

78. Faucett, R. L., and Miller, H. C.: Stomatitis in infants caused by B. mucosus capsulatus, Pediatrics **1:**458, 1948.

79. Feingold, M., and Gellis, S. S.: Cellulitis due to *Haemophilus influenzae* type b, New Eng. J. Med. **272:**788, 1965.

80. Ferro, E. R., and Richter, J. W.: Oral lesions of granuloma inguinale: Report of three cases, J. Oral Surg. **4:**121, 1946.

81. Finegold, S. M., Harada, N. E., and Miller, L. G.: Antibiotic susceptibility patterns as aids in classification and characterization of gram-negative anaerobic bacilli, J. Bact. **94:** 1443, 1967.

82. Finland, M.: The significance of mixed infections in pneumococcic pneumonia, J. A. M. A. **103:**1681, 1934.

83. Fish, E. W.: Bone infection, J. Amer. Dent. Assoc. **26:**691, 1939.

84. Fisher, A. M., and Abernethy, T. J.: Putrid empyema, with special reference to anaerobic streptococci, Arch. Intern. Med. **54:**552, 1934.

85. Fitzgerald, R. J., Parramore, M. L., and MacKintosh, M. E.: Antibiotic sensitivity of strains of *Veillonella,* Antibiot. Chemother. **9:**145, 1959.

86. Foster, C. F., and Young, W. G.: Tuberculous infection of a fractured mandible: Report of a case, J. Oral Surg. **28:**686, 1970.

87. Fothergill, L. D., and Wright, J.: Influenzal meningitis: The relation of age incidence to the bactericidal power of blood against the causal organism, J. Immun. **24:**273, 1933.

88. Fox, J., and Isenberg, H. D.: Antibiotic resistance of microorganisms isolated from root canals, Oral Surg. **23:**230, 1967.

89. Francis, T. C.: Recurrent aphthous stomatitis and Behçet's disease, Oral Surg. **30:**476, 1970.

90. Frazier, C. H.: Tetanus. In Keen, W. W. (ed.): Surgery, its principles and practice, Philadelphia, 1906, W. B. Saunders Co. vol. 1, p. 478.

91. Galloway, J. W., and Horne, N. W.: Primary tuberculosis infection of the gum of bovine origin: A case and a discussion, Brit. Dent. J. **95:**9, 1953.

92. Garrod, L. P.: Sensitivity of four species of *Bacteroides* to antibiotics, Brit. Med. J. **2:** 1529, 1955.

93. Georg, L. K., and Brown, J. M.: *Rothia, gen. nov.,* an aerobic genus of the family *Actinomycetaceae,* Int. J. Systematic Bact. **17:**79, 1967.

94. Georg, L. K., Roberstad, G. W., and Brinkman, S. A.: Identification of species of *Actinomyces,* J. Bact. **88:**477, 1964.

95. Georg, L. K., Roberstad, G. W., Brinkman, S. A., and Hicklin, M. D.: A new pathogenic anaerobic *Actinomyces* species, J. Infect. Dis. **115:**88, 1965.

96. Gerencser, M. A., and Slack, J. M.: Identification of human strains of *Actinomyces viscosus,* Appl. Microbiol. **18:**80, 1969.

97. Gibbons, R. J., and Macdonald, J. B.: Hemin and vitamin K compounds as required factors for the cultivation of certain strains of *Bacteroides melaninogenicus,* J. Bact. **80:** 164, 1960.

98. Gold, L., and Doyne, E. E.: Actinomycosis with osteomyelitis of the alveolar process, Oral Surg. **5:**1056, 1952.

99. Goldberg, M. H.: Gram-negative bacteremia after dental extraction, J. Oral Surg. **26:**180, 1968.

100. Goldberg, M. H.: Postoperative oral infection with *Pseudomonas aeruginosa,* J. Oral Surg. **24:**334, 1966.

101. Gordon, D. F., Jr.: Reisolation of *Staphylococcus salivarius* from the human oral cavity, J. Bact. **94:**1281, 1967.

102. Graykowski, E. A., Barile, M. F., Lee, W. B., and Stanley, H. R., Jr.: Recurrent aphthous stomatitis: Clinical, therapeutic, histopathologic and hypersensitivity aspects, J. A. M. A. **196:**637, 1966.

103. Green, M., and Fousek, M. D.: *Hemophilus influenzae* type b cellulitis, Pediatrics **19:**80, 1957.

104. Greenblatt, R. B., Dienst, R. B., and Baldwin, K. R.: Lymphogranuloma venereum and granuloma inguinale, Med. Clin. N. Amer. **43:**1493, 1959.

105. Griswald, D., and Herring, A. C.: Tetanus following dental extraction, Amer. J. Med. **7:**686, 1949.

106. Grodinski, M.: Ludwig's angina: An anatomical and clinical study with review of the literature, Surgery **5:**678, 1939.

107. Guggenheim, B.: Streptococci of dental plaques, Caries Res. **2:**147, 1968.

108. Guthof, O.: Ueber pathogene "vergrunende Streptokokken" Streptokokken-Befunde dentogenen Abszessen und Infiltraten im Bereich der Mundhöhle, Zbl. Bakt., I Abt., Orig. **166:**553, 1956.

109. Haight, T. H.: Erythromycin therapy of respiratory infections. I. Controlled studies on the comparative efficacy of erythromycin and penicillin in scarlet fever, J. Lab. Clin. Med. **43:**15, 1954.

110. Hall, I. C.: Bacterial factors in pyorrhea alveolaris. III. The isolation of *B. tetani, B. welchii* and three sporulating anaerobes from human saliva, J. Infect. Dis. **37:**87, 1925.

111. Hanks, M. E., and Bailey, J. H.: Oxidation-reduction potential requirements of *Cl. welchii* and other clostridia, Proc. Soc. Exp. Biol. Med. **59:**163, 1945.

112. Harvey, J. C., Cantrell, J. R., and Fisher, A. M.: Actinomycosis: Its recognition and treatment, Ann. Intern. Med. **46:**868, 1957.

113. Hecht, D. W., and Work, W. P.: Surgery for nonneoplastic parotid disease, Arch. Otolaryng. **92**:463, 1970.

114. Heilman, K. M., and Muschenheim, C.: Primary cutaneous tuberculosis resulting from mouth-to-mouth respiration, New Eng. J. Med. **273**:1035, 1965.

115. Heinrich, S., Pulverer, G., and Hanf, U.: Über das physiologische Vorkommen des *Bacteroides melaninogenicus* bei Mensch und Tier, Schweiz. Z. Path. Bakt. **22**:861, 1959.

116. Herberts, G., and Sandström, J.: Cervicofacial actinomycosis, Acta Otolaryng. **48**: 458, 1957.

117. Herrell, W. E.: Miscellaneous diseases. In Welch, H. (ed.): Principles and practice of antibiotic therapy, New York, 1954, Medical Encyclopedia, Inc., p. 591.

118. Hertz, J.: Actinomycosis: Borderline cases, J. Int. Coll. Surg. **34**:148, 1960.

119. Hewitt, L. F.: Oxidation reduction potentials in bacteriology and biochemistry, ed. 6, Edinburgh, 1950, E. S. Livingstone.

120. Hewitt, W. L., Seligman, S. J., and Deigh, R. A.: Kinetics of the synergism of penicillin-streptomycin and penicillin-kanamycin for enterococci and its relationship to L-phase variants, J. Lab. Clin. Med. **67**:792, 1966.

121. Hiller, B.: A membranous oropharyngitis, Med. J. Aust. **2**:649, 1935.

122. Hoffman, H.: Oral microbiology, Advances Appl. Microbiol. **8**:195, 1966.

123. Hoffman, M. A., and Finberg, L.: Pseudomonas infections in infants associated with high-humidity environments, J. Pediat. **46**: 626, 1955.

124. Holt, L. E., and McIntosh, R.: Holt's diseases of infancy and childhood, ed. 11, New York, 1940, Appleton-Century-Crofts, p. 1168.

125. Homans, J.: A textbook of surgery, ed. 5, Springfield, Ill., 1940, Charles C Thomas, Publisher p. 369.

126. Horsley, J. S.: Certain symbiotic bacterial infections producing gangrene with special reference to the principles of treatment, J. A. M. A. **98**:1425, 1932.

127. Howell, A., Jr., Murphey, W. C., III, Paul F., and Stephan, R. M.: Oral strains of actinomyces, J. Bact. **78**:82, 1959.

128. Howitt, B., and van Meter, M.: Lesions produced in rabbits by lactobacillus cultures, J. Infect. Dis. **46**:368, 1930.

129. Hoyne, R. M., Thompson, E. C., and Wilkinson, H. W.: Tetanus complicated by impacted dentures: Report of case, J. Oral Surg. **17**:59, 1969.

130. Hubbard, R. M.: Tetanus—difficult diagnosis, Oral Surg. **28**:348, 1969.

131. Hubbert, W. T., and Rosen, M. N.: *Pasteurella multocida* infection due to animal bite, Amer. J. Public Health **60**:1103, 1970.

132. Hughes, W. T., Jr., and Etteldorf, J. N.: Oropharyngeal tularemia, J. Pediat. **51**:363, 1953.

133. Hurst, V., and Fenderson, A.: Establishment of *Bacteroides melaninogenicus* as a component of the anaerobic oral flora, Bact. Proc.—1969, p. 103, Abstract M229, 1969.

134. Hylton, R. P., Samuels, H. S., and Oatis, G. W., Jr.: Actinomycosis: Is it really rare? Oral Surg. **29**:138, 1970.

135. Ikeda, T., Isoda, A., and Iidako, T.: A study on staphylococci isolated from the acute suppurative diseases in the oral area with reference to their comparison in pathogenicity, J. Nihon Univ. Sch. Dent. **6**:88, 1964.

136. Ingham, H. R., Sekon, J. B., Codd, A. A., and Hale, J. H.: A study *in vitro* of the sensitivity to antibiotics of *Bacteroides fragilis*, J. Clin. Path. **21**:432, 1968.

137. Intile, J. A., and Richert, J. H.: Cervicofacial actinomycosis complicated by meningitis, J. A. M. A. **181**:724, 1962.

138. Isenberg, H. D., Goldberg, D., and Sampson, J.: Laboratory studies with a selective enterococcus medium, Appl. Microbiol. **20**: 433, 1970.

139. Jackson, F. L., Goodman, Y., and Wong, P. C.: Investigation of the status of certain *Haemophilus*-like organisms hitherto classified as *Bacteroides corrodens*, Bact. Proc.—1969, p. 103, Abstract M232, 1969.

140. Jackson, G. G., Shih-Man, C., Barnes, M. W., and Finland, M.: Terramycin in pertussis: Clinical and laboratory studies, Ann. N. Y. Acad. Sci. **53**:422, 1950.

141. Jacobs, H. D.: Cavernous sinus thrombosis resulting from a mandibular alveolar abscess of a deciduous molar, J. Amer. Dent. Assoc. **27**:1641, 1940.

142. Jacobs, H. G.: Delayed tetanus simulating ankylosis of arthritic origin in the temporomandibular joint: Report of case, J. Oral Surg. **11**:157, 1953.

143. Jacobs, M. H.: Oral lesions in childhood, Oral Surg. **9**:871, 1956.

144. Johnson, E. E., Duvall, A. J., and Donaldson, J. A.: Infectious osteonecrosis of the maxilla, Arch. Otolaryng. **76**:558, 1962.

145. Johnson, W. S., Devine, K. D., Wellman, W. E., and Fischbach, J. E.: Ludwig's angina, Oral Surg. **16**:1023, 1963.

146. Jordan, H. V., Fitzgerald, R. J., and Faber,

J. E., Jr.: Studies on the aciduric oral micrococci, J. Dent. Res. **35**:404, 1956.

147. Jordan, H. V., and Keyes, P. H.: Studies on the bacteriology of hamster periodontal disease, Amer. J. Path. **46**:843, 1965.

148. Joske, R. A., and French, E. L.: Chronic brucella hepatitis with suppurative brucella parotitis occurring after antibiotic therapy, Med. J. Aust. **1**:589, 1953.

149. Keith, H. M., Weed, L. A., and Needham, G. M.: Nontuberculous acid-fast bacilli in cervical adenitis, Pediatrics **20**:688, 1957.

150. Keith, T. A., III, and Schreiner, A. W.: *Hemophilus influenzae* in adult bronchopulmonary infection, Ann. Intern. Med. **56**:27, 1962.

151. Kelstrup, J.: The incidence of *Bacteroides melaninogenicus* in human gingival sulci, and its prevalence in the oral cavity at different ages, Periodontics **4**:14, 1966.

152. Keudell, K. C., and Goldberg, H. S.: Dehydrogenase patterns in the study of *Bacteroides*, Appl. Microbiol. **19**:505, 1970.

153. Khosla, V. M.: Immediate bone graft following resection of mandibular osteomyelitic lesion, Oral Surg. **30**:29, 1970.

154. Killey, H. C.: Maxillo-facial injuries, Hosp. Med., May, 1968, p. 917.

155. Kirner, A., Gürtler, E., Ružička, A., and Galan, E.: Die bakteriologischen Befunde aus den submandibulären Abszessen, Deutsch. Stomat. **19**:434, 1969.

156. Klyhn, K. M., and Gorrill, R. H.: Studies on the virulence of hospital strains of *Pseudomonas aeruginosa*, J. Gen. Microbiol. **47**:227, 1967.

157. Knight, R. K., and Lehner, T.: Tuberculosis of the mouth, Guy Hosp. Rep. **117**:63, 1968.

158. Ködel, G., and Brühl, P.: Salmonellen in einer Epithelzyste am Oberkiefer—ein ungewöhnlicher Befunde, Schweiz. Mschr. Zahnheilk. **76**:33, 1966.

159. Kondo, W., and Onisi, M.: Ecological aspects of the human parotid saliva. II. The role of bacteria on the decreasing Eh of the parotid saliva, Bull. Tokyo Med. Dent. Univ. **7**:571, 1960.

160. Krause, F. W., Perry, W. I., and Nickerson, J. F.: Salivary catalase and peroxidase values in normal subjects and in persons with periodontal disease, Oral Surg. **11**:95, 1958.

161. Langenegger, J. J.: Actinomyces and their effects on oral tissues, J. Dent. Assoc. S. Afr. **20**:1, 1965.

162. Leake, D., and Leake, R.: Neonatal suppurative parotitis, Pediatrics **46**:203, 1970.

163. Ledingham, J. C. G., and Arkwright, J. A.: The carrier problem in infectious diseases, London, 1912, Edward Arnold, p. 213.

164. Leroux, L., and Hérard: Case of lupus of the nose and palate, Ann. Otolaryng. **13**:231, 1946.

165. Lester, W.: Chemotherapy of tuberculosis, Clin. Notes Resp. Dis. **9**(2):3, 1970.

166. Levinson, A., Marske, R. L., and Shein, M. K.: Tetanus in heroin addicts, J. A. M. A. **157**:658, 1955.

167. Lewin-Epstein, J., and Goldin, S.: Production of chronic osteomyelitis in the jaws of rabbits (a preliminary report). In: Oral Surg., Transactions of Second Congress International Association of Oral Surgeons, Copenhagen, June 22-24, 1965, p. 241.

168. Lewis, G. K.: The complex mandibular fracture, Amer. J. Surg. **97**:183, 1959.

169. Linsey, E. V.: Osteomyelitis of the jaws, Dent. Items Interest **68**:1064, 1946.

170. Macbeth, R.: Osteomyelitis of the maxilla, J. Laryng. **66**:18, 1952.

171. McCabe, W. R., and Jackson, G. G.: Gram-negative bacteria. I. Etiology and ecology, Arch. Intern. Med. **110**:847, 1962.

172. McCarthy, F. P.: Pyostomatitis vegetans: Report of three cases, Arch. Derm. **60**:750, 1949.

173. McCullough, N. B.: Human brucellosis, with special reference to the disease in the United States, Ann. N. Y. Acad. Sci. **70**:541, 1958.

174. Macdonald, J. B., Hare, G. C., and Wood, A. W. S.: The bacteriologic status of the pulp chambers in intact teeth found to be nonvital following trauma, Oral Surg. **10**:318, 1957.

175. McDonald, J. R., Henthorne, J. C., and Thompson, L.: Rôle of anaerobic streptococci in human infections, Arch. Path. **23**:230, 1937.

176. MacGregor, A. J.: Aetiology of dry socket: A clinical investigation, Brit. J. Oral Surg. **6**:49, 1968.

177. MacKee, G. M., and Cipollaro, A. C.: Skin diseases in childhood, ed. 2, New York, 1946, Paul B. Hoeber, Inc., p. 379.

178. McNamara, M. J., Hill, M. C., Balows, A., and Tucker, E. B.: A study of the bacteriologic patterns of hospital infections, Ann. Intern. Med. **66**:480, 1967.

179. McVay, L. V., and Sprunt, D. H.: Bacteroides infections, Ann. Intern. Med. **36**:56, 1952.

180. Magnus, K.: Epidemiological basis of tuberculosis eradication. 3. Risk of pulmonary tuberculosis after human and bovine infection, Bull. W. H. O. **35**:483, 1966.

181. Manning, E. L.: Pyogenic granulomas, Arch. Otolaryng. **70:**502, 1959.
182. Marcoux, J. A., Zabransky, R. J., Washington, J. A., II, Wellman, W. E., and Martin, W. J.: Bacteroides bacteremia, Minnesota Med. **53:**1169, 1970.
183. Markowitz, H. A., and Gerry, R. G.: Temporomandibular joint disease (concluded), Oral Surg. **3:**75, 1950.
184. Marsden, H. B., and Hyde, W. A.: Anonymous mycobacteria in cervical adenitis, Lancet **1:**249, 1962.
185. Martin, W. F.: Primary tuberculosis of the tongue, Southern Med. Surg. **99:**348, 1937.
186. Mashberg, A., Carroll, M. A., and Morrissey, J. B.: Gram-negative infections of the oral cavity and associated structures: Report of two cases, J. Oral Surg. **28:**376, 1970.
187. Mason, D. A.: Steroid therapy and dental infection: Case report, Brit. Dent. J. **122:**271, 1970.
188. Massler, M.: The oral flora in diabetics, J. Dent. Res. **28:**674, 1947.
189. Michman, J., and Sagler, F.: Changes in the anterior nasal spine and the alveolar process of the maxillary bone in leprosy, Int. J. Leprosy **25:**217, 1957.
190. Miller, J. K.: Human pasteurellosis in New York State, New York J. Med. **66:**2527, 1966.
191. Miller, J. L., and McGrath, D.: Functions of a dental clinic in a tuberculosis hospital, J. Oral Surg. **18:**154, 1960.
192. Miller, R. H., and Rogers, H.: Present status of tetanus, with special regard to treatment, J. A. M. A. **104:**186, 1935.
193. Moody, M. R., Young, V. M., Vermeulen, G. D., and Kenton, D. M.: *Pseudomonas aeruginosa*: Specific hemagglutinin levels against seven slime-layer antigens, Bact. Proc.—1970, p. 80, Abstract M38, 1970.
194. Moore, K., and Davis, G. H. G.: Taxonomy and incidence of oral corynebacteria, Brit. Dent. J. **106:**254, 1963.
195. Moorehead, F. B., and Dewey, K. W.: Tuberculosis of the mouth, Surg. Clin. N. Amer. **5:**931, 1925.
196. Morris, M. H.: Polyneuritis with facial diplegia following serum sickness in an adult, Med. Record **156:**420, 1943.
197. Morrison, W. W.: Diseases of the ear, nose and throat, New York, 1948, Appleton-Century-Crofts, p. 305.
198. Morse, D. R., and Hoffman, H.: Microbial diseases of the salivary glands, with special reference to mumps and acute and chronic sialadenitis, New York Dent. J. **36:**203, 1970.
199. Mouton, R. P., Stoop, J. W., Ballieux, R. E., and Mul, N. A. J.: Pneumococcal antibodies in IgA of serum and external secretions, Clin. Exp. Immun. **7:**201, 1970.
200. Murray, J. F., Finegold, S. M., Froman, S., and Will, D. W.: The changing spectrum of nocardiosis: A review and presentation of nine cases, Amer. Rev. Resp. Dis. **83:**315, 1961.
201. Neter, E.: A case of Ludwig's angina due to an esculin-fermenting hemolytic streptococcus (enterococcus), Arch. Path. **23:**295, 1937.
202. Newcomb, R. W., Ishizaka, K., and DeVald, B. L.: Human IgG and IgA diphtheria antitoxins in serum, nasal fluids and saliva, J. Immun. **103:**215, 1969.
203. Newman, C.: Removal of impacted molar assists in diagnosis of brucellosis, J. Amer. Dent. Assoc. **39:**754, 1949.
204. Nikiforuk, G.: The reducing property of saliva toward several oxidation-reduction indicator dyes, J. Dent. Res. **35:**377, 1956.
205. Norman, J. E. de B.: Cervicofacial actinomycosis, Oral Surg. **29:**735, 1970.
206. Ochs, C. J.: Pneumococcic stomatitis, J. Pediat. **28:**481, 1946.
207. Olinger, M. G.: Mixed infection in subacute bacterial endocarditis: Report of two cases, Arch. Intern. Med. **81:**334, 1948.
208. Ottens, H., and Winkler, K. C.: Indifferent and haemolytic streptococci possessing group-antigen F, J. Gen. Microbiol. **28:**181, 1962.
209. Parker, M. T., and Simmons, L. E.: The inhibition of *Corynebacterium diphtheriae* and other gram-positive organisms by *Staphylococcus aureus*, J. Gen. Microbiol. **21:**457, 1959.
210. Parkinson, R. H.: Tonsil and allied problems, New York, 1951, The Macmillan Company, p. 155.
211. Penhale, K. W.: Early diagnosis and treatment of osteomyelitis of the mandible, J. Amer. Dent. Assoc. **28:**288, 1941.
212. Pessin, S. B.: Tularemic pneumonia, pericarditis and ulcerative stomatitis, Arch. Intern. Med. **57:**1125, 1936.
213. Pike, E. B., Freer, J. H., Davis, G. H. G., and Bisset, K. A.: The taxonomy of micrococci and neisseriae of oral origin, Arch. Oral Biol. **7:**715, 1962.
214. Pine, L., and Hardin, H.: *Actinomyces israelii*, a cause of lacrimal canaliculitis, J. Bact. **78:**164, 1959.
215. Pine, L., Howell, A., Jr., and Watson, S. J.: Studies of the morphological, physiological,

and biochemical characters of *Actinomyces bovis,* J. Gen. Microbiol. **23**:403, 1960.

216. Pine, L., and Overman, J. R.: Determination of the structure and composition of the sulphur granules of *Actinomyces bovis,* J. Gen. Microbiol. **32**:209, 1963.

217. Place, E. H.: Diphtheria. In Cecil, R. L. (ed.): A textbook of medicine by American authors, ed. 6, Philadelphia, 1943, W. B. Saunders Co., p. 182.

218. Poston, M. A., and Menefee, E. E.: Acute brucellosis with bacteremia and oral lesions, treatment with immune human blood, New Eng. J. Med. **219**:796, 1938.

219. Prévot, A. R.: Manual of classification and determination of anaerobic bacteria, Philadelphia, 1966, Lea & Febiger.

220. Pritchett, I. W., and Stillman, E. G.: The occurrence of *Bacillus influenzae* in throats and saliva, J. Exp. Med. **29**:259, 1919.

221. Pulaski, E. J., and Keeking, W. M.: Acute suppurative parotitis: Report of two cases, New Eng. J. Med. **253**:1028, 1955.

222. Rabin, C. B., and Janowitz, H. D.: Actinomyces in putrid empyema, J. Thorac. Cardiov. Surg. **19**:355, 1950.

223. Ragheb, M.: Parotid infection caused by dryness of the mouth: Report of 3 cases after use of tranquilizers, Geriatrics **18**:627, 1963.

224. Raj, H., and Colwell, R. R.: Taxonomy, of enterococci by computer analysis, Canad. J. Microbiol. **12**:353, 1966.

225. Rattner, L. J.: Case of suspected oral nocardiosis, Oral Surg. **11**:441, 1958.

226. Ray, K. C., and Fuller, M. L.: Isolation of *Mycobacterium* from dental impression material, J. Prosth. Dent. **13**:93, 1963.

227. Read, T. T.: Tuberculous gingivitis, Univ. of Leeds, Med. J. **5**:25, 1956.

228. Reade, P. C., and Radden, B. G.: Chronic osteomyelitis of the maxilla associated with a Pseudomonas infection, Brit. Dent. J. **115**:246, 1963.

229. Reiss, F.: Cutaneous diphtheria: Two unusual cases with eruptions resembling lymphogranuloma venereum and ectodermosis erosiva pluriorificialis, Arch. Derm. Syph. **56**:216, 1947.

230. Richardson, R. L., and Jones, M. A.: Bacteriologic census of human saliva, J. Dent. Res. **37**:697, 1958.

231. Riddell, G. S.: Labial diphtheria, Brit. Med. J. **1**:818, 1950.

232. Robboy, S. J., and Vickery, A. L., Jr.: Tinctorial and morphologic properties distinguishing actinomycosis and nocardiosis, New Eng. J. Med. **282**:593, 1970.

233. Robins, A. B.: Detection of tuberculosis in New York, Arch. Environ. Health **4**:146, 1962.

234. Robinson, I. B., and Laskin, D. M.: Tetanus of oral origin, Oral Surg. **10**:831, 1957.

235. Rogosa, M.: The genus *Veillonella.* I. General cultural, ecological, and biochemical considerations, J. Bact. **87**:162, 1964.

236. Rogosa, M.: A selective medium for the isolation and enumeration of the *Veillonella* from the oral cavity, J. Bact. **72**:533, 1956.

237. Roistacher, S. L.: Ascending infections of the face, New York Dent. J. **19**:279, 1953.

238. Rosan, B., and Hammond, B. F.: Toxicity of *Lactobacillus casei,* J. Dent. Res. **44**:783, 1965.

239. Rosan, B., and Williams, N. B.: Serology of strains of *Streptococcus faecalis* which produce hyaluronidase, Nature **212**:1275, 1966.

240. Rose, S. S.: A clinical and radiological survey of 192 cases of recurrent swellings of the salivary glands, Ann. Roy. Coll. Surg. Eng. **15**:374, 1954.

241. Rosebury, T.: The aerobic non-hemolytic streptococci, Medicine **23**:249, 1944.

242. Rosen, S., and Weinstein, R. R.: Interrelationships among salivary reductase activity, certain oral bacteria and caries in man, J. Amer. Dent. Assoc. **67**:876, 1963.

243. Roth, G. D., and Flanagan, V.: The pathogenicity of *Rothia dentocariosa* inoculated into mice, J. Dent. Res. **48**:957, 1969.

244. Rubelman, P. A., Rebuck, J. F., and Loveman, C. E.: Postextraction acute cellulitis caused by *Salmonella choleraesuis*: Report of a case, J. Oral Surg. **19**:255, 1961.

245. Rud, J.: Cervicofacial actinomycosis, J. Oral Surg. **25**:229, 1967.

246. Runyon, E. H.: Anonymous mycobacteria in human disease, Med. Clin. N. Amer. **43**:273, 1959.

247. Salman, L., Harrigan, W. F., and Palladino, V. S.: Fatal bacterial endocarditis following tooth removal, Oral Surg. **30**:749, 1970.

248. Salyer, K. E., Votteler, T. P., and Dorman, G. W.: Surgical management of cervical adenitis due to atypical mycobacteria in children, J. A. M. A. **204**:1037, 1968.

249. Schenck, H. P.: Common infections of the pharynx and fauces, Med. Clin. N. Amer. **31**:1356, 1947.

250. Schroff, J.: Diseases of the salivary glands; sialography: Its application in the study and treatment of salivary gland infections, J. Amer. Dent. Assoc. **26**:861, 1939.

251. Schwabacher, H., Lucas, D. R., and Rimington, C.: *Bacterium melaninogenicum*—a misnomer, J. Gen. Microbiol. **1**:109, 1947.

252. Schweppe, H. I., Knowles, J. H., and Kane, L.: Lung abscess: An analysis of the Massachusetts General Hospital cases from 1943 through 1956, New Eng. J. Med. **265:**1039, 1961.

253. Sell, S. H.: The clinical importance of *Hemophilus influenzae* infections in children, Pediat. Clin. N. Amer. **17:**415, 1970.

254. Shengold, M. A., and Sheingold, H.: Oral tuberculosis, Oral Surg. **4:**239, 1951.

255. Shershin, P. H.: and Katz, S. S.: Diazepam in the treatment of tetanus: Report of a case following tooth extraction, Clin. Med. **71:** 362, 1964.

256. Ship, A. G., and Slater, H. L.: *Pasteurella multocida* infection of the hand with superimposed clostridial infection: A case report, Plast. Reconstr. Surg. **32:**564, 1963.

257. Shklair, I. L., Losse, F. L., and Bahn, A. N.: The isolation and incidence of *Pseudomonas aeruginosa* from human saliva, Bact. Proc.— 1963, p. 71, Abstract M68, 1963.

258. Silva, F.: A case of buccal localization of venereal granuloma, Urol. Cutan. Rev. **37:** 611, 1933.

259. Simmons, J. S.: Leprosy. In: The Oxford medicine, by various authors, New York, 1938, Oxford University Press, vol. 5, p. 387, 396(1)-396(36).

260. Sims, W.: A pathogenic lactobacillus, J. Path. Bact. **87:**99, 1964.

261. Slack, G. L.: The bacteriology of infected root canals and *in vitro* penicillin sensitivity, Brit. Dent. J. **95:**211, 1953.

262. Slack, G. L.: The resistance to antibiotics of micro-organisms isolated from root canals, Brit. Dent. J. **102:**493, 1957.

263. Small, I. A., and Kobernick, S.: Botryomycosis of the tongue: Report of a case, Oral Surg. **24:**503, 1967.

264. Smith, D. T.: Medical treatment of acute and chronic pulmonary abscesses, J. Thorac. Cardiov. Surg. **17:**72, 1948.

265. Smith, J. W.: Tetanus, Texas Med. **66:**52, 1970.

266. Socransky, S. S., and Gibbons, R. J.: Required role of *Bacteroides melaninogenicus* in mixed anaerobic infections, J. Infect. Dis. **115:**247, 1965.

267. Sparer, P. J., Sussman, A. A., and Goodman, M. H.: Ulcerative tuberculosis of the oral mucous membranes (tuberculosis orificialis), Arch. Derm. Syph. **39:**900, 1939.

268. Spink, W. W.: The nature of brucellosis, Minneapolis, 1956, University of Minnesota Press.

269. Spratt, J. S., Jr.: The etiology and therapy of acute pyogenic parotitis, Surg. Gynec. Obstet. **112:**391, 1961.

270. Sternberg, S., Hoffman, C., and Zweifler, B. M.: Stomatitis and diarrhea in infants caused by Bacillus mucosus capsulatus, J. Pediat. **38:**509, 1951.

271. Stetzer, J. J., Jr.: Acute infections of dental origin, Dent. Clin. N. Amer., July, 1957, p. 521.

272. Stevenson, A. E. M.: Actinomycosis of ovaries and fallopian tubes, J. Obstet. Gynaec. Brit. Comm. **64:**365, 1957.

273. Stones, H. H.: Oral and dental diseases, ed. 2, Edinburgh, 1951, Livingstone.

274. Sugg, J. Y., and Neill, J. M.: Loss of immune substances from the body. II. Diphtheria antitoxin in human saliva, J. Immun. **20:** 463, 1931.

275. Sutton, R. L., and Sutton, R. L., Jr.: Synopsis of diseases of the skin, St. Louis, 1942, The C. V. Mosby Co., p. 181.

276. Taplin, J., and Goldsworthy, N. E.: A study of 225 strains of *Staphylococcus* isolated from the mouth, Aust. J. Exp. Biol. Med. Sci. **36:**289, 1958.

277. Tarsitano, J. J., and O'Hara, J. W., Jr.: Rheumatic fever: In-depth appraisal with a discussion of penicillin, J. Amer. Dent. Assoc. **77:**1074, 1968.

278. Taylor, G. S.: Tetanus presenting primarily as trismus, Brit. J. Oral Surg. **8:**77, 1970.

279. Tefft, H. E., and Bibby, B. G.: Streptococci isolated from the mouth, J. Dent. Res. **19:** 285, 1940.

280. Thoma, K. H., and Goldman, H. M.: Oral pathology, ed. 5, St. Louis, 1960, The C. V. Mosby Co., p. 1352.

281. Thomas, C. G. A., and Hare, R.: The classification of anaerobic cocci, their isolation in normal human beings and pathological processes, J. Clin. Path. **7:**300, 1954.

282. Thompson, R. H. S., and Dubos, R. J.: Production of experimental osteomyelitis in rabbits by intravenous injection of *Staphylococcus aureus*, J. Exp. Med. **68:**191, 1938.

283. Torphy, D. E., and Ray, C. G.: *Pasteurella multocida* in dog and cat bite infections, Pediatrics **43:**259, 1969.

284. Treadway, C. R., and Prange, A. J.: Tetanus mimicking psychophysiologic reaction, occurrence after dental extraction, J. A. M. A. **200:**891, 1967.

285. Tstutsui, M., Utsumi, N., and Tsubakimoto, K.: Cellular components of staphylococci and streptococci in inflamed human gingiva, J. Dent. Res. **47:**663, 1968.

286. Tuberculosis in New York City 1969: A

report to the mayor and the citizens of the City of New York, New York, 1970, Tuberculosis and Respiratory Disease Association of New York.

287. Turner, P. L., and Clarke, T. W.: Temporomandibular arthropathy in serum sickness, Ann. Allerg. 1:115, 1943.

288. Tynes, B. S., and Frommeyer, W. B., Jr.: Bacteroides septicemia: Cultural, clinical, and therapeutic features in a series of twenty-five patients, Ann. Intern. Med. 56:12, 1962.

289. Unna, P. G.: The histopathology of the diseases of the skin, Walker, N. (trans.) Edinburgh, 1896, William F. Clay, p. 456.

290. van Reenen, J. F., and Coogan, M. M.: Clostridia isolated from human mouths, Arch. Oral Biol. 15:845, 1970.

291. Vener, H. I., and Bower, A. G.: Clinical tetanus: Treatment in 100 consecutive cases with a net mortality rate of 19 per cent, J. A. M. A. 116:1627, 1941.

292. Veys, E. M., and Claessens, H. E.: Serum levels of IgG, IgM, and IgA in rheumatoid arthritis, Ann. Rheum. Dis. 27:431, 1968.

293. Wade, W. M., Jr., Cocke, W. M., Jr., and Sture, V. J.: Neck mass caused by atypical mycobacteria: Report of case, J. Oral Surg. 27:137, 1969.

294. Walker, W. J., Massey, F. C., and Mostofi, F. K.: Streptomycin-resistant diphtheria, J. A. M. A. 135:771, 1947.

295. Walton, C. H. A., Graham, H. M., and Lansdown, L. P.: Acute ulcerative stomatitis, three unusual cases, Lancet 2:214, 1942.

296. Weidmann, G. M., and MacGregor, A. J.: Tuberculous osteomyelitis of the mandible: Report of a case, Oral Surg. 28:632, 1969.

297. Weinstein, L., and Wesselhoeft, C.: Penicillin in the treatment of tetanus: Report of two cases, J. A. M. A. 233:681, 1945.

298. Weiss, C., and Mercado, D. G.: Studies of anaerobic streptococci from pulmonary abscesses, J. Infect. Dis. 62:181, 1938.

299. Westenfelder, G. O., Feldman, J. L., Kyser, F. A., and Harding, H. B.: Microaerophilic streptococcal bacteremia, a rare course of febrile illness, Aerospace Med. 38:70, 1967.

300. Wheatcroft, M. G.: A comparative study of human serum and salivary antibody titers in cases of Brucella melitensis infections, J. Dent. Res. 36:112, 1957.

301. White, B.: The biology of pneumococcus, New York, 1938, The Commonwealth Fund.

302. WHO Expert Committee on Leprosy: Fourth report, Geneva, 1970, World Health Organization Techn. Rep. Ser., No. 459, 31 pp.

303. Whyte, H. J., and Kaplan, W.: Nocardial mycetoma resembling granuloma faciale, Arch. Derm. 100:720, 1969.

304. Williams, J. W., and McClure, C. W.: Tetanus. In: The Oxford medicine, New York, 1942, Oxford University Press, vol. 5, p. 203.

305. Williams, R. E. O.: Healthy carriage of Staphylococcus aureus: Its prevalence and importance, Bact. Rev. 27:56, 1963.

306. Wilson, G. S., and Miles, A. A.: Topley and Wilson's principles of bacteriology and immunity, ed. 3, Baltimore, 1946, The Williams & Wilkins Co., p. 1462.

307. Winslow, D. J.: Botryomycosis, Amer. J. Path. 35:153, 1959.

308. Wittwer, J. W., Toto, P. D., and Dickler, E. H.: Streptococcus mitis antigens in inflamed gingiva, J. Periodont. 40:639, 1969.

309. Woodburne, A. R., and Northrop, P.: Streptococcic hypertrophic gingivitis, Arch. Derm. Syph. 29:422, 1934.

310. Woodruff, P. S.: Tuberculosis and the dentist, Aust. Dent. J. 2:61, 1957.

311. Yarington, C. T., Jr., Sprinkle, P. M., and Gensler, S. W.: Granulomatous parotitis, West Virginia Med. J. 63:440, 1967.

312. Youmans, G. P., Youmans, A. S., and Parlett, R.: The incidence of hypersensitivity to mammalian and Battey PPD in medical and dental students, Amer. Rev. Resp. Dis. 82:114, 1960.

313. Zaias, N., Taplin, D., and Rebell, G.: Mycetoma, Arch. Derm. 99:215, 1969.

REFERENCES AND ADDITIONAL READINGS

Barksdale, L.: Corynebacterium diphtheriae and its relatives, Bact. Rev. 34:378, 1970.

Blair, J. D., Lennette, E. H., and Truant, J. P. (eds.): Manual of clinical microbiology, Bethesda, Md., 1970, American Society for Microbiology.

Cochrane, R. G., and Davey, T. F. (eds.): Leprosy in theory and practice, ed. 2, Bristol, England, 1964, Wright.

Cope, Z.: Actinomycosis, London, 1938, Oxford University Press.

Darzins, E.: The bacteriology of tuberculosis, Minneapolis, 1958, University of Minnesota Press.

Kauffmann, F.: Enterobacteriaceae, ed. 2, Copenhagen, 1954, Einar Munksgaard.

Prevention of rheumatic fever: Report of a WHO expert committee, World Health Organization Techn. Rep. Ser., No. 342, 1966.

Simon, H. J.: Attenuated infection, the germ theory in contemporary perspective, Philadelphia, 1960, J. B. Lippincott Co.

Spink, W. W.: The nature of brucellosis, Minneapolis, 1956, The University of Minnesota Press.

Whipple, H. E. (ed.): The staphylococci: Ecologic perspectives, Ann. N. Y. Acad. Sci. **128:**1, 1965.

Willis, A. T.: Anaerobic bacteriology in clinical medicine, ed. 2, Washington, D. C., 1964, Butterworths.

Wilson, G. S., and Miles, A. A.: Topley and Wilson's principles of bacteriology and immunity, ed. 5, Baltimore, 1964, The Williams & Wilkins Co.

4 / The spirochetes and Neisseria organisms

Both the spirochetes and *Neisseria* include a pathogenic species that is transmitted primarily by the venereal route. Both of these pathogens are responsible for widespread infection today existing in epidemic proportions in the United States and other parts of the world. According to the National Communicable Disease Center of the United States Public Health Service, approximately 1.5 million cases of gonorrhea probably occur annually in the United States. Recently, within a period of 12 years, the number of cases has risen by about 75%. Gonorrhea now affects more Americans each year than do measles, tuberculosis, hepatitis, whooping cough, and encephalitis combined.

Syphilis, in contrast to the recent epidemiologic course of gonorrhea, has not increased at as rapid a rate in recent years in some parts of the United States, and may have decreased in other parts of the country. The number of reported cases of primary and secondary syphilis for 1967 in the United States was 22,000, of which 56% occurred in local health districts that represented only 20% of the population. Unreported cases undoubtedly would add substantially to the total number of cases. Syphilis and gonorrhea are primarily diseases of the young adult, occurring most frequently among those between 15 and 30 years of age.[42]

Both of these venereal diseases come to the attention of the dentist, although syphilis is much more liable to cause lesions that are conspicuous or that may occur in the mouth or on the face.

TREPONEMA PALLIDUM: SYPHILIS

The origins of syphilis[41] are unknown, but its first notable appearance in modern times occurred in Europe at the end of the fifteenth century. It spread rapidly to pandemic proportions as a very acute disease, frequently fatal in the secondary stage. This extremely acute, severe form of syphilis apparently became rather quickly attenuated to the more chronic form seen today. The early lesions at that time were often confused with other venereal as well as nonvenereal diseases, particularly gonorrhea. This confusion was compounded by an experiment carried out upon himself by John Hunter in 1767. The specimen for self-inoculation came from a person suffering from both gonorrhea and syphilis, and Hunter assumed that the symptoms he suffered were all expressions of a single disease. His reputation was so great that he effectively delayed differentiation of syphilis from gonorrhea for 50 years.

Bacteriologic search for the etiologic agent began in the latter part of the nineteenth century, but the causative agent was not identified until 1905, when Fritz Schaudinn and Erich Hoffmann found a spiral organism in serum from a lesion of secondary syphilis. Complement fixation for serum diagnosis was introduced in 1906 by Wassermann. By 1909, with animal infection with the etiologic agent successfully accomplished, Paul Ehrlich began his systematic investigations with organic arsenicals that finally led to use of salvarsan. The basis for effective and rational medical treatment for syphilis was now finally established.[8]

Morphology.[44] The spirochete causing syphilis, *Treponema pallidum,* consists of from 8 to 20 tightly wound coils. The length of the microorganism varies between 8 and 20 μ, with a distance of 1 μ separating each coil. The depth between each crest and trough of each coil approximates 1 μ (Fig. 4-1).

Motility is of several types: rotation similar to the turning of a corkscrew; flexibility in which one or several coils may show mobility; and undulating progressive motion that rapidly moves the spirochete forward. The speed of progressive motion is dependent on the viscosity of the exudate. The more mucoid the exudate, the more motion is impeded and slowed; there may be more of a writhing and lashing motion with less forward progress.

Spirochetes in serous exudate obtained from a chancre and examined in moist preparation by the darkfield microscope may become elongated and lose some of their coils as the preparations are main-

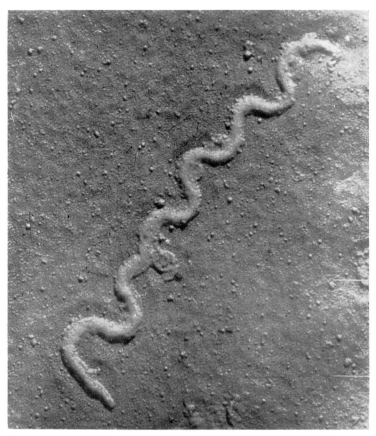

Fig. 4-1. *Treponema pallidum* seen in shadowed preparation through the electron microscope. (Courtesy Squibb Institute for Medical Research, E. R. Squibb & Sons, New Brunswick, N. J.)

tained at room temperature for 15 minutes or more.[37]

Staining. Spirochetes vary in the intensity with which they stain by Gram's method or with simple stains. Nonpathogenic strains such as *T. microdentium* may be readily stained by steaming with aqueous gentian violet (Fig. 4-2). *T. pallidum,* however, is more difficult to stain and requires special stains such as Fontana's silver stain or the use of carbolfuchsin following the application of a fixative solution and a mordant. Smears left overnight in Giemsa spirochete stain will stain *T. pallidum.* In tissue sections, spirochetes are nicely made visible by Levaditi's silver method.

Cultivation. It is still doubtful that *T. pallidum* has been ever cultivated. Noguchi reported the isolation of *T. pallidum* in an ascitic fluid or serum infusion broth medium containing pieces of sterile fresh guinea pig kidney. Other researchers have also reported the isolation of *T. pallidum.* Although several of these reportedly isolated strains morphologically resemble *T. pallidum,* these strains do not possess its pathogenicity. Some of these isolates are readily cultivable in such media as thioglycollate broth containing serum or ascitic fluid. Other strains are maintained through the periodic transfer of aspirated testicular material from a previously inoculated rabbit to a normal one. Among various isolates, the Reiter, Kazan, and Nichols strains have received the greatest attention. These strains are nonpathogenic for animals (except those transferred by testicular injection); yet they have antigenic components that react with serum from syphilitics and are used in the performance of serologic tests. Attempts to grow *T. pallidum* in tissue culture or the embryonated chicken egg have not been successful.[28]

Viability. Since *T. pallidum* is nonsporulating, it is readily destroyed when outside of the body: rapid drying causes its immobilization. In clinics, use of soap and hot water has, through the years, been considered adequate for destroying any spirochetes that may have inadvertently been transferred to the fingers. The ordinary washing procedure may be followed

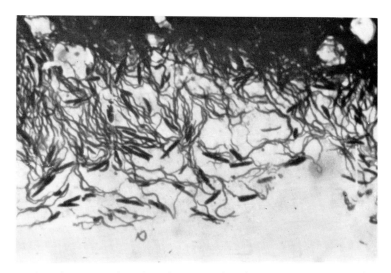

Fig. 4-2. Exudate from periodontal pocket stained with aqueous gentian violet and heat. Numerous oral spirochetes are present with a few fusiform bacilli (1,100 ×).

by immersing the hands in various germicides. Blood of donors used for transfusion should be tested serologically before it is administered to a recipient. The prevailing opinion is that *T. pallidum* in blood specimens dies within three days when the blood is kept at icebox temperature.[43]

Laboratory tests

Diagnostic procedures[21] are of two types: the examination of exudate by darkfield for the presence of spirochetes morphologically typical of *T. pallidum;* and examination of blood specimens for the presence of antibody.

Darkfield examination. Darkfield examination is performed by removing serous fluid with a fine capillary pipet from the suspected lesion or chancre. Specimens may also be obtained from swollen lymph nodes by aspiration of serous fluid by means of hypodermic needle and syringe. The fluid is gently expressed onto a slide, covered with a cover slip, and then examined by reflected light obtained by use of a darkfield condenser. The light bathes the surface of the spirochete so that it is somewhat like a balloon in the sky being lit by reflected moonlight (Fig. 4-3). The moist preparation permits study of

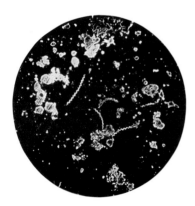

Fig. 4-3. *Treponema pallidum* as seen through darkfield microscope. (From Smith, A. L.: Principles of microbiology, ed. 5, St. Louis, 1965, The C. V. Mosby Co.)

the structure and form of the illuminated treponema and of its mode of motility. An experienced laboratory technologist is able to differentiate several types of spirochetes according to their length, the number of coils, depth of the coils, and the type of locomotion. However, lesions occuring in the mouth and on the lips present a problem. There is present in the mouth *T. microdentium*, which morphologically resembles *T. pallidum*. The person making the examination must qualify his observations with the statement that since *T. microdentium* is found in the normal mouth and resembles *T. pallidum*, no definite report is possible.[7]

Serologic tests. From several weeks to a month after the appearance of the hard chancre, there is generally enough antibody present in the patient's serum to be detected by a serologic test. Apparently there are two distinct types of antibodies: the Wassermann antibody or reagin, and a treponemicidal antibody.[21]

Wassermann test: complement fixation test. The principle of this serologic test is that a syphilitic individual develops an antibody (reagin) against the spirochete and that this reagin in vitro in the presence of a suitable antigen will fix or absorb complement into a reagin-antigen-complement complex. Since this complex cannot be detected by sight, a color indicator system is added containing an antigen, sheep red blood cells, and rabbit antisheep red blood cell antibody (produced by injecting rabbits with washed sheep red blood cells). Thus, if the patient's serum contains no reagin or antibody, the complement is not fixed but is free and can then become fixed into the indicator system. Such a reaction results in a hemolysis of the sheep red cells, which is observable as a clear red inklike colored solution in the test tubes. If the patient's serum contains reagin, then the complement becomes fixed in an antigen-reagin-complement complex. The indicator system consisting of the antigen sheep red cells and the rabbit anti-sheep red cell antibody can be activated only if complement is available. The sheep red blood cells therefore are not hemolyzed and remain as an opaque reddish suspension. The latter result, no hemolysis of sheep cells, is an indicator of a positive Wassermann reaction.

Flocculation-precipitin tests. Other procedures determining the presence of reagin are tests that do not require the presence of complement and are, therefore, more easily performed. Several of the more popular ones are the Kline, Kahn, and VDRL tests. These tests act on the principle that reagin will combine with an antigen and the complex will then form particles of sufficient size to be recognizable as a floccule or precipitate. The antigens used in these tests consist of cardiolipins extracted with absolute alcohol, plus cholesterol and lecithin. They can be obtained from various biological supply houses.

Antigen and antibody reaction. The antigen first employed in the Wassermann test was a suspension obtained by grinding and extracting the livers of syphilitic fetuses. Later, it was discovered that normal guinea pig's heart or beef heart, macerated and then extracted with alcohol, made an equally good antigen. Further sensitivity of the antigen could be obtained by the addition of cholesterol and lecithin. This cardiolipid antigen contains no spirochetes and is therefore a nonspecific antigen, yet it gives consistent results when used in performing the Wassermann test. Several explanations have been advanced to account for this apparent paradox. One is that the reagin actually is an antibody formed against some *T. pallidum* lipid substance; the second is that the reagin is a response to an autoantigen formed from the lipoidal denaturation of syphilitic disease tissue. False positive Wassermann reactions are known to occur in people with febrile diseases such as malaria, as well as in some alcoholics.

Such reactions indicate that substances are formed, in conditions other than syphilis, that react with the cardiolipid antigens and complement used in the Wassermann test.

Specimens of blood should preferably be collected before the patient eats and partakes of alcoholic beverages in order to eliminate possible false positives caused by the presence of chyle or alcohol in the blood. The specimens should be sent immediately to the laboratory to minimize the chances of the outgrowth of contaminants and the development of anticomplementary reactions.

Treponema pallidum immobilization test (TPI). A second type of antibody that is definitely treponemicidal in character and that will affect the motility of the syphilitic spirochete is also found in blood specimens. A *Treponema pallidum* immobilization test (TPI) has been devised in which the patient's serum, heat inactivated at 56° C. for 30 minutes as is done in the complement fixation (CF) or precipitin (Ppt) tests, is mixed with a suspension containing the Nichols strain of treponema grown in a suitable medium under anaerobic conditions. A control without the patient's serum will show active motility of spirochetes for as long as several days, whereas in the presence of luetic sera the spirochetes become immobile in hours. The test must be rigidly controlled since the spirochetes obtained from infected rabbits vary in their numbers and motility. Other factors inherent in the test require its performance by experienced technologists. Among other tests for the determination of this type of antibody are the *Treponema pallidum* complement fixation (TPCF), *Treponema pallidum* immune adherence (TPIA), and fluorescent treponemal antibody (FTA) tests.

Rapid plasma reagin card test (RPR Card Test). A simple procedure has been devised for the screening of blood specimens for the detection of syphilitic antibody. The results obtained have been identical in approximately 99% of instances with large series of specimens (thousands) examined by both the RPR Card Test[29] and the VDRL test. Use of the RPR Card Test in the clinic of an American dental school has shown that 1% of the patients admitted had syphilis.[20]

The RPR Card Test requires no apparatus such as a microscope, centrifuge, or test tubes. The necessary components for performing the test are readily available for purchase. The procedure for the test is as follows. A patient's finger is disinfected with 70% alcohol and punctured with a sterile lancet; three drops of blood are allowed to drop into the larger portion of a keyhole depression in a plasma collection slide. There it is mixed by means of a toothpick with heparin and a lectin, previously impregnated in the depression, which prevents clotting yet permits clumping of the red and white blood cells and allows the plasma to remain free. Tilting the slide permits the plasma to flow into the smaller portion of the keyhole depression from which it can be collected for the test. The test can be performed in 10 minutes or less; it provides a rapid method of screening migrant laborers and industrial plant personnel, and has been found practical in small laboratories and hospitals. Dental clinics are now using the test as a rapid and convenient means of screening patients, and its use in dental offices should be encouraged.

Biologic false positive reactions may occur with blood specimens from individuals ill with such diseases as infectious mononucleosis, virus pneumonia, vaccinia, and spirochetal diseases such as yaws, pinta, and bejel. However, such instances of false positive reactions are no greater than those obtained with the VDRL or other accepted screening procedures. All plasma specimens that give definite reactions must be confirmed by standard serologic procedures such as the Wassermann complement fixation test or the VDRL or other recognized precipitation methods.

Clinical course

The course of the infection[41] when acquired after birth may be divided into several stages. The spirochetes pass through the mucous membrane or skin into the tissue and are then carried by the bloodstream throughout the body. The infection now is systemic, only a few hours after exposure, although there is no clinical or serologic evidence to betray this situation.

Approximately three or four weeks, but as few as 10 days to as many as 90 days, after the treponemas have entered, there characteristically develops at the portal of entry a primary lesion, the hard chancre (Fig. 4-4). However, infection without a chancre is fairly frequent, and, moreover, the chancre may be easily overlooked by the patient in certain instances, particularly if it occurs in the genitourinary tract of a woman. The chancre persists for from one

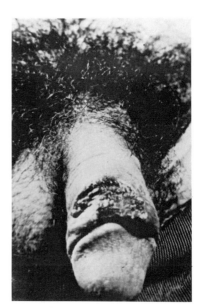

Fig. 4-4. Primary syphilis. Chancre of the penis appears as an ulcerous lesion with an indurated base. (Courtesy Dr. R. M. Montgomery, New York, N. Y.)

to five weeks and then heals spontaneously. Results of serologic tests for syphilis are usually negative when the chancre appears but become positive during the following one to four weeks. However, about half of the persons infected will be serologically normal during this stage.

About six weeks later (range of from two weeks to six months) the secondary stage (Fig. 4-5) develops, although in some cases the secondary stage may appear before the chancre has healed. In some cases the secondary stage may be so undeveloped that it escapes notice. Spontaneous healing occurs after from two to six weeks. A latent period then develops, but results of serologic tests are invariably positive. During this latent period, infection can be recognized only on the basis of results of serologic tests. Only the early period of less than a year produces sufficient infectious syphilis to be of epidemiologic importance. After four years of infection, relapsing infectious lesions of the kind seen during secondary syphilis are very rare. Latency may last a life time or be followed after a few years or 20 years or more by lesions of late syphilis. There is no way of predicting which patients will develop late lesions.

About one third of persons with untreated syphilis will develop the destructive syphilitic lesions of the late stage, and as many as 23% of untreated persons can be expected to die primarily as a result of the disease. Most of these deaths (more than 80%) will come from cardiovascular complications. Most of the remaining deaths are caused by involvement of the central nervous system.

Treatment

If therapy, usually with penicillin, is started before the chancre appears, it is likely that no lesion will be seen and that serologic test results will remain negative.

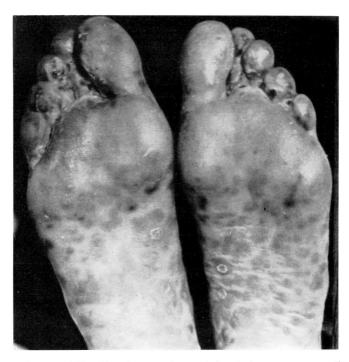

Fig. 4-5. Secondary syphilis. Macular-papular-pustular lesions appear on the feet. Early tentative diagnosis may be tinea pedis. (Courtesy Dr. R. M. Montgomery, New York, N. Y.)

If treatment occurs during the primary stage, before the serum becomes positive, then the chances are that the serum will remain negative and that the chancre will heal rapidly. If treatment does not begin until the secondary stage, from 90% to 95% of patients adequately treated will become serologically negative within 18 months. After the secondary stage, the effects of treatment upon the serologic reaction are variable. The longer a person's disease goes untreated, the longer adequate treatment takes to change the serologic reaction. If treatment begins two years or longer after infection, it may not be possible to obtain a negative serologic reaction at all.

Symptoms

Oral aspects of syphilis. In any phase of syphilis, the patient may be quite unaware that he has any surface lesions, even when they are easily observed in the mouth. These syphilitic lesions may, in other cases, be recognized as abnormalities, but incorrectly diagnosed. In one study of misdiagnoses in cases of extragenital syphilitic chancres, it was found that the following diseases had been named originally: tonsillitis, cellulitis, periapical abscess, infected submaxillary gland, submaxillary duct stone, gonorrheal stomatitis, tuberculosis, diphtheria, actinomycosis, aphthous ulcer, herpes zoster, and fusospirochetal infection. It is apparent, therefore, that the problem of diagnosis can be difficult. The following case history illustrates what may occur[36]: A 22-year-old soldier with complaints of painful gingiva and mild sore throat came into a U. S. Army dental dispensary for treatment. A lesion was found by the dentist that involved the interdental papilla between the maxillary left lateral and cuspid teeth. The rest of the mouth seemed normal. The dentist's initial impression was that this was a local inflammation from improper toothbrushing and massage. After eight days the lesion ap-

peared to be worse. At this point consultation with an oral surgeon was obtained. A total of six practitioners doing general dentistry, two oral surgeons, an otolaryngologist, and a general surgeon saw the patient without suspecting syphilis. Finally an oral pathologist examined biopsy material stained by a silver technique and saw spirochetes. This observation immediately suggested serologic study, which resulted in a definitive diagnosis of syphilis.

It is not surprising, therefore, that dentists as well as physicians have been known to acquire extragenital syphilitic infection from patients with unrecognized syphilis. There is some meager evidence indicating, in fact, that the dentist has suffered more in this respect than the physician. Figures from the Surgeon General's Office show that occupationally acquired syphilis has occurred about eight times more often among dentists than among physicians. Syphilitic infection transmitted from dentist to patient has also been known to occur.

Extragenital chancres. Extragenital chancres occur in from 4.5% to 12% of patients with primary lesions, with the lower incidence being characteristic of Negro series and the higher characteristic of white series. Chancre of the lips is the most common among these (Fig. 4-6), accounting for from 55% to 73% of extragenital cases. Other extragenital sites involved have been the mouth, hands, and breast. In the mouth, chancres have been reported on the tongue (5% to 14% of extragenital chancres), as well as to a lesser extent on the gums or tonsils. Transmission in these cases of extragenital infection may occur in kissing, by unusual sexual practices, by intermediate contact with drinking cups or glasses, eating utensils, the mouthpiece of musical instruments, or medical or dental instruments.

Secondary stage lesions. The oral lesions of the secondary stage sometimes precede the first eruption on the skin. The oral

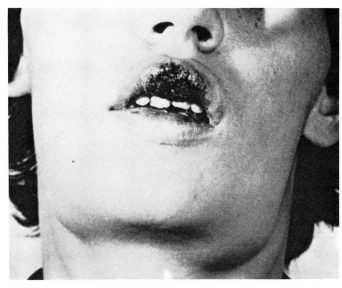

Fig. 4-6. Syphilitic chancre of the lip and lymphadenopathy. (Courtesy Dr. R. M. Montgomery, New York, N. Y.)

lesions, classically, consist of slightly raised, glistening, grayish-white, scaly, moist patches on the mucous membranes of the tonsils, soft palate, tongue, or cheek. The surface of these mucous patches is covered with a thin grayish membrane. Spirochetes swarm in these lesions and are highly infectious. In recent years, however, secondary syphilitic lesions of the mouth have been found that are atypical, a result of inadequate levels of antibiotic administered for a misdiagnosed infection.

Tertiary stage lesions. Oral lesions of the tertiary stage usually are not manifest for a year or so after the infection has started, but then they may last for years. The characteristic lesion is a tumor of granulomatous tissue referred to as a gumma. This late lesion may be single or multiple, and although the lips and the face are common sites for their appearance, the hard palate is the most common site[24] (Fig. 4-7). The nasal bones also appear to be especially liable to the development of syphilitic gummas. It has been suggested that localization in the inter-

maxillary bone may be the result of an anachoretic fixation of spirochetes at the apex of infected teeth. Treatment of the deformities resulting from syphilitic destruction of the palate is difficult. Dental prostheses help greatly by closing perforations that are large.[16]

In addition to the gumma of bone, two other forms of bone involvement in the tertiary stage are described: syphilitic osteomyelitis and ossifying syphilitic osteomyelitis. In syphilitic osteomyelitis extensive jaw involvement is more often found in the mandible than in the maxilla.[14] The clinical course in this type is characterized by pain, swelling, suppuration, and sequestration. This type often simulates in character the pyogenic osteomyelitis, which is more commonly found, but differs from it by a more progressive course, by a lack of improvement upon the usual form of treatment, and by a dramatic response to antisyphilitic drugs.[27] Radiographically, the syphilitic and pyogenic types of osteomyelitis resemble each other closely. They are seen as intrabony osteolytic areas with

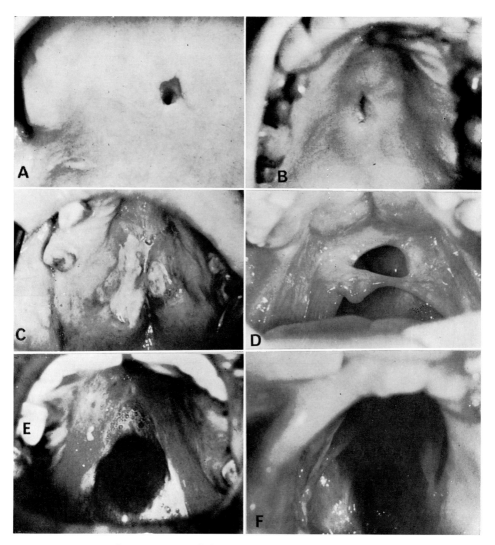

Fig. 4-7. A series of six gummas of the palate demonstrating different degrees of tissue destruction. In **A** there is a small area of destruction penetrating through mucosa and bone. In **B** the opening is not so deep, but the area of soft-tissue involvement is greater. In **C** there is extensive ulceration of palatal mucosa. In **D** there is soft palate involvement. In **E** and **F** the palatal destruction is extensive. (From Meyer, I., and Shklar, G.: Oral Surg. **23:**45, 1967.)

the regular radiopaque sequestra in them, and often with a marked periosteal osteoblastic response. The destructive process often proceeds to the point of pathologic fracture.

In ossifying syphilitic osteomyelitis the osteogenic reaction progresses to the point

that bony changes occur in the spongiosa, as well as in the periosteum. Because of this increased bone production, the disease may simulate osteogenic sarcoma radiographically.

Radiographic survey of bone involvement by syphilis in 67 known cases has

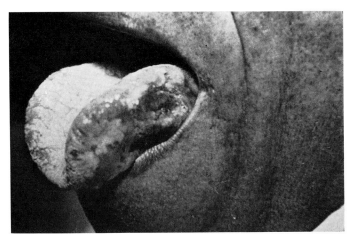

Fig. 4-8. Tertiary syphilis showing leukoplakia of the tongue and a cancerous lesion on the side of the tongue. (Courtesy Dr. R. M. Montgomery, New York, N. Y.)

shown that the tibia, clavicle, skull, and fibula were the most frequently involved. In two cases the mandible was involved, and in one case the facial bones.

Syphilitic glossitis develops in some cases of tertiary syphilis (Fig. 4-8). This affection may be divided into two groups: the superficial and the deep. The superficial type is usually associated with irritants such as smoking or drinking alcoholic beverages. The deep type consists of inflammatory tissue deep in the tongue that later causes scarring, fissuring, and the formation of irregular nodules on the tongue surface that give a highly characteristic picture. There is, commonly, marked enlargement of the tongue, so that it may fill up the entire mouth. An enlarged tongue, except in the case of edentulous patients, should suggest the possibility of syphilis.

The salivary glands rarely become involved at any stage of a syphilitic infection, but both secondary and tertiary lesions have been known to occur. Usually only the parotid gland is affected, but the other salivary glands may be involved, either alone or together with the parotid.

Congenital syphilis. In the United States 370 infants less than one year of age were

reported as having congenital syphilis in 1966.[13] Congenital syphilis[26] is an infection established by passage of the spirochete from mother to fetus through the placenta. Such an infection acquired before birth differs from an infection acquired in later years largely because it occurs in an immature and rapidly developing organism characterized by a general lack of resistance to infection. Syphilis in these early days of life is characterized by high mortality, in contrast to the marked chronicity of this infection in the adult. The most marked differences between congenital syphilis and syphilis acquired by an adult occur in the early stages of the infection. Practically all the lesions found in late syphilis in the adult may also occur as a result of old congenital syphilis. However, some differences are known. Keratitis, for example, which is common among children with congenital syphilis, is not common among those who are first infected after becoming an adult.

T. pallidum usually does not infect the fetus in a syphilitic mother before the fifth month of pregnancy. This immunity of the fetus is due in part, if not entirely, to the layer of Langhan's cells, which is intact until about the fourth month of gestation. The later the mother is infected, the shorter is the fetal period of infection, and thus the lesions at birth will be correspondingly less developed. In fact, there have been cases in which the mother's infection took place so late in pregnancy that the first visible symptoms in the infant did not appear until several weeks after birth. Not every syphilitic mother, however, gives the infection to her unborn child.

The conditions that first prompt the visit of a congenitaly syphilitic child to a clinic during the first two years of life include the following oral conditions: infiltration of the lips, sore mouth, and sores on the tongue. Clinical examination, however, shows that, actually, oral lesions are much more common than would be supposed from the complaints of the child.

The earliest lesions involving tissues that may come to the attention of the dentist develop in the very first two months of life; relatively few manifestations first appear as late as after the sixth month. These early lesions, in one series of cases studied, involved the lips of 80 out of 89 infants. The lesions about the lips develop into ulcerated fissures that eventually heal but leave scars radiating from the mouth. Known as rhagades, they are of considerable diagnostic value in patients to about 20 years of age, or when wrinkles begin to simulate these scars.

The dental lesions are a result of direct invasion of the tissue or organ by *T. pallidum*. Since calcification of the deciduous teeth is well developed by the time the treponemas have invaded the dental organs, these teeth are only minimally affected. Invasion by the treponemas of the permanent tooth buds may result in either complete failure of development of a tooth or the production of characteristic structural defects. Pathologic studies of dental tissues from congenitally infected fetuses indicate that on invasion of the dental organ by the treponemas, the inflamma-

tory reaction that follows results in tissue destruction. The ameloblasts appear to be more sensitive to this process than the odontoblasts. Treponemal effects upon local blood vessels supplying the dental buds also may be responsible for a part of the defects that arise.

The structure of the crown is usually altered according to the stage of calcification at the time of the start of the infection in the body. Delayed eruption and anomalies of shape, structure, and number of the teeth may occur. The most common manifestation is hypoplasia of the occlusal surfaces, usually of the first molars, and very commonly of all four first molars. There may also be an irregular, roughened surface, poorly developed cusps, and a dirty yellow color. These defective first molars are referred to as mulberry molars and are more or less characteristic and diagnostic of congenital syphilis.

Especially striking, and also of considerable diagnostic value, is the defect known as Hutchinson's teeth, since they were first described by Jonathan Hutchinson in 1856. These consist of the upper central incisors, which show crescentic notching at the incisal edge and a greater mesiodistal dimension at the gingival than at the incisal end of the crown. This gives a peg-shaped or screwdriver appearance to the tooth. These incisors usually appear to be wide apart. The disturbance is caused by a hypoplasia that results in the retraction of the middle lobe at the incisal edge (Fig. 4-9). In almost half of the cases in one investigation, the dental stigmata were found to occur on one side only. The changes are distinctive enough to allow diagnosis of congenital syphilis from the radiograms of unerupted teeth.[4]

Maxillary incisors that have been affected from congenital syphilis, when closely examined, may be graded into four groups[26] designated as: H[1], H[2], H[2-3], and H[3]. In the H[1] tooth the mesiodistal edges are parallel, or converge slightly, the in-

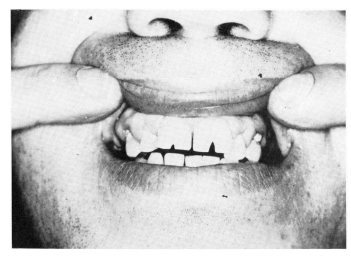

Fig. 4-9. Congenital syphilis is sometimes manifested by notched, bell-shaped incisors. (Courtesy Dr. I. W. Scopp, Veterans Administration Hospital, New York, N. Y.)

cisal edge is straight, and the corners are rounded. Such teeth are not diagnostic of syphilis but are sufficiently suggestive to justify a suspicion of the disease and a thorough search. The H^2 tooth is much narrower than H^1, or it may be barrel- or oat-shaped with a slightly concave incisal edge, or it may be shaped like a screwdriver or chisel. H^3 is the typical hutchinsonian tooth just described.

In some few cases there may also be complete absence of the upper lateral incisors, which increases the degree of malocclusion; when the upper lateral incisors are present, they may show narrowing toward the incisal edge.

In addition to the dental changes, congenital syphilis may also produce a peculiar open bite deformity. In this condition, there is no contraction of the anterior region to produce crowding of the teeth, nor is there evidence of failure of proper dental eruption. The deformity, rather, seems to be of the teeth, as well as their supporting bony structures, lacking in enough substance to bring them into proper occlusal relations.[34] There is a lack of development of the upper jaw that is common to all types of congenital syphilitic

faces in a greater or lesser degree, the so-called syphilitic facies.[30] The maxillary processes are foreshortened so that they must grow upwards and inwards in order to form the upper jaw, thus preventing approximation. The lower jaw thus seems to jut out, producing the dished appearance of the face.

A great proportion of syphilitic babies (approximately 70%) develop a rhinitis that is often of severity great enough to force mouth breathing for a long period, with possible undesirable effects upon oral structures, and especially the growing jaws.

In general, the dental deformities are the most important of the stigmata of congenital syphilis on account of their relative frequency and distinctive characteristics. Certain other lesions may also be observed that may aid in detecting congenital syphilis. These especially are the two other signs, which with the incisors are referred to as Hutchinson's triad: interstitial keratitis of the eyes and eighth nerve deafness. Because of the variety of visible stigmata, it is seldom necessary to make a presumptive diagnosis on the sign alone, but in all cases a study of the blood serum is necessary.

TREPONEMA PERTENUE: YAWS

Treponema pertenue is the etiologic agent of yaws[3] and is similar in its form and structure to *T. pallidum.* The initial lesion of the disease in most cases occurs on the feet or legs from three to four weeks after exposure. A painless red papule surrounded by an erythematous inflammatory zone becomes ulcerated and is called the "mother yaw." Darkfield examination of exudate from the lesion (yaw fluid) shows the presence of numerous spirochetes.

Similar to the syphilis chancre, the "mother yaw" heals and some individuals may have no subsequent syptoms and apparently are immune. Most of the diseased individuals, however, after a few weeks or months of freedom from symptoms, develop secondary lesions or "daughter yaws" of the skin and mucous membranes. Again, these lesions may disappear or may continue as ulcers, or a new exacerbation of lesions occurs. Papules and a hyperkeratosis are found frequently on the soles of the feet and the palms of the hands. Similar to the syphilitic syndrome, later sequelae may involve the bones and joints and appear as gummas of various organs and the skin, including the palate and nose.

Yaws is rarely found in temperate climates but is endemic to various parts of South and Central America, the West Indies, Africa, the Pacific Islands, and Australia. The tropic climate (high temperature and heavy rain fall) is apparently an ecologic factor. The disease occurs primarily in the lower socioeconomic strata that have poor hygienic conditions. The disease in most instances is nonvenereal and is transmitted by direct contact with lesions that occur primarily on the limbs and the face. Genital lesions are found in less than 5% of those affected with yaws. Countries to which the disease is endemic may have large numbers of the population infected, particularly children or young adults. Dissemination also occurs through flies feeding on the ulcers; the spirochetes are ingested into the fly's foregut and regurgitated into a bite of another human being.

Treatment with long-acting penicillin is very effective, often requiring only a single injection.

TREPONEMA CARATEUM: PINTA

The etiologic agent of pinta[22] is *T. carateum,* similar in structure and form to *T. pallidum.* Pinta begins as a papule on the skin that after a few months to a year is surrounded by an area of varying pigmentation. Since the disease is prevalent in Mexico, Colombia, Africa, parts of the Philippines, and the Middle East where the populations are predominately dark-skinned, the depigmented areas contrast vividly with the normal skin. As in syphilis, secondary and tertiary stages may develop. During the secondary stage, numerous papules as well as skin rashes and hyperpigmented and hypopigmented skin areas are observed. Tertiary lesions may appear several years later and often involve the palms of the hands and the soles of the feet where both papular and hyperkeratotic lesions occur. Disturbances in the circulation and central nervous system may accompany the skin lesions.

Pinta is not a veneral disease. It is transmitted by direct contact with lesions on various parts of the body or by the transportation of the treponema by flies feeding on the lesions and carrying the spirochete to another person. Both the Wassermann and the flocculation tests routinely used in the diagnosis of syphilis will give positive reactions. *T. carateum* has not been cultivated, and attempts to infect animals have not been successful.

Penicillin is very effective in treatment, as it is in yaws.

NEISSERIA

Neisseria constitutes a small group of closely related gram-negative, aerobic cocci found universally as bacterial parasites of the mucous membranes. Of the several species that have been described, two are highly pathogenic for man, *Neisseria gonorrhoeae* and *N. meningitidis;* but the normally saprophytic species that reside in the oral cavity and upper respiratory tract have a low degree of virulence, which may be expressed when an opportunity allows it.

Much of the bacteriologic study of the oral and upper-resiratory tract species has been motivated by the need to make an accurate identification of *N. meningitidis.* Most species of *Neisseria* grow best on media containing blood or serum; they are not active fermenters of sugars, as a rule; and they often have exacting temperature requirements for growth. Transformation experiments and DNA base determinations have shown that *Neisseria* species can be divided into two subgroups. One of these includes *N. gonorrhoeae, N. meningitidis, N. sicca,* and *N. flava.* The second subgroup, which consists of *N. catarrhalis, N. ovis,* and *N. caviae,* seems to have a close relationship to *Moraxella.*[12]

Some organisms of the *Neisseria* (*N. flava* group), which characteristically occur in the nasopharynx, produce pigmented colonies. The significant fermentation reactions useful for distinguishing the more clinically important species are given in Table 4-1, although it must be kept in mind that these reactions are frequently capricious. Certain strains of *N. meningitidis,* for example, may not ferment maltose, while other strains giving typical fermentation reactions for the meningo-

cocci cannot be placed in established serologic groups.

Neisseria gonorrhoeae: Gonorrhea

The gonococcus[11] was first described by Neisser (1879), when he observed it in the purulent secretion from patients with urethritis and newborn infants with conjunctivitis. The organism was first isolated in pure culture in 1885 by Bumm, who also succeeded in causing gonorrhea in human volunteers by inoculation of the pure culture.

The gonococcus, as typically seen in pus, occurs in large numbers as paired organisms in the cytoplasm of polymorphonuclear leukocytes. The adjacent sides of a pair are flattened, giving them a coffee-bean appearance; in diameter they range from 0.6 to 0.8 micron, while in length they range from 0.8 to 1.6 microns. Other cytologic features include the absence of spores, flagella, and capsule, and a negative gram-staining reaction.

In order to establish a diagnosis of gonorrhea, the demonstration of gram-negative diplococci within the polymorphonuclear leukocytes of the exudate (Fig. 4-10) is highly suggestive, but it is essential to isolate and identify the organism. Cultivation of the gonococcus is difficult, especially for initial isolation, requiring special enriched medium with the antibiotics vancomycin, colistimethate, and nystatin to suppress contaminants (Thayer-Martin medium) and an increased carbon dioxide concentrations (from 5% to 10%) in the atmosphere of a moist culture jar.[39]

Table 4-1. Fermentation reactions of some species of *Neisseria*

Species	Dextrose	Maltose	Sucrose	Levulose	Mannitol
N. gonorrhoeae	+	−	−	−	−
N. meningitidis	+	+	−	−	−
N. sicca	+	+	+	+	−
N. catarrhalis	−	−	−	−	−
N. flava	+	+	−	+	−

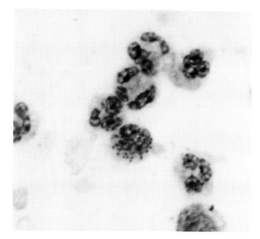

Fig. 4-10. Polymorphonuclear leukocyte with phagocytized gonococci.

Surface colonies on the plates are small, translucent, and grayish-white, but different strains of gonococci vary considerably in the size, consistency, and other physical properties of their colonies. Gonococci in culture do not have the typical form seen in the purulent exudate from patients, but may appear in somewhat oval pairs or as rounded individuals. Their positive indophenol oxidase reaction is useful for preliminary selection from primary plates of clinical specimens. This species is usually sensitive to penicillin.

Clinical picture

Genitourinary aspects. As a venereal disease, the organism is most commonly deposited directly upon the genitourinary mucosa during sexual intercourse. The bacterium penetrates into the tissue between the epithelial cells. On reaching the subepithelial connective tissue, it spreads either by direct continuity or through the lymphatic and blood vessels. The locally infected tissue develops an intense inflammatory reaction involving all the layers of the invaded site. There is an outpouring of polymorphonuclear leukocytes with phagocytized gonococci into the urethral lumen, in the case of the male, together with exuded blood serum and secreted

mucus. These are the constituents of the pus characteristic of the early stages of the disease. Additional symptoms are itching and burning in the urethra, and even great pain if the urethral inflammation is pronounced. Infection may extend into the bladder and if untreated, it passes to a chronic state in which the gonococci may be found in limited sites, but especially the prostate gland. In women, the urethra also is the most commonly infected initial site, but the more complex array of structures at subsequent risk makes the infection more widespread and the possible consequences quite serious. Since the structures at risk are within the abdomen, the infection is not as easily noted, and the subject may, in fact, be unaware of the disease. Chronic infections may progress through the entire genitourinary tract to involve the fallopian tubes and ovaries, from which site the peritoneum may be infected.

Oral aspects. Although the gonococcus usually infects the mucous membrane of the genitourinary tract, it is capable of directly infecting the oral mucosa under some circumstances. Normally, the oral mucosa has great resistance against gonorrheal infection, even in the case of newborn infants. Gonorrheal conjunctivitis, in contrast, acquired from the mother during birth, is such a frequent and serious infection that all states require prophylactic treatment with 1% silver nitrate of every infant's eyes immediately following birth. In recent years there has been some shift toward the use of penicillin or tetracycline solution for prophylaxis because of the chemical irritation from the silver nitrate, but it nevertheless remains the drug of choice.[1] Gonorrheal stomatitis rarely occurs among infants and may be overcome without difficulty or permanent scarring. In some instances gonococci have been cultured from oral specimens only to be found to have disappeared without treatment and without any apparent ill effects upon the infant.

Primary infection of the mouth, parotid gland, or the pharynx usually occurs in adults as a result of abnormal sexual practices (coitus *ab ore* or cunnilingus),[23] but it may occur by self-inoculation from a genital infection via the fingers. The incubation period for oral infections usually is accelerated, although it may vary from one to seven days. The oral lesions usually consist of round, slightly elevated, gray-white spots scattered over the tongue, soft palate, and cheeks. They vary in size from that of a pinhead to that of a pea. The lesions are eroded. The tongue is swollen, red, and dry; the oral mucosa has an itching and burning sensation; and the breath is foul. Infection of the parotid gland may occur secondarily, especially following surgery, but it is quite rare. Isolation of gonococci from the pharynx in some cases of pharyngitis has been reported, but in other instances gonococci have been isolated when no symptoms of pharynigitis are present.[31,38]

Diagnosis of gonorrheal stomatitis is possible from examination of oral smears taken at the onset of the disease and from the case history, in connection with the clinical findings.[5] Diagnosis, however, is complicated for these oral lesions by the presence of normally occurring nonpathogenic *Neisseria* organisms of the upper respiratory tract and oral cavity, so that for a confirmed diagnosis cultural studies in the bacteriologic laboratory for the causative agent must be undertaken. The organism is usually found to be sensitive to penicillin, although in recent years resistance has developed.

In the common genital infections, the gonococci have penetrated well below the surface epithelium by the time clinical symptoms have appeared. This is in from three to five days after exposure. The bacteria go on to invade the bloodstream and set up metastatic lesions. Most common among these is arthritis.[18] Before the advent of chemotherapy, roughly from 2% to 5% of individuals with gonorrhea developed arthritis.[9] In view of its present epidemic incidence and the large proportion of untreated cases, it is likely that a larger amount of gonococcal arthritis exists than is recognized. It has been estimated that perhaps as much as five times more gonorrheal arthritis occurs than all other types of acute bacterial arthritis combined. The age distribution of gonococcal arthritis corresponds closely with the period of greatest sexual activity, although the age range is quite great. In one large series of cases, 70% of the patients with this arthritis were between the ages of 20 and 39 years.

Gonococcal arthritis usually appears from one to three weeks after the acute genital infection, but it may appear concurrently or may not manifest itself for months or years after the genital attack. An arthritic infection starts with invasion of the synovial tissue by the gonococcus, although viable gonococci have been found in only from 25% to 30% of the synovial fluids examined bacteriologically. The knee is most commonly involved, but the temporomandibular joint is occasionally infected. There is some evidence perhaps indicating that the temporomandibular joint is especially apt to become involved if the primary gonorrheal infection is pharyngeal.[23]

In one series of fifty cases of gonococcal arthritis at the Johns Hopkins Hospital, two had involvement of the temporomandibular joint. Actually, any joint may be involved, and in most cases the infection is polyarticular. It occurs most often in the female, and often in the homosexual male. This pattern lies in contrast to the pre-antibiotic era when men with gonococcal arthritis often outnumbered women by as many as three to one.

The clinical symptoms at the onset of gonorrheal arthritis usually appear rapidly, being preceded by a chill and accompanied by fever. At first the process may be a polyarthritis, but shortly it localizes in one or, rarely, more joints, which becomes acutely swollen and inflamed. The tendons about the affected joints may also be involved, especially those of the small joints of the hands and feet. Symmetric joints usually are not affected. The joint fluid contains a high cell count with a preponderance of polymorphonuclear leukocytes; gonococci may often be recovered by bacteriologic culture techniques and less commonly be seen in smear.

In the case of gonococcal arthritis of the temporomandibular joint, local manifestations consist of spasms of the masseter muscles, difficulty in opening the mouth, and inflammatory signs in and around the involved joint.[17] The joint fluid is cloudy, polymorphonnuclear leukocytes are present, and culture yields *N. gonorrhoeae*.[23] In some cases perforation through the tympanic plate may occur, with exudation into the external auditory meatus; this condition may be mistaken for otitis media.[40] Untreated gonorrheal arthritis tends to progress to a destruction of the articular cartilage and to fibrous ankylosis of the joint.[35] Prompt and accurate diagnosis is necessary, including differentiation from Reiter's disease, to avoid this possibility. Intramuscular injection of penicillin is quite effective in treatment, especially if it is given before irreversible destruction of joint tissue has occurred.

A second form of gonococcal arthritis is recognized that is now more common than the metastatic type. It follows repeated gonococcal infections, but the pathogenesis is poorly understood. The onset tends to be less acute than the metastatic type, and there is a tendency for the involvement of symmetric joints. The clinical course tends to be chronic, and progressive involvement of new joints is common. Gonococci are never obtained from the joint fluid, and penicillin does not appreciably affect the course of this arthritis. It is consider by many investigators that this form is a manifestation of rheumatoid arthritis, with the gonococcus setting the process in motion. Management is that for rheumatoid arthritis in general.

Genital gonorrhea, in some few cases, may lead to secondary dermatologic infections with several possible types of lesions. One type consists of direct primary infection from the gonorrheal exudate, which leads to ulceration or an abscess-like process, often with considerable tissue breakdown; gonococci are readily demonstrable. Autoinfection of the mouth by way of the fingers is included in this group.

Another type of lesion is typically seen in what is referred to as the "gonococcal dermatitis syndrome."[6] In this case there are septic symptoms of fever from blood-borne gonococci. A dermatitis appears, accompanied by arthritis, as a result of small infarctions from the gonococci. The lesions usually are vesiculopustular, sometimes hemorrhagic, few in number, and they occur especially on the extremities. Gonococci either are not culturally demonstrable or are detected for only a short time. Immunofluorescent antibody techniques, however, will demonstrate gonococci in the skin lesions, although usually with distorted morphologic traits. The face is usually spared, but the oral cavity is among the sites that may be implicated. The tongue[6] may develop an ulcer at the same time that the patient becomes arthritic, acquires a skin rash, and feels a general malaise. Such symptoms, however, require careful study to determine whether or not syphilis is the real cause. The mucosa of either the soft palate or the hard palate may be affected by bloodborne gonococci.[2] In one such case, in which gonococci were grown from the blood, the soft palate was found to have a few small vesicles surrounded by an erythematous halo.

A third form of gonococcal dermatosis is so-called keratosis blennorrhagica, or gonorrheal keratosis.[33] This is a chronic inflammatory dermatosis occurring in conjunction with gonorrheal infection of the genital tract and the joints. It is characterized by an eruption of horny (hyperkeratotic), conical nodules, pustules, and thick, brownish crusts on various parts of the body. The oral and pharyngeal mucosae may develop intensely red, sharply circumscribed, hornlike, raised plaques. The oral lesions may involve the palate, gingiva, and cheeks.

Some investigators are of the opinion that these mucosal and dermatologic lesions include a localized allergic ("id") reaction to the bacterial antigens as a component in the pathogenesis of the lesions. Herpes labialis has been observed occasionally in general gonococcal infections and, in fact, occurs more frequently in such cases than it does in typhoid fever.

Extragenital cutaneous gonorrhea in adults may occur with no indication of genital infection. Such cases have included infection of the inframammary region, the thigh, the hand, and the glans penis (without concurrent urethritis). It is a remarkable fact that gonococci very rarely directly attack the skin.

The rare reports of gonococcal infection of the upper respiratory tract,[10] including the oral cavity, are puzzling in view of the great, uncontrolled, epidemic incidence of gonorrhea. It is possible in some cases that they have been overlooked or dismissed as a trivial "cold." Greater alertness to its possible occurrence, closer study of the oral cavity by microscopic and bacteriologic culturing methods, and more attention to obtaining a full case history may well result in a different epidemiologic judgment than holds at present.

Therapy[32]

For a quarter of a century, penicillin has been the recognized drug of choice for treatment for gonorrhea except in allergic persons. There has developed recently, however, a great rate of failure with existing recommended schedules because of increasing resistance to the antibiotic. At the present time, approximately 5 million units of penicillin are necessary in a single dose, whereas dosages of less than 100,000 units of penicillin had cured in the 1940s. In addition to increasing the amount of penicillin administered, trials in which probenecid is combined with penicillin are currently being made to retard penicillin excretion in the urine, thus intensifying its action.

Indigenous Neisseria organisms of the oral cavity

The saprophytic *Neisseria* organisms that occur in the oral cavity and upper respiratory tract present occasional problems when isolates may require differentiation from *N. gonorrhoeae* or *N. meningitidis*. Under some circumstances, also, these normally saprophytic bacteria have been identified as the only microorganisms present in extremely serious infections. Subacute bacterial endocarditis, for example, may be caused by *N. pharyngis* following the extraction of teeth.[15] Fatal purulent meningitis, with cerebral abscesses, has been reportedly caused by *N. crassus* in the case of a young adult with extensive oral sepsis[19]; the autopsy findings indicated that the brain infection had probably occurred by direct extension from the upper jaw. Infection of the parotid gland with *N. catarrhalis* has occurred following a blow from the fist upon the gland. A localized granulomatous infection of the tongue has been observed, with the typical appearance of botryomycosis, from which were isolated several typical oral bacteria, including *N. catarrhalis*. Very possibly, in this last case, the lesion resulted from a mixed infection, involving the interactions of the several bacteria present. There is suggestive evidence that in some instances of dental plaque that is pigmented, the color may be produced by certain oral chromagenic *Neisseria* organisms. Carious mouths appear to have a characteristic population of *Neisseria* organisms consisting of nonpigmented strains,[25] with abundant catalase, which fail to produce a copious amount of polysaccharide on 5% sucrose agar. Many of the strains isolated from noncarious mouths, on the contrary, produce copious polysaccharide on sucrose agar and are not as apt to produce catalase.

CITED REFERENCES

1. Benenson, A. S. (ed.): Control of communicable diseases in man, ed. 11, New York, 1970, The American Public Health Association.
2. Berman, L.: Über einen Fall von gonorrhöischer Keratose der Haut und Mundschleimhaut, Dermat. Z. **51**:420, 1928.
3. Butler, C. S.: Diagnosis and treatment of yaws, Int. Clin., series 40, **2**:1, 1930.
4. Cohen, M. M.: Dental stigmata in congenital syphilis, Dent. Radiogr. Photogr. **27**:24, 1954.
5. Copping, A. A.: Stomatitis caused by gonococcus, J. Amer. Dent. Assoc. **49**:567, 1954.
6. Cowan, L.: Gonococcal ulceration of the tongue in the gonococcal dermatitis syndrome, Brit. J. Vener. Dis. **45**:228, 1969.
7. Darkfield microscopy for the detection and identification of *Treponema pallidum*, bulletin 990, Public Health Service, 1962.
8. Dennie, C. G.: A history of syphilis, Springfield, Ill., 1962, Charles C Thomas, Publisher.
9. Dowling, H. F.: The acute bacterial diseases, their diagnosis and treatment, Philadelphia, 1948, W. B. Saunders Co., p. 241.
10. Fiumara, N. J.: Gonorrheal pharyngitis, New Eng. J. Med. **276**:1248, 1967.
11. Garson, W., and Thayer, J. D.: The gonococcus. In Dubos, R. J. (ed.): Bacterial and mycotic infections of man, ed. 3, Philadelphia, 1958, J. B. Lippincott Co.
12. Henriksen, S. D., and Bøvre, K.: The taxonomy of the genera *Moraxella* and *Neisseria*, J. Gen. Microbiol. **51**:387, 1968.
13. Herweg, J. C., Hoffmann, F. D., and Reed, C. A.: Pediatric use of the rapid plasma reagin (circle) card test, Pediatrics **40**:440, 1967.
14. Heslop, I. H.: Syphilitic osteomyelitis of the mandible, Brit. J. Oral Surg. **6**:59, 1968.
15. Hudson, R.: *Neisseria pharyngis* bacteriaemia in a patient with subacute bacterial endocarditis, J. Clin. Path. **10**:195, 1957.
16. Keogh, C., and King, A.: Syphilis of the mouth and upper respiratory tract, Practitioner **177**:691, 1956.
17. Kerr, D. A., Ash, M. M., Jr., and Millard, H. D.: Oral diagnosis, St. Louis, 1959, The C. V. Mosby Co., p. 260.
18. Kushner, I.: Gonococcal arthritis, Med. Times **98**:111, 1970.
19. Losli, E. J., and Lindsey, R. H.: Fatal systemic diseases from dental sepsis, Oral Surg. **16**:366, 1963.
20. Lucatorto, F. M., Katz, B. D., and Toto, P. D.: A rapid macroscopic screening test for syphilis. II. Further evaluation, J. Amer. Dent. Assoc. **73**:100, 1966.
21. Manual of tests for syphilis, bulletin 411, Public Health Service, 1969.
22. Marquez, F., Rein, C. R., and Areas, O.: Mal del pintoin in Mexico, Bull. W. H. O. **13**:299, 1955.
23. Metzger, A. L.: Gonococcal arthritis complicating gonorrheal pharyngitis, Ann. Intern. Med. **73**:267, 1970.
24. Meyer, I., and Shklar, G.: The oral manifestations of acquired syphilis, Oral Surg. **23**:45, 1967.
25. Morris, E. O.: The bacteriology of the oral cavity, Brit. Dent. J. **96**:259, 1954.
26. Nabarro, D.: Congenital syphilis, London, 1954, Edward Arnold (Publishers) Ltd.
27. Nathan, A. S., and Lawson, W.: Syphilitic osteomyelitis of the mandible, Oral Surg. **17**:284, 1964.
28. Pillot, J.: La culture des tréponemes, Ann. Inst. Pasteur **103**:231, 373, 1962.
29. Portnoy, J., Brewer, J. H., and Harris, A.: A rapid plasma reagin card test for syphilis and other treponematoses, Public Health Rep. **76**:645, 1962.

30. Robinson, R. C. V.: Congenital syphilis, Arch. Derm. **99**:599, 1969.
31. Schmidt, H., Hjørting-Hansen, E., and Philipsen, H. P.: Gonococcal stomatitis, Acta Dermatovener. **41**:324, 1961.
32. Schroeter, A. L., and Pazin, G. J.: Gonorrhea, Ann. Intern. Med. **72**:553, 1970.
33. Sherman, W. L., Blumenthal, F., and Heidenreich, J.: Blennorrhagic balanitiform keratoderma: Report of three additional cases, including one of buccal involvement, Arch. Derm. Syph. **39**:422, 1939.
34. Stathers, F. R.: Conditions of occlusion of teeth in congenital syphilis, J. Dent. Res. **13**: 196, 1933.
35. Steindler, A.: Pyogenic arthritis, Bull. N. Y. Acad. Med. **27**:101, 1951.
36. Steiner, M., and Alexander, W. N.: Primary syphilis of the gingiva, Oral Surg. **21**:530, 1966.
37. Syphilis, a synopsis, bulletin 1660, Atlanta, Georgia, 1968, Public Health Service.
38. Thatcher, R. W., McCraney, W. T., Kellogg, D. S., Jr., and Whaley, W. H.: Asymptomatic gonorrhea, J.A.M.A. **210**:315, 1969.
39. Thayer, J. D., and Martin, J. E.: Improved medium selective for cultivation of *N. gonorrhoeae* and *N. meningitidis,* Public Health Rep. **81**:559, 1966.
40. Thoma, K. H., and Goldman, H. M.: Oral pathology, ed. 5, St. Louis, 1960, The C. V. Mosby Co.
41. Thomas, E. W.: Syphilis: Its course and management, New York, 1949, The Macmillan Company.
42. Today's VD control problem, a joint statement, New York, 1968, American Social Health Association.
43. Turner, T. B., and Diseker, T. H.: Duration of infectivity of *Treponema pallidum* in citrated blood stored under condition obtaining in blood banks, Bull. Johns Hopkins Hosp. **68**:269, 1941.
44. Willcox, R. R., and Guthe, T.: *Treponema pallidum*: A bibliographical review of the morphology, culture, and survival of *T. pallidum* and associated organisms, Bull. W. H. O. **35**(suppl.), 1966.

REFERENCES AND ADDITIONAL READINGS

Fournier, A.: The treatment and prophylaxis of syphilis, ed. 2, New York, 1907, Rebman Company.

Holcomb, R. C.: Pinta, a treponematosis: Review of the literature, U. S. Naval Med. Bull. **40**:517, 1942.

Hudson, E. H.: Non-venereal syphilis: A sociological and medical study of bejel, Edinburgh, 1958, Livingstone.

Hudson, E. H.: Treponematosis, New York, 1946, Oxford University Press, Inc.

Hutchison, J.: Syphilis, New York, 1913, Funk & Wagnalls Co., Inc.

Jeans, P. C., and Cooke, J. V.: Prepubescent syphilis, New York, 1930, D. Appleton and Company.

Morton, R. S.: Venereal diseases, Harmondsworth, England, 1966, Penguin Books Ltd.

Youmans, J. B. (ed.): Syphilis and other venereal diseases, a symposium, Med. Clin. N. Amer. **48**: No. 3, 1964.

5 / Viruses, rickettsiae, and chlamydiae

VIRUSES

The developments in the methodology of human virology that have occurred in the past two decades have led to an enormous expansion of knowledge concerning these minute obligate intracellular parasites.[26] This new technology includes the electron microscope, a number of powerful biochemical techniques, cultivation in the embryonated egg and in tissue culture, and certain methods developed for the study of the bacterial viruses. This technology exposes many possibilities for experimental approaches in the study of the virus-host relationship among the animal viruses.

Notable among the advances thus made possible is the identification of a large number of previously unknown viruses. The first virus infection of animals was described in 1898. By 1910, only a handful of human diseases, notably smallpox, rabies, yellow fever, dengue, sandfly fever, and poliomyelitis, were known to be caused by viruses. By 1940, about 45 virus diseases were known. Within the past 20 years, in contrast to this slow start, more than 300 additional viruses have been uncovered.

Size and shape. The very small size of the viruses requires that they be studied with the electron microscope. It is found in this manner that there is wide variation in size among the different viruses, but that they may be similar in size within specific groups characterized by host or tissue spec-

ificities (Table 5-1). The shape of the virus may vary from the rod form of tobacco mosaic virus to the spheric form of poliovirus.

Structure. The virion (virus particle) structure consists of a central core, or nucleoid, containing either DNA or RNA, but not both. A protective coat of protein surrounds the core and is referred to as the capsid. The symmetrically distributed subunits of the capsid are the capsomeres, which are protein structures. Although a complete virus may consist simply of the nucleoid core and its capsid (the nucleocapsid), more complex virions also have a surrounding envelope.

Cultivation. Since viruses are obligate intracellular parasites, the culture methods used in the laboratory must rely upon living host cells, either the living animal, embryonated eggs, or tissue cultures. Each virus appears to invade a certain organ or tissue preferentially, and even to have a certain cell type in which it multiplies best. However, under suitable conditions, most viruses seem to be able to invade, multiply in, and even destroy a broad variety of tissue types. These special tissue requirements for a virus have resulted in the use of many different tissues for laboratory cultivations, among which currently are monkey, dog, or baby hamster kidney and human tracheal epithelium.

Multiplication. The viruses are not true

Table 5-1. Relative sizes of viruses*

	Approximate diameter (millimicrons)†
Red blood cells	7,500
Basophilic viruses	300 to 450
Poxviruses	250
Rabies virus	150
Syncytial viruses	100 to 140
Herpesviruses	110 to 120
Myxoviruses	100
Bacterial viruses	25 to 100
Adenoviruses	80
Reoviruses	75
Papovaviruses	45
Enteroviruses	28
Arborviruses	20 to 40
Hepatitis viruses	12 to 18
Certain plant viruses	17 to 30
Serum albumin molecule	5

*From Smith, A. L.: Principles of microbiology, ed. 5, St. Louis, 1965, The C. V. Mosby Co.
†1 millimicron = 1/1,000 micron. 1 micron = 1/1,000 millimeter

cells since they lack organelles such as ribosomes, and hence have no metabolism of their own. They must rely on the organelles, energy, and many of the enzymes of the host cell for their replication. The replication of the virion depends upon the genetic information in its nucleic acid core being inserted into the information that the host cell reads for its own activity. As a consequence, part of the host cell's synthetic capacity is taken over by the virion to produce virus particles. In a sense, therefore, the parasitized cell becomes a virus-producing factory.

Virulence. To the general virologist, the term "virulence" refers to the effect of the virus on the individual cell, whereas to the clinician it refers to the abnormal clinical effects of a viral infection. The difference in emphasis is important, for a large number of cells may become infected before clinical symptoms are apparent. It is estimated, for example, that in monkeys experimentally infected with poliovirus as many as 60% of the anterior horn cells supplying nerve fibers to a given muscle may be de-

stroyed before muscle weakness can be detected.

Effect of virus on the host cell. Invasion and multiplication of the virus within the host cell can cause either destruction, altered function, proliferation, or no change. Depending upon the physiologic condition of the cell, the same virus may cause any one of these effects.

Inclusions may be found in host cells infected by a virus. The inclusion body may be located within the nucleus or in the cytoplasm. Intranuclear inclusions have been found with such diseases as herpes simplex, zoster, yellow fever, and poliomyelitis. Intracytoplasmic inclusions may be found in the neuron cells of rabid animals and in smallpox lesions. Most viral inclusions are either eosinophilic or acidophilic when subjected to a polychrome stain. As a general rule, inclusion bodies may be considered to be colonies of viral particles, although not all cell inclusion bodies are produced by viruses.

Certain viral diseases evoke inclusion bodies that are diagnostic and have been named after their discoverers. Cytoplasmic inclusions found in smallpox and vaccinia are known as Guarnieri's bodies; the inclusions caused by rabies virus in neurons are Negri bodies; and the inclusions in the nuclei of epithelial cells infected by herpesvirus hominis are known as Lipschütz bodies.

Mutations. A certain proportion of the new virus particles produced in the host cells will contain genetic material slightly different from the others. New biologic properties may emerge from these changes that may significantly affect their virulence.

Stability of viruses. Resistance to heat, drying, and ultraviolet irradiation is an important factor in determining virus survival in nature. The infectivity of viruses generally disappears after heating at from 50° to 60° C. for 30 minutes, although there are some important exceptions. Serum hepatitis virus, for example, can withstand prolonged storage at elevated temperatures and under drying conditions; adenosatellite virus also has great resistance to heat. Smallpox virus in dried vesicle fluid and crusts has been known to cause the infection in many cases. In the dry state, viruses are more resistant to heat than in the normal hydrated state.

Diagnosis Nearly all viral pathogens require laboratory analysis for establishment of a firm diagnosis.[60] Three types of laboratory examinations are employed: (1) microscopy of tissues or cell spreads; (2) serologic tests to detect the presence of specific antibodies; and (3) isolation and identification of the etiologic agent. Of these procedures, microscopic examination is the simplest, the serologic tests are the most economic, and virus isolation is the most difficult and expensive.

Serologic methods of either complement fixation or hemagglutination inhibition techniques are probably the most readily available of the methods used for establishing a diagnosis of viral infection since they are technically feasible for any routine laboratory. It is necessary to obtain at least two blood samples in order to determine whether there is a rising titer or not since the presence of specific antibody is not necessarily the result of the current disease. The first sample is obtained as early as possible after the patient comes to the practitioner, and the second is obtained after convalescence.

Generally speaking, viral diagnostic tests are not requested because of the time lag between submission of the specimen and receipt of the laboratory report. There are times, however, when the diagnosis is prompt enough to be of practical value, such as when there is an effective vaccine available against such diseases as rabies, influenza, and poliomyelitis. Moreover, a diagnosis will aid the physician in the recognition and the management of similar cases in the future. Valuable basic epidemiologic and etiologic data are also obtained from laboratory diagnosis that are needed for the eventual control of virus diseases by vaccines.

Therapy. The most effective and economic procedure available for the prevention and control[62] of acute viral diseases is specific immunization by vaccines. Live-virus vaccines have generally been found to be most satisfactory if the antigenic types of the virus are few in number, if there is systemic invasion of the host, and if lifelong immunity follows natural infection as a rule. In those diseases in which the antigenic types of the causative virus are numerous and in which immunity is not lasting, control is best obtained by the use of killed-virus vaccines, especially in association with immunologic adjuvants that enhance the immune response.

Specific control of viral infections may possibly be attained by enhancement of host resistance. It has been found that virus-infected cells have a so-called interferon system, which is divisible into several components.[7] The cells produce a protein of low molecular weight, called interferon, which protects new and uninfected cells from viral infection by inducing the formation of an antiviral substance. This antiviral component of the interferon system may be a polypeptide or a protein. This body response is especially important since it is known that the conventional antibody immune mechanisms may have little to do with the early stages of recovery from viral infections. Interferon is operative within hours of infection and seems to provide the first line of defense to limit or to prevent viral infection. Most viruses are sensitive, but to varying degrees. Hopes of using interferon therapeutically, however, have not materialized because of the great cost of its production.

An alternative approach has been explored of finding an inducing substance that would stimulate the body to produce its own interferon. None of the many substances so far studied has given promise of being suitable for routine use. Currently, study has turned to uncovering the natural stimulus for interferon induction by viruses. It has been discovered that certain double-stranded ribonucleic acids are greatly active in inducing interferon and host resistance both in animals and in cells in culture. The possibility of using these ribonucleic acids therapeutically for virus infections is being actively explored, and there is hope that this approach will prove to be useful.

The great successes obtained in the chemotherapy for other microbial infections has stimulated an intensive search for chemicals that may be therapeutic for viral infections. At present, however, there are only three substances or classes of chemical substances for which claims of significant clinical effectiveness have been made. These are N-methylisatin-beta-thiosemicarbazone for the prophylaxis of smallpox, adamantanamine for prophylaxis of influenza, and metabolic inhibitors such as iododeoxyuridine for treating corneal infection incited by herpesvirus hominis.

The effectiveness of the last agent, however, does not appear to be significant.

PICORNAVIRUSES

The picornaviruses[76] are small RNA-containing viruses, with icosahedral symmetry, from about 15 to 30 nm. in diameter, which are found in both man and the lower animals. They are characteristically resistant to the action of either; inactivation of these viruses by heat occurs after one-half hour at 50° C. The picornaviruses of human origin have been subdivided into two major groups: (1) enteroviruses, which multiply in the human intestinal tract; and (2) rhinoviruses, which multiply in the upper respiratory tract.

Enteroviruses

The enterovirus group contains more than 60 members and consists of four subgroups, as follows: (1) polioviruses; (2) Coxsackie viruses, group A; (3) Coxsackie viruses, group B; and (4) ECHO viruses.

Polioviruses

The polioviruses (Fig. 5-1) are icosahedron particles about 28 nm. in diameter that consist of an RNA core and a protein shell. There are three types of naturally occurring "wild" viruses. Each of these types, established on immunologic grounds, has two type-specific antigens, one of which is infectious, and the other lacks RNA and is not infectious. There are group antigens, particularly common to types 1 and 2, but there is also some relationship between type 3 and the other two through an antigen common to all three.

Poliovirus is quite stable, being found viable after storage for several years at −70° C. Survival of the virus in human stools at room temperature varies from a day to several weeks, depending upon such factors as the amount of virus present, the pH and moisture content of the stool, and other conditions. The most active chemical

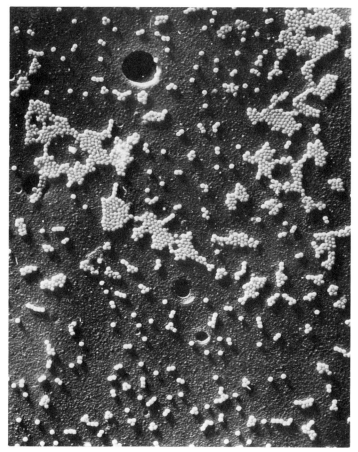

Fig. 5-1. Poliomyelitis virus, type II (79,000 ×). (Courtesy Parke Davis and Co., Detroit, Mich.)

disinfectants seem to be oxidizing agents. Free residual chlorine (0.2 to 0.3 ppm.) in water will kill the virus in 30 minutes. Polioviruses are inactivated by ultraviolet light.

Most strains of polioviruses have a very narrow host range. Primates are the only animals susceptible to all three types of virus, but some type 2 strains produce paralysis in mice, cotton rats, and hamsters, and some strains of types 1 and 3 have been adapted to mice. A major advance in cultivation was made in 1949 when Enders and co-workers succeeded in growing poliovirus in tissue culture with the aid of antibiotics to prevent bacterial growth. By means of tissue culture it has been possible to select variants that are practically without paralytic effects for primates.

Clinical picture. Poliomyelitis is an acute infectious disease with the ability to cause a wide range of clinical responses. The exposed person may have an inapparent infection without symptoms; a mild illness (abortive poliomyelitis); an aseptic meningitis (nonparalytic poliomyelitis), or in a small number of cases paralytic poliomyelitis, caused by invasion by the virus of the central nervous system and subsequent destruction of motor neurons in the spinal cord. The incubation period is from 7 to

14 days usually. Only about 1% of the infections are recognized clinically.

Pathogenesis. The exact site of multiplication during the initial infection of man is not known, but the evidence implicates the gastrointestinal tract, particularly the pharynx or small intestine. The lesions characteristic of human poliomyelitis are seen only in the central nervous system. The virus attacks only the neuron to cause various degrees of damage. Some neurons may die, while others recover. In fatal cases, the lesions occur mainly in the anterior horns of the spinal cord, although lesions in medulla and pons or other sites may also be found.

The portal of entry is the mouth. Virus in patients with poliomyelitis has been demonstrated in the pharynx, the gastrointestinal tract, the bloodstream, and the central nervous system. Possible routes of spreading from the primary sites of entry and multiplication are the bloodstream, the lymphatics, and the axons.

An infection results in the production of neutralizing antibodies for the infecting type, but paralytic poliomyelitis has been known to develop even when neutralizing antibodies are present to the infecting strain at the onset of the disease. Children in countries where paralytic poliomyelitis is rarely seen usually have a high antibody titer to all three types of virus at a very early age. In countries where there is epidemic paralytic poliomyelitis, antibody appears later in life and a small percentage of the population acquires it.

Diagnosis. Laboratory diagnosis of poliomyelitis rests upon isolation of the virus and results of serologic tests. Throat swabs, throat or nasopharyngeal washings, and feces may be used for demonstrating virus. Feces from early in the infection is the best source for the virus. At postmortem examination virus may be obtained from the central nervous system unless paralysis had set in which requires study of the intestinal contents for the best chance at isolation of the infective agent. Several serologic tests have been investigated for their utility in establishing the diagnosis, but the complement fixation tests are the most useful for routine diagnostic laboratories.

Epidemiology. At the present time, most cases of poliomyelitis occur in persons between the ages of 1 and 18 years in the temperate zones. Formerly, most individuals affected were less than five years of age. This shift in age distribution has been attributed to improved methods of sanitation. Poliomyelitis occurs throughout the world, including the tropics where it was at one time considered to be very rare. In the temperate zones the disease has tended to occur in late summer and autumn (July to September), but winter epidemics do occur.

Oral aspects. Careful studies have determined that subcutaneous or intramuscular injections of certain irritant substances may predispose one to or precipitate paralysis of the inoculated limb. Mixed diphtheria and pertussis vaccine with alum presents the greatest risk. If poliomyelitis is prevalent, elective tonsillectomy or dental extractions should be avoided to eliminate the possible risk of virus entering exposed nerve endings and causing the bulbar type of poliomyelitis. Teeth with caries or exposed pulps do not seem to be a portal of entry for the virus.

Involvement of the branches of the trigeminal nerve in poliomyelitis is rare.[133] The muscles of mastication were found to be involved in only 0.38% of a series of cases studied, while in another series 5.45% of the patients had the facial muscles affected. The masseter muscle may be paralyzed on either one side or both sides. If the muscle on only one side becomes paralyzed, facial asymmetry will develop consisting of hypertrophy of the masseter on the functioning side and atrophy of the masseter on the paralyzed side. Moreover, the angle of the jaw on the affected side becomes flattened. If these disturbed functions begin during the period of skeletal growth, they will also lead to asymmetric development of the parts of the zygomatic bones and mandible related to the origins and insertions of the muscles affected. Long-standing muscle disturbance may lead to temporomandibular joint pain and dysfunction, and even subluxation in some instances.

Prevention. The first effective vaccine consisted of killed virus (Salk vaccine), but its serious limitations have resulted in widespread adoption of the subsequently developed Sabin live attenuated virus vaccine. The number of paralytic cases in the United States today, since widespread use of live vaccine has become established, has fallen to less than 100 annually.

Coxsackie viruses, group A

These small RNA viruses, 28 nm. in diameter, are a large and antigenically heterogenous group, worldwide in their distribution, which are common causes of upper-respiratory tract infection, gastroenteritis, and other clinical syndromes. They were first isolated in 1948 from fecal specimens obtained from two paralyzed children in Coxsackie, New York, which accounts for their name. These first isolations were possible only because the fecal specimens had been inoculated into newborn mice. Certain strains of these viruses fail to produce disease in mice more than three days old.

On the basis of the lesions in newborn mice, it eventually became clear that two groups of Coxsackie viruses may be differentiated. Those in group A, consisting of at least 23 types, cause a diffuse skeletal myositis and flaccid paralysis, while those in group B, consisting of six types, cause encephalomyelitis, focal muscle lesions, myocarditis, hepatitis, pancreatitis, orchitis, and lesions in the fat pads and other organs. In man, group A viruses cause upper-respiratory tract infection, herpangina, aseptic meningitis, and flaccid paralysis simulating poliomyelitis. Group B in man causes pleurodynia (Bornholm disease), myocarditis, pericarditis, and aseptic meningitis. From 1.5% to 7.5% of healthy or nonspecifically ill persons in the United States show group A Coxsackie virus in their feces, especially those types associated with herpangina.

Herpangina. Herpangina is one of the principal manifestations of infection with group A viruses. It is a widely prevalent, self-limited disease that occurs especially in summer epidemics, mainly among infants and children. It was first described as a specific disease by Zahorsky in 1920, but its viral cause was not established until 1951.[66]

Herpangina has a sudden onset with fever lasting for several days, sore throat, anorexia, and sometimes vomiting. The pharynx is hyperemic. The mucosa of the mouth characteristically develops discrete grayish-white papulovesicular lesions (Fig. 5-2) from 1 to 2 mm. in diameter surrounded by an erythematous zone. The erythema becomes more intense during the next few days, and the vesicle becomes larger and is transformed into a shallow ulcer, usually not more than 5 mm. in diameter. On the average, about five such lesions occur in the mouth and persist for from four to six days. Most often, they are found on the anterior pillars of the tonsils, less often on the soft palate, uvula, tonsils, the pharyngeal mucous membrane, the posterior part of the buccal mucosa, or the tongue. However, various symptoms may develop that do not give this full picture of the infection, consisting of all gradations of fever, pharyngitis, headache, or myalgia. Acute parotitis and genital labial lesions may occur, but are rare.[65] The parotitis is difficult to differentiate clinically from mumps, and serologic study is necessary to establish the diagnosis.

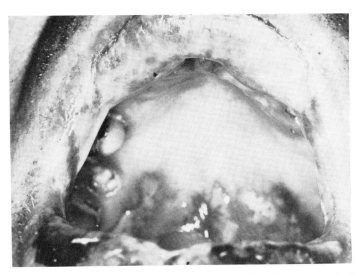

Fig. 5-2. Vesicular lesions of herpangina, incitant Coxsackie virus, group A. Such lesions, generally found about the soft palate area, may become confluent and ulcerous. (Courtesy Dr. I. W. Scopp, Veterans Administration Hospital, New York, N. Y.)

At least eight types of group A Coxsackie viruses may cause herpangina, including 1, 2, 4, 5, 6, 8, 10, and 22. Infection results in immunity only to the specific type involved, so that it is possible to have this clinical syndrome more than once. Moreover, a number of other Coxsackie viruses of the A type, the Coxsackie viruses of type B, and some ECHO viruses are capable of evoking herpangina symptoms.[30] Definitive etiologic diagnosis, therefore, requires isolation and identification of the virus from the patient.

Hand-foot-and-mouth disease. The Coxsackie group A virus infection hand-foot-and-mouth disease,[29] first reported from Toronto in 1957, has now been found in the United States, Australia, New Zealand, South Africa, and England. Clinically, the patient has cutaneous vesicular lesions of the hands and feet and vesicular-ulcerative lesions of the mouth and pharynx. The illness is generally mild and seldom lasts longer than a week. The incubation period appears to be from three to five days. Children appear to be affected more often than adults.

The disease may come to the attention of the practitioner first as a low-grade fever, but more often as a sore mouth. In some cases the only expression of the infection is a stomatitis,[1] but in other cases the stomatitis may be just the first of the lesions to appear.[85] The oral ulcers are superficial and usually follow the appearance of small vesicles on erythematous bases on the pharynx, soft palate, gingiva, buccal mucosa, tongue, or lips. Of these, the hard palate, tongue, and buccal mucosa are the most frequently affected areas. In contrast, the oral lesions of herpangina are confined to the posterior part of the mouth, occurring most often on the anterior portion of the fauces, the tonsils, the soft palate, and the uvula. Vesicles usually, but not always, also appear on the palmar surface of the hands and the plantar surface of the feet. Death from myocarditis is known to occur in severe cases.

Virus is found in the stools, salivary sediment, throat washings, and vesicle fluid. Coxsackie virus A16 is most commonly isolated,[90] but types A4, A5, A9, and A10 have been found, on occasion.[40]

There is some reason to suspect that hand-foot-and-mouth disease may be an occupational hazard for dentists. In a reported outbreak[119] in England, a presumptive infection that was diagnosed on clinical grounds only apparently was acquired by the dentist from a patient. Two children of the dentist subsequently became ill also.

Coxsackie viruses, group B

The group B Coxsackie viruses appear to cause more serious disease in man than the viruses of Coxsackie group A. Epidemic pleurodynia (Bornholm disease) is the characteristic clinical picture caused by the Coxsackie B viruses. It is most common during summer or fall. The chief symptoms are fever, excruciating chest pain, and respiratory distress. The illness is usually self-limited, and all patients recover. Relapses and complications may occur, however, and convalescence may be prolonged. Clinical diagnosis is difficult, if not impossible, so that laboratory studies are essential to establish the cause of the infection. The virus may be recovered from feces and throat washings. It occurs in various parts of the world in both epidemic and endemic forms.

In aseptic meningitis, the etiologic role of the group B viruses has been firmly established. All members of the group have been implicated. Headache, back and neck pain, pharyngitis, and myalgias are common symptoms. Signs of meningeal irritation are usually found. The illness is usually over by a week, although fatigue and irritability may last for several months. Definitive diagnosis cannot be established on the basis of clinical findings.

Experimental infection of young adult mice with a strain of Coxsackie B1 virus may result in acute parotitis and pancreatitis with necrosis.[131] Upon subsidence of the infection there is a partial regeneration of the parotid and pancreatic tissue. The virus is recoverable from the parotid tissue in high titer, multiplication apparently occurring by the second day after inoculation, and reaches its peak by the third day. The virus is demonstrable in the saliva and is still present in the parotid on the ninth day after infection. The other salivary glands show no lesions.

ECHO viruses (enteric cytopathogenic human orphan viruses)

The ECHO viruses were originally separated from the Coxsackie viruses by their lack of pathogenicity for infant mice. They are approximately the same size as the Coxsackie viruses and have the same resistance to ether. The most suitable method for isolation of these viruses from feces is in the first 7 to 10 days of illness by inoculation of tissue culture. At least thirty types have been differentiated on the basis of antigenic differences. The proportion of persons who carry these viruses decreases as age increases.

The ECHO viruses have been found to be associated with various clinical syndromes such as aseptic meningitis, upper-respiratory tract disease, summer diarrhea, and sometimes with paralysis resembling poliomyelitis or encephalitis. A febrile illness may occur in some cases in which maculopapular or other skin rash is present either alone or together with aseptic meningitis. Small papules or vesicles may appear on the pharynx or occasionally in the mouth on the soft palate or uvula that later ulcerate, but this occurs less often than with Coxsackie virus infections. The palatal lesions are either red or yellow-white and range from 3 to 5 mm. in diameter. A mild pharyngeal erythema is usually present. The clinical symptoms closely resemble those seen with group B Coxsackie viruses.

Rhinoviruses

The rhinoviruses,[100] or the "common cold" viruses, constitute a distinct, large group of picornaviruses that have been isolated from a great proportion of patients with acute but mild upper-respiratory tract infections and from those with moderately severe lower-respiratory tract infections. These are worldwide in distribution.

The rhinoviruses at present consist of more than 90 serotypes, and undoubtedly there are others. These viruses are easily distinguished from the enteroviruses, which share many of their biophysical and biochemical properties, by the fact that their infectivity is markedly reduced by exposure to pH 3.0 to 5.0 for three or four hours at 25 °C. They are ether stable and may be stored at −70° C. without suffering significant loss of infectivity. They multiply almost entirely in the upper respiratory tract rather than in the alimentary tract as do the enteroviruses. Shedding of rhinovirus occurs more frequently in the nasal secretions than in the oral secretions, and in the latter case it occurs principally during the illness.[39]

FOOT-AND-MOUTH DISEASE VIRUS: EPIZOOTIC STOMATITIS

Although foot-and-mouth disease, caused by one of the earliest recognized viruses, is found primarily in cloven-footed animals (cattle, sheep, goats, pigs), man may occasionally become infected.[75] The disease is widespread in Europe and Asia, but only sporadic outbreaks have occurred in the United States, Canada, and Mexico. These have been successfully eradicated by the most strenuous efforts.

Virus characteristics. This enterovirus, one of the smallest, is 23 nm. in diameter, contains a core of RNA, and is spheric in form. It is resistant to various chemicals such as ether, chloroform, and phenol but is destroyed in suspension by chlorine, iodine, potassium permanganate, or sodium hydroxide.

The virus can be inoculated into a variety of susceptible animals. The material containing the virus (blood, saliva, urine, fecal suspension, vesicle fluid, or tissue suspension) can be injected into the foot pads of a guinea pig or given intraperitoneally to suckling mice. The inoculum can be rubbed into the scarified lip or the mucosa of the tongue of the test animal. After an incubation period of several days vesicles appear in the mouth and throat and on the lips and foot pads of the diseased test animal. The infected mucosal cells become swollen and vesicular, and within several days they perforate and become ulcers. Healing eventually occurs without scar formation. An inoculum of vesicular fluid diluted to a million times may be sufficient to cause infection.

Transmission. The virus is highly infectious for animals but not for man. Dissemination may occur through contact with diseased cadavers or food and bedding contaminated by the saliva, feces, and urine of diseased animals, as well as by direct contact with vesicular fluid. It is quite resistant to environmental factors, is not readily destroyed by exposure to air, and remains viable for weeks on hay and fodder or on the hair of animals. Birds feeding on infected carcasses or feces may transport the virus to noncontaminated feeding areas. Man is occasionally infected with the virus by direct contact with diseased animals, by drinking the contaminated unpasteurized milk, by eating the meat of such animals or by laboratory contact with the virus.

Symptoms in man. The disease in man[44] is characterized by a mild course. It consists of an incubation period usually of from two to five days, which is followed by fever and vesicular eruptions of the mouth and pharynx and the skin of the palms, soles, fingers, and toes. Occasionally the virus may infect the conjunctiva. Excessive salivation may occur in some cases while the oral mucosa feels dry and hot. The infected epithelial cells contain intranuclear inclusion bodies that are found most frequently before vesiculation occurs. The neighboring tissue is infiltrated with polymorphonuclear leukocytes. The vesicles rupture in several days, liberate infectious blister fluid, and then become ulcers. Healing eventually occurs without scar formation. The illness seldom lasts for more than from 8 to 15 days.

Diagnosis. Diagnosis can be confirmed only by laboratory examination. The virus can be isolated in some cases from the blood serum or from vesicles. Complement fixation tests and antibody neutralization tests can be performed with tissue culture virus as an antigen. If paired sera samples are obtained, one at the beginning of the disease and the other several weeks later, the latter will show an increase in antibody titer.

Prevention. In view of the ease of dissemination of the virus, diseased animals should be quarantined and slaughtered and their carcasses incinerated or disinfected and buried. Neither milk nor meat of such animals should be consumed. Restriction of the transportation of animals from countries to which this disease is endemic has proved effective in controlling the disease in the United States.

Immunization. A formalized vaccine prepared from tissue cultures produces immunity of about six months' duration. A great difficulty that has been encountered in developing a satisfactory vaccine is that the virus occurs in seven types and a still uncertain number of subtypes.

MYXOVIRUSES

The myxoviruses[87] contain a core of RNA in the form of an helical nucleoprotein, which is surrounded by an ether-sensitive coat. Pleomorphic in shape, these viruses vary from 80 to more than 250 nm. in diameter. As the name indicates, this group has an affinity for mucins, and it includes the agents causing influenza, mumps, measles, and respiratory syncytial virus disease. Two subgroups have been established on the basis of the size of the RNA helix: 9 nm. for the orthomyxoviruses and 18 nm. for the paramyxoviruses.

Orthomyxoviruses: the influenza viruses
Influenza

Influenza is primarily an acute, infectious, respiratory disease that is highly transmissible and usually appears in epidemic form. Influenza virus occurs in three distinct types that are not antigenically related: A, B, and C. Types A and B are antigenically variable, whereas type C appears to be antigenically stable. Infections with types A and B are found in epidemics, while infections with the type C virus are usually associated with limited outbreaks or with sporadic cases.

The influenza virus is a round or ovoid particle about 110 nm. in its external diameter, and with a core of 70 nm. There are also found filamentous forms of the virus 1 μ or longer, which are most commonly found in newly isolated strains. The influenza viruses are able to cause agglutination of red blood cells through direct interaction with the surface of the erythrocytes. This involves the mucoprotein coating of the red blood cells, but numerous other mucoproteins in the body fluids and tissues are also able to react with the viruses.

Most strains are stable between pH 6.5 and 8.0. Commonly, the virus withstands storage at 4° C. for many days better than freezing at –20° C. Survival of the virus for many years may be obtained by storage at –70° C. or by lyophilization. Heat inactivation occurs at 56° C. after 30 minutes. Infectivity is also destroyed by formalin, ultraviolet irradiation, and ether.

Cultivation of the virus for primary isolation is by inoculation of the specimen into the amniotic and allantoic sacs of embryonated chicken eggs. The viruses of influenza also may be grown in cell cultures of embryonic chick and various mammalian tissues. Primary isolation of type

B virus appears to be better in cell cultures than in the embryonated egg.

Clinical picture. The incubation period is from 24 to 48 hours. The onset is usually abrupt and fever of 101° or 102° F. develops; there is also headache, muscle pains, chills, dry cough, nausea, substernal burning, and sometimes chest pain. There may be some evidence of conjunctival injection; a small proportion of the patients will have signs of pulmonary involvement with rales, friction rub, or change in breath sounds. The illness is sustained for about three or four days and then rapidly resolves. This is often followed by a period of a week or so of weakness. Complications such as influenza viral pneumonia are usually fatal, occurring primarily in persons with heart disease. Secondary bacterial pneumonia may also occur, and usually appears after the influenza symptoms have improved.

The oral mucosa may show very striking changes that seem distinctly characteristic in connection with influenza. The changes usually become fully developed during the first 24 hours of the disease. Sometimes there is a patchy, clearly limited enanthema on the soft palate; in some cases, the whole soft palate is inflamed a bright red along with the pharynx, tonsils, and pillars. Other persons show an easily bleeding hypertrophic gingivitis involving the whole gingiva. There may also be herpeslike ulcers (9% of cases), oval, patchy epithelial atrophy on the dorsum of the tongue, and total glossitis with severely hypertrophic fungiform papillae on the anterior third of the tongue. The most severe changes seen are hyperemia of the entire oral mucosa, with consequent desquamation of the epithelium and spontaneously bleeding ulcers. The oral symptoms may remain full-blown for about a week, but the redness may persist for some time, even into convalescence.

Pathogenesis. Influenza virus tends primarily to destroy ciliated respiratory epithelium of the nasal passages, trachea, bronchi, and bronchioles. The pneumonia that occurs usually is from bacteria, as a secondary process. There is edema of the lung, with the alveolar spaces filled with edema fluid. On recovery, the epithelium is progressively replaced by hyperplastic transitional epithelium, and, finally, normal epithelium develops.

Immunity after an attack may persist for several years, but has not been accurately evaluated. That there is a tendency for new subtypes to replace old ones and that many other vital agents are capable of inducing an influenzalike syndrome confuse clinical evaluation of the duration of immunity both from a natural infection and from a vaccine. Among normal adults or adults complaining of respiratory symptoms or chronic pulmonary disease, it has been found that 40% have salivary IgA active against the PR-8 strain of influenza virus. Some of these people with salivary influenza antibodies show a higher titer of the antibody in their saliva than in their serum.

Epidemiology. Influenza characteristically occurs in epidemics that develop rapidly. It occurs most commonly in the period from early autumn to late spring but may begin or extend during the warm season. In a given geographic area the peak of the epidemic may be reached in three weeks, and the entire occurrence may be completed within another three or four weeks. Morbidity is high since as many as from 20% to 40% of the general population may become ill. In most epidemics fatality is low, scarcely exceeding 1 per 10,000, and is usually the result of secondary bacterial infection of the lungs. In serious pandemics fatality is about 2% and may reach 10% or 20% among certain segments of the population. It is characteristic in pandemics that the same strain of the virus is involved throughout the world.

There is no specific treatment available against the virus, so that treatment is supportive and symptomatic. Rest in bed and aspirin and high fluid intake are useful. If secondary bacterial pneumonia occurs, antibiotic therapy may be required.

The most satisfactory course for handling the disease is by vaccination with the specific strain involved in the outbreak. When this is not possible, a polyvalent vaccine of influenza A virus (all subgroups) and influenza B is most frequently used. Annual booster shots are needed to maintain immunity. The usually limited supplies of vaccine during an epidemic require that only special groups in the population at increased risk should be vaccinated. These include the aged, cardiac patients, and people working with such patients.

Paramyxoviruses

The paramyxoviruses include the viruses causing mumps, measles, and Newcastle disease. They range in their outer diameter between 100 and 300 nm., being somewhat larger than the medium-sized orthomyxoviruses. Their nucleic acid is about four times greater in molecular weight than that of the orthomyxoviruses.

Mumps (epidemic parotitis)

The mumps virus has an average diameter of about 175 to 200 nm., although there is considerable variation in size. Only one antigenic type is known. The virus is able to lyse chicken, sheep, and human red blood cells in vitro, apparently by means of an enzyme. Hemagglutinating activity can also be demonstrated with chicken, human, and other red blood cells. Infectivity of the virus is destroyed when held at 56° C. for 20 minutes. Mumps develops in monkeys upon inoculation of the virus directly into the parotid gland or by instillation into Stensen's duct. The amniotic sac of the embryonated egg is an especially satisfactory medium for growth of the virus, but continued passage in this way greatly lowers its pathogenicity for man.

Live virus vaccine is currently derived from such cultures.

Pathogenesis and pathology. The portal of entry for the virus is thought to be the mouth or nose. Two theories have been suggested concerning the route by which the virus becomes established in the body. According to one theory the virus travels up Stensen's duct to the parotid gland where multiplication occurs. Invasion of the bloodstream follows, occurring early in the course of the disease; the generalized viremia is followed by infection of other organs. According to the second theory the primary site of viral replication is the superficial epithelium of the respiratory tract. This is then followed by a generalized viremia and localization in the salivary glands and other organs.

The salivary gland involvement is the most characteristic feature of mumps. The parotid gland becomes intensely hyperemic and edematous; the walls of the salivary ducts are swollen, and the ducts become obstructed. The virus appears to localize in the acinar cells of the parotid gland. The infected acini are scattered irregularly throughout the gland. The cytoplasm of the epithelial cells lining the parotid ducts also contains virus. Salivary IgA may play an important role in the infection. It has been shown that hemagglutination inhibition of mumps virus develops in whole saliva during the course of mumps infection.[96]

Clinical picture. The clinical course of mumps is usually quite characteristic if it takes the form of acute parotitis. The period of incubation is usually from 18 to 21 days. The onset is usually moderately acute, with malaise, increased irritability, headache, anorexia, muscle aches, chills, and a fever of from 101° to 102° F., together with pain and swelling of one parotid, or, in most cases (70%), both glands. Usually one gland swells before the other, which follows within one or two days. The skin over the affected glands is tense but not red. Pain is increased by movement of the jaw, and, in many cases, children have difficulty in eating because of the pain. The orifice of Stensen's duct, opposite the maxillary second molar tooth, is often red and swollen, and petechial hemorrhages may be present. No discharge can be obtained from the duct. In some cases, inflammation of the Stensen's duct orifice may be detected before the overt classic symptoms of mumps become apparent.

In severe cases the uvula and tonsils may be edematous and cause considerable difficulty in swallowing. The temperature varies from 100° to 104° F., and lasts for from two to four days. The pulse is characteristically slow. There is stomatitis and a fetid breath. Swelling of the gland is at its maximum within 48 hours and lasts for from 7 to 10 days.

The infection has a striking tendency to localize in other parts of the body and may avoid the parotid glands entirely. The submaxillary or sublingual salivary glands may be infected without the parotids being involved. The submaxillary gland may become infected first, and then it may be followed by the parotid, but it is extremely unusual for all three glands to be affected together. Infections of the central nervous system, thyroid, pancreas, testes, mammary glands, and ovaries are all possible, especially after puberty, so that mumps can be a quite serious infection for the adult.[61]

Diagnosis. Typical cases present such a characteristic picture that laboratory studies usually are not needed to establish the diagnosis. The possible difficulties in differentiating the disease, however, may pose serious problems even for the dentist. In one reported case, for example, tooth extraction was performed for an adult with unexplained pain in the molar region. Relief was not obtained, and only then did it become apparent that mumps was the cause of the pain.

When there is diagnostic difficulty, laboratory procedures may be very useful or even necessary. The most useful procedures include: (1) isolation of the virus from the patient's saliva, cerebrospinal fluid, or urine within four days of onset of the disease; and (2) search for a rising antibody titer by testing matched acute and convalescent sera by the complement fixation test.

Epidemiology. Mumps is an extremely contagious infection, worldwide in distribution, which occurs endemically throughout the year. The estimated annual incidence, from a Florida study, is 19.5 cases of mumps per 1,000 population.[86] The highest incidence during the year occurs in winter and spring. Children between the ages of 4 and 15 years contract the disease most frequently, while those less than two years of age rarely become infected. When mumps occurs in the aged, secondary infection with suppuration is more likely to develop than in the young.

During the first six months of life mumps antibodies are present that had been transferred from the mother during fetal life. Early resistance undoubtedly is at least partly the effect of this factor.[46]

Mumps is generally regarded as a mild disease, and this is borne out by the fact that approximately 30% or 40% of all infections produce no clinical signs of the infection. One attack usually results in permanent immunity, but instances of two or more attacks are known to occur. Nevertheless, some serious consequences from the infection are known to occur in some cases. About 1% of all cases of deafness in the United States have been ascribed to mumps. In those few instances when death occurs, most of these have been children less than five years of age, and especially less than one year of age. These deaths are, in most cases, caused by meningoencephalitis, pancreatitis, or nephritis.

Man is the only known reservoir of infection. Transmission probably occurs by direct contact, airborne droplets of saliva, or fomites contaminated with saliva. Salivary shedding of the virus may occur as early as the seventh day before the appearance of the clinical disease and may persist through at least the third day after onset of the clinical symptoms.[42] Virus excretion may occur through the saliva also in those persons with subclinical infections.

Mumps usually does not occur in epidemics except in gatherings of large numbers of susceptible people as in schools or military groups. These epidemics tend to continue throughout a whole season rather than to break out explosively. If upper-respiratory tract infection is also present at the same time, then the mumps outbreak tends to spread more rapidly and more widely than is the usual case.

Control. Live attenuated mumps virus vaccine in recent years has been administered to several million children in the United States.[129] Follow-up studies of many of these have shown that the pattern of mumps antibody persistence parallels that following natural mumps infection, and that these vaccinated children do not contract mumps when exposed to persons with the disease. The available evidence, therefore, indicates that the vaccine confers a lasting protection. No serious side effects have been noted, and spread of the live vaccine virus to susceptible children has not been demonstrated. In view of the occurrence of an average of 48 deaths from mumps annually in the United States, the occurrence of meningoencephalitis, the development of deafness, the risk of impaired fertility from orchitis, and the costs of time lost from the illness, use of the vaccine appears to be amply justified. It is especially indicated for certain groups known to be at high risk, such as persons from a rural area entering a camp that also includes urban dwellers.

Measles (rubeola)

The agent causing measles[23] is an RNA virus about 140 nm. in diameter, with the helical structure of a paramyxovirus. The virus is relatively labile, being destroyed by heating at 56° C. for 60 minutes or by exposure to ultraviolet irradiation, and is rapidly inactivated upon exposure to ether.

Measles virus was first isolated in cell cultures in 1954. It grows in primary human and monkey kidney cells, and produces cytopathic effects in continuous cell lines from a large number of animals. The most characteristic features of the cytopathic effect are the formation of multinucleated giant cells, together with the formation of eosinophilic cytoplasmic and intranuclear inclusion bodies.

Clinical picture. Measles is a highly communicable disease that is most commonly seen among children in the first five years of life, although it may strike individuals of all ages. The incubation period is symptomless and extends from the time of infection to the first appearance of catarrhal symptoms. It averages from 9 to 11 days. The prodromal period, or period of invasion, begins on about the tenth day after infection. The early symptoms closely resemble those of a common cold and include mild fever, headache, malaise, increased irritability, and fatigue. There is usually marked anorexia; vomiting or diarrhea may occur. With an increase in the catarrhal inflammation, lacrimation and photophobia develop. The conjunctivae become red, and there is sneezing, nasal discharge, and a hard, dry cough. The face appears swollen, which, with the watering eyes and puffed lids, gives a characteristic woebegone expression to the face.[115]

Examination of the oral mucosa at this time may show Koplik's spots,[93] which occur in more than 90% of all cases. These are small, slightly elevated, pinpoint, white or bluish-white spots surrounded by dark-red areolae. They commonly occur on the buccal mucous membrane opposite the molar teeth, around the papilla of the parotid duct, and inside the lips, and are best seen by direct daylight. The number varies from two or three at first to many, which may coalesce and involve whole areas of the mucosa. They cannot be wiped off; a scraping examined microscopically shows only epithelium and detritus. They appear from one to four days before onset of the skin rash and disappear in from two to five days without leaving a mark. They never occur in scarlet fever, or in other exanthematous diseases, and are easily distinguishable from thrush or from aphthae.

As Koplik's spots increase, a mottled red rash develops over the entire oral mucous membrane, particularly that of the soft palate. This enanthema sometimes precedes Koplik's spots and at times is accompanied by a fine transitory eruption on the skin of the face. The mouth feels so sore that a young child or infant struck by measles who has been breast fed may refuse to suck at the breast.[92] There is marked loss of weight; malnutrition develops as a consequence. The infected child's mouth becomes dry and ulcerated and, because of the disturbed nutrition, may develop noma.[57] This highly destructive process that commonly ends in death has not occurred in European and American cases in recent years but is still encountered in the preindustrial countries of Africa.

The moderately elevated temperature persists for one or two days, falls to normal, and then rises sharply as the skin rash develops. There appears a dry, metallic cough that is persistent. After about two days the rash begins to fade, and rapid improvement occurs. A slight pigmentation may remain for two or three weeks. Desquamation usually begins with the fading and is especially marked on the face, neck, and thighs.

Epidemiology. Measles is endemic through the world, with epidemics occurring regularly at about two- or three-year intervals. The epidemic outbreaks appear following an accumulation of susceptible children in the population. By 20 years of age, more than 80% of the population have had an attack of measles. The greatest incidence occurs in late winter and spring.

The virus is thought to be transmitted through the air during the prodromal catarrhal period when the patient is sneezing or coughing.

Control. Measles is one of the most serious of the common diseases of childhood in countries with relatively high standards of hygiene, both because of the encephalitis that occurs in one case of every 1,000 and because of the complications from secondary infections.[27] It had become imperative in recent years, therefore, to develop an effective vaccine. Intensive study has now established that control is best achieved by means of live attenuated vaccine obtained from cultures in chick embryo cells, although cultures from dog kidney cells may be satisfactory. Since the widespread use of measles vaccine was instituted, the number of cases of measles had dropped to 5% of the earlier incidence.[81] The vaccine fails to provide protection, however, in an infant who is still showing maternal antibodies, so that if vaccine is given in the first few months of life, it should be followed about six months later by a second vaccination.

Pseudoparamyxovirus
Rubella (German measles)

The agent of rubella[102] is a pseudoparamyxovirus that was first isolated in 1961. This virus is a moderately large one, measuring about from 150 to 200 nm. in diameter, and is of the RNA type. It is relatively sensitive to heat, to extremes of pH, and to chemical agents. Heating at 56° C. rapidly inactivates the virus. Preservation is most suitable at –60° C. A pH less than 6.8, or of 8.1 or greater, inactivates the virus. Ether and chloroform destroy infectivity.

Many tissue culture systems are capable of supporting growth of the virus. For isolation from clinical specimens, African green monkey kidney cells are the most satisfactory. The virus produces a cytopathic effect in established cell lines.

Prevention today is possible by active

immunization with live attenuated rubella virus vaccine. The antibody levels attained from vaccination are lower than those resulting from the natural infection, but they nevertheless remain substantial for at least one year and may afford protection for as many as three years. Children of kindergarten and early elementary grades are vaccinated first in a community campaign for vaccination since this group is the major source for the dissemination of virus in a community.[91]

Clinical picture. The first clear picture of rubella was drawn by Wagner in 1835, although it had been recognized as early as the fifteenth century. Only man develops full-blown rubella, although other primates can be infected.

Rubella[115] is typically a childhood disease consisting of some swollen posterior auricular, sublingual, and cervical lymph glands, a little fever, and a transient rash. Among the prodromal symptoms is a faintly marked, pinpoint, rose-red enanthema of the soft palate. The skin eruption generally begins on the fourteenth day after exposure in most natural infections. It usually starts on the hairy part of the head, and often on the ridge of the nose and the upper lip; from these parts it spreads very rapidly, reaching the buttocks in a few hours. The rash fades rapidly when it is fully developed, an important point distinguishing rubella from measles. Another point useful in differentiating from measles is that Koplik's spots in the mouth do not occur in rubella. In about one third of the patients, the onset of the exanthema is accompanied by a soreness of the gums that lasts for a day or two.[19] The skin eruption lasts only two or three days. As a rule, the child does not feel ill, and an adult patient can scarcely believe he is suffering from an infectious disease. This latter case, nevertheless, can be disastrous if the adult is a pregnant woman.

Congenital rubella syndrome. In 1941, Gregg[54] of Australia reported an epidemic of congenital cataracts among 78 infants born following maternal rubella infection acquired during the 1940 rubella epidemic in Australia. These infants were poorly nourished, less than the normal birth weight, and more than half had congenital heart disease. Continued studies in later years made it apparent that these were the effects of the teratogenic action of the virus during fetal development. The targets most vulnerable to the virus are the eye, heart, ears, and brain, but dental and oral effects have been noted also.

Evans[43] found in his Australian cases that there was delayed eruption of the teeth, hypoplasia of the enamel, aplasia of the upper and lower incisors, and a high incidence of caries. It appeared that in his cases the dental changes were associated with rubella in the mother during the first three months of pregnancy. Histologic study in a later investigation indicated some conspicuous dental defects were present. These consisted of aplasia of the primordia of the first molars and other permanent teeth, malposition of the incisors, and hypoplasia of the enamel of the upper incisors. In a more recent study in the United States it was found that the maxillary teeth exhibit abnormalities more frequently than the mandibular teeth in cases of congenital rubella infection, and that, of the maxillary teeth, the second molar was the most frequently affected. Of the children with congenital rubella who were studied, 44% gave some evidence of having had the dentition affected. Cleft of the soft palate has also in some cases been attributed to rubella of the fetus.

The mechanism of rubella action in producing a teratogenic effect is not known. It is possible that the virus affects only those cells that are most rapidly multiplying at the time the embryo is affected. Rather than a specific tissue affinity, the virus may possess a more general affinity for cells while they are in the particular biochemical state required for rapid proliferation. At any rate, it appears that the fetus during early pregnancy is highly vulnerable to the rubella virus, for cases of damage are known when the mother had had rubella prior to the pregnancy and was then exposed to rubella in the first trimester without developing any sign of illness.

It appears that, as far as teratogenic effects of viruses are concerned, only the viruses of rubella, herpes simplex, and cytomegalovirus are known to exhibit this effect. In the case of congenital anomalies caused by infection of the fetus by toxoplasma and treponema, the effects primarily result from specific destructive pathologic lesions, such as inflammation and necrosis, rather than from an effect on organogenesis. It is also known that smallpox, mumps, varicella, infectious hepatitis, vaccinia, poliomyelitis, Coxsackie group B, and other enteroviruses may all cause abortion or stillbirth, especially when the disease is severe and occurs early in pregnancy.[104] Most recently, the Australian antigen found in blood serum from patients with hepatitis has been associated with Down's syndrome (see viral hepatitis section).

HERPESVIRUS

The herpesviruses[71, 77] are a group of at least twenty medium-sized icosahedron viruses that contain a DNA nucleoid. The complete virion, consisting of nucleic acid core, capsid, and envelope, has a diameter of about 180 nm., but the naked virion (virus particle without envelope) has a diameter of only about 110 nm. and contains 162 capsomeres. These viruses are rapidly inactivated by ether. Cell localization is in the nucleus of host tissue cells, where multiplication occurs. Intranuclear eosinophilic inclusion bodies are formed.

The herpesviruses have been separated into four divisions on the basis primarily of cytopathology and host range. The first division includes the viruses infecting man (herpesvirus hominis), monkey (herpesvirus simiae), pig (herpesvirus suis), and the viruses causing varicella and zoster (varicella-zoster virus). The second division contains the various salivary gland viruses (cytomegaloviruses). Group 3, the third division, consists of certain avian viruses such as those causing pigeon disease and cormorant disease. The fourth division is a miscellaneous group that includes equine abortion virus and the orphan virus of lumpy skin disease.

Herpesvirus hominis: herpes simplex

Serologic studies of various isolated strains of herpesvirus hominis have shown that they fall into two distinct antigenic groups referred to as type 1 and type 2. Type 1 strains cause infections of the mouth, while type 2 strains are responsible for herpes genitalis. The type 2 strains, in addition to antigenic differences from type 1, also exhibit differences in cytopathogenic effect in rabbit kidney tissue culture, have lower levels of infectivity, and have greater instability. The type 2 strains are considerably more neurotrophic in laboratory animals than are the type 1 strains.

Clinical picture. Herper simplex infection[111] occurs in two forms: primary and recurrent. Primary herpetic infection with overt clinical symptoms occurs most frequently in infants after six months of age and in young children to five years of age, but it is not unknown among adolescents and adults (Fig. 5-3). In only about 15% of the population in a normal, uncrowded environment, however, does the first invasion of the virus lead to clinical symptoms. The most common clinical manifestation of primary infection is an acute gingivostomatitis. The prodromal period of from three to five days is characterized by irritability, pharyngitis, a rise in temperature, and lymphadenopathy of the submental, submaxillary, and superficial cervical nodes. The gingiva and adjacent mucosa then become intensely red and edematous, and in certain areas may cover the teeth. The entire mucous membrane of the mouth and tongue may become involved to a more or less great extent. The lesions become vesicles that rupture, and the roof then collapses. After the roof membrane is rubbed off, a true ulcer is present. Sometimes the first lesions appear in the tonsillar region and may be mistaken for a bacterial sore throat. The stomatitis lasts about seven days on the average. Scarring does not occur with healing of the ulcers.

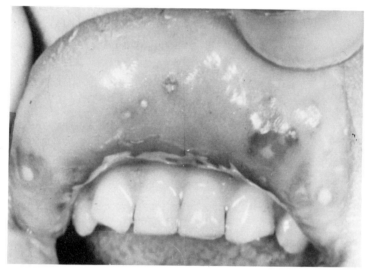

Fig. 5-3. Primary herpetic stomatitis. Numerous vesicles are evident on mucosa of lip. Some become ulcerous and are surrounded by reddened zones of inflammation. (Courtesy Dr. M. Wheatcroft, Houston, Tex.)

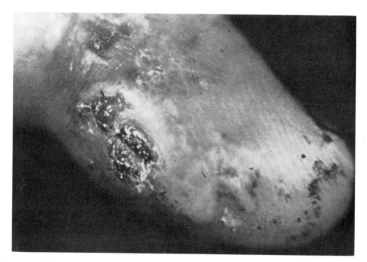

Fig. 5-4. Encrusted herpetic lesions on left index finger of a dental student. These lesions appeared following contact with a patient having multiple fever blisters of the lip and oral mucous membrane. (From Blechman, H., and Pascher, F.: Oral Surg. **12:**185, 1959.)

Next in frequency to stomatitis is herpetic infection of the skin. Skin lesions may develop from stomatitis either on the face or on fingers that are sucked. The most important form of skin infection is involvement of eczematous skin by the herpesvirus. This clinical condition may vary in severity from an extremely mild to a fatal illness. Primary herpes simplex infections of the dentist's fingers (Fig. 5-4) have been reported a number of times in recent years[9] as a result of treating patients with recurrent herpes lesions of the lips or following trauma to the finger. Such primary infections occur most commonly on the terminal portion of the index finger. Frequently, the paronychial region is involved. The onset is abrupt, with development of local irritation, tenderness, edema, and erythema followed by the appearance of deep-seated vesicles. After from 10 to 14 days, the vesicles become dry and crusted, and the edema subsides. The lesions are usually gone in about three weeks. A problem in differentiating from bacterial pyoderma, particularly that caused by staphylococci, is presented that requires laboratory studies for a clear diagnosis.

Vulvovaginitis[67] as the primary genital form of herpetic infection occurs at almost any age. Type 2 of the virus is found in the genital infections of both male and female, whereas type 1 is characteristically found in the other localizations for primary infections. The genital lesions are rather similar to those seen in the mouth.

After there have been one or more exposures to the virus of herpes simplex, a balance is established between the host and the only latently active but permanently established virus. The host's antibody titer develops to a point of balance at which the virus is held in check without any lesions. When host resistance is reduced from either local or systemic causes, such as from sunburn, fever, menstruation, allergy, or emotion, then the recurrent lesions, usually the so-called cold sores or fever blisters, will appear. These carriers can spread their chronic virus to susceptible persons either from an overt lesion such as a fever blister or even from the saliva during apparent good health. The incidence of healthy carriers less than two years of age is 20%, while among adults it is 2.5%.

Recurrent lesions are usually evoked by some form of stress such as an upper-respiratory tract infection, menstruation, fever, or an allergic reaction. Most commonly, these lesions are found about the mouth (Fig. 5-5). They occur almost ex-

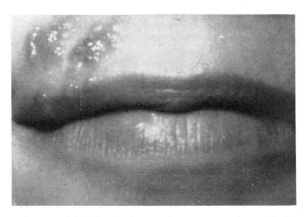

Fig. 5-5. Recurrent herpes labialis. Early vesicle stage is shown before ulceration and encrustment occur. (Courtesy Dr. M. Wheatcroft, Houston, Tex.)

clusively on the border of skin and mucous membrane, and consist of grouped thin-walled vesicles on an erythematous base. The vesicle is preceded by a prodrome of from 24 to 48 hours, marked by a peculiar hyperesthesia and burning sensation in the region of the forming lesion. Persons who suffer frequent episodes of cold sores can predict the onset of a lesion from 12 to 24 hours before the actual appearance of any pathologic changes. The adjacent lymph nodes are nearly always swollen and moderately sensitive to pressure.

Recurrent intra-oral lesions may occur at any age, but most commonly among middle-aged and older adults. The lesions are almost always located on oral mucosa that is tightly bound to periosteum. The hard palate, near the posterior aspect at the reflections of the vault, is the most common location, followed by the attached gingiva or alveolar ridge of the maxilla or mandible.[128] The lesions are small, discrete, and usually 1 mm. or less in diameter. They occur in clusters, first as vesicles filled with a clear fluid, and then as punctate ulcers with a red base upon rupture of the vesicles.

Recurrent lesions may also affect the eye, most commonly involving the conjunctiva and cornea. Repeated attacks of the infection may result in blindness. Almost one third of cases of trigeminal neuralgia have been associated with herpes simplex. The symptoms may imitate zoster of the trigeminal ganglion. It is considered possible that herpes simplex virus infects the gasserian ganglion or the fifth cranial nerve. However, attempts to isolate virus from the gasserian ganglion have not been successful.

Pathology. Herpetic lesions are superficial, consistently involving the epithelium and adjacent lamina propria. The damage to the tissues caused by herpes simplex virus is a result of cellular changes brought about by multiplication of the virus within the nucleus of the cells in the epidermis.

The changes are easily observed in ordinary histologic sections. There is an acute infiltration of leukocytes and a vascular engorgement of the dermis. Vesicle formation appears in the prickle-cell layer of the epidermis.

Basophilic feulgen-positive material fills the nucleus of the swollen infected cells (Lipschütz bodies), and on examination with the electron microscope this is found to consist essentially of a mass of virus. Later in the development of the parasitic process, only a small eosinophilic and feulgen-negative body remains in the center of an empty nucleus. Multinucleate giant cells are found in the fluid of the vesicle that result from amitotic nuclear division in epithelial cells. These are of great help in diagnosis since they are present in simple smears made from the vesicles of infected epithelium. Nevertheless, since identical changes occur in zoster-chickenpox lesions, virus isolation or serologic tests are necessary if it is desired to distinguish the precise cause of the infection.

Epidemiology.[110] Among adults in a low socioeconomic group of Philadelphia, neutralizing serum antibodies are found in 63%, and the same incidence occurs in infants to four months of age. This latter finding is not surprising since passive transfer of antibodies occurs in utero. From four months of age to two years the incidence of positives drops to 5%, but clinical cases of infection in this susceptible group do not appear commonly until one year of age. By five years of age the rate of infection is the same as that among the adults in the community.

The average incubation period appears to be seven days, although it may be as short as two days and as long as twelve days.

The greatest reservoir of infection appears to be among children with an inapparent infection. Shedding of virus may occur from the upper respiratory tract or through the feces, apparently from swallowed virus. In one group of children in a children's home, it was found that virus shedding occurred in episodes lasting as long as five months in some cases, and separated by intervals of nonshedding of from 2 to 45 months. The mechanism of spread may be either by conveyance through the air or by direct contact. In the adult the rare primary infection can usually be traced to physical contact of some sort. In one unusual case a young adult woman incurred a primary herpetic gingivostomatitis after 10 years of marriage to a man who had recurrent attacks of herpes labialis when she started to massage her gums vigorously on her dentist's orders. Teething in the infant leads to traumatized gums that might open an entrance for the virus.

Diagnosis. Definitive diagnosis in the primary herpetic infections should include demonstration of the virus by culture, increase during convalescence in the amount of specific circulating antibody, and demonstration of a typical histologic picture. These points are of particular importance in differentiating recurrent herpetic lesions in or about the mouth from a variety of superficially similar lesions of still undetermined cause that are referred to by a variety of designations such as aphthous ulcers (Fig. 5-6), Behcet's syndrome, Reiter's syn-

drome, Stevens-Johnson syndrome, erythema multiforme, and periadenitis mucosa necrotica recurrens.

Therapy. In the case of primary herpes, only symptomatic treatment for the local lesions and antibiotics for secondary bacterial infections are useful in the clinical management.[51] Recurrent herpes simplex may also be treated symptomatically, but some small success has also been claimed for use of the antiviral agent idoxuridine (0.1%). Some investigators have reported that this chemical reduces the severity of the disease when applied early, during the papule and early vesicle stages, but recent observations[79] have found no useful effect.

Varicella-zoster virus: chickenpox and zoster
Chickenpox

The virus of varicella[78] (chickenpox) is a member of the herpesvirus group. Morphologically it is identical with herpes simplex virus, including a central core of DNA and a diameter of about 200 nm. In parasitized cells it is the cause of acidophilic intranuclear inclusion bodies.

The disease caused by the virus is a mild, highly contagious exanthematous infection. There is an incubation period of about two weeks, following which there

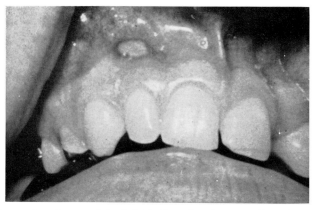

Fig. 5-6. Aphthous ulcer in mucolabial fold. The ulcer has a yellowish center surrounded by an inflammatory zone. (Courtesy Dr. M. Wheatcroft, Houston, Tex.)

develops malaise and fever, then a skin eruption. The skin lesions progress from a macule to a vesicle and may then become pustular. They usually occur first on the trunk and then on the face and hairy scalp, and then spread rapidly, within a few hours, over the entire body. They are usually most abundant on the back and shoulders. Crops of the lesions break out in succession during the next three or four days, and they may be observed in all stages of development. Occasionally, the virus may cause encephalitis about from 5 to 10 days after the rash.

In about half the cases[5] enanthema may occur in the mouth, usually occurring before the exanthema.[122] The oral lesions are found especially on the gingiva, hard or soft palate, buccal mucosa, tonsils, and the pharynx, while in rare instances the tongue may show numerous ruptured vesicles. Additional mucosal lesions may occur on the conjunctiva, in the nose, prepuce, urethral meatus, vulva, or anus. In the mouth, the lesions look like small canker sores or aphthae since the vesicles rupture quickly after their appearance. They seem to give very little pain, as the children affected seldom complain at chewing or swallowing.[115] The characteristics of these oral lesions are helpful in differential diagnosis. Parotitis has been reported occasionally; sometimes both parotid glands may be infected. In severe attacks, laryngitis is not uncommon.[11]

Most children have but one attack of chickenpox, but cases of two or even three attacks are known to occur. Mortality is very low. In mild cases, the whole infection is over in six or seven days. In more severe cases, with many vesicles and repeated crops, the illness may last from 17 to 21 days. Such cases are the only ones that may leave a mark. These marks, however, although few in number, are most likely to occur upon the face. Secondary pyogenic infection may occur at the sites of some of the lesions.

Epidemiology. Chickenpox is very readily transmitted to a susceptible host. The route of infection is not known with certainty, but apparently the disease is passed on by droplets or droplet nuclei, since air disinfection by ultraviolet light significantly reduces the spread of the infection. Patients are infectious from 24 hours before the eruption to six or seven days afterwards. The most common age for infection is from two to six years, although the disease has been reported in newborn infants. Epidemics of chickenpox may be started by a patient suffering from herpes zoster.

Zoster ("shingles")

Varicella and zoster are different clinical manifestations of infection with the same virus.[13] Varicella is the expression of a primary infection whereas zoster is the expression of an infection in a person with only a partial immunity from a previous infection. It is not known whether the virus in this latter case had been reintroduced into the host or whether it had been latent and was simply reactivated.

Zoster is a relatively rare disease that is the clinical manifestation of a posterior root ganglion of a spinal nerve or an extramedullary ganglion of a cranial nerve.[88] The disease is characteristically preceded by general malaise for several days. It is then followed by burning, pruritus, acute neuralgic pain, and then vesicular eruption in the area of anatomic distribution of the peripheral sensory nerves arising in the affected root ganglion (Fig. 5-7). Vesiculation is primarily on one side, although bilateral involvement may occur. The cutaneous or mucosal vesicle is thought to be a result of the peripheral migration of the virus from the ganglionic focus to a location in the epithelial cells. Virus has been shown to be present in the vesicles.

The trigeminal nerve was involved in 16% of the cases in one large series of cases analyzed, the cervical nerves in 25%, the

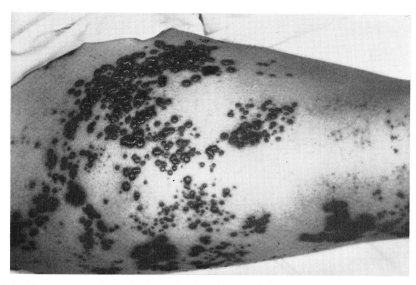

Fig. 5-7. Herpes zoster (shingles) on the leg of an adult. Lesions are generally localized to areas innervated by a specific sensory nerve and root ganglion. The etiologic agent is probably the varicella virus. (Courtesy Dr. R. H. Montgomery, New York, N. Y.)

dorsal spinal nerves in 48%, the lumbar nerves in 9%, and the sacral nerves in 2%. Of the cranial nerves, the ophthalmic division of the trigeminal nerve was involved most often, followed by the maxillary and mandibular divisions. With involvement of the ophthalmic division of the trigeminal nerve, one of the most serious forms of the disease, the eyelids, the cornea, and skin of the forehead will develop lesions. The corneal lesions may be permanent and may result in blindness. Involvement of the maxillary or mandibular divisions of the trigeminal nerve may result in lesions on the oral mucosa or skin, or both. The most common intra-oral sites are the anterior portion of the tongue, the soft palate, and the cheek. There are cases known which suggest that bone changes of the mandible occurred from involvement of the mandibular division. In some cases all three divisions of the trigeminal nerve may be involved, either on one side[12] or bilaterally.[28] Multiple involvement of the fifth, seventh, eighth, ninth, and tenth cranial nerves may occur also.[84, 88] Zoster of the second

and third cervical ganglia is not uncommon.

Dermal vesicles may persist as long as 10 days, but those in the oral cavity may last only a matter of hours. The oral vesicles are indistinguishable from those of herpes simplex. Upon rupturing, the oral vesicle leaves an eroded area within an erythematous ring. The erosion takes on a yellow-gray, cheesy coating and becomes acutely painful. They heal more quickly than the dermal lesions and rarely leave a scar.

Zoster may occur after the infliction of oral trauma such as the surgical removal of teeth, and after subgingival scaling and oral prophylaxis.[70]

Although zoster most often affects sensory ganglia and nerves, there may be involvement of motor nerves. If the motor part of the facial nerve is involved, paralysis may precede or follow the zoster eruption. The soft palate may be affected by palsy resulting from involvement of the levator palati; secretory function disturbance may lead to a dry mouth. The anterior two thirds on one side of the tongue may be involved along with facial paralysis on the same side.[73] Usually, the course of the disease is rapid, being resolved within a few days. In rare cases, however, especially of aged and debilitated persons, there may be prolonged neuralgia and motor palsy. The disease affects adults more commonly than children, and men more than women. Second attacks of zoster do occur, but are rare.

Diagnosis. Zoster usually can be diagnosed[112] on the basis of the case history and the unilateral distribution of the skin and mouth lesions.[20] In the case of an outbreak occurring only in the mouth, smear preparations from the lesions will aid in the diagnosis if acidophilic intranuclear inclusion bodies are present in the epithelial cells.

Treatment. If the case is mild, then acetylsalicylic acid by mouth and a topically applied lotion that dries the lesions may be satisfactory. When the pain is very severe, rather heavy sedation may be necessary. Antibiotic therapy may be indicated if secondary bacterial infection of the lesions has occurred.

Cytomegaloviruses: salivary gland virus disease

Salivary gland virus disease[48] is an important human disease occurring as an acute or chronic infectious condition with single or multiple organ localization. It is produced by a herpeslike virus that causes distinctive inclusions in the cell nucleus. The inclusions are most commonly found in ductal and acinar epithelium of the salivary glands.

The disease is one of the causes of developmental malformations in the fetus. Most reported cases, however, involve abortions, stillborns, prematurity, and newborn infants presumably infected in utero by the mother carrying the virus within her salivary glands. In children the disease may occur as an acute, fulminating, and fatal infection, with jaundice or anemia, or

it may be mild, with recovery as the outcome. In the adult it may occur as a fatal illness, often with pneumonitis frequently associated with an antecedent hematologic disturbance.

The cytomegaloviruses are closely similar to and therefore are grouped among the herpeslike viruses. They have a DNA core and measure 113 nm. in diameter. They multiply within the cell nucleus. They are heat-labile, unstable at a pH less than 5, and are ether-sensitive. The virus may be inactivated by heating at 56° C. for 30 minutes. The infectivity of a virus cell suspension is maintained after exposure to room temperature, 37° or 40° C. for three hours. Hemagglutinin and hemadsorption activity have not been demonstrated. Antigenically distinct species-specific cytomegaloviruses have been isolated from several animals, but notable among these are such domesticated animals as the guinea pig and the mouse.

The virus is worldwide in occurrence. Approximately 50% of the women of childbearing age have serologic evidence of previous infection. Their antibody is transferred to the infant, but it is relatively infrequent in young children. In the 5- to 10-year-old age group, 15% were found to have antibody in London, England, and Rochester, New York. In London, among persons older than 35 years, on the other hand, 54% were found to be serologically positive for the virus.

The transmission of virus most likely occurs by means of saliva and urine, since it is found in both of these excretions. If infection of the infant occurs from the mother before birth, the chances are great for spread of the infection to other persons in the immediate environment. The laboratory findings on isolation of virus from saliva and urine have provided confirmation of the previously suspected chronicity and great prevalence of subclinical salivary gland infection, and suggest that persistent urinary tract infection occurs with nearly equal frequency.

In about half the cases of neonatal infection it is possible to find pathognomonic exfoliated cells with large nuclear inclusions in the urine sediment. The best method for establishing the diagnosis, however, is by direct isolation of the virus from the urine. The virus grows in a variety of human fibroblastic cultures.[127] Cytopathic effects on the tissue culture cells are characteristic enough to allow tentative identification of the virus.

Infectious mononucleosis

Infectious mononucleosis[83] is an acute infectious disease of unknown origin characterized by malaise, chill, fever, generalized myalgia, enlargement of the lymphatic glands, and changes in the blood, especially lymphocytosis and the appearance of heterophile antibodies. The disease is commonly self-limiting and ends in complete recovery. While three distinct clinical types have been described, actually any combination of these may occur. These principal forms of the infection are as follows: (1) In the glandular type, which has a prominent feature enlargement of the lymphatic glands, sore throat is often present. The most common occurrence is between the ages of 5 and 15 years. (2) The anginose type, characterized by a membrane over the throat or in the oral cavity, occurs between 15 and 30 years of age and is less common than the glandular type. (3) The febrile type, which occurs most typically in adults, is seen sometimes in children.

The oral lesions found in patients having infectious mononucleosis are not uncommon, but they are quite variable and may present a problem in differential diagnosis to the oral surgeon.[4] Acute stomatitis with associated gingivitis may be found in about one quarter of the cases, and in half of these cases with stomatitis the oral symptoms are the first clinical symptoms. The oral membrane, present in only a few cases, may be either extensive or present as small patches. The presence of peri-coronitis, in which the inflammatory process extends beyond the retromolar area and is accompanied by involvement of the lymphatics, has sometimes led to the detection of the disease. A few patients may have multiple pinpoint petechiae distributed irregularly in the soft palate mucosa, usually near the junction with the hard palate. Involvement of the major salivary glands is rare. Edema of the oral and pharyngeal mucosa and lymphoid hyperplasia may be so marked as to cause dysphagia. The oral lesions, in some instances, have been the initial stimulus for one's entertaining the diagnosis of infectious mononucleosis.

In recent years, several investigators have studied the hypothesis that infectious mononucleosis is caused by a herpes-type virus.[38] The highly suggestive evidence that has accumulated to date is as follows:

1. Antibody, as demonstrated by immunofluorescence and complement-fixation, first appears in some individuals after they have clinical infectious mononucleosis; all sera obtained from infectious mononucleosis patients before their illness do not contain demonstrable antibody.
2. Only serologic negative persons develop infectious mononucleosis.
3. Long-term, leukocyte cultures, some containing herpes-type virus, can be obtained with greater ease from infectious mononucleosis patients than from healthy persons.
4. Increases in antibody can be demonstrated during the course of infectious mononucleosis.
5. Antibody levels are higher in patients with active infectious mononucleosis than in controls.

Herpes-type virus and Burkitt's lymphoma

In 1961, a series of cases of a highly malignant lymphoma with distinctive characteristics was described[21] in children living in equatorial Africa, a tumor now referred to variously as African lymphoma syndrome, nonleukemic lymphoma, or

Burkitt's tumor or lymphoma. Although Burkitt's tumor is endemic only to regions of tropical Africa and New Guinea, more recently similar but sporadic cases have been discovered in other parts of the world, including the United States.[108] The tumor occurs in the jaw in more than half the cases. The gross enlargement of the jaw in these instances is associated with loosening of teeth and replacement of bone by tumor. Other patients may have tumor masses in the salivary glands and cervical areas.

There is accumulating epidemiologic evidence that Burkitt's lymphoma has an infective cause. It has been found that virus-like particles occur in specimens of bone marrow and lymph nodes from lymphoma patients and that on the basis of electron microscopy these appear to be herpes-type virus particles, referred to as EB virus (Epstein-Barr virus). EB virus is also present in cultured neoplastic cells from Burkitt's tumor. It is undetermined at present, however, whether this virus plays an important role in the causation of the tumor or whether it is merely a passenger, being carried along in the progress of the tumor.[59]

The evidence available indicates that any virus responsible for the disease most probably is an agent normally widespread in the population, which causes lymphomas in only very few of the infected subjects. This situation may be related to the observation that active host resistance in conjunction with chemotherapy of the tumor correlates positively with the serum IgG levels. High levels of antibodies to the Epstein-Barr virus are present in persons with Burkitt's lymphoma, infectious mononucleosis, and carcinoma of the post-nasal space.

PAPOVAVIRUSES

The papovaviruses[41] are double-stranded DNA viruses that multiply in the cell nucleus but are also seen in the cyto-plasm. They are spheres from 40 to 55 nm. in diameter; highly stable to heat, to prolonged storage at -70° C., to formalin, and to ethyl ether. These viruses are of particular interest because of the association of certain members of this group with the development of tumors in a number of animals, including rabbits, cattle, and man.

Verruca vulgaris (common wart)

The tumorous growth verruca vulgaris, which commonly occurs on the fingers, hands, knees, and plantar surface of the feet of schoolchildren, has been known for several decades to be caused by a virus. Since it is autoinoculable, the growths may appear on the face, both in the bearded area and about or in the mouth.[49] Small, eosinophilic, intranuclear inclusion bodies are seen in sections of tissue taken from the lesions. Viral antigen is found located at the periphery of nuclei in epithelial cells from the lesion, near the skin surface, and patients with warts have specific antibody for human papovavirus. The warts may be removed by electrodesiccation or by excision under local anesthesia.

Laryngeal papilloma is the benign lesion of the larynx most frequently found clinically, with the exception of inflammatory polyps. Evidence is accumulating to support the viral origin of these lesions. Inoculation of papilloma from the human larynx into experimental animals has yielded lesions. Accidental inoculation of human beings similarly has resulted in lesions. In one reported case of a young boy, the surgeon injured a point on the upper lip of the patient with the operating instrument after removing a papilloma from the larynx. After 3½ months, several small flat warts appeared at the injured site and then spread over the whole face. It is a common observation that children with laryngeal papilloma develop warts at the corners of the mouth and on the face and hands. Apparently there is autoinoculation of the skin from the laryngeal lesions. Treatment with a vaccine of bovine wart virus[68] has been reported to have some success. A wide variety of surgical and physical therapeutic measures have been developed but none of these is entirely satisfactory.

Polyoma virus

In 1951, Ludwik Gross of the Veterans Administration Hospital in the Bronx, New York,[55] found that a mouse leukemia virus filtrate injected into newborn mice less than 16 hours old caused the development of parotid gland tumors. In most instances the submaxillary glands were not involved. Further study showed that the filtrate actually contained two distinctly different viruses, one of which caused leukemia and the other, parotid gland carcinoma. Certain dental lesions have also been noted in these infected mice. The second molars show coronal hypoplasia, and the third molars are missing; the incisor teeth are either deformed or missing.

The virus is rather small, averaging about 30 nm. in diameter in ultrathin sections of infected tissue, and is observed in very large numbers in the nuclei of infected cells, often in almost crystalline geometric arrays. Only occasionally is it found in the cytoplasm. The particles have no external membrane and consist of a homogeneous spheric mass of low density. It has been established in monkey kidney cell cultures and in mouse embryo cell cultures. The latter tissue culture system has been especially useful since these cells show cytopathogenic effects from the infection, a fact which has greatly aided laboratory studies.

ADENOVIRUSES

The adenoviruses[80] are a large family of DNA viruses ranging in size from 70 to 100 nm. This group shares a common group-specific, complement-fixing antigen and has the properties of ether resistance, cytopathogenicity for certain tissue cultures, and lack of pathogenicity for small laboratory animals. The adenoviruses occur in many animals, which include the dog, chicken, mouse, opossum, monkey, chimpanzee, and man. Thirty-one serotypes have been isolated from man alone. In tissue culture, the adenoviruses typically grow only in cells of the host species or closely related species, and preferably in epithelial cells. They usually cause respiratory, intestinal, and conjunctival diseases in man, but occasionally have been also associated with other acute diseases such as encephalitis, meningitis, and hepatitis.

The adenoviruses, and especially types 3, 4, 7, 7a, and 14, are of particular interest as the agents causing acute respiratory disease (ARD). The clinical course of this infection occurs in three phases. In the initial phase, or incubation period, which lasts two or three days, the patient is free of clinical symptoms. The second phase, which lasts four or five days, is the stage of acute respiratory illness. At this time, the patient appears only mildly ill. There are symptoms of fever, headache, and anorexia. The throat is sore, the voice hoarse, and a nonproductive cough is present; pharyngeal and nasal symptoms are prominent. The palate, pharyngeal wall, and tonsils show varying degrees of infection. There is a slight prominence of the vessels of the soft palate. Petechiae may be noted in some cases about the base of the uvula. Oral and pharyngeal lymphatic hypertrophy without exudate may be seen. Cervical adenopathy may be present, and rarely the conjunctivae may be inflamed. The third phase of adenovirus respiratory infection is the period of convalescence.

Cases have been reported with various other oral involvements by adenoviruses. Parotitis with cervical adenitis has been found that yielded adenovirus on cultivation. Oral mucosal lesions initially diagnosed as herpetic stomatitis have in a few instances failed to yield herpes simplex virus or enterovirus, but evidence for adenovirus was obtained upon cultivation. Early symptoms of an adenovirus respiratory infection of infants have sometimes been mistakenly attributed to teething.

One of the outstanding characteristics of infection with certain adenoviruses is the persistence of the virus in pharyngeal lymphoid tissues in a latent state. It has been well established that enlarged tonsils and adenoids frequently harbor these viruses. In one study 26% of the tonsils examined and 58% of the adenoids yielded adenoviruses.[69] These were either type 1, 2, or 5, all of which are relatively innocuous. After puberty the incidence of these infections lessens sharply.

It is estimated that adenoviruses are responsible for some 5% of the respiratory tract infections seen in children. The peak incidence occurs for children from 6 to 12 months old, among whom adenoviruses are isolated from 10% to 15% of those with respiratory infections. In adults adenoviruses account for only 1% or 2% of all respiratory infections. The incidence of adenovirus infections varies according to the season of the year; it is greatest in the spring and summer and least in autumn.

Some cases of acute respiratory infections are accompanied by gastroenteritis. Diarrhea is a common symptom in children especially as a secondary effect from the primary respiratory infection. In some epidemics, the gastroenteritis may be the most prominent symptom.

Effective vaccine has been developed, but it is not used at present because it has been found that type 7 adenovirus is tumorigenic in hamsters and that the vaccine may be contaminated with simian virus 40 which also is tumorigenic in hamsters.

VIRAL HEPATITIS

Viral hepatitis[58] is a highly communicable disease commonly found in all parts of the world. In typical cases there is a pre-icteric and an icteric stage, but cases without jaundice are very common, especially in children. A post-icteric stage is also recognized. Inapparent (symptomless) infections are also very common.

Clinical picture. The characteristic signs of viral hepatitis include malaise, arthralgia, nausea, vomiting, abdominal distress, liver enlargement, and jaundice. Typically, the duration of the illness is usually between two and eight weeks, but may be longer. Attacks are more severe in the old than in the young, in whom the disease may be very mild and brief. Mortality varies from about 0.2% in some outbreaks to as much as 20% or even 50% among very elderly persons. There is no specific treatment, but gamma globulin has been claimed by some clinicians to be useful.

Diagnosis. Laboratory diagnosis, until recently, depended upon biochemical tests for serum glutamic oxalacetic transaminase and serum glutamic pyruvic transaminase, which are not specific for viral hepatitis. There is now available, however, an immunoelectroosmophoretic screening test that is useful for the detection of carriers of the recently identified antigen associated with the disease.

It is recognized that hepatitis may be caused by a wide variety of infectious agents, including viruses such as yellow fever, Coxsackie, and herpes simplex, and bacteria such as leptospires. However, it is also apparent that when the known agents have been identified there still remain many cases caused by viral agents that have resisted cultivation in spite of intensive efforts.

Recently, nevertheless, significant progress has been made toward identifying antigens in the blood serum associated with viral hepatitis.[82] A specific blood antigen has been found as a precipitin band in sera obtained from an Australian aborigine, referred to as Australian antigen or Au(1), which is present in nearly 50% of patients from whom blood was obtained early in the course of acute viral hepatitis. This antigen could not be detected in any other type of liver disease studied, including infectious mononucleosis, Laennec's cirrhosis, hepatoma, chlorpromazine hepatitis, and miscellaneous liver disorders. Ultracentrifugation of Au(1)-positive serum has yielded fractions that were found to contain viruslike particles when examined in the electron microscope. These particles are from 18 to 21 nm. in diameter and agglutinate when antibody to Australian antigen is added. This is the size that had been expected on the basis of ultrafiltration of human serum from patients with hepatitis and the use of human volunteers to test the ultrafiltrates. It is highly probable that Au(1) is the actual viral particle.

Epidemiology. It has been found that the general population of the United States has a low frequency of Au(1), that is, 1 per 1,000, but certain groups gave a much higher incidence. Blood donors in prison have a 2% rate, and professional donors have a rate of 1.5%. The presence of Au(1) in the blood of persons having acute hepatitis is usually transient. In most patients it is no longer detectable two or three weeks after onset of clinical disease, and may be present for as short a period as one day. In chronic cases, however, which exhibit an impaired immunologic mechanism, principally a defect in delayed tissue hypersensitivity, Au(1) may be detected for years. Patients with Down's syndrome, particularly, have shown this prolonged carrier status.[15] The high incidence of chronic carriage of Australian antigen by individuals with Down's syndrome makes such patients of special concern to the attending dentist, but, in addition, these mongoloids have been found to suffer from an increased incidence of prenatal dental anomalies and advanced periodontal disease.[114]

Epidemiologic evidence indicates that there are probably at least two antigenically different viruses that account for the major number of cases of viral hepatitis, of which Au(1) seems to be associated with only one, serum hepatitis. Serologic studies of blood sera gathered from people all over the world indicate that, in fact, there may possibly be more than two.[16] These remain to be identified. At present, there seem to be two forms of viral hepatitis well differentiated on the basis of length of incubation. Au(1) is associated with serum hepatitis, which has an incubation period of from 41 to 108 days, while a distinctively different agent may be associated with infectious hepatitis, which has an incubation period of from 30 to 38 days.[116]

Transmission. Transmission of viral hepatitis can occur in several ways. The virus occurs in the feces during the pre-icturic phase and persists for one or two weeks after onset of jaundice. Any fecal-to-oral route will carry the virus, including contamination of water, food, or milk. Virus circulating in the blood of carriers or patients with acute cases may be transferred to another person by contaminated needles and syringes or surgical instruments.

There is a certain accumulation of evidence on transmission of viral hepatitis through dental procedures, although this is a quite difficult point to prove conclusively.[22] In one study published in 1956[47] of 57 patients with viral hepatitis discharged from the medical service of an American hospital, 15 had a history of an injection by a dentist during the preceding one to six months. Of these, thirteen had had injections preceding extraction of teeth, and two had had injections in connection with cavity preparations. The increasing popularity of single-use needles and syringes, and other disposable equipment, has been effective in reducing the likelihood of transmission of viral hepatitis among patients. Medical and paramedical personnel, however, have continued to be at risk, for the danger of accidental exposure to used instruments still exists because of careless and improper practices in discarding them.[25] Several reports have indicated that dentists may acquire hepatitis.[123, 126] Nevertheless, the available evidence indicates that hepatitis is not an occupational risk for dentists. Among Danish dentists the frequency of hepatitis does not appear to be significantly greater than it is for lawyers.[10]

It is wise, however, for the dental practitioner to observe certain precautions to minimize the risk of acquiring viral hepatitis. Used needles should always be discarded into autoclavable metal containers designated specifically for this use. Needles should never be thrown into wastebaskets, paper bags, or other easily punctured containers from which nursing or maintenance personnel may accidently suffer injury while handling and transporting the refuse.[24]

POXVIRUSES

Members of the poxvirus[18] group resemble one another in the pathogenesis of the diseases they produce. Moreover, the mature virus particles of these viruses contain a brick-shaped central body, or nucleoid, which has its own coat and which in turn is surrounded by an outer layer of protein. The genome consists of very large molecular weight DNA. There is a common internal antigen among the members of this group. In the electron microscope, the poxviruses have a size of from 200 to 250 nm. by from 250 to 320 nm. The poxviruses consist of five subgroups,[74] each of which has several members. Of special dental interest among them are smallpox, vaccinia, and molluscum contagiosum.

The viruses of both variola and vaccinia are resistant to desiccation for months at room temperature. Lower temperatures are withstood for years. In the moist state, these viruses are destroyed within 10 minutes at 60° C. Phenol (1%) inactivates the viruses in 24 hours at 37° C.

Variola (smallpox)

At one time smallpox was a common and often fatal disease. It has now been placed under effective control, but cases are not unusual in the Far East and are still breaking out sporadically in the West European countries and the United States.

Smallpox is an acute, extremely contagious disease. After an incubation period of about 12 days, there is a gradual or sudden onset of fever, malaise, headache, and prostration. Then the temperature falls and a skin eruption appears that passes through the stages of macule, papule, vesicle, pustule, and crust.

The skin lesions begin on the scalp and face and then gradually pass downward over the body. At the same time enanthema appear on the mucous membranes of the mouth, fauces, and throat. The lesions in the mucous membranes show a general resemblance to those of the skin. The mucosal eruptions are most abundant upon the soft palate. It may begin here, often before the appearance of any lesions upon the skin, with the formation of a papule that develops into a vesicle, which in turn ruptures to form a deep, white erosion. The rupture takes place so early that it is unusual to find unruptured lesions at autopsy. Deep and superficial necroses of the soft palate and the pharynx may occur. Glossitis is sometimes seen, noma less frequently. Parotitis occurs in a few severe infections.

Experimental infection[17] of the inner side of the lower lip and the soft palate of the monkey *Macacus cynomologus* with the variola virus provokes a self-limiting lesion at the site of inoculation, which may be followed by a general cutaneous eruption and a constitutional reaction. The mucous membrane lesion runs a course very similar to that seen in the skin. Histologic study also indicates cell changes in the mucosa similar to those seen in the skin. The lesions in the mouth differ from the skin lesions by the absence of a crust, which indicates that vesicular and pustular stages do not develop. Also, in contrast to the skin, the mucosal lesions are more exudative and proliferative than necrotic. A general exanthema is much less likely to develop upon inoculation of the mucosa rather than the skin. Moreover, the constitutional reaction is not as marked upon mucosal inoculation. On testing the skin of the monkey to infection by variola virus following variolation of the mucous membrane, it is found that its immunity is lower than that produced by variolation of the skin. It has been suggested that this relative inefficiency of the oral mucosa is the result of washing out by continually flowing saliva of the virus from the open superficial lesion created by the variolation.

Epidemiology. Smallpox is worldwide in distribution, ranging from sporadic to endemic to epidemic. The disease is endemic to parts of Asia, Africa, and South America, and is a continual threat to all countries. The World Health Organization began in 1967 an intensified program of smallpox eradication, including all but two of the countries where the disease is endemic. There has been a marked decrease in the incidence of smallpox since the first year of the program, and these efforts are still continuing.[118]

Transmission occurs by contact with a sick person, but the contact need not be intimate. Airborne transmission takes place over short distances, especially within closed spaces. An outbreak via this route occurred in an hospital in Meschede, Germany, in 1969, which resulted in four deaths among the 20 cases that developed.[2] Indirect transmission occurs through articles or persons freshly contaminated. Effective control may be obtained by immunization with a vaccine of vaccinia virus.

Vaccinia virus: vaccination against smallpox

By the latter part of the eighteenth century persons in many places were aware that cowpox inoculation appears to protect against smallpox. The English physi-

cian Edward Jenner, however, produced the scientific basis for present practice when he published his study, *An Inquiry into the Causes and Effects of the Variolae Vaccinae*, in the summer of 1798. By 1800 the practice he recommended of inoculation with cowpox virus had spread to most parts of Europe and to America.

Vaccine of the vaccinia virus for human use is usually produced by inoculating scratches upon the shaved abdomens of calves. The virus is harvested by scraping off the vesicle walls and contents and then emulsifying this material in glycerol. If stored at −10° C., the vaccine retains its activity for a very long time, but at room temperature it is useful for only little more than a week.

Vaccination is performed by inserting the fully potent virus preparation into the superficial layers of the skin by the multiple pressure method. The reaction of the skin must be watched to make certain that the inoculation is satisfactory. When the maximum diameter of redness at the site of inoculation occurs in less than three days, it represents an early reaction; between three and seven days, an accelerated reaction or vaccinoid reaction; and after seven days, vaccinia. Practically all primary vaccinations should result in vaccinia. The vaccinia reaction indicates previous absence of immunity; the accelerated reaction with vesicle formation indicates some persisting protection from previous vaccination. Early reactions indicate existing protection only if produced by a fully potent vaccine. Immunity is usually maintained by vaccination every three to five years.

Complications from vaccination are rare. They include: (1) encephalitis, (2) disseminated vaccinia, (3) eczema vaccinatum, (4) vaccinia gangrenosum, and (5) secondary infection.

Eczema vaccinatum may follow a recent attack of either herpes simplex or chickenpox. In such cases the mucous membranes of the mouth, tongue, and oral pharynx may develop aphthous ulcers.[63] Implantation vaccinia of the tongue has been observed in persons who either have kissed the inoculation lesion of a child "to make it better" or have bitten the inoculation lesion of another person.[106] The vaccinia lesions can be disseminated by the vaccinated person over other parts of his own body by scratching the inoculation site first, and then another part of the body. These autoinoculations occur especially on the hands, face, and vulva.

Secondary infections are quite rare, but among the possible conditions that may result in such cases is suppurative parotitis. An extremely serious form of disseminated infection arises if the vaccinated person has a defect in his immunity mechanisms, such as agammaglobulinemia or a dysgammaglobulinemia. These persons fail to develop antibodies to the virus, and the disease then becomes progressive and may cause death. The use of hyperimmune vaccinial gamma-globulin has been life-saving in such a situation.

Molluscum contagiosum

The virus of molluscum contagiosum[103] is a member of the paravaccinia group. These viruses differ significantly morphologically from the other poxviruses in that they are smaller and more ovoid, and in that their surface structure has a criss-cross pattern produced by the crossing of two sets of parallel threads, rather than a beaded mulberrylike arrangement.

Molluscum contagiosum is a benign superficial disease, first described by Bateman of England in 1814, whose viral nature was recognized and demonstrated in 1904 by Juliusberg. The disease is of special interest because it is one of the very few tumors of man definitely known to be caused by a virus. The infection produces a typical pearly wartlike tumor lying wholly within the skin epithelium that appears after an incubation period of from

two to seven weeks. The lesions have a central umbilication from which creamy sebaceouslike material can be expressed. Infections of the human oral mucosa, eyelids,[124] and face are known to occur.

RABIES VIRUS: HYDROPHOBIA

The highly virulent virus causing rabies[45] is one of the larger neurotropic viruses, being from 100 to 150 nm. in diameter. It is rapidly inactivated by formalin, relatively resistant to phenol, and destroyed by ultraviolet irradiation. The virus remains viable for months or years when stored at from −56° to −72° C. or when desiccated while in the frozen state and refrigerated. It grows in embryonated duck or chicken egg, mouse brain tissue culture, and hamster kidney tissue culture. The virus consists of a single antigenic type, although small immunologic differences have been found between strains coming from cattle and dogs. Strain differences have also been found in the ability to invade the salivary glands.

Clinical picture. The incubation period is usually from four to six weeks, occasionally shorter or longer, depending upon the extent of laceration from the bites, the site of the wounds in relation to the richness of nerve supply, and other factors. The onset of the disease in man is marked by a feeling of apprehension, headache, fever, malaise, and indefinite sensory changes often referred to the site of a preceding local wound. The disease results in an almost invariably fatal encephalitis. Its course consists of paralysis, with spasms of the muscles of deglutition when swallowing is attempted; then delirium and convulsions follow, and death ensues from respiratory paralysis. The usual duration is from two to six days, although it may be longer.

Epidemiology. Rabies is primarily a disease of animals that rarely occurs in man. It is found throughout the world except in Australia, New Zealand, Hawaii and other Pacific Islands, some of the West Indies, Great Britain, and the Scandinavian peninsula. Its urban occurrence is caused primarily by dogs, whereas rural rabies occurs primarily among wild biting animals, with sporadic disease occurring among dogs and domestic livestock. The disease in dogs and most biting animals may be communicable for from three to five days before onset of the clinical signs, and during the course of the disease. Bats may shed virus for many months.

The reservoirs for the virus include many wild and domestic Canidae, including the dog, fox, coyote, wolf, as well as the cat, skunk, raccoon, and other biting mammals. Vampire and fruit-eating bats are infected in Central America and Mexico; insectivorous bats in the United States, Canada, Europe, and the Middle East. The source of infection in rabies of man is the saliva of rabid animals.

Laboratory diagnosis. The biting animal should not be destroyed, in order to facilitate diagnosis. Symptoms of the disease should be watched for, and when the animal is killed impression smears are made of Ammon's horn. Giemsa stain and fluorescent antibody both are useful for study of the smears. The fluorescent technique may be used also for identifying virus in the salivary glands of infected animals. The virus itself may be isolated by intracerebral inoculation of mice and the identification of Negri bodies in the mouse brain.

Treatment. A combination of rabies antiserum and vaccine has been found to give better results than either alone. The vaccine is effective in exposed persons because the extended incubation period allows time for the body to respond with its own production of antibody if the virus was not deposited too close to the central nervous system and if the vaccine is given early enough for the body to develop active immunity. The course of treatment consists of administering vaccine soon after

injury, usually on 14 consecutive days; in severe or multiple bites sometimes for 21 days.

The development of a satisfactory vaccine began with Pasteur's original method of emulsifying dried spinal cord from rabbits infected with fixed rabies virus. In recent years, with new methods of cultivation, a number of other types of vaccine have been developed. These include the Flury strain chicken embryo vaccine and the duck embryo vaccine. Such preparations are especially good because they do not have large amounts of nerve tissue.

BACTERIOPHAGES

Viruses that infect bacteria are known as bacteriophages. Mature bacteriophages are found in nature outside the bacteria as, for example, in sewage. Some phages on entering the microbial cell replicate rapidly, causing lysis of the cell upon completion of the replication period, and are known as virulent phages (Figs. 5-8 and 5-9). On the other hand, temperate phages may reside within the microbial cell in a relationship that is not apparently destructive to either, and these phages may multiply together with the bacterial nucleus. Such an association, known as lysogeny, may induce variations in the metabolism of the bacterial cell. A notable instance of this is the case of diphtheria bacillus infected with the prophage B, which causes an alteration in the bacillus that leads to the release of exotoxin; diphtheria bacilli not infected do not produce exotoxin.

Phage types have been isolated that cause lysis only of particular strains of microbial species. This fact is used in epidemiologic investigations as a means of determining the specific strain of the etiologic agent. Thus an outbreak of summer diarrhea among children may be traced to a food handler who is a carrier of *Salmonella*. The *Salmonella* isolated from the fecal specimens of the children and the food handler are lysed by the same phage

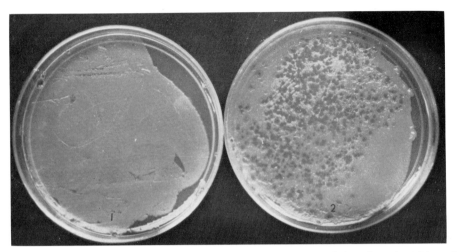

Fig. 5-8. Bacteriophage activity. *1,* Nutrient agar (control) is seeded with *Escherichia coli.* *2, E. coli* mixed with phage is seeded on medium. Absence of growth areas (plaques) is the result of lysis of the *E. coli* by the phage. (Courtesy Dr. S. Schaefler, New York, N. Y.)

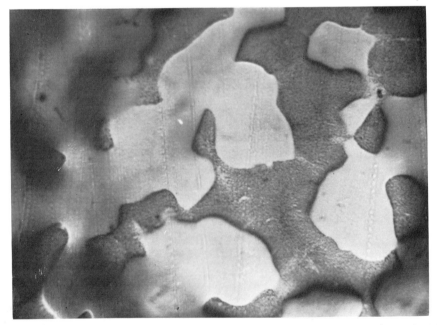

Fig. 5-9. Areas of plaque magnified 40 x. Clear areas are zones wherein the *Escherichia coli* was lysed or destroyed by the bacteriophage. (Courtesy Dr. S. Schaefler, New York, N. Y.)

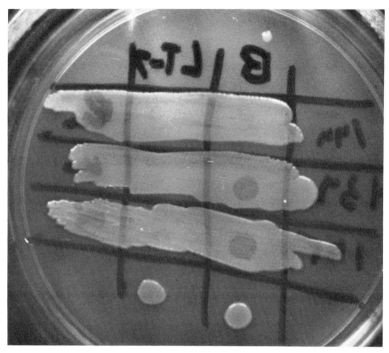

Fig. 5-10. Phage typing. Three strains of *Salmonella typhimurium* are streaked on nutrient agar, and a phage is inoculated in drops onto the three streaks. The two lower strains give similar lysis areas with the same phage, indicating they are similar types. (Courtesy Dr. S. Schaefler, New York. N. Y.)

type and thus identified as the same strain (Fig. 5-10).

Oral bacteriophages

As a rule, bacterial viruses have been found for any group of bacteria that is examined closely enough. It is only in recent years, however, and only after great effort, that phages have been found for some of the typical oral bacteria. In the case of several other of the oral microorganisms, no demonstration of phage has yet been made, but the probabilities are good that eventually these intracellular parasites will be found in them also.

The oral tissues appear to have some special reactions to ingested phage. In experiments with coliphage T3 in white mice,[64] it was found that a viremia follows rectal instillation and that the virus is intensively concentrated in the salivary gland and then excreted in the saliva. Salivary excretion of the virus is much reduced when the virus is introduced into the body by intramuscular injection. Aspiration of coliphage during anesthesia of the mice also results in the appearance of the virus in the salivary gland.

Lactobacillus phage

The first phage active on lactobacilli was reported in 1934, and was found to be active on *Lactobacillus acidophilus* and *L. bulgaricus*. A phage parasitizing *L. casei* has been isolated from sewage in Japan[99] and South Africa[36] and from saliva in the United States.[89] The phages active on *L. casei* have octahedral or icosahedral heads and possess collars. Additional phages have been found[37] in sewage that are active on *L. fermenti* and possess icosahedral heads and sheathed tails ending in baseplates and pins. Temperate phages have been found for *L. salivarius*, *L. casei*,[109] and *L. fer-*

menti. Temperate *L. fermenti* phages have a small hexagonal head and a long unsheathed tail ending in a star-shaped structure. It is seen, therefore, that there is a structural difference between phages active on heterofermentative and homofermentative lactobacilli, which is also reflected in serologic studies showing that the two groups of phages are serologically distinct.[37]

Neisseria phage

Throat washings and lysogenic chromogenic strains of *Neisseria* have yielded phages[101] that parasitize chromogenic *Neisseria,* including those isolated from the mouth, and that may be separated into five groups on the basis of serologic and host-range characteristics. All phages within a group seem to be serologically identical. A remarkable feature of these phages is the extremely limited host range of each phage. Electron micrographs indicate that the phage head is polyhedral and that the tail has a retractable sheath. Survival in storage is poor at any temperature; a few viral particles survive at least 16 months when lyophilized.

Staphylococcal phage

The characteristics of the phage parasitizing the staphylococci[130] allow such precise identification of host strains that they have proved to be extremely useful for epidemiologic studies of hospital infections. Staphylococci found in the oral cavity of man exhibit remarkably stable phage strain specificity; a single phage type may be found to persist for at least 14 months. Staphylococcal phages have been detected in excised tonsils and diseased submaxillary salivary gland (sialolithiasis with chronic inflammation).

Streptococcal phage

Virulent strains of phage active against oral enterococci have been isolated from sewage and from the small intestine of the rat. Temperate phages have been found in both oral and nonoral strains of enterococci.[97] Phages for group D streptococci (enterococci) have been found with high specificity for *Streptococcus faecalis* Lancefield's serotype 19, but the phage receptor site involved in the cell wall has not been identified.[125] Cariogenic strains of *Streptococcus mutans* have been found to be lysogenic.[53]

Bacteroides phage

Phage preparations active against *Bacteroides distasonis* and *B. tumidus* have been isolated from raw sewage.[107]

RICKETTSIAE

The rickettsiae[35] are obligate intracellular parasites, ranging in size for length from 0.3 to 0.6 μ by 0.3 μ in width. Although of small size, they differ significantly from the viruses because they have a typical bacterial cell wall, possess most of the typical bacterial enzymes, and are susceptible to chloramphenicol and the tetracyclines. They are now considered to be true bacteria.

The rickettsiae stain gram-negative. Laboratory cultivation is usually carried out in the embryonated chicken egg, tissue culture, or laboratory animals. Rickettsial resistance to various deleterious agents resembles that of the more delicate bacterial vegetative cells. These microorganisms are distinctive for being transmitted to man by arthropod vectors, which may be their natural host. Indeed, arthropods harbor a wide variety of rickettsiae, only a few of which are known to produce disease in man.

The human infections caused by rickettsiae can be divided into several groups that include the typhus fevers, spotted fevers, tsutsugamushi disease, Q fever, and trench fever.

Diagnosis by isolation of the rickettsiae is technically difficult so that this approach is of limited usefulness. For ordinary practical purposes, serologic tests serve adequately for confirmation of the clinical diagnosis. Serology is based upon the Weil-Felix test, which utilizes certain strains of *Proteus vulgaris* in an agglutination reaction. During the patient's convalescence, a rise in the agglutination titer is of prime significance for establishing the diagnosis for spotted fevers, with the exception of rickettsialpox and Q fever. The complement fixation test with purified type-specific yolk sac antigens clearly differentiates the rickettsial diseases occurring in the United States.

Treatment is a complex clinical problem and consists of specific antibiotic therapy and supportive care. The effective antibiotics are chloramphenicol and the tetracyclines. Supportive treatment requires measures to correct fluid electrolytic and nutritional deficiencies. In severely ill patients pyogenic complications, which include otitis media and parotitis, may develop, but these usually respond to use of the antibiotic combined with ordinary indicated surgical measures.[132]

Rickettsialpox

Among the spotted fevers is rickettsialpox,[132] a usually mild infection first reported from a single housing development in Kew Gardens Hills, Queens, New York, in 1946,[113, 121] which is of dental interest because of the oral lesions that may occur.

Rickettsialpox (Kew Gardens spotted fever) is a nonfatal, self-limited, acute illness caused by *Rickettsia akari,* which is transmitted from mouse to man by mites. Following its initial recognition in New York, it was also reported in New England, Philadelphia, and Cleveland. Approximately 200 cases a year are known to occur in the United States.

R. akari is similar to the other rickettsiae in its morphologic and biologic characteristics. It is antigenically related to but distinct from *R. rickettsii,* the etiologic agent of Rocky Mountain spotted fever. Guinea

pigs that have recovered from rickettsialpox have a partial protection against spotted fever. No serologic relationship exists with epidemic typhus, scrub typhus, or Q fever; the Weil-Felix reaction with *Proteus* strains OX19 and OX2 is negative.

Clinical picture. The primary lesion[6] occurs at the site of inoculation by the rodent mite, and may be found on any part of the body, including the face and lips. The primary lesion is a firm red papule which develops into a vesicle that then shrinks and dries to form a black eschar. The regional lymph nodes become enlarged and tender. Systemic effects, evident about a week after inoculation, consist of chills, fever, sweat, backache, headache, sore throat, and muscular pain.

From one day to a week of onset of fever, a diffuse skin rash develops. At first the rash is maculopapular, and then vesicles develop in the summit of the papules. They dry to form black crusts, which ultimately fall off, producing scars. The spleen may be enlarged and there may be general lymphadenopathy. A significant number of patients may develop eruptions on the face or may have transient oral mucosal lesions[31] that may be present for less than 48 hours. In view of the ease with which the oral lesions are missed, because they are so fleeting, it is probable that they occur more often than has been reported.[105] The oral lesions are found on the lip, tongue, buccal mucous membrane, hard and soft palates, and pharynx. They are very much like those on the body surfaces, consisting of vesicles 2 mm. in diameter, surrounded by a zone of erythema.[52]

CHLAMYDIAE

The chlamydiae are a large group of microorganisms formerly thought to be viruses because of their small size and obligate intracellular habitat. Today, however, it is known that they resemble the bacteria more closely than the viruses.

Among the characteristics that have led to the present view of their nature are the following: (1) these microorganisms contain both RNA and DNA, while viruses have only a single nucleic acid; (2) they multiply by binary fission, but viruses never do; (3) they are bound by a cell wall of the bacterial type; (4) they contain ribosomes, whereas viruses do not; (5) they exhibit a variety of enzymes that perform metabolic activity; and (6) antimicrobial drugs inhibit their growth. Moreover, the chlamydiae show distinct size and morphologic similarities to the rickettsiae, notably in regard to the limiting envelope and the protoplasmic inclusions.[3] Since the chlamydiae, as the rickettsiae, are gram-negative, it is possible that they are descended from the gram-negative bacteria.[94]

The pathogens in this group include the agents of psittacosis (parrot fever), trachoma, and lymphogranuloma venereum. This latter infection, as its name indicates, is a venereal disease, but it is capable of causing oral lesions.

Lymphogranuloma venereum

The agent of lymphogranuloma venereum is an obligate intracellular parasite just large enough to be seen in the light microscope. It is found only in man and is transmitted almost exclusively by sexual intercourse. The infection is characterized by a chronic granulomatous lesion. The primary lesion usually appears from 7 to 12 days after exposure and usually consists of a herpetiform vesicle on the genitals. Upon rupturing, the vesicle heals without scarring. From one week to two months later, swelling and tenderness of the regional lymph nodes occurs which may go on to suppurate. Upon healing, the lymph nodes form scar tissue that may block lymphatic channels, thus resulting in edema.

The infection is widespread throughout the world, especially in tropic and subtropic areas. It is endemic to the southern part of the United States and occurs most commonly among the lower social classes. It is usually contracted during the age of greatest sexual activity and is most frequent among the sexually promiscuous, including homosexuals. There is no pronounced difference in incidence between the sexes, and all races are liable to contract the infection.

Oral contact with the genitalia in abnormal sexual relations with a person infected venereally may result in a primary and, if untreated, a chronic infection of the mouth and its associated cervical lymph nodes.[14] The lips, cheeks[120] oral mucosa, tongue, floor of the mouth, soft palate, and uvula are among the oral structures that may become diseased.[32, 34] The pharynx and larynx may also become infected.[95]

The tongue is the most frequently infected oral site in primary infections. The lingual lesion is painless and vesicular. Sometimes, in well-developed cases, the tongue is enlarged, exhibiting areas of scarring and retraction of tissue. Deep grooves may be seen on the dorsum, with zones that are intensely red.[33]

Some puzzling problems in diagnosis with oral lesions have been found to be due to lymphogranuloma venereum. In one reported case,[117] an osteitis of the mandible that simulated pyogenic osteomyelitis because of drainage into the mouth developed from cervical lymph node infection. There is some reason to suspect that certain cases of elephantiasis of the lips, a swelling caused by inflammation and obstruction of the lymphatic vessels, may be produced by lymphogranuloma venereum. One such suspicious case has been reported that was apparently precipitated in a middle-aged man by dental treatment.[98]

For diagnosis, specimens are collected of pus aspirated from a suppurating lymph node, or of lymph node biopsy material. The yolk sac of embryonated eggs or the cerebrum of mice is used for cultivation.

A presumptive diagnosis is usually made from the allergic reaction to the intradermal injection of killed organisms (Frei test) or by a complement fixation test, but the result of neither test is conclusive.[72]

Treatment is with the tetracyclines, which, however, have little effect upon any scarring that may have developed.

CITED REFERENCES

1. Adler, J. L., Mostow, S. R., et al.: Epidemiologic investigations of hand, foot, and mouth disease, Amer. J. Dis. Child. **120**:309, 1970.
2. Airborne transmission of smallpox, W. H. O. Chron. **24**:311, 1970.
3. Armstrong, J. A., and Reed, S. E.: Fine structure of lymphogranuloma venereum agent and the effects of penicillin and 5-fluorouracil, J. Gen. Microbiol. **46**:435, 1967.
4. Banks, P.: Infectious mononucleosis: A problem of differential diagnosis to the oral surgeon, Brit. J. Oral Surg. **4**:227, 1967.
5. Barker, L. F.: The clinical diagnosis of internal diseases, New York, 1919, D. Appleton & Co., vol. 1, p. 419.
6. Barker, L. P.: Rickettsialpox: Clinical and laboratory study of twelve hospitalized cases, J.A.M.A. **141**:1119, 1949.
7. Baron, S.: The biological significance of the interferon system, Arch. Intern. Med. **126**:84, 1970.
8. Barsh, L. I.: Molluscum contagiosum of the oral mucosa, Oral Surg. **22**:42, 1966.
9. Bart, B. J., and Fisher, I.: Primary herpes simplex infection of the hand: Report of case, J. Amer. Dent. Assoc. **71**:74, 1965.
10. Baunøe, J.-H.: Hepatitishyppighed hos danske tandlaeger, Tandlaegebladet **63**:407, 1959.
11. Beardsley, E. J. G.: Chickenpox. In McCrae, T. (ed.): Modern medicine, ed. 3, Philadelphia, 1925, Lea & Febiger, vol. 2, p. 90.
12. Benedek, T.: Herpes zoster opthalmicus successfully treated with aureomycin, Milit. Surg. **108**:491, 1951.
13. Blank, H., Eaglstein, W. H., and Goldfaden, G. L.: Zoster, a recrudescence of VZ virus infection, Postgrad. Med. J. **46**:653, 1970.
14. Bloom, D.: Lymphogranuloma inguinale of the tongue and cervical glands, Arch. Derm. Syph. **28**:810, 1933.
15. Blumberg, B. S., Gerstley, B. J. S., Sutnick, A. I., Millman, I., and London, W. T.:

Australia antigen, hepatitis virus and Down's syndrome, Ann. N. Y. Acad. Sci. **171**:486, 1970.
16. Blumberg, B. S., Sutnick, A. I., London, W. T., and Millman, I.: Australia antigen and hepatitis, New Eng. J. Med. **283**:349, 1970.
17. Brinkerhoff, W. R., and Tyzzer, E. E.: Studies upon experimental variola and vaccinia in Quadrumana, Philipp. J. Sci. **1**:239, 1906.
18. Briody, B. A.: Poxvirus. In Prier, J. E., Jr. (ed.): Basic medical virology, Baltimore, 1966, The Williams & Wilkins Co., p. 403.
19. Brown, B. L.: Soreness of the gums in rubella, New Eng. J. Med. **250**:726, 1954.
20. Burket, L. W.: Oral medicine, diagnosis and treatment, ed. 5, Philadelphia, 1965, J. B. Lippincott Co., p. 118.
21. Burkitt, D. P., and O'Conor, G. T.: Malignant lymphoma in African children. I. Clinical syndrome, Cancer **14**:258, 1961.
22. Burton, W. E.: Changing requirements for sterilization, J. Prosth. Dent. **14**:127, 1964.
23. Bussell, R. H., and Karzon, D. T.: Measles-canine distemperrinderpest group. In Prier, J. E., Jr. (ed.): Basic medical virology, Baltimore, 1966, The Williams & Wilkins Co., p. 313.
24. Byrne, E. B.: Prevention of viral hepatitis as an occupational hazard of medical personnel, Med. Times **95**:243, 1967.
25. Byrne, E. B.: Viral hepatitis: An occupational hazard of medical personnel; experience of the Yale–New Haven Hospital, 1952 to 1965, J.A.M.A. **195**:362, 1966.
26. Cabasso, V. J.: Virology: Some of its tools and achievements, BioScience **17**:796, 1967.
27. Cabasso, V. J., Levine, S., Markham, F. S., and Cox, H. R.: Prospects for measles immunization with reference to the relationship between distemper and measles viruses, J. Pediat. **59**:324, 1961.
28. Campbell, R. M.: Bilateral herpes zoster of the trigeminal nerve, Lancet **1**:1066, 1936.
29. Cawson, R. A., and McSwiggan, D. A.: An outbreak of hand-foot-and-mouth disease in a dental hospital, Oral Surg. **27**:451, 1969.
30. Cherry, J. D., and Jahn, C. L.: Herpangina: The etiologic spectrum, Pediatrics **36**:632, 1965.
31. Colman, R. S.: Rickettsialpox—a new rickettsial disease with oral manifestations, Oral Surg. **3**:1257, 1950.
32. Costello, M. J., and Cohen, J. A.: Lymphogranuloma venereum affecting simulta-

neously cervical and inguinal lymphatic glands: Report of a case, Arch. Derm. Syph. **41:**557, 1940.

33. Coutts, W. E., Opazo, L., and Montenegro, M.: Digestive tract infection by the virus of lymphogranuloma inguinale, Amer. J. Dig. Dis. **7:**287, 1940.

34. David, V. C., and Loring, M.: Extragenital lesions of lymphogranuloma inguinale, J.A. M.A. **106:**1875, 1936.

35. Davis, B. D., Dulbecco, R., Eisen, H. N., Ginsberg, H. S., and Wood, W. B., Jr.: Microbiology, New York, 1967, Harper & Row, Publishers.

36. deKlerk, H. C., and Coetzee, J. N.: The characterization of a series of lactobacillus bacteriophages, J. Gen. Microbiol. **32:**61, 1963.

37. deKlerk, H. C., and Coetzee, J. N.: The fine structure of Lactobacillus bacteriophages, J. Gen. Microbiol. **38:**35, 1965.

38. Diehl, V., Henle, G., Henle, W., and Kohn, G.: Demonstration of a herpes group virus in cultures of peripheral leukocytes from patients with infectious mononucleosis, J. Virol. **2:**663, 1968.

39. Douglas, R. G., Cate, T. R., Gerone, P. J., and Couch, R. B.: Quantitative rhinovirus shedding patterns in volunteers, Amer. Rev. Resp. Dis. **94:**159, 1966.

40. Duff, M. F.: Hand-foot-and-mouth syndrome in humans: Coxsackie A10 infections in New Zealand, Brit. Med. J. **2:**661, 1968.

41. Eddy, B. E.: Oncogenic viruses. In Prier, J. E., Jr., (ed.): Basic medical virology, Baltimore, 1966, The Williams & Wilkins Co., p. 471.

42. Ennis, F. A., and Jackson, D.: Isolation of virus during the incubation period of mumps infection, J. Pediat. **72:**536, 1968.

43. Evans, M. W.: Further observations on dental defects in infants subsequent to maternal rubella during pregnancy, Med. J. Aust. **1:**780, 1947.

44. Faaborg-Andersen, K.: Foot-and-mouth disease in man, Acta Otolarying. **39:**282, 1951.

45. Fernandes, M. V.: Rabies. In: Prier, J. E., Jr., (ed.): Basic medical virology, Baltimore, 1966, The Williams & Wilkins Co., p. 543.

46. Florman, A. L., and Karelitz, S.: The fate of mumps antibodies following their passage through the placenta, J. Immun. **71:**55, 1953.

47. Foley, F. E., and Gutheim, R. N.: Serum hepatitis following dental procedures, Ann. Intern. Med. **45:**369, 1956.

48. Frankel, J. W., and Prier, J. E., Jr.: Cytomegalovirus. In Prier, J. E., Jr., (ed.): Basic

medical virology, Baltimore, 1966, The Williams & Wilkins Co. p. 465.

49. Frithiof, L., and Wersäll, J.: Virus-like particles in papillomas of the human oral cavity, Arch. Ges. Virusforsch. **21:**31, 1967.

50. Gordon, J. E. (ed.): Control of communicable diseases in man, ed. 10, New York, 1965, American Public Health Association.

51. Graykowski, E. A., and Holroyd, S. V.: Therapeutic management of primary herpes, recurrent labial herpes, aphthous stomatitis, and Vincent's infection, Dent. Clin. N. Amer. **14:**721, 1970.

52. Greenberg, M., Pelliteri, O., Klein, I. F., and Huebner, R. J.: Rickettsialpox—a newly recognized rickettsial disease. II. Clinical observations, J.A.M.A. **133:**901, 1947.

53. Greer S., Hsiang, W., and Zinner, D. D.: Viruses of cariogenic streptococci, International Association for Dental Research, Forty-eighth General Meeting, 1970, Program and Abstracts, Abstract 160, p. 88.

54. Gregg, N. M.: Congenital cataract following German measles in mother, Trans. Ophthal. Soc. Aust. **3:**35, 1941.

55. Gross, L.: Pathogenic properties and "vertical" transmission of the mouse leukemia agent, Proc. Soc. Exp. Biol. Med. **78:**342, 1951.

56. Habel, K.: The nature of viruses and viral diseases, Med. Clin. N. Amer. **43:**1275, 1959.

57. Harries, E. H. R.: Prognosis in measles, Lancet **1:**677, 1936.

58. Havens, W. P., Jr.: Infectious hepatitis and serum hepatitis. In Prier, J. E., Jr., (ed.): Basic medical virology, Baltimore, 1966, The Williams & Wilkins Co., p. 566.

59. Henle, W.: Evidence for viruses in acute leukemia and Burkitt's tumor, Cancer **21:**580, 1968.

60. Herrmann, E. C., Jr.: Experience in providing a viral diagnostic laboratory compatible with medical practice, Mayo Clin. Proc. **42:**112, 1967.

61. Hilleman, M. R.: The control of viral diseases with special reference to mumps, rubella, and interferon, Clin. Pharmacol. Ther. **9:**517, 1968.

62. Hilleman, M. R.: Toward control of viral infections of man, Science **164:**506, 1969.

63. Hoffman, I. L.: Atypical eczema vaccinatum, U. S. Armed Forces Med. J. **3:**885, 1952.

64. Hoffmann, M.: Tierversuche zur Schleimhautpassage und Resorptionsvirämie von T₃-Phagen nach oraler, trachealer und rektaler Gabe, Zbl. Bakt., 1 Abt., O. **198:**371, 1965.

65. Howlett, J. G., Somlo, F., and Kalz, F.: A

new syndrome of parotitis with herpangina caused by the coxsackie virus, Canad. Med. Assoc. J. **77**:5, 1957.

66. Huebner, R. J., Cole, R. M., et al.: Herpangina: Etiological studies of a specific infectious disease, J.A.M.A. **145**:628, 1951.

67. Hutfield, D. C.: Herpes genitalis, Brit. J. Vener. Dis. **44**:241, 1968.

68. Irvine, E. W., Jr., Irvine, E. S., and Moffitt, O. P., Jr.: Treatment of laryngeal papillomas with bovine wart vaccine, Cancer **14**:636, 1961.

69. Israel, M. S.: The viral flora of enlarged tonsils and adenoids, J. Path. Bact. **84**:169, 1962.

70. Jarabak, J. P.: Herpes zoster of the mandibular division of the trigeminal nerve: Report of a case, J. Oral Surg. **17**:57, 1959.

71. Jawetz, E., Melnick, J. L., and Adelberg, E. A.: Review of medical microbiology, ed. 9, Los Altos, Calif., 1970, Lange Medical Publications, p. 405.

72. Jawetz, E., Schachter, J., and Hanna, L.: Psittacosis-lymphogranuloma venereum- trachoma group of agents. In Blair, J. E., Lennette, E. H., and Truant, J. P. (eds.): Manual of clinical microbiology, Bethesda, Md., 1970, American Society for Microbiology, p. 594.

73. Jepsen, O.: A case of lingual herpes zoster with homolateral facial paralysis, Acta Otolaryng. **39**:172, 1951.

74. Joklik, W. K.: The poxviruses, Bact. Rev. **30**:33, 1966.

75. Jones, T. C.: Foot-and-mouth disease in western Germany during 1951, Milit. Surg. **111**:180, 1952.

76. Kalter, S. S.: Picornavirus. In Prier, J. E., Jr., (ed.): Basic medical virology, Baltimore, 1966, The Williams & Wilkins Co., p. 207.

77. Kaplan, A. S.: Herpesvirus. In Prier, J. E., Jr., (ed.): Basic medical virology, Baltimore, 1966, The Williams & Wilkins Co., p. 427.

78. Katz, S. L., Medearis, D. N., Jr., and Enders, J. F.: Some recent advances in varicella and measles. In Rose, H. M. (ed.): Viral infections of infancy and childhood, New York, 1960, Paul B. Hoeber, Inc., p. 215.

79. Kibrick, S., and Katz, A. S.: Topical idoxuridine in recurrent herpes simplex, Ann. N. Y. Acad. Sci. **173**:83, 1970.

80. Klein, M.: Adenovirus. In Prier, J. E., Jr., (ed.): Basic medical virology, Baltimore, 1966, The Williams & Wilkins Co., p. 385.

81. Krugman, S.: Present status of measles and rubella immunization in the United States: A medical progress report, J. Pediat. **78**:1, 1971.

82. Krugman, S., and Giles, J. P.: Viral hepatitis: New light on an old disease, J.A.M.A. **212**:1019, 1970.

83. Leibowitz, S.: Infectious mononucleosis, New York, 1953, Grune & Stratton, Inc.

84. Leider, M., and Contreras, M. A.: Herpes zoster, Arch. Derm. **75**:397, 1957.

85. Levin, S., Measroch, V., Pech, W., and Malherbe, H. H.: Hand-foot-and-mouth disease, S. Afr. Med. J. **36**:502, 1962.

86. Levitt, L. P., Mahoney, D. H., Jr., Casey, H. L., and Bond, J. O.: Mumps in a general population: A sero-epidemiologic study, Amer. J. Dis. Child. **120**:134, 1970.

87. Lief, F. S.: Myxoviruses. In Prier, J. E., Jr., (ed.): Basic medical virology, Baltimore, 1966, The Williams & Wilkins Co., p. 246.

88. McGovern, F. H., and Fitz-Hugh, G. S.: Herpes zoster of the cranial nerves, Virginia Med. J. **79**:250, 1952.

89. Meyers, C. E., Walter, E. L., and Green, L. B.: Isolation of a bacteriophage specific for a *Lactobacillus casei* from human oral material, J. Dent. Res. **37**:175, 1958.

90. Miller, G. D., and Tindall, J. P.: Hand-foot-and-mouth disease, J.A.M.A. **203**:827, 1968.

91. Moghadam, H.: Rubella and its prevention, Canad. J. Public Health **61**:379, 1970.

92. Morley, D. C.: Measles and measles vaccine in pre-industrial countries. In Heath, R. B., and Waterson, A. P., (eds.): Modern trends in virology 1, London, 1967, Butterworths, p. 141.

93. Moser, P.: Measles. In Pfaundler, M., and Schlossmann, A., (eds.): The diseases of children, ed. 2, Philadelphia, 1912, J. B. Lippincott Co., vol. 2, p. 243.

94. Moulder, J. W.: The psittacosis group as bacteria, New York, 1964, John Wiley & Sons, Inc.

95. Myerson, M. C.: Lymphogranuloma venereum of the hypopharynx and larynx, J.A.M. A. **117**:1877, 1941.

96. Nakao, T., Chiba, Y., and Chiba, S.: Hemagglutination inhibition activity for mumps virus in saliva, Tohoku J. Exp. Med. **100**: 369, 1970.

97. Natkin, E.: Isolation of bacteriophages active against oral enterococci, International Association for Dental Research, Forty-fourth General Meeting, 1966, Program and Abstracts, Abstract 68, p. 54.

98. Netherton, E. W., and Curtis, G. H.: Elephantiasis of the lips and of the male genitalia, with special reference to syphilis and lymphogranuloma venereum as etiologic factors, Arch. Derm. Syph. **41**:11, 1940.

99. Onose, H., Sasaki, I., and Kim, T. E.: Iso-

lation of lactobacilliphage and its biological characteristics, J. Nihon Univ. Sch. Dent. **10:**75, 1968.

100. Person, D. A., and Herrmann, E. C., Jr.: Experiences in laboratory diagnosis of rhinovirus infections in routine medical practice, Mayo Clin. Proc. **45:**517, 1970.

101. Phelps, L. N.: Isolation and characterization of bacteriophages for *Neisseria*, J. Gen. Virol. **1:**529, 1967.

102. Plotkin, S. A.: The virology of rubella, Amer. J. Med. Sci. **253:**356, 1967.

103. Rake, G., and Blank, H.: The relationship of host and virus in molluscum contagiosum, J. Invest. Derm. **15:**81, 1950.

104. Rambar, A. C.: Effect of maternal virus infections on the fetus, Illinois Med. J. **136:**261, 1969.

105. Rose, H. M.: The clinical manifestations and laboratory diagnosis of rickettsialpox, Ann. Intern. Med. **31:**871, 1949.

106. Rzeszutko, R.: Vaccina implantata linguae, Czas. Stomat. **15:**51, 1962.

107. Sabiston, C. B., Jr., and Cohl, M. E.: Bacteriophage virulent for species of the genus *Bacteroides*, J. Dent. Res. **48:**599, 1969.

108. Sachs, R. L.: Burkitt's tumor (African lymphoma syndrome) in California, Oral Surg. **22:**621, 1966.

109. Sakurai, T., Takahashi, T., and Arai, H.: The temperate phages of *Lactobacillus salivarius* and *Lactobacillus casei,* Japan. J. Microbiol. **14:**333, 1970.

110. Scott, T. F. McN.: Epidemiology of herpetic infections, Amer. J. Ophthal. **43:**134, 1957.

111. Scott, T. F. McN.: Infection with herpes simplex virus, GP **12:**58, 1955.

112. Servais, R.: Le zona bucco-facial, Acta Stomat. Belgica **62:**463, 1965.

113. Shankman, B.: Report on an outbreak of endemic febrile illness, not yet identified, occurring in New York City, New York J. Med. **46:**2156, 1946.

114. Shapiro, B. L.: Prenatal dental anomalies in mongolism: Comments on the basis and implications of variability, Ann. N. Y. Acad. Sci. **171:**562, 1970.

115. Shaw, H. L. K.: Infectious diseases of infancy and childhood, New York, 1928, D. Appleton and Co., p. 34.

116. Shulman, N. R., Hirschman, R. J., and Barker, L. F.: Viral hepatitis, Ann. Intern. Med. **72:**257, 1970.

117. Slaughter, W. B.: Lymphogranuloma venereum, with special reference to head and neck lesions: Collective review, Surg. Gynec. Obstet. **70:**43, 1940.

118. Smallpox eradication: The first three years, W. H. O. Chron. **24:**301, 1970.

119. Southam, J. C., and Colley, I. T.: Hand, foot and mouth disease, Brit. Dent. J. **125:**298, 1968.

120. Stokes, J. H., and Guthrie, M.: A case for diagnosis (lymphogranuloma venereum of the face?), Arch. Derm. Syph. **60:**123, 1949.

121. Sussman, L. N.: Kew Gardens' spotted fever, New York Med. **2:**27, 1946.

122. Swoboda, N.: Varicella. In Pfaundler, M. and Schlossmann, A. (eds.): The diseases of children, ed. 2, Philadelphia, 1912, J. B. Lippincott Co., vol. 3, p. 330.

123. Thompson, J. L., Jr., Sutliff, W. D., Hennessey, T. P., and Norman, S. L.: Transmission of viral hepatitis by dental procedures, J.A. M.A. Ala. **23:**45, 1953.

124. Thygeson, P.: Viral infections of the eye and adnexa, Trans. Amer. Acad. Ophth. Otolaryng., p. 411, 1958.

125. Timperley, W. R., Horne, C. H. W., and Stewart-Tull, D. E. S.: A bacteriophage specific for *Streptococcus faecalis* Lancefield's serotype 19, J. Path. Bact. **91:**631, 1966.

126. Trumbull, M. L., and Greiner, D. J.: Homologous serum jaundice: An occupational hazard to medical personnel, J.A.M.A. **145:**965, 1951.

127. Vonka, V., and Benyesh-Melnick, M.: Interactions of human cytomegalovirus with human fibroblasts, J. Bact. **91:**213, 1966.

128. Weathers, D. R., and Griffin, J. W.: Intraoral ulcerations of recurrent herpes simplex and recurrent aphthae: Two distinct clinical entities, J. Amer. Dent. Assoc. **81:**81, 1970.

129. Weibel, R. E., Buynak, E. B., Whitman, J. E., Jr., Leagus, M. B., Stokes, J., Jr., and Hilleman, M. R.: Jeryl Lynn strain live mumps virus vaccine, J.A.M.A. **207:**1667, 1969.

130. Williams, R. E. O., and Rippon, J. E.: Bacteriophage typing of *Staphylococcus aureus,* J. Hyg. **50:** 320, 1952.

131. Wilson, W. B., and Cheatham, W. J.: Parotitis in weanling mice produced by coxsackie B-1 (Conn.-5) virus, Amer. J. Path. **41:**415, 1962.

132. Woodward, T. E.: Rickettsial diseases in the United States, Med. Clin. N. Amer. **43:**1507, 1959.

133. Young, A. H.: Bulbar poliomyelitis involving the muscles of mastication, Oral Surg. **25:**24, 1968.

REFERENCES AND ADDITIONAL READINGS

Andrewes, C. H., and Pereira, H. G.: Viruses of vertebrates, ed. 2, London, 1967, Baillière Tindall & Cassell Ltd.

Debré, R., Duncan, D., Enders, J. F., et al.: Poliomyelitis, Geneva, 1955, World Health Organization.

Diagnostic procedures for viral and rickettsial infections, ed. 4, New York, 1969, American Public Health Association.

Dixon, C. W.: Smallpox, London, 1962, J. & A. Churchill Ltd.

Fenner, F.: The biology of animal viruses, New York, 1968, Academic Press, Inc.

Fenner, F., and White, D. O.: Medical virology, New York and London, 1970, Academic Press Inc.

Hahon, N. (ed.): Selected papers on the pathogenic rickettsiae, Cambridge, Mass., 1968, Harvard University Press.

Horsfall, F. L., Jr., and Tamm, I. (eds.): Viral and rickettsial infections of man, ed. 4, Philadelphia, 1965, J. B. Lippincott Co.

Smith, W. (ed.): Mechanisms of virus infection, London and New York, 1963, Academic Press, Inc.

6 / Mycology

Although fungal diseases do not figure prominently among the causes of death, it is well recognized that mycotic infections are very widespread and of very high incidence, affecting millions of persons throughout the world.[2] Moreover, in recent years the common use of antibacterial chemotherapeutic agents and corticosteroids has contributed significantly to the steadily rising clinical importance of fungal infections. Dentists, as well as physicians, must therefore be alert to their possible occurrence.

Fungal diseases[48] fall into two distinct groups, the superficial infections and the deep or systemic infections. Two points are particularly noteworthy regarding their general characteristics: (1) The fungi causing superficial mycoses are normally parasites of man and animals, while the fungi causing the deep mycoses are believed to live normally as saprophytes and are less well adapted for a parasitic role. (2) The course of superficial mycoses follows a pattern similar to that of most bacterial and virus diseases; the incubation period is relatively short, the onset of the disease is sudden, and the symptoms are initially severe but decrease in severity with time, so that spontaneous healing may occur. Deep mycoses, on the other hand, have a protracted incubation period, the symptoms are insidious in their onset, and the course of the disease becomes increasingly severe, not infrequently ending in death in the era before modern antifungal therapy ap-

peared. Both types of fungal disease induce an allergic state in the patient.[47]

For effective therapy, the first requirement is to make the correct diagnosis. Definitive diagnosis of a fungal infection depends primarily upon identification of the causative fungus on the basis of its morphologic characteristics, both in the microscope and on the Petri plate. Morphologic criteria, especially those of the reproductive structures, form the basis for differentiation into genus, species, and variety. The commonly occurring significant morphologic structures are shown in Fig. 6-1. The following key identifies the illustrated structures[73]:

1. Microconidia in clusters (French, *en grappes*)
2. Microconidia along hypha (French, *en thyrse*)
3. Macroconidium *(Trichophyton)* (French, *fuseau*)
4. Spiral
5. Intercalary chlamydospore
6. Macroconidium *(Microsporum)*
7. Nodular organ
8. Pectinate body
9. Macroconidia *(Epidermophyton)*
10. Racquet mycelium
11. Arthrospores
12. "Tuberculate" chlamydospore
13. *Aspergillus*
    A. Conidiophore
    B. Sterigmata
    C. Conidia
14. *Penicillium*
    A. Conidiophore
    B. Sterigmata
    C. Conidia
15. Sporangium

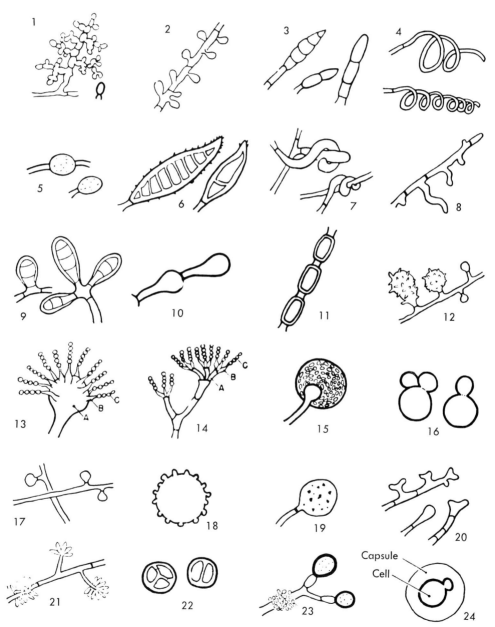

Fig. 6-1. Morphological characteristics of fungi; see text for key. (From Methods for medical laboratory technicians, TM8-227-AFM160-14, Washington, D. C., 1951, U. S. Government Printing Office, p. 501.)

16. Single budding cell
17. Lateral conidia
18. Multiple budding cell
19. Cell containing granules
20. Favic chandeliers
21. Conidia (*Sporotrichum*)
22. Ascospore
23. Terminal chlamydospore (*Candida albicans*)
24. Encapsulated cell

THE SUPERFICIAL MYCOSES (DERMATOMYCOSES)

In the older medical writings on the dermatomycoses, classification of the etiologic agents was based upon clinical rather than upon mycologic characteristics. On the basis of the types of parasitic relationship to the tissues, two main divisions have been described. The most important group is the keratinolytic fungi; these are the organisms causing ringworm and include the genera *Microsporum, Trichophyton,* and *Epidermophyton.* They all contain an enzyme capable of digesting keratin, and therefore they directly invade the keratin of the stratum corneum, hair, and nails. Moreover, they never invade the living layers of the epidermis.[97]

Among the diseases in this group are tinea capitis (ringworm of the scalp), tinea corporis (ringworm of the body), tinea cruris (ringworm of the groin), tinea pedis (ringworm of the feet), tinea barbae (ringworm of the beard), and tinea unguium (ringworm of the nails). Several species of the dermatophytes can cause clinical lesions of the same body surface that are almost identical in their characteristics, although significant differences may be found in their responses to therapeutic agents.

The second group of fungi causing superficial infections does not have keratinolytic enzymes. These grow in the interspaces between keratinized cells rather than in the cells themselves. Therefore, they are more easily reached with topical medicaments and are more controlled with therapeutic agents. Most prominent among the diseases in this group is tinea versicolor, but trichomycosis axillaris is also a common infection belonging to this group.

Although classification on the basis of clinical characteristics has a certain usefulness for practitioners, it is recognized today that the etiologic agents must be classified on the basis of their cultural characteristics and that taxonomic designations must be made according to the rules of botanical nomenclature.

The dermatophytes are Fungi Imperfecti since the sexual phase in their life cycle is unknown and their classification therefore is impossible by the classic criteria of sexual reproduction. Recourse has necessarily been made to other morphologic and physiologic characteristics such as the type of macroconidia, gross colony form, pigment production, and various physiologic tests. On these grounds, several species have been recognized in the three keratinolytic genera of dermatophytes.

Infection with the keratinolytic dermatophytes usually results in skin hypersensitivity, while circulating antibodies in the blood appear to be either less frequent in occurrence or more difficult to demonstrate. The keratinolytic dermatophytes contain a group-specific antigen, trichophytin, which is used for skin hypersensitivity testing. A positive reaction indicates a present or past infection. The reaction is of the delayed type, resembling the tuberculin reaction, and may last for as long as seven days. Secondary, widespread eruptions may occur during the course of an infection, referred to as dermatophytids, which are remote from the site of the infection and which are a result of the generalized hypersensitivity. The hands are a frequent site for dermatophytids when an infection of the feet is present. It is thought that spores or pieces of mycelium from the infection enter the bloodstream and finally lodge in the sensitized skin where they induce the local delayed allergic response.

The tissue changes at the infection site

are compounded from the hypersensitivity reactions and the reactions from the materials produced by the parasite that have a local primary irritating effect. If the tissue reaction is mild, as in the case of *Trichophyton rubrum* infections, the parasite may persist indefinitely; if the reaction is acute, however, then the parasite may be rejected and spontaneous cure may result.

Keratinolytic dermatophytes: species and infections

The genus *Microsporum* contains species that invade the hair and skin but rarely the nails. The fungus characteristically gives rise to numerous fusiform macroconidia produced singly at the ends of the hyphae, and also produces a few microconidia along the sides of the hyphae. *Microsporum audouini* causes ringworm of the scalp, although it occasionally may infect glabrous skin. It has been isolated from the deep type of ringworm of the beard, a mycotic dermatitis rarely seen in the United States, which develops slowly and produces nodular thickenings and kerionlike swellings. The lesions as a rule develop slowly until they become confluent and form diffuse boggy infiltrations with abscesses. Usually they are limited to one part of the face or neck in men, especially the maxillary and submaxillary regions, but they may spread over almost the entire bearded area. The mustache region of the upper lip is rarely involved. The superficial form of tinea barbae, in contrast, is caused by species of *Trichophyton*.

M. audouini is of worldwide distribution, but it especially favors large cities. It is endemic to Europe, and until World War I it occurred only sporadically in the United States. By World War II, however, epidemics began to appear in the United States. Children who have not reached puberty are especially liable to infection by this species. Tinea capitis is commonly transmitted by contact from child to child.

The fungus, on direct examination of the infected hair, appears as a mosaic sheath of spores around stubby hairs. The spores are round and small and appear in large numbers in these specimens. The active site of proliferation of the organisms is just above the hair root where the final stages of keratinization take place. Most infections limited to the hair undergo spontaneous cure. In infections of glabrous skin, segmented mycelium may be apparent, but it cannot be distinguished from those of *Trichophyton* and *Epidermophyton*.

The genus *Trichophyton* contains several species that parasitize hair, skin, and nails. This genus is more difficult to characterize than is *Microsporum* since spores are not found in some forms. Species, therefore, are artificially grouped by colony rather than microscopic morphologic traits. Nutritional characteristics are of great value in identifying certain species. Microconidia are numerous and develop either from the sides of hyphae (*en thyrses*) or in grapelike clusters (*en grappe*); macroconidia are rare or lacking in some species.

Trichophyton rubrum (synonym *T. purpureum*) grows initially as a cottony, pure white colony on the surface of cornmeal dextrose or Sabouraud's glucose agar, but it later develops a velvety surface with a rose-purple or reddish color on the back of the colony. The pigmentation may spread into the agar and into the surface mycelium. This dermatophyte is a very common cause of superficial fungus infections, and the incidence of infections by it is increasing rapidly.[107] In northern New York State, it is the most common agent found, accounting for one third of all superficial fungus infections studied during a period of 15 years. *Trichophyton* infections in this region occurred at an average age of 30 years and were found three times more often among males than females.

T. rubrum infections cause only slight tissue reactions, which frequently leads to their being overlooked and is the reason for their being difficult to treat effectively. The lesions of the skin and nails that it causes are chronic processes that are rarely cured even with griseofulvin. Infections of the feet by *T. rubrum*, for example, if the nails are involved (onychomycosis), have a discouraging rate of cure, with continuous treatment lasting 10 months or more.[86] On the hands, dry chronic ringworm involving the palmar rather than the dorsal surface is caused almost only by *T. rubrum*. The infection may spread to one fingernail or more. These infections were almost never cured before griseofulvin became available, and the infection still presents a formidable problem in therapy.

T. rubrum is also involved in both superficial and deep-seated forms of tinea barbae. The superficial form is a condition characterized by a mild pustular folliculitis that results in a loosening of the beard hairs to the point at which they can be easily pulled out.[5] The skin between the follicles usually shows scaling. If the hairs are broken off, the fungus is *T. violaceum*. Tinea barbae of the deep type may sometimes be difficult to diagnose, and leads to confusion with possible dental lesions. In one case[63] lumps under the skin of both cheeks of a middle-aged white man were diagnosed by a physician as having started from a "gum" condition, and he treated the patient by an injection of penicillin. Failure to respond prompted his visit to a dentist, who found the gingivae were in good condition. Later, attention from three other physicians was required before the correct diagnosis of tinea barbae produced by *T. rubrum* was attained. The overall incidence of tinea barbae is low when the face is kept clean-shaven and the skin is given conventional hygienic care.[66]

Infection of the facial skin by *T. rubrum*, with involvement of the vermilion border of the lips, has been observed in conjunction with infection of fingernails, toenails, and the skin of the hands and arms.[94] *T. rubrum* also has been reported to cause an infection first apparently limited to the vermilion border of the upper lip, and then with spread to the lower lip, which raised some questions of a possible dental causation.[84] *Candida albicans* was found associated with the dermatophyte in this case. There have also been reported infections of the lip with *T. violaceum*[10] and *T. verrucosum*.[80]

The species *T. mentagrophytes* (synonym *T. gypseum*) is a highly pleomorphic fungus, which characteristic has led to a rich accumulation of synonyms for what seems to be a continuous series of a single species. This fungus occurs naturally on small mammals, and human infection can often be traced to contact with these. It is the commonest cause of dermatophytosis of the foot (athlete's foot), but may also cause follicular infection of the scalp and onychomycosis. Colonial morphologic traits on culture medium fall into four general types: (1) Most frequently found is a fluffy colony that becomes flat, velvety, and yellowish buff in color as it develops. (2) A white fluffy colony with aerial mycelium is largely vegetative. (3) A granular, powdery, light tan to yellow colony has a velvety surface that turns fluffy with age. (4) A white colony, at first fluffy, becomes compact with surface irregularities upon aging. Scrapings of diseased skin show numerous conidia (Fig. 6-2).

T. mentagrophytes causes the acute vesicular and intertriginous type of tinea pedis, whereas the dry, subclinical type is usually caused by *T. rubrum*. The feet are among the most common sites of fungus infection. The specific areas involved are the interdigital spaces, the sole (Fig. 6-3), and the lateral aspect of the foot. This distribution is the result of several anatomic, physiologic, and mechanical factors. The weight of the body exerts excessive pressure on the skin of the sole during walking. Perspiration loosens the tissue and thus makes it highly susceptible to infection in the presence of

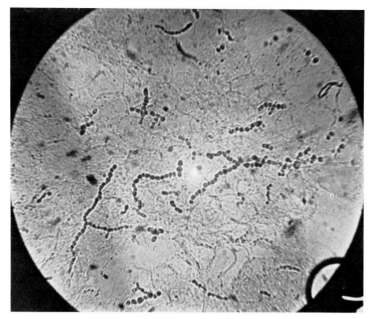

Fig. 6-2. Spores (conidia) *Trichophyton mentagrophytes* isolated. Moist preparation of skin scraping prepared with 10% potassium hydroxide shows numerous conidia. (Courtesy Dr. R. M. Montgomery, New York, N. Y.)

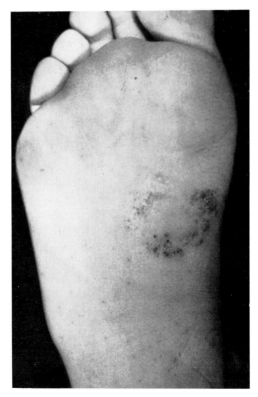

Fig. 6-3. Tinea pedis. Vesicles and encrusted ulcers appear on the sole of foot. *Trichophyton mentagrophytes* was isolated. (Courtesy Dr. R. M. Montgomery, New York, N. Y.)

excessive moisture and heat. Deformities of the feet may be a contributing factor.[86]

Mycotic infections of the toenails are generally, but not always, associated with tinea pedis. In some instances the nails alone may be infected. The most common type of infection consists of discolored, brittle, eroded, free nail plates, caused by the infection starting on the recessus sub-unguinalis. The entire nail may be affected by gradual extension of the infection. It then loses its luster, becoming opaque and uneven. Other, less common, reactions of the nails may be: (1) thickening, discoloration, and curving of the nail plate; (2) separation, thinning, and discoloration of the nail plate; and (3) a white-yellow discoloration of the nail plate, sometimes forming longitudinal streaks and usually caused by *T. mentagrophytes*. The first two forms are caused by either *T. rubrum* or *E. floccosum.*

Diagnosis. It is desirable to determine the etiologic agent of mycotic skin infections for epidemiologic purposes, to determine the proper therapeutic approach, and to establish a more reliable prognosis than would otherwise be possible.

Direct mounts are made of skin and nail scrapings, placed on a slide with 10% sodium hydroxide solution, and then covered with a coverslip. Slight heating of the preparation allows the mycelia to be readily recognized. Specimens are also placed on the various special media available.[86]

Sabouraud's dextrose agar has been traditionally used, but several more effective media are now available. Among these, dermatophyte test medium (DTM) is especially useful.[72] This is a differential and selective medium containing glucose, phenol red, cycloheximide, gentamicin, and chlortetracycline.[99] Ink blue medium (IB) is also effective and contains glucose, ink blue, chloramphenicol, and cyclohexi-mide.[110]

Therapy. Therapy for dermatomycoses and onychomycoses caused by *T. menta-*

grophytes, *T. rubrum,* or *E. floccosum* is strongly dependent upon use of griseoful-vin.[87] Topical treatment with Whitfield's ointment is also instituted to reinforce the effects of the antibiotic. For onychomycosis, debridement of the nails with a nail file or glass slide, followed by painting with tincture of iodine is useful. The average duration of treatment when the onychomycosis is caused by *T. mentagrophytes* is six months, whereas it is 10 months if the infection is caused by *T. rubrum.* For tinea pedis, treatment may last for six weeks on the average if *T. mentagrophytes,* seven weeks if the fungus is *E. floccosum,* and eight weeks if it is *T. rubrum.* Relapse is apt to occur with *T. rubrum,* but not with *T. mentagrophytes.*

The species *Trichophyton schoenleini* is found in the countries of the Mediterranean littoral, the Balkans, and scattered areas throughout Europe and the Far East. Infections found in the United States usually involve families who have recently immigrated. This fungus causes favus, a characteristic infection of the scalp that produces scutula (cuplike structures) from the infected hair follicles. The organism forms a slow-growing colony that is heaped, compact, waxy, and smooth with many irregular folds; it is yellowish-white to light brown.

Trichophyton tonsurans commonly causes *Trichophyton* ringworm infection of the scalp in Europe, although in an increasing number of instances it is being seen in the southern part of the United States. The infection is most common among children, but it may persist into adult life. This organism may also infect the nails or smooth skin. It has been known to cause an infection of the cheeks, extending down to the upper lip, which lesion resembled lupus erythematosus.[34] *T. ton-surans,* occurring as the *acuminatum, crateriforme,* and *cerebriforme* varieties, grows on the surface of agar as a creamy white colony, although some strains may be yellowish or violet. The surface of the colonies is fine and powdery in character. Slide cultures show the presence of many round to oval microconidia that occur either at the tips of the hyphae or along the sides.

The genus *Epidermophyton* has only one species, *E. floccosum,* which is pathogenic for man. It invades the skin and nails but not the hair. Among the infections it causes is an eczema of the crural region and a few of the cases of intertriginous dermatophytosis of the foot. This organism is found widely distributed but is most common in the tropics.

The genus is characterized by the production of numerous oval to club-shaped, multiseptate macroconidia in clusters or coming off directly from the hyphal walls. No microconidia are produced by this genus. Chlamydospores and racquet hyphae are seen in the mycelium. *E. floccosum* grows on Sabouraud's glucose agar as a powdery, greenish-yellow colony that develops a white, cottony aerial mycelium in about three weeks. The surface of the colony is irregularly folded with radial furrows. This fungus exhibits only slight pathogenicity with the guinea pig.

Nonkeratinolytic dermatophytes: species and infections

Tinea versicolor[68] is a fungal skin infection commonly found throughout the world. The causative agent has been referred to as *Malassezia furfur,* but it is questionable whether or not the organism has ever been cultured, and it is probable that it is simply a variant of *Pityrosporon orbiculare,* a normal resident of the skin. The disease is extremely chronic but ordinarily symptomless. The patient complains chiefly because of the cosmetic effect. Tinea versicolor is not contagious, and attempts to transmit it experimentally have failed.

The lesions of tinea versicolor typically occur as multiple, slightly scaling, macular patches ranging from whitish to fawn-color to brown, which accounts for the term "versicolor." The upper trunk, front and back, is most frequently affected, but the lesions may extend onto the extremities and the lower abdomen. When the lesions are scraped with a curet, a fine, branny scale is obtained which has abundant yeastlike and filamentous organisms. These are easily seen in wet mounts made with potassium hydroxide solution.

Topical treatment with various preparations, such as an ointment of sulfur and salicylic acid, induces only a temporary response. Recurrence is the usual experience regardless of the therapeutic regimen adopted. Use of griseofulvin is not effective.

Trichomycosis axillaris is a fungus infection of the axillary and pubic hairs caused by *Nocardia tenuis.* The hair shaft, in this infection, becomes covered with a yellow, red, or black nodular coating continuous along the hair. The delicate mycelia are embedded in the mucilaginous material of the hair coating. The cortex of the hair is invaded. The hair appears lusterless and brittle, and breaks easily. Treatment consists of shaving the hair and then applying lotion or ointment containing neomycin and bacitracin to the involved region.

THE DEEP MYCOSES

The fungi causing deep mycoses are a heterogeneous group which allow few generalizations. The very name for the group is misleading since some of the members are able to cause cutaneous lesions as well as lesions of the viscera. *Candida albicans* constitutes an intermediary form between the dermatophytes and the fungi causing deep infections, although it is primarily a pathogen that prefers the skin and mucosa rather than the deeper organs.[65]

Candida: candidiasis (moniliasis)

More than thirty species of the genus *Candida*[96] have been described. These rather primitive fungi are members of the family *Cryptococcaceae,* being widely scattered in nature and frequently isolated from other than animal sources. Man is a natural but not exclusive habitat for these yeastlike forms. Infection with *Candida* is a relatively frequent mycosis, of worldwide distribution.[105]

Of the several different species of fungi that have been cultivated from the human mouth, the *Candida* species have attracted the greatest amount of study because they are frequently present in substantial numbers and because they are opportunistic pathogens capable of causing very serious deep infections as well as quite annoying superficial infections.[53] *Candida* species with the same potentialities as those in the mouth occur on the other exposed mucosal surfaces of the body as well as upon the skin. The most pronounced pathogenic species among these parasitic forms is *Candida albicans*, although there is good experimental evidence for the pathogenicity of *C. tropicalis, C. stellatoidea, C. pseudotropicalis,* and *C. viswanathii.* There is also

reason to suspect that *C. parapsilosis, C. guilliermondi,* and *C. krusei* also may be pathogenic for man.

C. albicans[18] has been isolated from clinical specimens, carriers, soil, vegetation, and foods. It is unicellular and reproduces by blastospores, which are formed by simple multiple budding. Cells obtained directly from a lesion stain grampositive. The blastospores are oval to round, varying from 2 to 4 μ in diameter. *C. albicans,* in contrast to the other *Candida* species, has a marked tendency to form large, thick-walled spores (Fig. 6-4), referred to as chlamydospores, when placed on special media such as cornmeal agar. The chlamydospore is from 7 to 8 μ in diameter and usually arises at the ends of the pseudomycelia. It is an important morphologic character in the identification of *C. albicans.* The pseudomycelium of *C. albicans* appears under semi-anaerobic conditions and consists of elongated cells that may remain end-to-end in chains. Blasto-

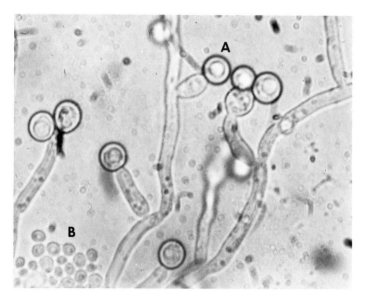

Fig. 6-4. *Candida albicans.* Phase contrast of colony grown on cornmeal agar (1,100 x) shows pseudomycelium with attached large refractile chlamydospores, *A,* and small blastospores, *B.*

spores are clustered in bunches along the pseudomycelium at the points where the pseudomycelial cell-ends abut upon each other.

On Sabouraud's agar or a similar medium, the colonies appear smooth, moist, and creamy in color. These are typically medium-sized (1.5 to 2 mm. in diameter) yeastlike colonies, soft in consistency, which rather quickly send filaments into the depth of the agar. A distinct yeasty odor develops after four or five days. If allowed to continue growth for six weeks, giant colonies form, a single one of which will occupy a large part of a conventional-sized Petri plate (Fig. 6-5).

Candida species grow readily on a simple agar medium containing peptone and dextrose, maltose, or sucrose. Their isolation from the usual clinical specimens that have many normally present bacteria is aided by the addition of an antibiotic such as streptomyin or chloramphenicol to the simple medium. A considerable number of other special media have been developed that may allow differentiation or selection. Among these, the Pagano-Levin medium[82] is particularly useful as a means of quickly differentiating several species of *Candida* on the basis of tetrazolium salt reduction.[4] The tetrazolium is reduced to a red formazan by liberated dehydrogenases. *C. tropicalis* grows on the medium with a deep red color, whereas *C. albicans* does not reduce the tetrazolium and appears in its usual colonial color. Colonies of other

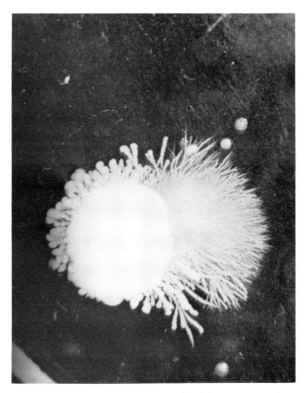

Fig. 6-5. Giant colony, *Candida albicans* 1 month old on cornmeal agar. Smooth white surface growth consists almost entirely of yeastlike cells (blastospores). Hairlike projections beneath surface of agar medium contain pseudomycelium and attached blastospores and chlamydospores.

Table 6-1. Differential diagnosis of species *Candida**

Species	Sabouraud's broth	Glucose	Maltose	Sucrose	Lactose
C. albicans	No surface growth	AG†	AG	A	—
C. tropicalis	Surface film thin with bubbles	AG	AG	AG	—
C. pseudotropicalis	No surface growth	AG	—	AG	—
C. krusei	Wide surface film	AG	—	—	—
C. parakrusei	No surface growth	AG‡	—	—	—
C. stellatoidea	No surface growth	AG	AG	—	—
C. guilliermondi	No surface growth	—	—	—	§

*Modified from Martin, D. S., Jones, C. P., Yao, K. L., and Lee, L. E., Jr.: J. Bact. **34:**99, 1937.
†A = acid, G = gas
‡Occasionally acid only
§Occasionally acid and gas at 25° C. for 20 days

species of *Candida* produce lighter shades of red. *C. krusei* is similar in color to *C. albicans,* but its growth is much drier, as well as wrinkled and flat. Moreover, a bismuth glycine glucose yeast extract agar (Bacto-BiGGy agar) has also been developed that facilitates the detection, isolation, and differentiation of *C. albicans.*

Fermentation reactions with glucose, maltose, sucrose, and lactose are valuable in determining the species of *Candida* (Table 6-1), but this is a time-consuming and expensive procedure receiving only limited application in the diagnostic laboratory.

Animal pathogenicity. Laboratory studies[52] of candidiasis to determine the mechanisms of pathogenicity and to provide a model system for studies of therapeutic agents are subject to difficulties because of the relatively low pathogenicity of *C. albicans* and of the other, even less active, species of *Candida.* Special procedures have been necessarily developed to establish animal infections in the laboratory. Among these are inoculation by the intravenous route, the use of a very high dosage of the yeast, lowering of host resistance by cortisone or antibiotics, low temperature, radiation, mucin, or the production of alloxan diabetes.[78]

Mice, guinea pigs, and rabbits have been the animals commonly used in experimental studies, but the rabbit is the most useful among these. In mice it has been found that infection by the intravenous route results in a disseminated candidiasis characterized by inflammation, abscesses, and granulomas, which are most prominent in the heart, kidney, brain, and spleen. If the animal is injected by the subcutaneous or intraperitoneal route, disseminated infection does not develop. Intravenous injection of the rabbit kills in four or five days. Lesions of the kidneys and brains are especially prominent in these cases. Candidiasis of the oral mucosa and the mucocutaneous border of the mouth of rabbits has been produced by feeding the animals both tetracycline and packed cells of *C. albicans.*[46] The mucocutaneous lesions of thrush in the healthy host may be obtained if physical damage is produced in the mucosa.

Clinical picture.[112] *Candida* organisms are opportunists commonly found as saprophytes in the oral cavity, intestine, vagina, and bronchial secretion. The normal oral, intestinal, and vaginal mucous membranes, in fact, are able to support comparatively large populations of *Candida* without any apparent ill effects. However, when there is an altered metabolism such as in diabetes or iron-deficiency anemia, a breakdown or lack of normal body defense mechanisms as in acute leukemia or hypogammaglobulinemia, or a marked disturbance in the normal balance in the surface microbiota

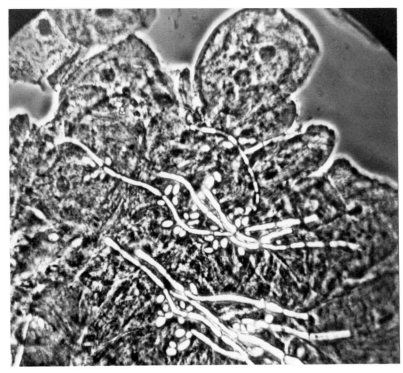

Fig. 6-6. Phase contrast of oral mucosal scraping showing pseudomycelium and blasto-spores of *Candida albicans* together with many squamous epithelial cells. (Courtesy Dr. M. Wheatcroft, Houston, Tex.)

caused by the use of broad-spectrum antibiotics, these fungi can cause characteristic infections that may be quite serious, or even life-threatening. The infection in man may be divided into two main groups: the superficial infections and the deep infections. The latter fortunately are rare for they are often fatal. The superficial infections, affecting mucous membranes and the skin, are common.

The infection of the oral cavity referred to as thrush, oral moniliasis, or acute pseudomembranous candidiasis is caused by *C. albicans*.[25] The disease may start in any part of the mouth as a swelling or primary ulcer, or as a lesion secondary to some other oral abnormality. It may occur at any age but is predominantly a disease of infancy and old age. Apparently, passive immunity obtained from the mother plays a

role in the occurrence of infantile thrush for it occurs more often in the bottle-fed than in the breast-fed baby. Antibody transferred through the placenta from mother to fetus presumably also plays a role in protecting the infant against thrush.[17] This immunity is probably produced by IgG since IgA and IgM do not cross the placenta in quantity.[36]

In the newborn, thrush typically appears between the sixth and tenth days of life in the form of white, curdy, adherent patches. The white patches contain numerous desquamated epithelial cells and microorganisms that tend to adhere to a reddened, inflamed mucosa. It is also seen that pseudomycelia and blastospores both are present (Fig. 6-6), in contrast to blastospores alone in the normal healthy mouth. If the infection extends to the pharynx, bronchi, esophagus, or through the bloodstream to vital body organs, then the disease becomes much more serious. In the adult, oral candidiasis tends to become chronic and the thrush membrane is thicker and less friable than it is in the infant. Sometimes large areas of the mouth are involved, and the plaques may ulcerate. There is an incidence of thrush of some 4% among all infants, and approximately 10% among elderly debilitated hospital patients.[60] Terminal patients suffering from tuberculosis or cancer are especially liable to develop thrush.

Chronic oral hyperplastic candidiasis (candidal leukoplakia)[23] is a condition difficult to differentiate clinically from leukoplakia, but quite different from thrush. It consists of white, firm, persistent plaques in the mouth, most commonly involving the cheek, lips, and tongue. Hyphae are invariably present, but only in the superficial part of the epithelium. Most of the hyphae grow at right angles to the surface, and yeast forms are seen only on the surface. Chronic inflammatory changes are

present in the corium. These patients have both serum and saliva antibodies against *C. albicans*. Similar chronic lesions, but involving a granulomatous tissue reaction, may occur in the skin. In contrast to the chronic lesions without granuloma, there is almost always present in these cases a generalized cutaneous anergy; there is a failure of the skin to respond to intracutaneously administered antigens.[43] The lesions may persist for as long as two decades. They are difficult to treat, although nystatin tablets used for from three to five months may clear them in some cases, or at least bring about some improvement.

Candidiasis confined to the lips (candidal cheilitis) apparently develops only upon damage to the mucosa of the lip by sunburn or windburn. A mixed flora is always present in these lesions.[33] The need to differentiate this syndrome from cancer or other possible diseases must be kept in mind.

In the condition referred to as perlèche, or angular cheilitis,[22] the corners of the mouth are characterized by cracking and

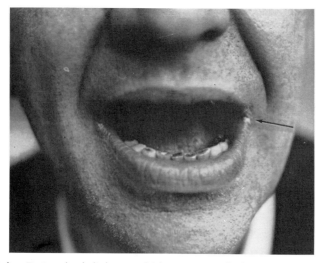

Fig. 6-7. Perlèche. Patient had diabetes which was controlled under insulin therapy during which *Candida albicans* previously present in mouth decreased in numbers and perlèche lesions disappeared.

fissuring from infection with *C. albicans* (Fig. 6-7), although bacteria may also play a role. The lesions extend from the oral mucosa to the mucosa of the lips, and on to the skin of the face. The mucosa of the lips is thickened and somewhat macerated, and the lesion is most marked in this area. Overclosure of the bite in patients wearing dentures may contribute to the development of perlèche by irritating the skin folds at the corners of the mouth, but more commonly these facial fissures are created by placing the maxillary incisor teeth too far posteriorly in the denture. A habit of licking the sides of the mouth may also be a factor in evoking perlèche. Angular cheilitis caused by *C. albicans* in many cases can be differentiated in the clinic from a bacterial infection by everting the cheek and inspecting the buccal mucosa for the presence of a white plaque radiating from the margins of the fissure. The white plaque is absent if the cheilitis is caused by gram-positive cocci. In this last case the fissures do not usually extend onto the buccal mucosa

and the surface of the lesion is usually crusted.

It appears that angular cheilitis is closely associated with denture stomatitis,[61] the most common form of oral candidiasis, and it usually clears up when the denture stomatitis is treated successfully. In denture stomatitis, also known as denture sore mouth or chronic atrophic candidiasis, the mucosa of the palate underlying a full upper denture becomes diffusely inflamed. The inflammation may occur in patches or it may spread to involve the whole area covered by the denture. Women have a significantly higher incidence than men. Direct smears of the mucosa taken immediately upon removal of the denture usually show hyphae. Cultures of the mucosa (Fig. 6-8) yield heavy growth of *Candida* colonies that may even become confluent. Denture stomatitis in some cases may be the forerunner of oral thrush.

Intertriginous regions such as under female breasts, under the arms, in the inguinocrural and intergluteal folds, or between the fingers (Fig. 6-9) or toes are

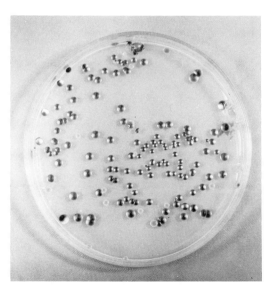

Fig. 6-8. *Candida albicans* growing on BiGGY agar, isolated from scrapings from inflamed area under upper denture case.

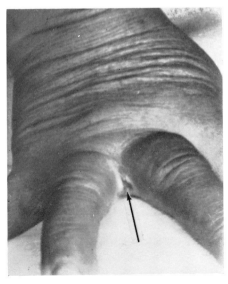

Fig. 6-9. Intertriginous lesion between the fingers; etiologic agent is *Candida albicans.*

also at risk of infection from *C. albicans*.[33] These lesions are characterized initially by vesicles, followed by fairly well demarcated and dusky-red inflamed and moist patches of the skin whose outer epithelial cells tend to exfoliate rapidly. The intertriginous lesions between the fingers consist of soggy, whitish, erythematous, scaly lesions in the webs of the fingers. The lesions between the toes often yield *C. albicans* associated with *S. aureus* and occasionally *E. coli*. Most probably, the pyogenic bacteria are the primary agents causing the infection, and *C. albicans* has only a secondary role.

C. albicans may cause infection of the nails (onychomycosis), but this disease is probably preceded by a chronic parony-chia[69] caused by the same organism. The infection originates in the sulci unguis, and the matrix becomes secondarily infected. Fully developed candidal infection of the nail is indistinguishable from that caused by species of *Trichophyton* or *Epidermophyton*. The nails show transverse ridges and finally become thickened, distorted, and brownish.

Respiratory tract infections with *C. albicans* may be either bronchopulmonary or pulmonary. Bronchopulmonary candidiasis is not uncommon and produces symptoms of a bronchitis. The infection is limited to the bronchial tree, and peribronchial tissue is little affected. The infection may last for years with little affect upon the general health. It has been observed that bronchial candidiasis, with asthma, may follow the appearance of so-called denture sore mouth (chronic oral candidiasis).[55] Apparently, the oral infection in such cases spreads to the respiratory tract. Simultaneous treatment for both the respiratory tract and oral lesions results in disappearance of all the lesions and recovery of the patient. In pulmonary candidiasis, involvement of the lung parenchyma occurs. It is a slowly progressing disease with a persistent, productive cough. The sputum characteristically is mucoid, tenacious, and gelatinous, with the odor of bread or yeast. If the disease is severe, it may mimic advanced pulmonary tuberculosis.[93]

The saprophytic *Candida* resident in the vagina may, under certain circumstances, cause a vaginitis,[104] especially if the person has diabetes mellitus, is pregnant, or is taking broad-spectrum antibiotics by mouth. In most cases the infection is mild, characterized by a vaginal discharge and local pruritus. Vaginal carriage in the pregnant woman may result in transmission to the infant during birth or shortly after, resulting in oral thrush of the infant.

In the male a urethritis caused by *Candida* or a venereal candidiasis of the glans penis and prepuce of the sexual partners of women with vaginal thrush has been noted in several reports.[45] These latter male patients generally are uncircumcised, and some have marked phimosis. Their symptoms consist of mild irritation around the glans penis and the mucosa of the prepuce; often there is a slight seropurulent discharge.

Clinical manifestations of anaphylactic hypersensitivity such as eczematoid dermatitis of the face may develop during an infection with *C. albicans*.[39] Certain cases of miliaria (acute inflammation of the sweat glands, which are characterized by the sudden appearance of small papules and vesicles, and by itching and burning) may be hypersensitive reactions to *C. albicans* infection. The moniliid, a sterile vesicular or exudative lesion which appears on the hands following the development of candidiasis elsewhere in the body, is also a form of candidal hypersensitivity.

Generalized candidal infections of the body are most often caused by the direct inoculation of the organism into the bloodstream through intravenous infusions or vascular catheters, and only a few hematogenous infections are secondary to blood-vessel invasion from the gastrointestinal tract.[71] There is a tendency for *C. albicans* and *C. tropicalis* to localize more fre-

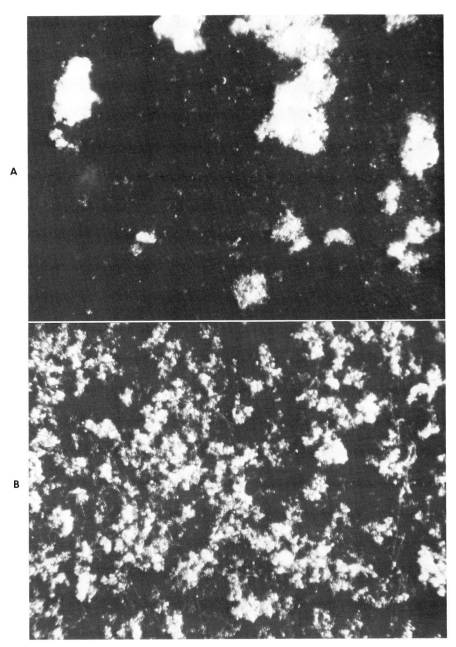

Fig. 6-10. A, Agglutination of *Candida albicans* with adsorbed antiserum; strong reaction, with large clumps. **B,** Agglutination of *Candida tropicalis* with adsorbed *C. albicans* antiserum, weak reaction, with small clumps.

quently in the kidney than in any other tissue in these generalized infections. The tendency for some persons to develop disseminated candidiasis may possibly be the result of a sharp reduction in the property of normal blood plasma or serum to kill *C. albicans*, as determined by an in vitro test. This loss of candidacidal ability has been noted especially in patients suffering from candidiasis in the presence of liver disease, azotemic renal disease, diabetes acquired before the age of 50 years, or leukemia.

Diagnosis. Clinical specimens may include swabs, skin or mucosal scrapings, sputum, and other forms; these may be stored for as long as 10 weeks in the laboratory without fear that suspected yeasts may not retain viability. Microscopic examination of original material from a lesion caused by *C. albicans*, mounted in potassium hydroxide solution on a slide, should show a tangled mass of pseudohyphae, as well as a variable number of blastospores, since the pseudohyphal phase is the invasive state of this fungus. This is an important point even if cultures are positive for *Candida*.

The tetrazolium reaction on Pagano-Levin culture medium is a rapid and convenient means for the preliminary identification of *C. albicans*. On eosin methylene blue agar, in an atmosphere of 10% carbon dioxide at 37° C., clinical specimens will yield characteristic colonies of *C. albicans* that can be positively identified within from 24 to 48 hours.[106]

A rapid laboratory procedure useful for identification consists of determining whether so-called germ tubes are formed.[100] These are filamentous outgrowths of the blastospore or chlamydospore that appear after exposure to blood serum for four hours at 37° C. The production of chlamydospores, usually in great numbers, upon suitable medium is a property useful for presumptive identification also.[31] A quite rapid presumptive test for the identifica-

tion of *C. albicans* is slide agglutination of the culture by adsorbed *C. albicans* antiserum (Difco). Strong and rapidly clumping reactions occur if the culture is *C. albicans* (Fig. 6-10, *A*), while slow and less pronounced clumping indicates that the culture is *C. tropicalis* (Fig. 6-10, *B*).

Definitive identification of the isolated culture is a difficult technical procedure. The biologic point that must be established is the formation of chlamydospores and pseudohyphae. In some instances it may be necessary to resort to fermentation studies for identification.

All cases should arouse a suspicion of some underlying systemic disorder for which a thorough search should be undertaken. Diabetes mellitus, particularly, should be kept in mind since the earliest manifestation of this metabolic disturbance may be the development of candidiasis.[33] If an underlying factor is discovered, its correction may well lead to a clearing of the candidal infection without further specific treatment.

Specific treatment. Superficial lesions of the oral cavity or skin were, in the past, treated successfully with a 1% gentian violet solution. Today, however, nystatin[113] topically applied in the form of a troche three or four times a day for one or two weeks is the agent of choice for oral lesions since in some cases gentian violet may produce a superficial necrosis (so-called gentian violet burn) or unsightly staining. Amphotericin B also may be used (Fig. 6-11), especially if the patient has difficulty with the strong and unpleasantly bitter flavor of nystatin. In the case of denture stomatitis, the denture should not be worn during treatment to allow exposure of the tissue to the drug. When both *C. albicans* and gram-positive cocci are found in the fissures of angular cheilitis, neomycin ointment should be prescribed in addition to nystatin tablets. Chronic candidal infections treated with nystatin for a dec-

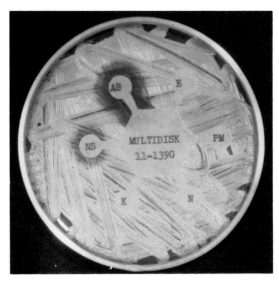

Fig. 6-11. *Candida albicans* reaction to amphotericin B at a concentration of 25 μg (disc AB), and nystatin at a concentration of 25 units (disc NS). The culture was isolated from a patient with denture sore mouth.

ade or more have yielded cultures of the yeast that have an increased resistance to nystatin and cross-resistance to amphotericin B, but at present the development of antibiotic resistance by *Candida* does not appear to be a serious matter.[16]

Intertriginous candidiasis has been most successfully treated with iodochlorhydroxyquin (Vioform)[33]; nystatin apparently has not been effective. Candidal infections of the skin with an allergic component have been successfully treated with candicidin, a polyene antibiotic currently under investigation.[39] In the case of candidal paronychia, therapy consists of potassium permanganate soaks and applications of nystatin ointment or amphotericin B lotion to the affected parts. Venereal candidiasis may require circumcision of the male and vaginal treatment of his sexual partner before cure can be obtained.[45]

Geotrichum: geotrichosis

Various species of *Geotrichum*,[19] which is placed in the family Moniliaceae, have been isolated especially from lesions in the respiratory tract, oral cavity, and intestinal tract, although they have also been found in every part of the body. The most commonly identified species is *Geotrichum candidum*. Since *Geotrichum* is often present in the alimentary tract[30] without evidence of infection, it is considered to be an opportunist that becomes pathogenic for seriously debilitated persons or patients receiving immunosuppressive treatment.

The fungus appears as oblong or rectangular cells, 2 by 6 μ, or as large spheric cells to 10 μ in diameter. Cultures from sputum, pus, or feces are made on Sabouraud's glucose agar plates incubated at room temperature and at 37° C. for at least two weeks. At 37° C., the colony largely grows into the agar, with a smaller central growth upon the surface. At room temperature, the fungus initially appears as a soft and creamy colony which then becomes dry, tough, and membranous. It is easily picked up from the medium with a loop. The rectangular arthrospores formed from segmenting hyphae characteristically germinate by a germ tube from one corner. Most species do not grow well at 37° C.

Oral lesions of geotrichosis are indistinguishable clinically from those of candidiasis.[26] Only mycologic study, especially direct examination of material from the lesion, can differentiate the two. Mixed infections may occur which involve both *Geotrichum* and *Candida* species. Rarely, similar lesions may be caused by *Saccharomyces cereviseae*.[89]

Geotrichum may cause a chronic infection of the tonsils with symptoms, including a slight sore throat, that are seldom acute or severe.[20] Bronchial geotrichosis is the most commonly recognized form of the infection. The patient has a chronic bronchitis with a persistent cough and the production of a mucoid or gelatinous sputum with occasional streaks of blood. There is little or no rise in temperature.

Treatment is similar to that for candidiasis. Both nystatin and amphotericin B are effective.

Cryptococcus neoformans: cryptococcosis

Cryptococcosis,[13] referred to as torulosis in the older medical writings, is a subacute or chronic fungal disease involving the lungs, the central nervous system, and occasionally other organs such as the skin or tongue.[57] It was first described late in the nineteenth century, but it was not until 1916 that the disease was differentiated from other deep mycoses.

The etiologic agent is *Cryptococcus neoformans* (synonym *Torula histolytica*), a monophasic, yeastlike, round to oval fungus that is easily cultured on all the usual media. It produces only yeastlike colonies on the various media at either room temperature or 37° C.; neither mycelia nor sexual spores have been observed. The yeast cells are gram-positive and are approximately 4 to 6 μ in diameter in culture, but may vary to 10 μ or more. Reproduction is by multilateral asexual budding. The cytoplasm contains numerous vacuoles and granules. Sugars are fermented slowly with the formation of acid and no gas, but this biochemical character is not distinctive. The cells are surrounded by a capsule in the tissues or spinal fluid and sometimes on blood agar. The capsule is one of the most outstanding characteristics of the genus, usually ranging in size from 1 to 2 μ in culture. The thickness of the capsule increases with age, however, and may be varied according to the amount of carbohydrate in the medium. Glistening, cream-colored colonies generally appear in several days on glucose blood agar or Sabouraud's glucose peptone agar. With continued incubation the color may become a deep tan or orange.

The genus *Cryptococcus* has been divided into four distinct serologic groups with a minimal degree of cross-agglutination or precipitation between them. The fungus is capable of evoking protective antibodies in the body, and experimental studies with laboratory animals indicate that a dead cryptococcal vaccine may effect substantial protection against ordinary lethal challenge.

Epidemiology. Cryptococcosis[3] is more prevalent than the available data would indicate. Many cases are either misdiagnosed or not reported. In general, cryptococcosis occurs almost twice as often in males as in females. Two thirds of the patients are between the ages of 30 and 60 years. The fungus and the infection have been found in every part of the world. Pathogenic strains have been recovered from peach juice, soil, and pigeon excreta. The most suitable habitat, however, is in areas frequented by birds.

As many as 50 million viable cells of *C. neoformans* have been found per gram of dried pigeon droppings. These apparently are both an enrichment and a selective medium for the proliferation of *C. neoformans* because of their high content of creatinine. It has been reported that among various yeasts and yeastlike microorganisms *C. neoformans* apparently is the only species that can assimilate and use creatinine as a source of nitrogen.

Human pathogenicity. Lowering of the host's natural resistance by trauma, diabetes mellitus, Hodgkin's disease, reticuloendothelial system diseases, leukemia, or the administration of steroids may result in lesions in human beings. Inhalation of windblown dust containing the fungus may cause lesions of the lungs, which appear to be the usual portal of entry. Apparently, variation in the host's defenses plays an important role, since probably everyone at one time or another carries the organism although only very few become ill. Normal human serum inhibits the growth of *C. neoformans*, but the infection itself provokes only a minimal immunologic response.

Lung infection appears to be the most frequent lesion to develop. Its symptoms consist of fever, cough, and pleural pain. Roentgenograms may show small or large involved lung areas. The lesions may be confined to the lungs for months or even years, simulating tuberculosis in some cases. In some instances dissemination of *C. neoformans* from the lungs occurs by the bloodstream, and, most seriously, establishes foci of infection in the central nervous system. *C. neoformans* is the most frequent cause of fungal meningitis in man. The symptoms include violent and persistent headache, dizziness, double vision, mental aberrations, irritability, and stiffness of the neck, which require differentiation from brain tumor or meningeal tuberculosis.

Lesions of the skin occur that may be primary following trauma but usually are associated with the disseminated disease. The skin lesions may be acneiform, with papules, nodules, abscesses, ulcers, superficial granulomas, and plaques resembling ecchymosis. Skin manifestations occur in about 15% of cases of cryptococcosis in one reported series of cases.

Oral lesions. Lesions of the oral cavity[21] generally occur in persons who have a systemic debilitating disease such as leukemia. Ulcers may occur on the hard or soft palate, in the maxillary antrum, on the tongue, on the gingiva, about a painful loose tooth, or in the tooth socket after extraction of a tooth. These ulcers may become secondarily infected by members of the indigenous flora. Biopsy material of such lesions shows a marked lymphocytosis with some neutrophiles and the presence of encapsulated cryptococci.

Histopathology. On initial invasion of the body, *C. neoformans* is a bland and inert agent, producing no perceptible necrosis or inflammation. The early lesions[76] are gelatinous, consisting of masses of organisms derived from multiplication of the fungus. With their continued residence in the tissue, the lesion becomes granulomatous since the organisms are phagocytosed by giant cells, while macrophages and lymphocytes accumulate. A neutrophilic response and abscess formation develop in only a few cases. Compression effects from growth of the fungus appear to play a role in the pathogenicity of the infection also. The changes in the tissue apparently depend more upon the duration of the infection than upon the virulence of the cryptococci. The *C. neoformans* cells accumulated in the tissue aggregations may become necrotic en masse, which bears only a superficial resemblance to the caseation in tuberculosis, which is based upon the death of reacting tissue cells.

Experimental pathogenicity. Intraperitoneal injection of mice[62] with a saline suspension of culture results in death from generalized cryptococcosis in from 10 days to a few weeks. The organism invades the brain, lung, and kidney. The characteristic lesion consists of cysts containing many cryptococci of various sizes, some budding, others not. Often in experimental animals, and occasionally in human beings, the organisms become calcified. The calcified cells finally rupture. In mice, brain infection evokes less of an inflammatory reaction than occurs in other tissues, which fact, it has been suggested, may account for the relatively high incidence of brain infection by this organism.

Diagnosis. Smears, cultures, examination of tissue, and a correlation of the clinical features are used to establish the diagnosis of cryptococcosis. Diagnosis from histologic examination of tissue may be made with relative ease if the organisms are readily demonstrable. In these cases they are single budding or simple, ovoid to spheric, thick-walled, yeastlike, from 5 to 12 μ in diameter, and surrounded by a thick, refractile, gelatinous capsule that may reach from 50 to 60 μ in diameter. It usually stains poorly with hematoxylin and eosin. The capsule then is often seen only as a clear or unstained halo around the fungus cell. Intracerebral inoculation of the mouse is the easiest and quickest method for diagnosis. Death occurs in from five to eight days. Immunologic techniques such as agglutination, precipitation, complement fixation, or skin tests have been used for the diagnosis of cryptococcosis, but their lack of reliability has restricted their value in routine diagnostic procedures.

Treatment. Amphotericin B has been invaluable in treatment for cryptococcal meningitis as well as for lesions of the lungs, skin, and oral mucosa.[44] Before amphotericin B was available more than 86% of patients with cryptococcal meningitis died within one year of diagnosis, with 70% of the deaths occurring within three months of diagnosis.

When the cryptococcal lesions are confined to the lung, cure by lung resection may occur. In such cases amphotericin B therapy is started before surgery to inhibit the development of cryptococcal meningitis.[102]

Coccidioides immitis: coccidioidomycosis

Coccidioides immitis is a diphasic yeastlike microorganism which in its parasitic form in tissues appears as a sac or spherule containing some small yeast cells. The diameter of the spherules varies from 10 to 70 μ, and the small endospores are approximately 2 to 5 μ in diameter. When the spherule grows larger, it ruptures and liberates the endospores. No budding occurs in the spherule stage.

The mycotic disease coccidioidomycosis,[50] the primary form of which is respiratory, was at one time considered to occur infrequently and to be usually fatal. However, it is now recognized that many animals as well as human beings become infected by the etiologic agent, *C. immitis*, and recover after having mild symptoms that simulate "flu" and last at most several weeks. It has been estimated that some 10 million persons have had coccidioidomycosis.[111] The disease has been called by various names, including desert fever, desert rheumatism, valley fever, and San Joaquin fever.

When the fungus is grown on Sabouraud's medium at room temperature, a septate, white, cottony, fluffy mycelium appears within a week which later changes to a dark cream or brown color. The aerial hyphae tend to form into many arthrospores that easily become free from the mycelium. Cultural examination of this microorganism is a dangerous procedure and instances of laboratory infection have been reported. Minor air currents from the movement of a Petri dish or its cover are sufficient to disseminate the arthrospores into the surrounding air where they are inhaled by the laboratory worker. Masks and gloves need to be worn, and the culture is carried in well-stoppered tubes rather than in Petri dishes.

Transmission. The natural habitat of *C. immitis* is the alkaline arid or semiarid soil of the southwestern United States, specifically Arizona, California, New Mexico, Nevada, Utah, and parts of Texas. The fungus and the infection are also found in other countries of the Western Hemisphere, including Argentina, Venezuela,

Honduras, and Guatemala. Sporadic cases have been reported also from Italy. It has been suggested that during the summer months in such areas the topsoil may reach a temperature of from 60° to 70° C., which persists for several months and inhibits proliferation of microbial life in the topsoil; but *C. immitis* remains viable in the deeper soil. With the advent of the rainy season when the soil becomes saturated with moisture, *C. immitis* proliferates and again appears in the topsoil in large numbers. Then the topsoil dries and is windblown; the blastospores are readily disseminated into the air, and individuals inhale them with dust particles. In World War II 6,000 cases were diagnosed in soldiers.[37]

Man-to-man transmission is known to occur. In one series of cases, six infections occurred from a patient with coccidioidal osteomyelitis whose dressings were changed infrequently without adequate attention to preventing germination of the spherules on the plaster cast, which had been soiled with spherule-containing exudate.

Pathogenicity. Pulmonary lesions are usually the result of primary infection. Apparently, the symptoms that occur may be severe in some individuals, while in many others they may simulate influenza. Symptoms such as pains in the joints and muscles, a fever of from 100° to 103° F., and probably a slight cough, or subclinical symptoms may occur and then subside in several weeks. Some individuals, however, have a chronic pulmonary form of the infection that may be confused with tuberculosis (Fig. 6-11). In 2 of 1,000 cases of primary infections, *C. immitis* may be disseminated by the hematogenous route and cause metastatic lesions in other organs and bones, especially the ribs and the small bones of the hands and feet. In some instances, meningitis may occur.

The mucous membranes of the lips and nose as well as the skin of the face may develop lesions secondary to the primary lung lesions.[40] Usually the cutaneous le-

sions start as small superficial pustules that are soon replaced by papillomatous nodules. The papillomas are friable and pressure causes the expulsion of purulent material. *C. immitis* may be easily demonstrated in a potassium hydroxide slide preparation of this pus. Ulcers or granulomatous lesions may occur in the oral cavity.[115]

The white race seems more resistant to the disease than the darker Indian, Mexican, or black races.

Diagnosis. Coccidioidomycosis may be diagnosed by microscopic examination of clinical specimens, culture, animal inoculation, cutaneous tests, and serology.

Cutaneous tests are made with coccidioidin, an antigen prepared from cultures of *C. immitis*. When injected intracutaneously into sensitized individuals, it produces an erythematous reaction. Many individuals, residents of the endemic areas, give positive reactions without having any apparent symptoms. This may mean that at some time in the past there was infection and subclinical symptoms. In persons with severe symptoms, a low titer or a negative complement reaction is considered a favorable sign.

Treatment. Persons with mild symptoms recover with little treatment or none. Those having severe cases may benefit from long periods of treatment with amphotericin B and supportive measures. Lesions of the head and neck leave unsightly puckered scars upon healing which may require surgical correction.

Blastomyces dermatitidis: North American blastomycosis

North American blastomycosis[92] (Gilchrist's disease) is a chronic granulomatous disease first described by Gilchrist in Baltimore in 1894 as a localized skin infection. The systemic form was first reported in 1902. It subsequently became apparent that there are two forms of the infection: a primary cutaneous form and a pulmonary form that has a tendency for dissemination. Usually, the cutaneous manifestations are a result of dissemination from a primary pulmonary infection. True primary cutaneous blastomycosis is an extremely rare condition.

Blastomyces dermatitidis is a diphasic fungus that in sputum, pus, or exudates occurs in the parasitic yeast stage as large, thick-walled cells, from 8 to 25 μ in diameter, which give rise to buds. The buds are characteristically single and broad based. In culture on blood agar at 37° C., round budding forms are found whose appearance is identical to those found in tissue or in lesion discharges. Soft, waxy, wrinkled colonies not unlike those of *Mycobacterium tuberculosis* are seen. On Sabouraud's glucose agar at room temperature, the fungus grows out as a white to light brown filamentous colony. It consists of branching septate hyphae with lateral or terminal conidia. These spores develop as small projections that gradually enlarge. The cell wall of these projections is at first thin, but slowly begins to thicken, giving the appearance of chlamydospores. These conidia are smooth-walled, in contrast to those of *Histoplasma capsulatum*, which can resemble *B. dermatitidis* very closely when cultured on Sabouraud's agar.

Clinical picture. The exact manner of infection has not been conclusively defined. It is in all probability, however, thought to be by inhalation. The pulmonary disease begins with fever and symptoms of upper-respiratory tract infection resembling influenza; it progresses gradually with fever, weight loss, cachexia with cough, and purulent sputum. The disease may persist for years. The fungus sometimes may invade the chest wall and produce multiple sinuses. The sputum usually has numerous yeastlike budding cells of *B. dermatitidis*.

The cutaneous form of the disease is characterized by a papule that ulcerates and spreads slowly outward for months or even years, leaving an irregular, crested ulcer with a granulomatous base and an elevated verrucous border containing minute abscesses. The center of the ulcer heals with a thin scar. The lesions are usually on exposed parts of the body such as the face, hands, wrists, feet, and ankles.

Oral lesions occur infrequently. They have been reported occurring on the tongue,[79] gingivae,[27] mandible,[74] hard palate,[28] lips,[32] and oral mucosa.[28] It is significant that some patients with blastomycosis first sought medical or dental attention because of their oral lesions. In one case, "toothache" was an initial symptom.[12] The dentist, instead of the physician, thus may well be the first to see the patient with blastomycosis.

Epidemiology.[41] North American blastomycosis is a relatively common mycotic disease in the north central and southeastern states of the United States. Kentucky has the greatest frequency of reported cases. Occasional cases have been reported in other parts of the world, including Canada, Mexico, Central and South America, South Africa, Tunisia, Uganda, India, Australia, and Europe. About two thirds of the patients are between 15 and 45 years of age, and there is a marked prevalence of the disease in males.

The available evidence indicates that the soil is a natural reservoir for *B. dermatitidis*, although it is difficult to isolate the organism from it. Unsterilized soil, in fact, will yield positive cultures for only two weeks, after seeding with yeast cells of *B. dermatitidis*, which may help account for the relative infrequency of clinical cases of blastomycosis compared to either histoplasmosis or coccidioidomycosis. Person-to-person transmission seems to occur but rarely; direct mechanical transmission has been reported. In one case, for example, cutaneous infection of a finger followed the bite of a dog.

Experimental animal pathogenicity. In the laboratory it has been shown that guinea pigs, mice, and hamsters are susceptible to North American blastomycosis when infected with material containing the organism. The most sensitive of the animals is the white mouse when injected intraperitoneally. Subcutaneous inoculation of the hamster results in cutaneous blastomycosis, with no conclusive evidence of subsequent hematogenous spread. This is suggestive of clinical findings of primary cutaneous infection in man.[12] Blastomycosis has been reported to occur as a natural infection in the dog and the horse.

Diagnosis. The diagnosis of blastomycosis is made by culturing or by finding the characteristic budding forms of the fungus in the lesions. Sputum or bronchial washing is studied directly by means of potassium hydroxide solution mounts. The specimen is inoculated on Sabouraud's agar for incubation at room temperature, and on blood agar plates for incubation at 37° C. If the culture presents difficulties in identification, it is injected intraperitoneally into mice. Fatal infection will ensue usually in about two or three weeks. Necropsy of the animal will show large caseous nodes in the mesentery, and tubercles in the spleen, liver, and lungs. The typical tissue phase of the fungus will be present in these organs.

Biopsy of the lesion may be desirable since differentiation from a low-grade squamous cell carcinoma may be necessary if the site of involvement is the skin or mucous membrane. Since the fungus is irregularly distributed through the tissue, extensive search for the typical fungal cells may be necessary, but culturing is also needed in any case. Tuberculosis may present a problem in differential diagnosis.

Skin testing has utilized as antigen heat-killed yeast phase cells or a filtrate from a synthetic broth culture. Intradermal injection in the positive case results in a localized edematous reaction, which reaches its peak in from 24 to 48 hours and then rapidly fades. Since the skin reaction is positive in fewer than half the cases estab-

lished by means of culture, it is not satisfactory for diagnosis with the individual patient, but in surveys it does supply information useful for the epidemiologist.

Treatment. Amphotericin B is the drug of choice. The response ranges from marked improvement in some cases to apparent cure in others. General measures of nursing care, rest, good nutrition, and appropriate surgical measures are still necessary.[81] Mortality has been lowered to 5% since amphotericin B became available, whereas previously it had been as great as 75% for the disseminated form. Isolated solitary lesions may be removed surgically with complete success. It is important to establish the diagnosis as early as possible to assure the greatest success in therapy. Unfortunately, physicians seldom consider North American blastomycosis among the diagnostic possibilities, and the disease has been present for as many as 15 years before diagnosis was established.

Blastomyces brasiliensis: South American blastomycosis

South American blastomycosis[83] is a fungal disease, first reported in Brazil in 1908 by Lutz, and by Splendor in 1909. It is characterized by chronic granulomatous lesions in various internal organs and lymph nodes, as well as on the skin and mucous membranes. The disease is endemic to rural Brazil, particularly in the São Paulo, Rio de Janeiro, and Minas Gerais areas, but occurs also, to a lesser extent, in Argentina, Venezuela, Peru, and Colombia. All these areas are similar in that they lie within subtropic or tropic forest zones. Among cases discovered in the United States the patients have a history of having been in South America. The highest incidence is in adults aged from 20 to 30 years; the infection is ten times as common in males as in females.

The etiologic agent is a diphasic fungus, *Blastomyces brasiliensis*. The parasitic or yeast phase occurs both in vivo and in vitro on glucose blood infusion agar at 37° C. The colonies are smooth and white or tan. The mycelial phase develops at room temperature on Sabouraud's glucose agar. The colonies at this temperature are white or yellowish, wrinkled, and firm; as the colony ages, it turns brown. Fluffy aerial mycelia develop which carry blastospores and some chlamydospores. The characteristic multiple buds on these blastospores (Fig. 6-12) differentiate this species from the agent causing North American blastomycosis, which reproduces by single buds.

Transmission. B. brasiliensis is thought to inhabit soil and vegetative material, but the microorganism has not been isolated from these niches. Direct transmission from man to man probably does not occur. It is not entirely clear why the disease is so sharply limited to South America.

Clinical picture. The single most characteristic clinical finding is enlarged and draining lymph nodes. Lymphadenopathy with draining sinuses seldom develops in North American blastomycosis. Another difference is that South American blastomycosis almost always includes oral lesions, whereas they occur rarely in the North

American disease. Lesions on the skin occur most commonly as primary lesions around the mouth or nose. They may, however, be secondary, the result of hematogenous spread. The lesions ulcerate and become papulopustular and encrusted; the edges are uneven and raised. Attempts at central healing may result in the formation of scar tissue.

The lungs may become primarily involved or they may become infected secondarily, following infection of the oral cavity. Lung symptoms may include fever, rales, and cough; in some instances the sputum may be tinged with blood. False diagnoses of tuberculosis have been made as a consequence. Symptoms related to disease of the lung or mucous membranes or both are the usual cause for seeking treatment.

Oral lesions. Infections of the oral cavity[54] in the past had often been considered to be primary, but there is increasing evidence now that the primary infection occurs in the lungs through inhalation of the fungus and that the oral lesions constitute secondary involvement.[88] Nevertheless, oral lesions do occur very frequently and form

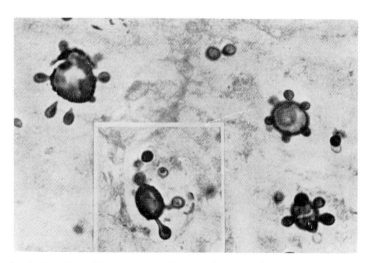

Fig. 6-12. South American blastomycosis. Spores showing characteristic multiple budding (Gomori's methenamine silver nitrate stain; 1,680 ×, reduced 3/10). (From Joseph, E. A., Mare, A., and Irving, W. R.: Oral Surg. **21:**732, 1966.)

an important diagnostic feature for detecting the disease.

The oral lesions may involve almost any of the structures of the mouth or oropharynx including the tonsils, the mucosa of the lips, cheeks, the soft and hard palates, the gingivae, or the tongue. The infection may also appear in the oral cavity as a tooth socket granuloma following extraction, secondary to pulmonary infection.[90] The disease in the oral cavity appears first as a small papule on the mucosal surface which becomes an ulcer surrounded by an erythematous zone. The pharyngeal lesions may go on to complete destruction of the epiglottis, vocal cords, and uvula. The cervical lymph nodes may become infected, then necrotic, and give rise to sinus tracts opening onto the skin. The anterior oral mucosal lesions may extend onto the skin where they form encrusted papulopustular lesions. The fungus may enter the root canal of a carious tooth to form an apical granuloma. From this site the organism may gain access to the body, and it gives rise to a generalized infection.[7]

Periodontal infection may develop with loosening and loss of the teeth. An infiltrative process usually arises in the tissues of the lips, cheeks, and nose that severely reduces facial movements and almost completely suppresses movement of the mandible. At times the face has a more or less elephantiasic appearance.[29] There may be a continual flow of saliva from the angles of the mouth as the mouth may be held partially open.[83]

Immunology. The immunologic mechanisms of the body react very sluggishly to infection by B. brasiliensis. Most patients have circulating antibodies detectable by either complement fixation or immunodiffusion techniques. An intradermal test with culture antigens or antigens prepared from pus has not yielded uniform results, but some investigators consider it useful for both diagnosis and prognosis. The reaction is negative in the severe cases.

Diagnosis. Sputum samples are examined both directly in the microscope and by culture at 37° C. and room temperature. Every effort must be made to obtain the fungus in pure culture in order to establish a definitive diagnosis. Cultures are kept for at least one month before being discarded, since growth may not appear for several weeks. Scrapings from skin or oral mucous membrane lesions are studied microscopically in potassium hydroxide mounts and by culture also. Biopsied tissue examined histologically may alone allow establishing the diagnosis. Infected material may be inoculated into guinea pigs and mice. The infection may require five or six weeks to become apparent. The lesions are found scattered through the mesentery, on the spleen, liver, and diaphragm.

Treatment. Before the sulfonamides appeared, South American blastomycosis was usually fatal. Following the introduction of the sulfonamides it was found that large doses of sulfathiazole, sulfadiazine, and sulfamerazine given for at least five years results in control of the infection; today amphotericin B is preferred for advanced cases or for cases that have developed an idiosyncracy toward the sulfonamides. Early therapy is essential to reduce mortality and to minimize permanent tissue damage.

Histoplasma capsulatum: histoplasmosis

Histoplasma capsulatum was first observed in sections of tissues taken at postmortem examination from lesions by Darling in 1905 in the Panama Canal Zone. Because its size and appearance resembled the Leishman-Donovan bodies of kala-azar, he believed it to be a protozoan organism. The first case to be described in the United States was in 1926.

It was eventually established that histoplasmosis[24] is a deep mycosis, with a preference for the reticuloendothelial system, caused by a diphasic fungus that in the tissue phase appears as a small, oval, yeastlike encapsulated cell, from 3 to 5 μ in diameter. It is found especially within phagocytic reticuloendothelial cells or within mononuclear leukocytes in the peripheral blood.

H. capsulatum was first cultivated in 1933. It develops in the mycelial phase on Sabouraud's medium in the laboratory at room temperature. In this phase it develops on culture medium as a white, fluffy colony that later becomes brownish. Later, as the medium is depleted of nutrients, chlamydospores develop that have several spiked projections about the periphery of the cell. These tuberculated chlamydospores are quite characteristic, distinguishing H. capsulatum from the other fungi that form chlamydospores. On blood agar slants at 37° C., H. capsulatum grows in the yeast form. The fungus is very resistant to physical influences. It has been kept in dried sterile soil for four months and in ice for more than one year, and it is viable after heating at 62° C. for 10 minutes or 45° C. for 30 minutes.

Epidemiology.[1] The number of individuals who have been infected by H. capsulatum is estimated to be in the millions. The reason for this large number is not difficult to understand in view of the repeated recoveries of the fungus from soil contaminated by avian droppings, especially from chickens and pigeons. In the United States the disease is endemic to large areas of the country, being found especially in the drainage basin of the Mississippi River, where 30% or more of the population gives a positive skin reaction to histoplasmin. The disease is known to occur throughout the world but has a relatively high incidence in Panama, the Philippines, Argentina, Brazil, Honduras, and Java in addition to the United States. Transmission from man to man is not known to occur. In adults the disease seems to have some predilection for males, since it affects four males to every female infected. In children the sex ration is 1 to

1. The organism is airborne and enters the body by inhalation. Epidemiologic data indicate an incubation period of from 5 to 15 days.

Clinical picture. Histoplasmosis may vary from an asymptomatic or mild and self-limited infection of the lungs to an acute fulminating disease or a chronic and long drawn-out disease with lung calcifications. Cough, chest pains, fever, loss of weight, and lack of strength are the complaints usually encountered, although more than 95% of patients with only localized involvement have either subclinical symptoms or a mild respiratory illness. The most severe cases usually occur in young children or in elderly persons with some debilitating disease. In a few cases the disease may spread to other parts of the body.

Among the extrapulmonary lesions, ulcerations of the skin and mucosa occur the most frequently.[11] The mucosa of the gastrointestinal tract may be affected in different degrees, even to the point of being massively involved from the mouth to the rectum, especially in patients 40 years of age or older. The cells of the reticuloendothelial system, especially the spleen and bone marrow, are parasitized upon the systemic dissemination of the fungus.

The oral lesions are usually secondary, derived from bloodborne organisms rather than from the sputum. On rare occasions the oral lesions may be the primary and only manifestation of the disease.[58] The most common gross lesion of oral histoplasmosis is one shallow ulcer or more with indurated borders on the tongue.[49] Other lesions, but nodular in character, may appear on other soft oral tissues, including the fauces, tonsils, buccal mucosa, hard or soft palate, gingiva, or lips. About half the patients with disseminated histoplasmosis will have such lesions, which may be quite painful and may in part be the cause of the bad breath present in many of these patients. Laryngeal involvement not uncommonly accompanies oral lesions, with symptoms of hoarseness.[14]

Diagnosis.[64] Any chronic ulcerative lesion involving the pharynx, tongue, or larynx with a palpable spleen and liver may be suggestive of histoplasmosis. Unfortunately, some oral lesions are treated symptomatically over a long period for such conditions as "poorly fitting denture," "ulcerative stomatitis," or "trench mouth"[71,] [109] before serious efforts are made to obtain a definitive diagnosis. The infection may also mimic tuberculosis, syphilis, Hodgkin's disease, or other fungal diseases so that a difficult problem in differential diagnosis is involved.[85]

Biopsy will demonstrate the fungus in some but not all of the tissue specimens (Fig. 6-13). The periodic acid–Schiff stain is useful for differentiating *Histoplasma* from *Leishmania* in tissue since the capsules of *Histoplasma* stain intensely, while the outer membranes of *Leishmania* do not stain. The tissue reaction may vary from inflammatory to the true granulomatous reaction typical for fungal disease, depending upon the vigor of the body defenses. Definitive diagnosis, however, is based upon the isolation and identification of *H. capsulatum* from cultivation of tissue, blood, or sputum in the laboratory. Blood agar cultures incubated at room temperature yield the greatest number of positive results. The mycelial phase of the fungus developing on Sabouraud's agar at room temperature differs from other pathogenic fungi by the formation of large, thick-walled, tuberculate chlamydospores.

Serologic procedures for identification of specific circulating antibodies, and the skin test for histoplasmin sensitivity are useful techniques.

Treatment. Amphotericin B is the most effective antibiotic available and is the drug of choice in spite of its toxicity.[35] For badly debilitated patients, supportive measures are important. Since oral lesions are almost always a consequence of systemic infection, intensive intravenous administration of amphotericin B is usually necessary for their treatment.[15]

Phycomycetes: phycomycosis

Phycomycosis,[59] also known as mucormycosis, is a rare disease caused by phycomycetes, such as *Rhizopus oryzae*, which

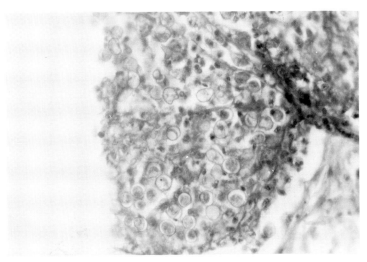

Fig. 6-13. Histoplasmosis. Lesion of lung (1,100 ×) shows numerous yeastlike cells (blastospores) present in tissue. (Courtesy Dr. McClendon, Houston, Tex.)

ordinarily are not pathogenic. These fungi, however, may be opportunists that are particularly apt to establish themselves if the body defenses are impaired by such states as malnutrition, incipient or uncontrolled diabetes or leukemia, or if the patient's disease has been overtreated with antibiotics, antileukemic drugs, and cortisone. Diabetes mellitus is particularly significant in laying the basis for infection for between 40% and 50% of the patients who have it. There has been increased frequency of this infection in recent years, with the increasing use of the newer chemotherapeutic agents and with the prolongation of life in spite of continued disease. In this latter case, body defenses become increasingly inadequate.[59]

Experimental studies have shown that acute alloxan-induced diabetes in rabbits increases the severity of mucormycosis and activates quiescent foci in previously infected animals.[59] Histologic examination of the tissues from these animals indicated a failure to mobilize leukocytes, which, in turn, seemed to be related to a decrease in mast-cell degranulation. There are suggestive observations in human diabetes, especially if acidosis is present, that there is a defect in the mobilization of polymorphonuclear leukocytes. Moreover, normal human serum has the ability of inhibiting growth of mucor in vitro, but serum from patients with diabetes or leukemia and cirrhosis is either defective or lacking in this property.

Phycomycetes occur normally in soil, manure, and fruits, and they are commonly known as bread molds. Their spores are easily wafted into the air, and their inhalation or ingestion may then lead to infection of the mouth, sinuses, lungs, or gastrointestinal tract. These fungi consist of branching nonseptate hyphae with occasional small sporangiophores from 2 to 3 μ in diameter. In pathologic tissue they characteristically appear as broad, nonseptate branching hyphae regardless of the particular species involved. The infection is not known to be transmitted from man to man.

In infections of the head and neck, a characteristic triad includes involvement of the oral cavity, maxillary sinus, and orbit of the eye.[70] Oral lesions have been usually reported as a large ulcer in the hard palate,[42] a result of sloughs of both soft and bony tissues. These lesions characteristically develop from initial sites of infection above in the maxillary sinuses, which also extend upward into the orbit and cerebrum. Local tissue damage in some cases appears to be an important factor in determining the site of invasion. In one case, for example, the suspected portal of entry was the unhealed socket of a recently extracted tooth.[108]

Successful treatment of phycomycosis is possible only upon early recognition of the disease. In such cases the survival rate is at least 53%. It is necessary to establish rapid control of the underlying condition that has made infection possible and to administer amphotericin B, which is the antibiotic of choice.[103] Surgical drainage and debridement of all necrotic tissue are additional important measures that must be taken.[101]

The fungus *Rhinosporidium seeberi,* a phycomycete, is the etiologic agent of rhinosporidiosis, an infection predominantly involving the mucous membrane of the nose and nasopharynx but occassionally affecting other sites, such as the lips, palate, uvula, maxillary antrum, parotid gland, tonsil, and skin. The infection is usually limited to the surface epithelium, but it may sometimes be disseminated systemically and the organism can then be found in any part of the body. The infection is chronic and is characterized by polyps or by papillomatous lesions. It occurs most often in India and Ceylon, but sporadic cases have been reported from all over the world, including the United States and many of the South American countries. Children and young adults are most frequently infected, and males more often than females.

Rhinosporidiosis is rarely fatal, unless it becomes disseminated throughout the body. In some cases of localized infection, simple excision suffices to eliminate the infection.

Attempts to cultivate the fungus have not been successful for most investigators, and when success was claimed, the results appear to be questionable.

Sporotrichum: sporotrichosis

Sporotrichosis[95] is a chronic mycotic disease generally beginning as a primary lesion on a finger; then secondary nodular lesions develop along the lymphatic channels and regional lymph nodes so that the infection may extend and involve the entire arm. The infection was described originally by Schenck in 1897.

The etiologic agent is *Sporotrichum schenckii*, an aerobic fungus that is diphasic. In the parasitic stage in the tissues, the fungus is difficult to observe because of its small size, from 1 to 2 μ. At times it is found in phagocytes in the form of small, cigar-shaped spores.

S. schenckii grows readily in standard culture media. When the microorganism is cultivated on glucose blood infusion agar at 37° C., yeastlike colonies develop that are smooth and of a creamy consistency. The cells are elongated and cigar-shaped, and vary in size between 1 and 5 μ. When it is grown at room temperature on Sabouraud's glucose agar, a septate mycelium develops with lateral and terminal projections that contain groups of pear-shaped microconidia, from 1 to 5 μ in diameter. In older cultures chlamydospores may be present.

Transmission. *S. schenckii* is worldwide in distribution, but the disease has been found most frequently in the north central United States and in France. The organism is found in soil and on plant life and rotting wood. The disease is particularly prone to occur in agricultural workers and florists and also in South African miners who work in environments with extremely high relative humidities where rotting wood shores the walls of mines. The microorganism is found in sphagnum moss and is also the etiologic agent of carnation rot. The thorns of certain plants may cause trauma to the fingers, and these small areas of injury may then become contaminated with the yeastlike microorganism. In some cases mechanical transmission may occur from the bite of the rat, mouse, mule, chicken, parrot, dog, horse, or mosquito.[75] *S. schenckii* has been isolated from the normal oral cavity of man.

Clinical picture. Cutaneous inoculation sporotrichosis accounts for most of the clinically recognized cases.[67] Florists are particularly prone to infection by this route since they are exposed daily to dirt, moss, carnations, and barberry thorns. The lesion in such individuals generally begins on a finger as an indurated ulcer that does not heal. Infection proceeds along the regional lymph channels as a red line to the lymph nodes and thus extends up the arm. Subcutaneous indurated nodules unattached to the skin may appear and are known as sporotrichotic chancres. These may ulcerate and the lesions appear in various colors. The skin of the face has been known to become infected. In some instances the mucosal surfaces of the nose and mouth are involved.[8] Oral lesions occur in some individuals probably as a result of self-contamination from the fingers. The lesions may appear as nodules that later ulcerate and then become secondarily infected. Oral sporotrichosis is usually a consequence of cutaneous rather than systemic infection. The lungs rarely become diseased. *S. schenckii* may be disseminated via the bloodstream to other organs and to the skin.

Diagnosis. Culture of the clinical specimen is the most trustworthy method for obtaining a diagnosis. Serologic techniques are not as valuable as cultivation.

Treatment. Potassium iodide therapy, an old method, starts with 10 drops three times a day of a 10% solution and increases daily by 5 drops until 30 drops three times a day are administered. This is generally the limit before toxicity occurs. Such treatment has been consistently found to be effective. Amphotericin B, however, is today the therapy of choice for systemic sporotrichosis in spite of its highly toxic effect upon the kidneys. Surgical excision may be effective if the infection is localized.[98]

Aspergilleae: Aspergillosis, penicillosis

Aspergillus is a widely distributed genus of blue-green fungi that include the molds seen on damp bread and are the most common contaminants seen in the microbiology laboratory. Among the species described as pathogenic for man are *A. fumigatus, A. nidulans, A. flavus,* and *A. niger.* Of these, *A. fumigatus* is now being increasingly recognized as a producer of disease in man.

The aspergilli grow well at room temperature on Sabouraud's dextrose agar. Initially, within the first 24 hours of cultivation, the colonies appear as white filamentous surface growths, but during the second 24 hours they become green to dark green or green-black as the spores are produced. Microscopically the aspergilli are characterized by conidiophores that expand into large vesicles. The vesicles are covered with sterigmata bearing long chains of conidiospores.

Aspergillus conidiospores are present everywhere in the atmosphere. When they deposit upon damaged or debilitated tissue, they may germinate and grow to cause a mycotic infection. Aspergillosis[114] most often affects the ear, skin, sinuses, bronchi, or lungs, but it can affect the bones, meninges, and almost any other organ of the body. In recent years, with the development of more accurate and sensitive diagnostic methods, there has been an increasing recognition of aspergillus infections. In all likelihood, however, there has also been an actual absolute increase in aspergillosis as a consequence of ecologic disturbances from antibacterial chemotherapeutic agents. The lesions, at microscopic examination, are found to be a chronic inflammatory granulomatous reaction that includes giant cells containing septate mycelial filaments. Polymorphonuclear leukocytes and macrophages are present.

Several cases have been reported with aspergillosis of structures of direct interest to the dentist. Most common among these is infection of the maxillary sinus. The course of this disease is slow and progressive; clinically, the initial symptoms are like those of chronic suppurative sinusitis. Laceration of the right side of the face in one reported case led to an infection which started in the pre-auricular area of the face and spread to the infra-orbital area and over the mandibular area in spite of x-ray therapy and surgical excision. Both the parotid gland and the maxillary sinus were invaded later.[6]

From Japan[56] has been reported a case of *Aspergillus* infection of the periodontal tissues and dental pulp, diagnosed on the basis of histologic sections. In this instance it was considered that the infection probably was opportunistic, becoming possible because the normal ecologic balance of microorganisms in the oral cavity had been profoundly affected by antibiotic therapy for pulmonary tuberculosis. In disseminated aspergillosis, the tongue and palate have been found to be involved in a small percentage of cases. These lesions produce intense local pain and oral bleeding. *A. fumigatus* and *A. niger* were isolated as the only organisms present in extensive curdlike plaques on the oral mucosa which had been clinically diagnosed as oral candidiasis in a child 19 months of age.[38] *A. niger* has been implicated by some authors in localized infections of the tongue dorsum, which appeared black apparently from the presence of conidiospores.

In France, the practice of allowing pigeons to take masticated food directly out of the mouth of their master has been considered to be a possible route by which aspergillosis may be acquired from an infected bird.[9] The reality of these infections, referred to as "pigeon-fancier's disease" or "pseudotuberculosis aspergillina," has in recent years been questioned[105] because of the difficulty in establishing with certainty that the isolated fungus did come directly from the avian lesion and not from aerial contamination.

Diagnosis. Cultivation at room temperature of the fungus from clinical specimens is necessary to establish a firm diagnosis. A negative culture, however, does not necessarily rule out this diagnosis. An agar-gel double-diffusion serologic test with standardized carbohydrate antigens has proved valuable in detection of the infection and as a guide in therapy. This procedure is especially useful because of the wide distribution of aspergilli in nature, which makes any cultural isolation from a clinical specimen open to question as a possible contaminant unless serologic evidence is also obtained. Biopsy of the involved tissue is often diagnostic. Typical biopsy material shows evidence of chronic inflammation. Broken fragments of hyphae with numerous small, round, dark green spores are seen.

Therapy. Recognized treatment today consists of systemic use of amphotericin B if the infection is deep. If necessary, radical surgery must be resorted to in order to save the patient's life. Potassium iodide solution by mouth in massive doses is still useful, and recent reports indicate a favorable response may be obtained if griseofulvin is used. Successful therapy may be determined from a decrease in blood serum titer; relapse is indicated by a reappearance of serologic reactions.

Penicillium and Aspergillus. These fungi are members of the tribe aspergilleae. While *Aspergillus* has been recognized as an opportunistic fungus, *Penicillium* has not been usually considered as capable of acting as an infective agent. It now appears, however, that this view is incorrect since a fatal infection involving the brain has now been observed that began upon extraction of a loose left maxillary deciduous tooth.[77]

CITED REFERENCES

1. Ajello, L.: Comparative ecology of respiratory mycotic disease agents, Bact. Rev. **31:** 6, 1967.
2. Ajello, L.: Geographic distribution and prevalence of the dermatophytes, Ann. N. Y. Acad. Sci. **89:**30, 1960.
3. Ajello, L.: Occurrence of *Cryptococcus neoformans* in soils, Amer. J. Hyg. **67:**72, 1958.
4. Allison, R. T.: An evaluation of Pagano-Levin medium in a quantitative study of *Candida albicans*: Preliminary communication, J. Med. Lab. Techn. **24:**199, 1967.
5. Andrews, G. C., and Domonkos, A. N.: Diseases of the skin for practitioners and students, ed. 5, Philadelphia, 1963, W. B. Saunders Co., p. 263.
6. Arons, M. S., Lynch, J. B., Lewis, S. R., Larson, D. L., and Blocker, T. G., Jr.: Hemifacial resection for rare inflammatory diseases of the parotid gland, Amer. Surg. **32:** 469, 1966.
7. Artagaveytia-Allende, R. C.: Some biological characteristics of the pathogenic fungi named *Paracoccidioides brasiliensis* and *Paracoccidioides cerebriformis*, J. Dent. Res. **28:**242, 1949.
8. Banks, H. S.: Sporotrichosis resembling diphtheria, Lancet **2:**270, 1946.
9. Barker, L. F.: The clinical diagnosis of internal diseases, New York, 1919, D. Appleton & Co., vol. 1, p. 308.
10. Batchvarov, B.: Chéilite trichophytique, Bull. Soc. Franc. Derm. Syph. **47:**15, 1940.
11. Baum, G. L., Schwarz, J., Slot, W. J. B., and Straub, M.: Mucocutaneous histoplasmosis, Arch. Derm. **76:**4, 1957.
12. Bell, W. A., Gamble, G. E., and Garrington, G. E.: North American blastomycosis with oral lesions, Oral Surg. **28:**914, 1969.
13. Benham, R. W.: The genus Cryptococcus, Bact. Rev. **20:**189, 1956.
14. Bennett, D. E.: Histoplasmosis of the oral

cavity and larynx, Arch. Intern. Med. **120:** 417, 1967.

15. Boden, R. A.: Disseminated histoplasmosis with an oral lesion, Oral Surg. **23:**549, 1967.
16. Bodenhoff, J.: Resistance studies of *Candida albicans,* with special reference to two patients subjected to prolonged antimycotic treatment, Odont. T. **76:**279, 1968.
17. Brody, J. I., and Finch, S. C.: Candida-reacting antibody in the serum of patients with lymphomas and related disorders, Blood **15:** 830, 1960.
18. Brown-Thomsen, J.: Variability in *Candida albicans* (Robin) Berkout. I. Studies on morphology and biochemical activity, Hereditas **60:**355, 1968.
19. Carmichael, J. W.: *Geotricum candidum,* Mycologia **49:**820, 1957.
20. Castellani, A.: Miscellaneous mycological notes, Ann. N. Y. Acad. Sci. **93:**147, 1962.
21. Cawley, E. P., Grekin, R. H., and Curtis, A. C.: Torulosis, a review of the cutaneous and adjoining mucous membrane manifestations, J. Invest. Derm. **14:**327, 1950.
22. Cawson, R. A.: Denture sore mouth and angular cheilitis, Brit. Dent. J. **115:**441, 1963.
23. Cawson, R. A., and Lehner, T.: Chronic hyperplastic candidiasis—candidal leukoplakia, Brit. J. Derm. **80:**9, 1968.
24. Christie, A.: The disease spectrum of human histoplasmosis, Ann. Intern. Med. **49:** 544, 1958.
25. Cohen, L.: Oral candidiasis, Oral Surg. **20:** 316, 1965.
26. Conant, N. F., Martin, D. S., Smith, D. T., Baker, R. D., and Callaway, J. L.: Manual of clinical mycology, Philadelphia, 1944, W. B. Saunders Co., p. 89.
27. Crich, A.: Blastomycosis of the gingiva and jaw, Canad. Med. Assoc. J. **26:**662, 1932.
28. Curtis, G. H., and Netherton, E. W.: Cutaneous blastomycosis: Report of two cases, one being a mucocutaneous form, Cleveland Clin. Quart. **14:**47, 1947.
29. DaFonseca, O., filho: Deep skin and pulmonary mycosis in Brazil. In Sternberg, T. H., and Newcomer, V. D. (eds.): Therapy of fungus diseases, an international symposium, Boston, 1955, Little, Brown and Company, p. 56.
30. Davies, R. R., and Leese, M.: Filamentous fungi in the transient flora of the alimentary tract, Sabouraudia **6:**324, 1968.
31. Dawson, C. O.: Identification of *Candida albicans* in primary culture, Sabouraudia **1:** 214, 1962.

32. DePalma, A. T., Hardy, S. B., and Erickson, E. E.: Blastomycotic ulcer of the lower lip, Amer. Surg. **24:**919, 1958.
33. Donald, G. F., Burry, J. N., and Brown, G. W.: Candidiasis: Reflections on the problems of clinical assessment and treatment, Aust. J. Derm. **8:**197, 1966.
34. Drouhet, E., and Robin, J.: Mycose cutanée simulant un lupus érythémateux provoquée par *Trichophyton tonsurans* var. *acuminatum,* Bull. Soc. Franc. Derm. Syph. **76:**502, 1969.
35. Epstein, S., and Magnin, G. E.: Diagnosis: Generalized histoplasmosis involving tongue and pharynx, Arch. Derm. **82:** 133, 1960.
36. Esterly, N. B.: Serum antibody titers to *Candida albicans* utilizing an immunofluorescent technic, Amer. J. Clin. Path. **50:**292, 1968.
37. Forbus, W. D., and Bestebreurtje, A. M.: Coccidioidomycosis: A study of 95 cases of the disseminated type with special reference to the pathogenesis of the disease, Milit. Surg. **99:**653, 1946.
38. Fox, E. C., and Ainsworth, G. E.: A contribution to the mycology of the mouth, Brit. Med. J. **2:**826, 1958.
39. Fox, J. L.: Candicidin therapy in mixed mycotic-allergic skin lesions, Curr. Ther. Res. **8:**12, 1966.
40. Frauenfelder, D., and Schwartz, A. W.: Coccidioidomycosis involving head and neck, Plast. Reconstr. Surg. **39:**549, 1967.
41. Furculow, M. L., Chick, E. W., Busey, J. F., and Menges, R. W.: Prevalence and incidence studies of human and canine blastomycosis, Amer. Rev. Resp. Dis. **102:**60, 1970.
42. Georgiade, N., Maguire, C., Crawford, H., and Pickrell, K.: Mucormycosis and palatal sloughs in diabetics, Oral Surg. **17:**473, 1956.
43. Goldberg, L. S., Bluestone, R., Barnett, E. V., and Landau, J. W.: Studies on lymphocyte and monocyte function in chronic mucocutaneous candidiasis, Clin. Exp. Immun. **8:** 37, 1971.
44. Gordon, M. A., and Lapa, E.: Serum protein enhancement of antibiotic therapy in cryptococcosis, J. Infect. Dis. **114:**373, 1964.
45. Haley, L. D.: Comments on yeasts seen in the medical mycology laboratory, Trans. N. Y. Acad. Sci., Ser. II, **21:**708, 1959.
46. Hazen, E. L., Brown, R., and Little, G. N.: Moniliasis in experimental animals: Prophylaxis and therapy with nystatin. In Sternberg, T. H., and Newcomer, V. D. (eds.): Therapy of fungus diseases, an international symposium, Boston, 1955, Little, Brown and Co., p. 199.

47. Henrici, A. T.: Characteristics of fungus diseases, J. Bact. **39:**113, 1940.

48. Hildick-Smith, G., Blank, H., and Sarkany, I.: Fungus diseases and their treatment, Boston, 1964, Little, Brown and Co.

49. Hiley, P., and Fields, J.: *Histoplasma* ulcer of the tongue, J. A. M. A. **200:**1130, 1967.

50. Huppert, M.: Recent developments in coccidioidomycosis, Rev. Med. Vet. Mycol. **6:**279, 1968.

51. Hurley, R.: Effect of route of entry of *Candida albicans* on the histogenesis of the lesions in experimental candidosis in the mouse, J. Path. Bact. **92:**578, 1966.

52. Hurley, R.: Experimental infection with *Candida albicans* in modified hosts, J. Path. Bact. **92:**57, 1966.

53. Hurley, R.: The pathogenic candida species: A review, Rev. Med. Vet. Mycol. **6:**159, 1967.

54. Joseph, E. A., Mare, A., and Irving, W. R., Jr.: Oral South American blastomycosis in the United States of America, Oral Surg. **21:**732, 1966.

55. Keeney, E. L.: Candida asthma, Ann. Intern. Med. **34:**223, 1951.

56. Kobayakawa, Y., Kawamoto, M., and Moro, I.: On the Aspergillus infection in the dental pulp and periodontal tissues, J. Nihon Univ. Sch. Dent. **6:**100, 1964.

57. Kuykendall, S. J., Ellis, F. H., Jr., Weed, L. A., and Donoghue, F. E.: Pulmonary cryptococcosis, New Eng. J. Med. **257:**1009, 1957.

58. Lamb, J. H.: Combined therapy in histoplasmosis and coccidiodomycosis: Methyltestosterone and meth-dia-mer-sulfonamides, Arch. Derm. Syph. **70:**695, 1954.

59. Landau, J. W., and Newcomer, V. D.: Acute cerebral phycomycosis (mucormycosis), J. Pediat. **61:**363, 1962.

60. Lehner, T.: Oral thrush, or acute pseudomembranous candidiasis, Oral Surg. **18:**27, 1964.

61. Lehner, T.: Symposium on denture sore mouth. II. The role of Candida, Dent. Pract. **16:**138, 1965.

62. Levine, S., Zimmerman, H. M., and Scorza, A.: Experimental cryptococcosis (torulosis), Amer. J. Path. **33:**385, 1957.

63. Loewenthal, K., and Rein, R. L.: Tinea barbae of the kerion type produced by *Trichophyton purpureum:* Report of a case, Arch. Derm. Syph. **64:**194, 1951.

64. Loosli, C. G.: Histoplasmosis, some clinical, epidemiological and laboratory aspects, Med. Clin. N. Amer. **39:**171, 1955.

65. Lorincz, A. L.: Candidiasis. In Yaffee, H. S.

66. Ludwig, J. S.: Sycosis barbae due to *Trichophyton rubrum* (*purpureum*), Arch. Derm. Syph. **68:**216, 1953.

67. Lynch, P. J., Voorhees, J. J., and Harrell, E. R.: Systemic sporotrichosis, Ann. Intern. Med. **73:**23, 1970.

68. McGinley, K. J., Lantis, L. R., and Marples, R. R.: Microbiology of tinea versicolor, Arch. Derm. **102:**168, 1970.

69. Marten, R. H.: Chronic paronychia, a mycological and bacteriological study, Brit. J. Derm. **71:**422, 1959.

70. Martinez, M. G., and Robinson, L. H.: Mucormycosis of the head and neck: A report of three cases, Oral Surg. **24:**381, 1967.

71. Merchant, R. K., Louria, D. B., Geisler, P. H., Edgcomb, J. H., and Utz, J. P.: Fungal endocarditis: Review of the literature and report of three cases, Ann. Intern. Med. **48:**242, 1958.

72. Merz, W. G., Berger, C. L., and Silva-Hutner, M.: Media with pH indicators for the isolation of dermatophytes, Arch. Derm. **102:**545, 1970.

73. Methods for medical laboratory technicians, TM8-227-AFM160-14, Washington, D. C., 1951, U. S. Government Printing Office, p. 501.

74. Mincer, H. H., and Oglesby, R. J., Jr.: Intraoral North American blastomycosis, Oral Surg. **22:**36, 1966.

75. Moore, J. J., and Davis, D. J.: Sporotrichosis following mouse bite, with certain immunologic data, Trans. Chicago Path. Soc. **10:**284, 1918.

76. Moore, M.: Cryptococcosis with cutaneous manifestations: Four cases with a review of published reports, J. Invest. Derm. **28:**159, 1957.

77. Morriss, F. H., Jr., and Spock, A.: Intracranial aneurysm secondary to mycotic orbital and sinus infection: Report of a case implicating *Penicillium* as an opportunistic fungus, Amer. J. Dis. Child. **119:**357, 1970.

78. Mourad, S., and Friedman, L.: Pathogenicity of Candida, J. Bact. **81:**550, 1961.

79. New, G. B.: Blastomycosis of the tongue, J.A.M.A. **68:**186, 1917.

80. O'Mahony, J. B.: Tinea of the lip, Dent. Pract. **18:**325, 1968.

81. O'Neill, R. P., and Penman, R. W. B.: Clinical aspects of blastomycosis, Thorax **25:**708, 1970.

82. Pagano, J., Levin, J. D., and Trejo, W.: Diagnostic medium for differentiation of species of *Candida*, Antibiotics Annual, 1957-

(ed.): Newer views of skin diseases, Boston, 1966, Little, Brown and Co., p. 131.

1958, New York, 1958, Medical Encyclopedia, Inc., p. 137.

83. Perry, H. O., Weed, L. A., and Kierland, R. R.: South American blastomycosis, Arch. Derm. Syph. **70:**477, 1954.

84. Pokowitz, W., and Hoffman, H.: Infection of the lips by *Trichophyton rubrum,* Oral Surg. **30:**201, 1970.

85. Reddy, P., Gorelick, D. F., Brashear, C. A., and Larsh, H.: Progressive disseminated histoplasmosis as seen in adults, Amer. J. Med. **48:**629, 1970.

86. Reiss, F., and Kornblee, L.: Common mycotic infections of the lower extremities, New York State J. Med. **63:**548, 1963.

87. Reiss, F., Kornblee, L., and Solowey, C.: Survey of long-term therapeutic results with griseofulvin in superficial fungus infections in 111 patients, New York J. Med. **61:**3631, 1961.

88. Restrepo, A., Robledo, M., Gutiérrez, F., Sanclemente, M., Castañeda, E., and Calle G.: Paracoccidioidomycosis (South American blastomycosis): A study of 39 cases observed in Medellín, Colombia, Amer. J. Trop. Med. Hyg. **19:**68, 1970.

89. Rippon, J. W.: Medical mycology: The pathogenic fungi and the pathogenic actinomyces. In Burrows, W.: Textbook of microbiology, ed. 19, Philadelphia, 1968, W. B. Saunders Co., p. 735.

90. Salman, L., and Sheppard, S. M.: South American blastomycosis, Oral Surg. **15:**671, 1962.

91. Satyanarayana, C.: Rhinosporidiosis, with a record of 255 cases, Acta Otolaryng. **51:**348, 1960.

92. Schwarz, J., and Baum, G. L.: Blastomycosis, Amer. J. Clin. Path. **21:**999, 1951.

93. Scott, P. W.: A possible case of pulmonary moniliasis, Amer. Rev. Tuberc. Pulmon. Dis. **77:**329, 1958.

94. Shannon, J., and Raubitschek, F.: Tinea faciei simulating chronic discoid lupus erythematosus, Arch. Derm. **82:**268, 1960.

95. Singer, J. I., and Muncie, J. E.: Sporotrichosis, New York J. Med. **52:**2147, 1952.

96. Skinner, C. E., and Fletcher, S. W.: A review of the genus *Candida,* Bact. Rev. **24:**397, 1960.

97. Strauss, J. S.: The treatment of superficial ringworm infections, Med. Clin. N. Amer. **42:**1375, 1958.

98. Takaro, T.: Mycotic infections of interest to thoracic surgeons, Ann. Thorac. Surg. **3:**71, 1967.

99. Taplin, D., Zaias, N., Rebell, G., and Blank, H.: Isolation and recognition of dermatophytes on a new medium (DTM), Arch. Derm. **99:**203, 1969.

100. Taschdjian, C. L., Burchall, J. J., and Kozinn, P. J.: Rapid identification of *Candida albicans* by filamentation on serum and serum substitutes, Amer. J. Dis. Child. **99:**212, 1960.

101. Taylor, C. G., Alexander, R. E., Green, W. H., and Kramer, H. S., Jr.: Mucormycosis (phycomycosis) involving the maxilla, Oral Surg. **27:**806, 1969.

102. Taylor, E. R.: Pulmonary cryptococcosis: Analysis of 15 cases from the Columbia area, Ann. Thorac. Surg. **10:**309, 1970.

103. Taylor, R., Shklar, G., Budson, R., and Hackett, R.: Mucormycosis of the oral mucosa, Arch. Derm. **89:**419, 1964.

104. Timonen, S., Salo, O. P., Meyer, B., and Haapoja, H.: Vaginal mycosis, Acta Obstet. Gynec. Scand. **45:**232, 1966.

105. Vanbreuseghem, R.: Mycoses of man and animals, J. Wilkinson (trans.), Springfield, Ill., 1958, Charles C Thomas, Publisher.

106. Vogel, R. A., and Moses, M. R.: Weld's method for the rapid identification of *Candida albicans* in clinical materials, Amer. J. Clin. Path. **28:**103, 1957.

107. Warin, R. P.: Fungal infections of the skin, Brit. Med. J. **2:**1307, 1966.

108. Wasserman, A. J., Shiels, W. S., and Sporn, I. N.: Cerebral mucormycosis, Southern Med. J. **54:**403, 1961.

109. Weed, L. A., and Parkhill, E. M.: The diagnosis of histoplasmosis in ulcerative disease of the mouth and pharynx, Amer. J. Clin. Path. **18:**130, 1948.

110. Wiegand, S. E., Ulrich, J. A., and Winkelmann, R. K.: Diagnosis of superficial pathogenic fungi: Use of ink blue agar method, Mayo Clin. Proc. **43:**795, 1968.

111. Wilson, J. W., and Bartok, W. R.: Immunoallergic aspects of coccidioidomycosis, Int. J. Derm. **9:**253, 1970.

112. Winner, H. E., and Hurley, R.: *Candida albicans,* London, 1964, J. & A. Churchill Ltd.

113. Wright, E. T., Graham, J. H., and Sternberg, T. H.: Treatment of moniliasis with nystatin, J.A.M.A. **163:**92, 1957.

114. Young, R. C., Bennett, J. E., Vogel, C. L., Carbone, P. P., and DeVita, V. T.: Aspergillosis: The spectrum of the disease in 98 patients, Medicine **49:**147, 1970.

115. Zeisler, E. P.: Chronic coccidioidal dermatitis: Report of an unusual case, Arch. Derm. Syph. **25:**52, 1932.

REFERENCES AND ADDITIONAL READINGS

Dalldorf, G. (ed.): Fungi and fungous diseases, a symposium of the Section of Microbiology, The New York Academy of Medicine, Springfield, Ill., 1962, Charles C Thomas, Publisher.

Emmons, C. W., Binford, C. H., and Utz, J. P.: Medical mycology, ed. 2, Philadelphia, 1970, Lea & Febiger.

Fiese, M. J.: Coccidioidomycosis, Springfield, Ill., 1958, Charles C Thomas, Publisher.

Lewis, G. M., Hopper, M. E., Wilson, J. W., and Plunkett, O. A.: An introduction to medical mycology, ed. 4, Chicago, 1958, Year Book Medical Publishers, Inc.

Marples, M. J.: The ecology of the human skin, Springfield, Ill., 1965, Charles C Thomas, Publisher.

Moss, E. S., and McQuown, A. L.: Atlas of medical mycology, ed. 2, Baltimore, 1960, The Williams & Wilkins Co.

Negroni, P.: Histoplasmosis, diagnosis and treatment, revised ed., McMillen, S. (trans.), Springfield, Ill., 1965, Charles C Thomas, Publisher.

Pillsbury, D. M., Shelley, W. B., and Kligman, A. M.: Dermatology, Philadelphia, 1956, W. B. Saunders Co.

Recent advances of human and animal mycology, Proceedings of the International Dermatologic Symposium, Bratislava, Czechoslovakia, Oct. 4-6, 1966, Bratislava, 1967, Publishing House of the Slovak Academy of Sciences.

Wilson, J. W.: Clinical and immunologic aspects of fungous diseases, Springfield, Ill., 1957, Charles C Thomas, Publisher.

Wolstenholme, G. E. W., and Porter, R. (eds.): Systemic mycoses, a Ciba symposium, Boston, 1967, Little, Brown and Co.

7 / Periodontal disease

Diseases affecting the periodontium are unique in that they occur in an unusually complex oral environment within a diverse group of specialized tissues. Many types of infectious, neoplastic, and degenerative diseases occur in the tissue components that support the teeth. However, the most common form of periodontal disease to be discussed in this chapter is of the inflammatory type. This type consists of gingivitis, periodontitis, and acute necrotizing ulcerative gingivitis.

The prevalence of these periodontal diseases is attested to by the fact that by the age of 45 years from 97% to 100% of the population is afflicted. Fig. 7-1 documents further the importance of these diseases by indicating that inflammatory periodontal disease is the major cause of tooth loss in the adult population. These diseases occur in the soft and the hard tissues of the mouth only in the presence of teeth. The gingiva is the tissue that is altered; more specifically, the junction where the gingiva meets the tooth is the primary area of pathologic change. Marked differences in the prevalence of these diseases in populations throughout the world suggest that they are not the result of one cause. In most instances prevention of and treatment for inflammatory periodontal disease involves minimizing the bacterial masses residing in juxtaposition to the periodontium.

Discussion of the etiology of these three diseases requires knowledge of the host, the bacteria, and the interrelationship between the two in the gingival crevice. The microbial content of the gingival crevice is the result of interactions of microorganisms with each other and with the host. The development of these diseases may be understood by comparing the macrostructure and microstructure of the periodontium in health and in disease. Being viable tissues, some of the host cells are constantly being replaced, and the morphologic traits observed are the result of tissue destruction and repair.

NATURE OF THE PERIODONTIUM

Following complete eruption of a tooth into the oral cavity, a fiber system exists which connects the alveolar bone to the cementum, the cementum to the gingiva, and the cementum of one tooth to another. These are the gingival ligament, the alveolodental ligament, and the transseptal ligament, respectively (Fig. 7-2). The ultrastructure of these connecting elements consists of gingival and periodontal fibers that extend into the cementum as parallel bundles of calcified and uncalcified collagen fibers. These fiber bundles may be further subdivided into groups, according to their connections. The gingival ligament includes the three groups of fibers connecting the cementum to the gingiva and the ligamentum circulare. The latter is a circular group of fibers encircling the tooth. The fibers of the main supporting group, the alveolo-

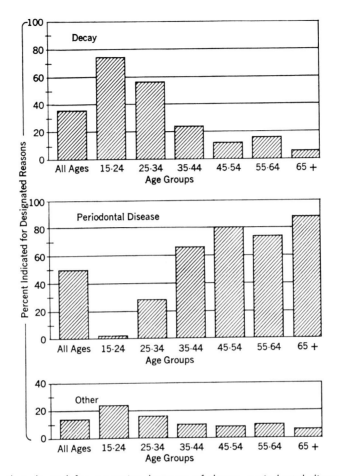

Fig. 7-1. Teeth indicated for extraction because of decay, periodontal disease, and other reasons. (From Pelton, W., Pennell, E., and Druzina, A.: J.A.D.A. **49:**441, 1954. Copyright by the American Dental Association. Reprinted by permission.)

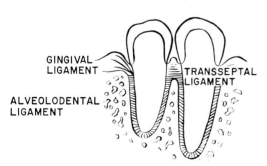

Fig. 7-2. A diagram of the periodontal ligament. Three major fiber components of the periodontium anchor the tooth to the jaw.

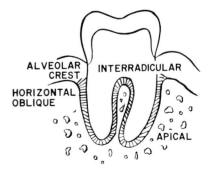

Fig. 7-3. Alveolodental ligament. Groups of fibers of the alveolodental ligament run from the cementum to the crest of the alveolar bone, horizontally and obliquely to the alveolar bone, and at the apical and interradicular region of the root to the bone.

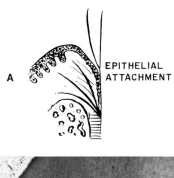

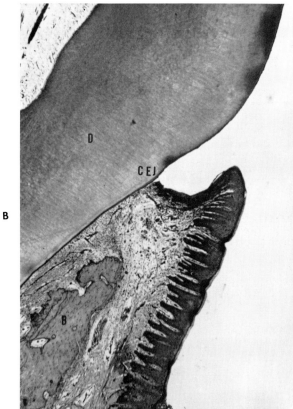

Fig. 7-4, A, Epithelial attachment. The base of the gingival crevice contains some epithelial cells which have a fibrous attachment to cementum. This is located at the cemento-enamel junction in health, and these cells are located at the base of the crevice. **B,** Photomicrograph of the gingival crevice area. Note the position of the epithelial attachment at the cementoenamel junction and the lack of rete pegs and keratinization on the sulcular wall. *D,* dentin; *B,* bone; and *CEJ,* cementoenamel junction. (Histologic section courtesy Dr. S. Arnim, Houston, Tex.)

dental ligament, include the alveolar crest, horizontal, oblique, apical, and interradicular fibers (Fig. 7-3).

The epithelium surrounding the neck of the tooth is well keratinized, except for the inner wall of the shallow crevice that surrounds the tooth (i.e., the gingival crevice). In gingival health, a depth of from 0 to 2 mm. can be measured from the most coronal aspect of the gingiva (i.e., the free margin of the gingiva) to the zone where the epithelial cells attach to the cementum surface. A group of epithelial cells some five to six cells deep, which is called the epithelial cuff or epithelial attachment, is found at this junction (Fig. 7-4). Experimental animal studies concerning the rate at which these epithelial cells turn over indicate that this critical area is renewed every four to seven days. Recent electron-microscopic findings demonstrate an attachment between sulcular epithelial cells and the enamel or cementum which establishes a barrier at the neck of the tooth be-

tween the external environment of the oral cavity and the host internal environment. This attachment consists of hemidesmosomes and a cementing layer (Fig. 7-5).

Another epithelial area, which is not keratinized, is found apical to the contact point in the interdental papilla. This is called the gingival col. Since it is thought that the presence of keratin affords additional protection to the epithelium, this col area may be a zone of susceptibility to bacterial penetration.

A stratified squamous epithelium covers most of the attached gingiva. The epithelial cells are connected to each other by fine structures called desmosomes or intercellular bridges. The material between the cells is called the intercellular cementing substance and chemically contains such acid mucopolysaccharides as hyaluronic acid and chondroitin-sulfuric acid. The tissue beneath the gingival epithelium is typical connective tissue and contains cells,

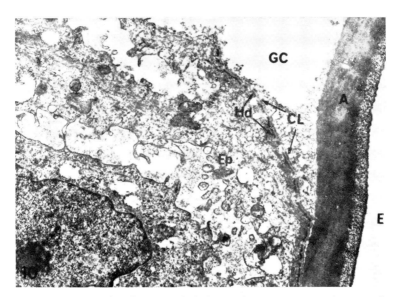

Fig. 7-5. Electronmicrograph of the epithelial attachment in man, showing the fibrous attachment from the cells to the cementum. *A*, type A cuticle; *E*, enamel space; *GC*, gingival crevice; *CL*, basement lamina adjacent to tooth; *Hd*, hemidesmosome; *Ep*, cell of epithelial attachment. (From Listgarten, M. A.: Am. J. Anat. **119:**162, 1966.)

fibers, and vessels embedded in a viscous ground substance. The connective tissue of the periodontal ligament also contains groups of epithelial cells surrounded by an outer argyrophilic limiting membrane; these cell groups are also called the epithelial rests of Malassez. Chemically, the ground substance contains submicroscopic fibers as well as high and low molecular weight components. The latter may be derived from plasma in the case of albumin, globulin, hormones, inorganic ions, glucose, and water. Locally formed high molecular weight molecules include polysaccharide protein complexes containing acid mucopolysaccharides, heteropolysaccharides, and sialic acid. The physiologic properties of the ground substance are related to these mucoproteins. Most of the fiber structure is made up of a fibrous protein called collagen. The precursors of these fibers are produced by fibroblasts. Macrophages, mast cells, and mesenchymal cells are found here in addition to fibroblasts. Another feature of the periodontium is the presence of unusually large numbers of plasma cells in the subepithelial connective tissues; these cells have long been associated with antibody production and in at least one experimental animal are known to produce antibodies at this local level.

Physiologic studies of the gingival crevice area have shown the movement of fluid out of this area. Analysis of the fluid has shown several host products that could have biologic activity, and the presence of polymorphonuclear leukocytes and globulin as well as several enzyme systems has been reported. Increased flow is associated with inflammation, and inert particles are removed from this zone. The permeability of the sulcular epithelium is seen at passage of systemically administered fluorescent compounds from the body outward in this fluid. Large plasma protein molecules and leukocytes enter the oral cavity by this route.

The epithelium is also in contact with saliva, another environmental fluid, containing an array of biologically active cells and enzymes. The antibacterial properties of this fluid may be factors in stabilizing the oral flora.

A well-studied example of a salivary antibacterial system is the peroxidase-hydrogen peroxide-thiocyanate system, which combination inhibits a wide variety of bacteria (Fig. 7-6). The peroxidase in saliva may be derived from leukocytes or may be of salivary gland origin; hydrogen peroxide is thought to be supplied endogenously by bacteria; and the thiocynate component varies with the diet and, in some instances, with the introduction of tobacco smoke. Individually each component is ineffective; however, antibacterial activity is demonstrable when all three are present.

Inherent resistance or susceptibility to bone resorption has been postulated as an important variable in inflammatory periodontal disease; but little is known regarding the factors that contribute to these properies of the host. Ultimately the local tissue resistance must be dependent upon cell metabolism and, therefore, adequate nutrition. The cells of the periodontium derive their nutrition from the circulatory system. The requirements for energy sources and the building blocks for the life and maintainnance of these tissue cells are similar to those of other cells.

Some systemic factors such as aging, severe psychiatric disturbances, and advanced metabolic diseases have been correlated with the severity of periodontal disease. An additional influence of hormones on the oral epithelium makes the periodontium respondent to changes in the endocrinologic status throughout the host's life. A classic example of this is the marked increase in response to local irritants by a woman's gingiva during her pregnancy. Other host changes that could affect the gingival crevice area are alterations in humoral and cellular antibacterial activities. Phagocytosis, antibody production, lyso-

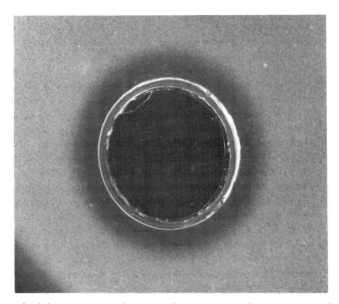

Fig. 7-6. Zone of inhibition surrounding a well containing saliva in a pour plate inoculated with *Lactobacillus acidophilus*.

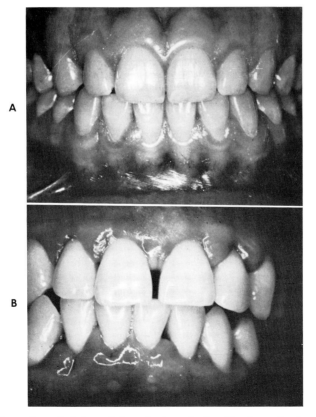

Fig. 7-7. Surface characteristics of the gingivae in health, **A**, and when moderately inflamed, **B**. Note the alteration in gingival color, shape, and texture.

zyme content, or simply the mechanical flushing properties in the gingival crevice may all effect a reduction of the bacterial masses in this area and thus be important local defense mechanisms of the gingivae.

Two important features present in the development of gingivitis, periodontitis, and acute necrotizing ulcerative gingivitis are, first, the presence of marked inflammation and, second, a deepening of the space surrounding the tooth which results in the formation of a periodontal pocket.

Clinically, one diagnoses the presence of gingivitis and periodontitis by inspecting and probing the gingivae and the gingival crevice. A bluish red color rather than coral pink color coupled with swelling and loss of the normal contour of the gingivae are seen in both diseases. Also, early stages of gingivitis may be recognized by a loss of the pebbly or stippled texture of the

gingiva. The crevice depth increases because of swelling of the tissues, and bleeding is elicited upon probing (Fig. 7-7).

Histologically, these surface changes and signs of inflammation in the gingivae are accompanied by proliferation in length of the epithelial attachment. The sulcular epithelium is characterized by rete peg proliferation, acanthosis, and ulceration in the most advanced stages. Degeneration of the fiber apparatus may be seen as a disruption of the gingival fibers and the ligamentum circulare associated with polymorphonuclear leukocytic infiltration. Later, a round cell infiltrate (plasma cells and lymphocytes) is found in the periodontal ligament and subepithelial connective tissue.

In gingivitis, by definition, the epithelial attachment is located at the cementoenamel junction. A spectrum of change occurs in the clinical appearance of the gingiva

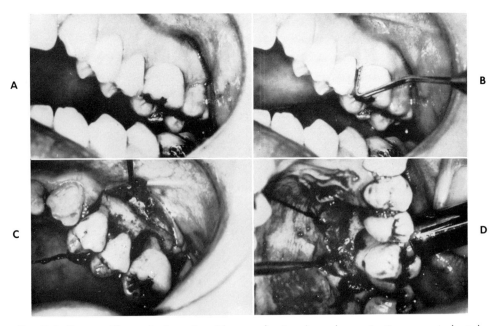

Fig. 7-8. The maxillary gingiva, **A,** with a probe in place demonstrating a periodontal pocket, **B.** When a mucoperiosteal flap is raised, a defect in the bone is seen from the buccal, **C,** and the palatal view, **D.** (Courtesy Dr. D. Carman, Lexington, Ky.)

from the most subtle early stages of gingivitis to more marked alterations in longstanding gingivitis. As the overwhelming irritation of the bacteria remains, the inflammatory process spreads to involve the deeper structures. The transseptal fibers disintegrate and the epithelial attachment proliferates apically. Simultaneously, it becomes detached from the tooth at the most coronal level and a periodontal pocket is created. Development of a periodontal pocket is pathognomonic of periodontitis. The inflammatory infiltrate now is seen concentrated in the loose perivascular connective tissue that envelopes the interdental blood vessels which extend across the interdental bony septa. Bone resorption occurs in the interdental region, forming cuplike deformities (Fig. 7-8). Continued progression of periodontitis results in generalized resorption of supporting alveolar bone along with the progressive loss of periodontal ligament attachment.

The pathogenesis of advanced periodontitis is seen clinically as a deepening of the pocket associated with exudate and a progressive increase in tooth mobility. Roentgenographic findings depict the loss of crestal bone and the relative amount of root that retains the tooth (Fig. 7-9).

ROLE OF BACTERIA IN THE INFLAMMATORY PERIODONTAL DISEASE

A great deal of incriminating data from various lines of clinical and experimental investigation of inflammatory periodontal disease in man suggests that bacteria are the prime etiologic factors. Obviously, the response of the host to the parasitic insult is also important in the pathogenesis of inflammatory periodontal disease.

Epidemiology

The most useful information comes from epidemiologic studies that show a linear relationship between the lack of good oral hygiene and the occurrence of gingivitis or periodontitis (Fig. 7-10). This relationship seems to be the same irrespective of race,

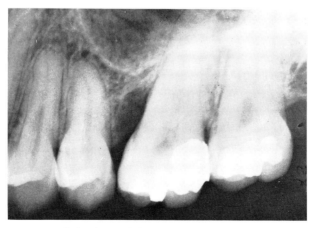

Fig. 7-9. Roentgenogram of the bony defect depicted in Fig. 7-8. A reduced surface area of periodontal support is suggested on the mesial surface of the first molar. (Courtesy Dr. D. Carman, Lexington, Ky.)

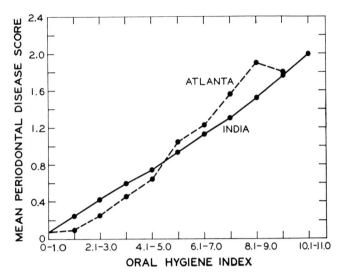

Fig. 7-10. The oral hygiene index compared with periodontal disease scores for 11- to 17-year-old males in urban and rural India and Atlanta, Georgia. (From Greene, J. C.: J. Dent. Res. **39**:308, 1960.)

diet, climate, and other population variables. However, marked differences in prevalence exist between populations, suggesting that control of this complex disease may be possible.

Studies of the uncalcified material adhering to the tooth surface have shown it to contain concentrations of bacteria approaching packed cell preparations.* Thus, the material quantitated in the hygiene studies is almost wholly bacterial in nature.

Empirically, dentists have long recognized the importance of the bacterial masses associated with the tooth surface in relation to both destructive periodontal disease and caries. Methods and instruments have been devised to minimize the mass of bacteria that collects above the gingival margin as plaque and in the gingival crevice as debris. Treatment for periodontal disease and caries control have as their basis the concept of minimizing the bacterial population at the surface of the

teeth through cleansing procedures. The common clinical finding of a dramatic improvement in the status of the gingivae following the institution of rigorous oral hygiene procedures is convincing information regarding the role of the bacterial masses residing near the periodontium.

Oral ecology

The establishment and maintenance of a characteristic group of microorganisms occur within the oral cavity as on external surfaces of the body. This is relatively constant in spite of the routine introduction of other organisms from the extraoral environment. Furthermore, certain sites of the oral cavity harbor different populations of microbes. For example, when comparing the sites of growth of the two oral organisms *Bacteroides menalinogenicus* and *Streptococcus salivarius*, one finds the gram-negative anaerobe *B. melaninogenicus* in the gingival sulcus, but rarely in the supragingival plaque or on the tongue. On the other hand *S. salivarius* is rarely found in the gingival crevice; it is found more

---

*The bacterial pellet obtained following centrifugation of a bacterial culture.

Table 7-1. Distribution of bacteria in various sites of the oral cavity*

	Plaque	Tongue	Gingival crevice
Mean percentage of total cultivable B. melaninogenicus	0.32	0.42	4.5
Mean percentage of facultative streptococcus S. salivarius	0.66	55	0.47

*Adapted from Gibbons, R. J., Kapsimalis, B., and Socransky, S. S.: Arch. Oral Biol. 9:102, 1964.

Table 7-2. Percentage of total cultivable bacteria per unit mass of debris from the gingival crevice versus periodontal pocket*

Characteristics of microbiota	Anaerobes	Facultative	Gram-positive	Gram-negative	Cocci	Rods
Normal crevice	59.7	40.3	70.2	29.8	42.7	57.3
Periodontal pocket	49.0	51.0	72.7	27.3	51.7	48.3

*Adapted from Gibbons, R. J., Socransky, S. S., Sawyer, S., Kapsimalis, B., and Macdonald, J. B.: Arch. Oral Biol. 8:287, 1963.

often in plaque and is the major component of the bacterial flora of the tongue (Table 7-1).

Comparative studies of the bacteria associated with the periodontium have been made on quantitative and qualitative bases. Bacteria obtained from a healthy gingival crevice were compared with those from a periodontal pocket. The total number of bacteria as determined by microscopic count of a unit mass of debris removed from the normal gingival crevice was found to be 10^{11} per gram, wet weight, while the total aerobic and anaerobic viable counts were found to be $352 \pm 78 \times 10^8$ and $197 \pm 69 \times 10^8$ per gram, wet weight, respectively. This is not markedly different from the numbers of viable bacteria found in debris obtained from a periodontal pocket. The total mass of debris collected from the periodontal pocket, however, is approximately fourfold greater than that material obtained from the normal sulcus. Only the spirochete counts showed a slightly but statistically greater number per milligram, wet weight of debris.

Qualitatively, the percentage of pre-

Table 7-3. Comparison of the indigenous bacteria in plaque and debris*

Organism	Logarithm of bacterial count per gram	
	Plaque	Debris from gingival crevice
Streptococci		
facultative	10	9 to 10
anaerobic	+	9 to 10
Neisseria	10	+
Veillonella	+	7 to 8
Lactobacilli	0 to 6	0 to 5
Bacteroides	–	8 to 9
Fusobacteria	+	7 to 8
Treponema, Borrelia		7

*Adapted from Sognnaes, R. F., editor: Chemistry and prevention of dental caries, Springfield, Ill., 1962, Charles C Thomas, Publisher.

dominant cultivable organisms per unit mass of gingival crevice debris is also similar in health and disease. Table 7-2 shows the predominant cultivable organisms from the gingival crevice area in health and disease.

This composite of microorganisms inhabiting the gingival crevice area is differ-

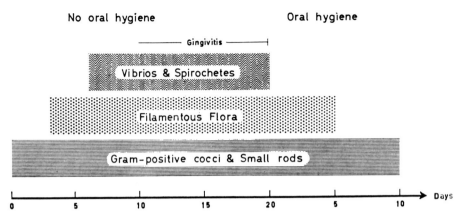

Fig. 7-11. Trends in the changes in the microflora of the gingival margin during the periods of no oral hygiene and oral hygiene. (From Löe, H., Theilade, E., and Jensen, S.: J. Periodont. **36:**183, 1965.)

ent in makeup from the organisms found in plaque (Table 7-3). Plaque contains many facultative streptococci, *Neisseria,* and lactobacilli. Crevice debris is different in that anaerobic streptococci, *Veillonella, B. melaninogenicus,* fusobacteria, and spirochetes are found in great numbers. However, upon the cessation of oral hygiene procedures, the mass of bacteria surrounding the tooth increases. Concomitantly, the plaque material shifts in its bacterial population, and the more apical portion of the plaque resembles gingival crevice debris. This change is accompanied by the development of reversible gingivitis. Fig. 7-11 shows the types of bacterial changes that are noted in the development of experimental gingivitis. Motile gram-negative anaerobes become more numerous and there is an increase in the mass of bacteria.

These changes may reflect the anaerobic conditions which the mass of undisturbed proliferating bacteria creates. Even within normal plaque, a stratification of the bacterial population occurs, the anaerobes being found close to the inner tooth surface and the facultative types being found nearer the external surface of the plaque.

Bacterial characteristics

A greater abundance of bacteria seems to be associated with the periodontal pocket than with the healthy gingival crevice. When one examines the biologic properties of these organisms, it is apparent that they possess destructive capabilities. The following characteristics may be present singly or together in order for the bacteria to initiate a change in the periodontium. No one bacterium can be said to be the etiologic agent in these diseases. It is known that bacteria that live in close association with the periodontium contribute to some of the following categories. In a recent review article, Socransky has concluded that "the mechanism by which microorganisms lead to the destruction of the periodontium is unclear."[18] A greater reducing physicochemical environment has been described for periodontal pockets versus the normal gingival crevice.[7]

Infectivity. Several human infections have been described that are associated with bacterial components similar to those of the gingival crevice area. These have been termed the fusospirochetal infections and include the human bite wounds, noma, tropical ulcer, and the lung abscess.

Gingival crevice debris has the ability to initiate a transmissible infection when inoculated subcutaneously into a number of experimental animals. Some twenty-two different types of oral organisms are found in such infections. One minimum infective combination of these bacteria that has been described includes four organisms: two bacteroides, one of which was *B. melaninogenicus;* a motile gram-negative anaerobe rod; and a facultative diphtheroid. Noticeably absent from the minimum combination are fusobacteria and spirochetes. One of the bacteria, *B. melaninogenicus,* has been shown to be essential for the production of this experimental mixed anaerobic infection; the different strains of this organism vary in their ability to produce infections. This experimental infection produced by gingival crevice bacteria is unique in that it is composed of oral anaerobes whose interactions are nutritionally symbiotic.

When a mixed anaerobic infection was produced in the guinea pig as an assay system, the dosages of gingival crevice debris from normal gingival sulci and periodontal pockets which infect 50% of the animals were found to be similar. Thus, when comparing approximately equal masses of crevice bacteria collected from a healthy crevice and from a periodontal pocket, there does not seem to be a marked difference in the bacterial numbers, types, and virulence. Potentiation of these mixed anaerobic infections has been possible through the addition of various compounds such as the epinephrine and mucin. The fact that other potentiating substances act as foreign bodies suggests an important role of calculus in the pathogenesis of the periodontal pocket. The property of synergism in infections produced by an oral anaerobic streptococcus has been examined, and the bacterial enzyme hyaluronidase has been shown to be an intermediary in the synergistic process. Tissue destruction has also been associated with the implantation of other oral bacteria in animals.

Enzymic activity. A variety of enzymes associated with the crevicular bacteria of man has been described. Conceptually, the presence of a bacterial enzyme capable of degrading a substrate that is known to be a component of the host suggests that oral bacteria have the potential ability to alter or destroy host tissue components. Table 7-4 lists the types of enzymes that have been reported to be associated with isolates or mixtures of oral bacteria. The bacterial source, the enzyme, and its host substrate are listed for comparative purposes.

Depolymerization of hyaluronic acid of the intercellular cementing substance could allow the separation of the epithelial cells. This separation might aid the penetration of bacteria or their products into the tissues or alter the water balance of the connective tissue. Another aid in bacterial progression into the tissues could result from bacterial chondroitin sulfatase's degrading the chondroitin-sulfuric acid of the ground substance. Alteration of tissue function would accompany the action of the former enzymes. The presence of neuraminidase in oral bacteria allows speculation about the destruction of neuraminic acid, another major component of connective tissues.

Regarding proteases, the effect of a bacterial collagenase could be great since the major fibrous protein of the periodontal fiber system, bone, and connective tissues is collagen. There appears to be collagenase of both host origin and bacterial origin in the gingival crevice area. These enzymes differ in that the latter is active only under anaerobic or reducing conditions (Fig. 7-12). This bacterial collagenase is produced by the gram-negative anaerobe *B. melaninogenicus,* and its collagenolytic activity is not as great as that of clostridial collagenase.

Toxic factors. Components of the oral flora are also known to possess endotoxin. This type of toxin is commonly found in

Table 7-4. Enzymic activities associated with members of the oral microbial flora*

Types of bacteria	Enzymes produced	Substrates
Staphylococci	Hyaluronidase	Hyaluronic acid
	Coagulase	Plasma clot
	Gelatinase	Gelatin
	Hemolysin	Erythrocyte
Streptococci	Hyaluronidase	Hyaluronic acid
	Streptokinase	Fibrin, fibrinogen
	Streptodornase	Nucleoprotein
	Hemolysin	Erythrocytes
	Beta glucuronidase	Glucuronidic linkages
	Proteases	Proteins
Diphtheroids	Hyaluronidase	Hyaluronic acid
	Chondroitin sulfatase	Chondroitin-sulfuric acid
Fusobacteria	Proteases	Proteins
	Sulfatase	Arylsulfates
Bacteroides melaninogenicus	Collagenase	Collagen
	Gelatinase	Gelatin
	Proteases	Protein
Gram-negative cocci	Proteases	Protein
	Neuraminidase	Sialic acid

*From Schultz-Haudt, S. D.: Int. Dent. J. **14:**401, 1964.

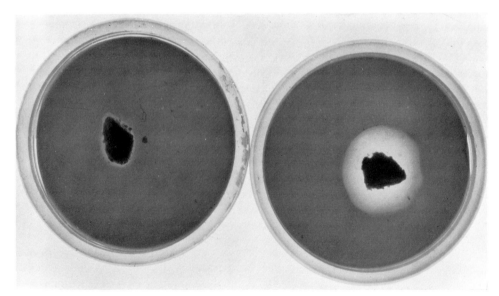

Fig. 7-12. The area of lysis around a collagen gel is great when the *Bacteroides melanino-genicus* sample is tested in an atmosphere of 95% heavy hydrogen and 5% carbon dioxide (right). When tested in air, no activity is seen (left). Other proteases are ineffective in lysing this collagen gel.

gram-negative bacteria and is ordinarily isolated as a complex of lipid, polysaccharide, and proteinlike substance. Increases in the gingival crevice exudate endotoxin have been associated with an increased degree of inflammation as assessed clinically[16] and histologically.[17] Recently, more precise measurements of various portions of the periodontal endotoxin pool also indicated a rise in the level of detectable endotoxin in states of greater clinical inflammation.[15] Among the unique and varied biologic activities associated with this material, several experimental pathologic changes have been brought about in the oral tissues of experimental animals by the administration of endotoxin. Single submucosal injections, combined local and systemic injections, or local and systemic injections combined with catecholamines all have the ability to cause destruction of the oral tissues of experimental animals. In addition, administration of endotoxin can alter the host's reaction to the inoculation of oral bacteria. A diphasic effect on the phagocytic ability of host leukocytes can be brought about with endotoxin. Other alterations on the cellular level have been attributed to the introduction of endotoxin. For example, upon the inclusion of endotoxin with mammalian cells in vitro, a shift of cellular metabolism to a more glycolytic type has been described. Conceivably, interactions with circulating endotoxin released from the endotoxin pool of the intestines could occur at the gingival level and result in tissue damage.

Toxic products of bacteria have been postulated to be of importance in the pathogenesis of periodontal disease. Among these indole, skatole, other amines, and ammonia are known to be produced by the members of the oral flora. Their concentration in vivo in the oral tissues and their direct effect, if any, on those tissues are unknown.

Bacteria in diseased tissues. Since the crevicular epithelium is usually ulcerated

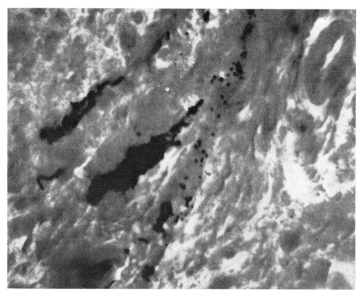

Fig. 7-13. Photomicrograph demonstrating perivascular infiltration of microorganisms in diseased gingiva stained by Gomori's methenamine-silver nitrate method (675 ×). (From Haberman, J.: J. Periodont. **30:**192, 1959.)

within the periodontal pocket, it is not surprising that several investigators have described the presence of bacteria or their antigenic products in the subepithelial tissues of inflamed gingivae. Fig. 7-13 shows spotty foci of bacteria in the perivascular tissues, which are associated with chronic inflammation. Also, viable filamentous bacterial forms have been isolated from diseased gingival samples. In addition to the presence of bacteria, another source of bacterial irritation could come from the diffusion of bacterial substances into the subepithelial tissues from extragingival sites.

Host response to oral organisms. The ability of oral bacteria to act as potent antigens allows one to postulate the involvement of an antigen-antibody interaction in the cause of periodontal disease. Low levels of circulating serum antibodies are found against most oral organisms. Furthermore, bactericidal activity has been reported in the human sera against human oral gram-negative organisms. It is known that the antibody response to endotoxins from these organisms is the IgM, immunoglobulins. The mechanism of bacterial action could initiate the inflammatory response by means of antigen-antibody reactions. The release of hydrolytic leukocytic enzymes is increased by bacterial derivatives. If this is true in the periodontal tissues, the actual mediators of bone resorption and soft tissue destruction may be the biologically active compounds derived from such host cellular components as lysosomes. Furthermore, the ability of cell-free extracts of oral bacteria to sensitize experimental animals suggests hypersensitivity in the host-parasite relationship in the oral cavity. The experimental production of periodontitis in a nonhuman primate by the repeated application of an antigenic material lends support to the hypothesis that allergic phenomena are involved in the development of periodontal destruction.[13] Much investigation is under way which postulates periodontal

disease as a type of allergy or at least as being aggravated by an allergic component.[3] Inferential data showing an increase in allergic reaction to *Actinomyces* with increasing periodontal inflammation would support this concept.[12] The process of inflammation and activation of the immune response has been demonstrated upon injection of oral endotoxin into oral mucosa.[2] Microbial antigens that may be involved in causing periodontal disease have been categorized as (1) the mucopeptide layer of the cell wall of gram-positive bacteria, (2) endotoxin, and (3) proteins.[1]

Calculus production. Dental calculus is a mineralized material that forms on and is firmly adherent to the surfaces of teeth occlusal and apical to the free margin of the gingiva. When in contact with the oral tissue, calculus is usually associated with tissue inflammation. Studies of the development of calculus have shown the progressive histochemical and bacteriologic alteration of dental plaque to this mineralized state.

The formation of calcium phosphate crystals occurs until as much as 80% of the dry weight of the calculus is inorganic matter. Table 7-5 shows the incidence and abundance of calcium phosphate types in dental calculus. Hydroxapatite is the most common type of crystal found. The percentages of types of organic components found in calculus are listed in Table 7-6. Studies of the in vivo formation of supragingival calculus have described a cuticlelike membrane that attaches to the enamel surface first. This cuticular material, better termed the acquired pellicle, is thought to be derived from saliva and serves to localize microorganisms on the surface of the teeth. The in vivo development of the pellicle is not altered by antibiotics.

Histologic studies show that the types of microorganisms gradually shift from the coccoid and rodlike types in the early stages of calculus formation to the fila-

Table 7-5. Incidence and abundance of calcium phosphates in four hundred thirty-seven dental calculus specimens*

Component	Percentage of incidence	Percentage of abundance
Hydroxyapatite	99.5	55.3
Whitlockite	80.7	24.2
Octocalcium phosphates	94.8	20.0
Brushite	43.6	8.9

*From Rowles, S. L.: Dent. Pract. **15**:3, 1964.

Table 7-6. Organic components of calculus (6% to 28% of total components of calculus)*

	Percentage organic
Carbohydrate	12 to 20
Proteins	36 to 40
Lipid	0.2

*Adapted from Theilade, J.: Int. Dent. J. **16**:211, 1966.

Table 7-7. Relative prevalence of certain groups of organisms isolated from developing and mature calculus*

Organism isolated	Age of plaque (days)		
	2	28	90
Streptococci	50.4% (26.7–59.3)	50.2% (17.7–81.1)	16.5% (3.4–31.8)
Actinomyces naeslundii	1.3% (0.0–6.8)	11.5% (0.0–38.2)	26.6% (0.0–67.7)
Actinomyces israelii	0	0	0
Filamentous forms including Bacterionema matruchotii Leptotrichia buccalis	2.8% (0.0–15.3)	4.4% (0.0–5.7)	6.2% (0.0–23.0)

*Adapted from Howell, A., Jr., Rizzo, A., and Paul, F.: Arch. Oral Biol. **10**:310, 1965.

mentous forms at seven days. This older plaque in the process of forming calculus contains a mass of microorganisms embedded in a homogenous intermicrobial matrix. In contrast, studies on the cultivable bacteria of calculus indicate that the *Streptococcus* is one of the predominant forms cultivable for as many as four weeks of precalculus development. Table 7-7 lists the percentages of *Actinomyces naeslundii*, *A. israelii*, and filamentous forms cultivable from calculus samples of different ages.

Interestingly, viable and nonviable forms of the former *Actinomyces* species as well as *Bacterionema matruchotii* and other bacteria have the ability to mineralize when placed in animals. Further studies of *B. matruchotii*, an aerobic filamentous orga-

nism isolated from dental plaque, have shown the presence of a calcifiable cell-free substance in this organism. In vitro intracellular calcification has also been shown with oral filamentous organisms. Current understanding of the actual calcification process is incomplete. The epitaxic concept, which is the most popular, postulates the development of a primary seed of salt crystal that forms in the proper spatial framework of an organic matrix. Further calcification takes place by crystal growth in which calcium and phosphate ions are derived from saliva. Organic materials derived from other sources may be involved since the presence of neither viable nor nonviable bacteria is mandatory for calculus formation. Germ-free animals on special diets develop calculus; however, the extent of calculus formation is increased in animals with a conventional flora. Some animal studies show a marked diminution in the amount of calculus formed when antibiotics are administered systemically, but in rodent studies this relationship was not found.

Various agents have been tested for their ability to lessen calculus formation in man. Some such as antimicrobial agents, enzymes, and chemicals have been directed against the plaque while others such as decalcifying and complexing agents have been directed against the salts of calculus. At the present time none of these has been shown safe and effective.

A direct cause-effect relationship between calculus and gingival inflammation has been obvious in view of the fact that removing this accretion and smoothing the root surface result in a dramatic lessening in the degree of inflammation. The gingival irritation produced by calculus may be both mechanical, in the sense of chronic wounding, and bacteriologic in nature. The attachment of this deposit to the root surface is extremely strong, and its extent is usually to the base of the periodontal pocket; thus, it is difficult to remove. The following four types of attachment that physically bind calculus to teeth have been described: (1) the organic matrix of calculus is attached to acquired pellicle; (2) the pellicle is absent and the calculus matrix is attached to minute irregularities in the cementum surface; (3) organisms have penetrated into the cementum and are continuous with the organisms in the calculus matrix; and (4) calculus is located in areas of cementum resorption. The bacterial invasion of the cementum and dentin with subsequent calcification may occur in the most inaccessible areas of the root surface. Nevertheless, the removal of subgingival calculus is the sine qua non of successful periodontal therapy. Since plaque precedes calculus, the minimizing of the bacterial population through effective oral hygiene procedures and through the eradication of periodontal pockets greatly lessens the further extent of calculus formation.

Any factor in the oral environment that aids in plaque formation will invariably aid in calculus formation. Therefore such things as salivary flow rate and mouth breathing influence the ease with which the bacterial masses collect around the cervical area of the teeth. If left undisturbed, this material calcifies. Curiously, however, people with higher viscosity values of saliva tend to form less calculus than do control subjects. The role of salivary mucins in this calculus formation is unknown. The oral flora is capable of removing sialic acid from these mucoproteins.

Preliminary clinical trials have found that use of a dextranase mouthwash reduces the dry weight of plaque available.[9] In carefully controlled clinical experiments other proven methods of reducing plaque formation have included use of mouth rinses of the antibiotic vancomycin and the disinfectant chlorhexidine.[10] Intense research activity has focused on the subject of plaque formation. The development of plaque seems in part related to the production of an extracellular polysaccharide. Clinical studies and laboratory investigations point to sucrose as an especially important source for the bacterial production of this nondialyzable extracellular material. Furthermore, in animal studies, plaque that developed in primates fed by tube, metabolized glucose in a manner different from that of plaque that formed in primates exposed to dietary carbohydrate.[5] This material, dextran, demonstrates an avidity for hydroxyapatite as well as salivary polymers[11] and probably aids greatly in the localization of the bacterial mass on the tooth surface. Other mechanisms of plaque adherence that have been studied are specific adhesive interactions among bacteria[4] and sorption to enamel or acquired pellicle surface.[20]

Experimental animal periodontal disease

A number of experimental animals have been used in the study of periodontal disease. The marmoset, a nonhuman primate, is known to experience periodontal changes analogous to periodontitis in man and appears to be a model fruitful for further studies.[8] The rodents in particular have served as laboratory tools for the investigation of the bacteriologic aspects of this chronic disease.

The clear demonstration of the production of hamster periodontal disease by transmission of bacteria unequivocally affirms that, at least in this experimental situation, periodontal disease is bacterially induced. The causative agent was shown to be an aerobic branching filamentous organism. Dietary sucrose was essential for production of this disease, whose progression could be retarded by the use of antibiotics. A similar lessening in the severity of a periodontal syndrome in the rice rat has been accomplished by the addition of antibiotics to the diet. Furthermore, the microorganisms responsible for the periodontal syndrome in the rice rat are readily transmitted to other animals. Genetic differences in the host's susceptibility to the periodontal syndrome are apparent.

Experiments utilizing the gnotobiotic mouse have demonstrated an enhanced destruction of the periodontium upon the introduction of the major components of the human flora. A less severe alteration of the alveolar bone and periodontium is seen in the germ-free mouse. The lack of inflammatory response suggests this latter situation is not analogous to periodontitis in man. Further studies with mice have shown that histologic signs of periodontal disease required not only bacteria but an irritant as well.

Acute necrotizing ulcerative gingivitis

Acute necrotizing ulcerative gingivitis (ANUG) is an interesting disease defined by clinical criteria. This disease occurs suddenly, and only recurrent episodes make it appear chronic. Characteristically, the interdental papillae become necrotic, although the other marginal gingival tissue may also necrotize. The interdental lesion is associated with pain, bleeding, and membrane formation (Fig. 7-14). The creation of soft tissue deformities in the interdental area occurs upon healing, and if the tissue structure is left in this condition, gingivitis or periodontitis usually develops. ANUG is sometimes confused with primary herpetic gingivostomatitis because of the pain and acute symptoms. However, the specific type of interdental papillary necrosis and lack of temperature rise and malaise should suggest its diagnosis.

The important role of bacteria in the manifestation of this disease is shown by the dramatic response of the affected area to local debridement. The use of oxygenating mouthwashes is also thought to aid in treatment for the acute symptoms. Use of antibiotics topically or systemically produces a marked improvement in symptoms within 24 hours. British investigators have reported the successful use of a trichomonacide in the management of the acute phase of necrotizing gingivitis.[6]

Characteristically, smears of material from the interdental ulcerative zone show many large spirochetes and fusiform bacilli in addition to leukocytes and some erythrocytes (Fig. 7-15). It is curious that, at careful microscopic and bacteriologic examination, the debris covering the interdental area shows, on a wet weight basis, quantitative and qualitative similarity to gingival crevice debris. Also, on a wet weight basis, the median infective dose (I.D.$_{50}$) of such bacterial mass does not differ markedly from gingival crevice debris in its ability to produce the experimental mixed anaerobic infection.

Biopsy materials of the ulcerative interdental lesion show inflamed tissue covered by a layer of necrotic cells that contain bacteria. A layer of polymorphonuclear

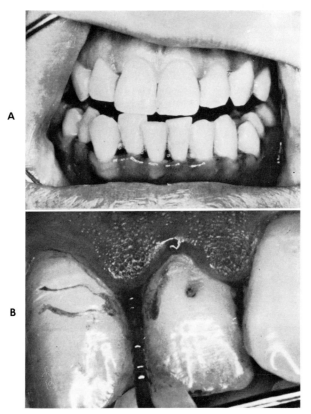

Fig. 7-14. Interdental ulceration characteristic of acute necrotizing ulcerative gingivitis, **A.** The soft tissue craterlike deformity in the gingival papilla is seen following cessation of the acute stages, **B.**

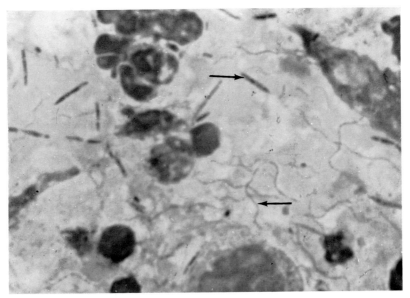

Fig. 7-15. A gram-stained smear of material obtained from an interdental ulceration reveals many types of bacteria, including large spirochetes and fusobacteria (arrows).

leukocytes covers this, and a layer of bacterial plaque is on the external surface.

Similarly, an electron photomicrograph of a thin section of this interdental ulcer has shown these four zones of the ulcer: There is an outer bacterial layer similar morphologically to gingival debris; beneath this is a layer of polymorphonuclear leukocytes mixed with bacteria; internal to this, necrotic epithelial cells are interspersed with a layer of large spirochetes of unusual internal structure. This layer of spirochetes abuts upon the viable tissue cells, and these same bacteria may be seen intercellularly (Fig. 7-16).

Currently, most authorities consider ANUG noncontagious. The peculiar epidemiologic pattern of incidence of this disease is not proof in itself but is only suggestive of an infectious agent. Studies in army populations and university students show an increased incidence in times of stress. A possible common nutritional lack may be responsible for the description of a high incidence in the Indian and African populations; these latter studies show that both ANUG and noma commonly occur in the younger age groups. This finding has not proven true in the studies of American and European populations in that the disease is seldom, if ever, seen in persons younger than 13 years and older than 30 years.

A clinically apparent alteration of the host has been further defined by psychiatric and physiologic studies of ANUG patients. Personality analysis of these patients has disclosed a common pattern of acute anxiety related to a life situation. Comparison of the response of the autonomic nervous system in ANUG patients with the response of a control population has shown a characteristic dominance of the sympathetic nervous system in ANUG patients. This evidence, coupled with the clinical impression that there is a certain type of personality associated with the ANUG patient, suggests that while bacteria may be involved in the pathogenesis of ANUG, a host alteration is also necessary for the development and manifestation of this disease.

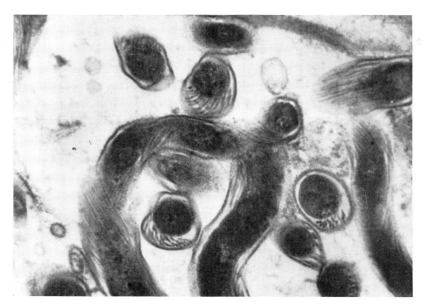

Fig. 7-16. Electron photomicrograph of the interdental ulcer associated with acute necrotizing ulcerative gingivitis. Notice the dense layer of large spirochetes between the cells of the host. (From Listgarten, M. A.: Arch. Oral Biol. **9:**97, 1964.)

Theories as to the mechanism of interaction of the host with the bacteria have involved the central nervous system— adrenal axis. Stress as measured by amount of free 17-hydroxycorticosteroids in the urine seems to be increased in patients suffering with necrotizing gingivitis as compared with that of normal patients and patients with the usual forms of periodontal inflammation, that is, gingivitis and periodontitis.[14]

ORAL PHYSIOTHERAPY

As with all diseases, prevention is far more desirable than treatment. The effect of tooth cleansing procedures in beagle dogs has been studied for a period of years and its effect on the periodontium recorded. Fig. 7-17 depicts the mouth of a dog that had its diagonally opposite quadrants cleaned daily. Notice the marked periodontitis on the uncleaned quadrants of the mouth.

In man, the daily physical removal of bacteria through tooth cleansing procedures is both the basis of prevention and the treatment for gingivitis and periodontitis. Yet all brushing methods are predicated on the patient's ability to recognize a clean tooth surface versus a plaque-covered surface. The following technique has been developed and is known to be effective. The patient chews a tablet containing a nontoxic vegetable dye, after which areas of the tooth surface covered by a film of plaque stain red. This is readily differentiated from clean areas of the tooth because no stain is visible on a clean tooth surface (Fig. 7-18). The patient is instructed to direct the bristles of the brush

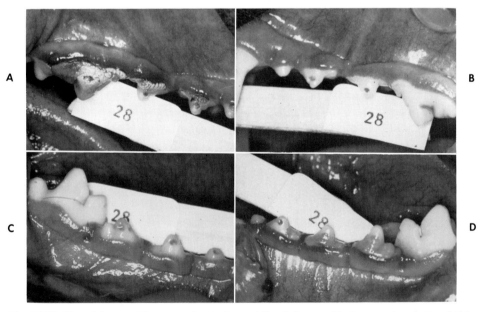

Fig. 7-17. The right maxillary quadrant, **B,** and the left mandibular quadrant, **C,** of this beagle dog have been brushed daily for 1½ years. Note the lack of inflammation or clinical signs of periodontal disease. Contrast this with the maxillary left, **A,** and mandibular right quadrants, **D,** which have not been cleaned. Gingival erythema, alterations in gingival form, and bacterial plaque are quite evident in the uncleaned areas. These signs of periodontitis are accompanied by radiographic evidence of bone loss. (Courtesy Dr. S. R. Saxe, Lexington, Ky.)

to these areas of stain and to brush or scrub the area until the stain is removed.

The critical zone of the oral cavity that requires cleaning is the gingival crevice area. By one's purposely directing the bristles of the brush into this area and scrubbing, the gingival crevice is physically debrided of the bulk of the bacterial masses. The interproximal areas are especially difficult to clean adequately. If the embrasure space is small, the use of dental floss is most effective once the patient has been instructed how to move the floss across the mesial and distal surfaces of the teeth. Interdental stimulators are also a great aid not only in helping to remove the bacterial mass in the interproximal area but also in compressing the interdental tissues. This is associated with increased keratinization of the gingival papilla and may thereby increase the tissue's defensive barrier. This pressure on the tissue helps to flush the crevice of fluid and thus aids the removal of bacteria from this important zone of the periodontium. Presumably, the gingival sulcus is the area where the periodontal tissues are chronically and intimately associated with the deleterious aspects of the oral flora.

A pressurized stream of water may also be used in areas of the mouth. Although this serves as an aid in flushing out food particles and in diluting toxic products, the plaque is not completely removed. This

and other adjuncts have been advocated in order to physically disengage the bacterial mass from the root surface. It is this phase of treatment which is carried out by the patient that is the prerequisite for successful periodontal therapy. Simultaneously, an effective program of caries control is initiated since caries, too, is a complex, bacterially induced disease. The reductive effect of an antimicrobial mouth rinse on dental plaque, calculus, and gingivitis has opened promising adjunctive procedures in the clinical practice of preventive periodontics.[19]

Treatment for gingivitis and periodontitis involves primarily the removal of calculus and plaque from the root surfaces. By itself, trauma from occlusion does not result in pocket formation. The presence of both occlusal traumatism and large collections of bacterial irritants results in rapid and extensive destruction of the periodontium. Once pocket formation occurs, it is necessary to alter the soft and possibly the hard tissues of the periodontium in such a way as to eliminate the periodontal pocket. The excision of this tissue results in a greater clinical crown, and, therefore, accessibility to a far greater surface area of the tooth can be maintained. The aim of eradication of the periodontal pocket is the establishment of a healthy periodontium at a more apical position on the tooth. If the patient is able to clean the root surfaces, the progressive destruction

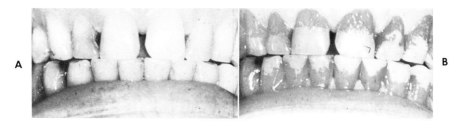

Fig. 7-18. Compare a tooth surface before, **A,** and after the use of a vegetable dye as a staining medium for the plaque, **B.** (From Arnim, S. S.: J. Periodont. **34:**229, 1963.)

of periodontal disease is arrested and preservation of the natural dentition is aided. It may be significant that the areas in the dentition that are least accessible to cleaning are the same areas where periodontal disease first appears as gingivitis and also where the destructive process advances to the greatest extent in the form of periodontitis. These are the interproximal areas.

Undoubtedly, inflammatory periodontal disease is the result of a myriad of influences of both local and systemic origins. At the present time, however, the local bacterial factors appear to be the most important; for when the bacterial population in apposition to the peridontium is minimized, the progressive destruction of the supporting structures of the teeth is prevented.

CITED REFERENCES

1. Bahn, A.: Microbial potential in the etiology of periodontal disease, J. Periodont. **41**:603, 1970.
2. Berglund, S., Rizzo, A., and Mergenhagen, S.: The immune response in rabbits to bacterial somatic antigens administered via the oral mucosa, Arch. Oral Biol. **14**:7, 1969.
3. Bickley, H.: Allergy and oral disease, J. Periodont. **41**:302, 1970.
4. Bladen, H., Hageage, G., Pollock, F., and Harr, R.: Plaque formation in vitro on wires by gram-negative oral organisms (Veillonella), Arch. Oral Biol. **15**:127, 1970.
5. Bowen, W.: The microbiology of gingival-dental plaque. Recent findings from primate research, International Conference on Dental Plaque, Warner-Lambert Co., Morris Plains, N. J., 1969.
6. Glenwright, H., and Sidaway, D.: The use of metronidazole in the treatment of acute necrotizing gingivitis, Brit. Dent. J. **121**:174, 1966.
7. Kenney, E. B., and Ash, M.: Oxidation reduction potential of developing plaque, periodontal pockets and gingival sulci, J. Periodont. **40**:630, 1969.
8. Levy, B.: The nonhuman primate as an analog for the study of periodontal disease, J. Dent. Res. **50**:246, 1971.
9. Lobene, R.: A clinical study of the effect of dextranase on human dental plaque, J. Amer. Dent. Assoc., **82**:132, 1971.
10. Löe, H.: Human research model for the production and prevention of gingivitis, J. Dent. Res. **50**:256, 1971.
11. McHugh: Salivary-induced aggregation of plaque bacteria, Symposium on Dental Plaque, Dundee, Scotland, 1969.
12. Nisengard, R., and Bentuer, E.: Immunologic studies of periodontal disease V IgG type antibodies and skin test responses to actinomyces and mixed oral flora, J. Periodont. **41**:149, 1970.
13. Ranney, R. R., and Zander, H.: Allergic periodontal disease in sensitized squirrel monkeys, J. Periodont. **41**:12, 1970.
14. Shannon, J., Kilgore, W., and O'Leary, T.: Stress as a predisposing factor in necrotizing ulcerative gingivitis, J. Periodont. **40**:240, 1969.
15. Shapiro, L., Lodato, F., Courant, P., and Baker, E.: Endotoxin content of dental plaque, sulcular fluid, gingiva and saliva, International Association for Dental Research, 1971, Abstract 323.
16. Simon, R., Goldman, H., Ruben, M., and Baker, E.: The role of endotoxin in periodontal disease, J. Periodont. **41**:81, 1970.
17. Simon, R., Goldman, H., Ruben, M., and Baker, E.: The role of endotoxin in periodontal disease, J. Periodont. **42**:210, 1971.
18. Socransky, S. S.: Relationship of bacteria to the etiology of periodontal disease, J. Dent. Res. **49**:203, 1970.
19. Stallard, R., Volpe, A., Orban, J., and King, W.: The effect of an antimircrobial mouthrinse on dental plaque, calculus and gingivitis, J. Periodont. **40**:9, 1969.
20. Van Houte, J., Gibbons, R. J., and Banghart, S. B.: Adherence as a determinant of the presence of *Streptococcus salivarius* and *Streptococcus sanguis* on the human tooth surface, Arch. Oral Biol. **15**:1025, 1970.

REFERENCES AND ADDITIONAL READINGS

Arnim, S.: The use of disclosing agents for measuring tooth cleanliness, J. Periodont. **34**:227, 1963.

Bibby, B.: The role of bacteria in periodontal disease, J. Tenn. Dent. Assoc. **40**:1, 1960.

Brandtzaeg, P.: Local factors of resistance in the gingival area, J. Periodont. Res. **1**:19, 1966.

Brill, N.: The gingival pocket fluid, Acta Odont. Scand. **20**, 32(suppl.):1-115, 1962.

Carlson, J., and Egelberg, J.: Effect of diet on early plaque formation in man, Odont. Rev. **16**:112, 1965.

Cohen, B.: Morphological factors in the pathogenesis of periodontal disease, Brit. Dent. J. **107**:31, 1959.

Courant, P. R., and Bader, H.: *Bacteroides melaninogenicus* and its products in the gingiva of man, J. Amer. Soc. Periodont. **4**:131, 1966.

Courant, P. R., Paunio, I., and Gibbons, R. J.: Infectivity and hyaluronidase activity of debris from healthy and diseased gingiva, Arch. Oral Biol. **10**:119, 1965.

Dick, D. S., and Shaw, J.: The infectious and transmissable nature of the periodontal syndrome of the rice rate, Arch. Oral Biol. **11**:1095, 1966.

Fodor, J. T., and Ziegler, J. E.: A motivational study in dental health education, J. S. Calif. Dent. Assoc. **34**:203, 1966.

Fullmer, H. M., and Gibson, W.: Collagenolytic activity in gingivae of man, Nature **209**:728, 1966.

Gibbons, R. J., and Banghart, S. B.: Synthesis of extracellular dextran by cariogenic bacteria and its presence in human dental plaque, Arch. Oral Biol. **12**:11, 1967.

Gibbons, R. J., Berman, K. S., Knoettner, P., and Kapsimalis, B.: Dental caries and alveolar bone loss in gnotobiotic rats infected with capsule forming streptococci of human origin, Arch. Oral Biol. **11**:549, 1966.

Gibbons, R. J., and Macdonald, J. B.: Degradation of collagenous substances by *Bacteroides melaninogenicus*, J. Bact. **81**:614, 1961.

Gibbons, R. J., Socransky, S. S., Sawyer, S., Kapsimalis, B., and Macdonald, J. B.: The microbiota of the gingival crevice area of man. II. The predominant cultivable organisms, Arch. Oral Biol. **8**:281, 1963.

Glickman, I.: Clinical periodontology, ed. 3, Philadelphia, 1964, W. B. Saunders Co.

Glickman, I.: Occlusion and the periodontium, J. Dent. Res. **46**(suppl.):53, 1967.

Going, D. H.: Hypersensitivity in guinea pigs to oral fusospirochetal organisms, J. Dent. Res. **44**:1358, 1965.

Goldhaber, P., and Giddon, D. B.: Present concepts concerning the etiology and treatment of acute necrotizing ulcerative gingivitis, Int. Dent. J. **14**:468, 1964.

Greene, J. C.: Oral hygiene and periodontal disease, Amer. J. Public Health **53**:913, 1963.

Howell, A., Jr., Rizzo, A., and Paul, F.: Cultivable bacteria in developing and mature human dental calculus, Arch. Oral Biol. **10**:370, 1965.

Jordan, H. V., and Keyes, P. H.: Studies on the bacteriology of hamster periodontal disease. Amer. J. Path. **46**:843, 1965.

Klebanoff, S. J., Clem, W. H., and Luebke, R. G.: The peroxidase-thiocyanate-hydrogen peroxide antimicrobial system, Biochim. Biophys. Acta **117**:63, 1966.

Landy, M., and Braun, W.: Bacterial endotoxins, New Brunswick, N. J., 1964, Rutgers University Institute of Microbiology.

Listgarten, M. A.: Electron microscopic study of the gingiva-dental junction of man, Amer. J. Anat. **119**:147, 1966.

Listgarten, M. A., and Socransky, S. S.: Ultrastructural characteristics of a spirochete in the lesion of acute necrotizing ulcerative gingivastomatitis (Vincent's infection), Arch. Oral Biol. **9**:95, 1964.

Löe, H., Theilade, E., and Jensen, S. B.: Experimental gingivitis in man, J. Periodont. **36**:177, 1965.

Macdonald, J. B.: On the pathogenesis of mixed anaerobic infections of mucous membranes, Ann. Roy. Coll. Surg. Eng. **31**:361, 1962.

Mergenhagen, S. E.: Nature and significance of somatic antigens of oral bacteria, J. Dent. Res. **46**(suppl.):46, 1967.

Mergenhagen, S. E., Hampp, E. G., and Scherp, H. W.: Preparation and biological activities of endotoxins from oral bacteria, J. Infect. Dis. **108**:304, 1961.

Mergenhagen, S. E., Thonard, J. C., and Scherp, H. W.: Studies on synergistic infections. I. Experimental infections with anaerobic streptococci, J. Infect. Dis. **103**:33, 1958.

Richardson, R. L.: Effect of administering antibiotics, removing the major salivary glands, and toothbrushing on dental calculus formation in the cat, Arch. Oral Biol. **10**:245, 1965.

Rizzo, A. A., Martin, G. R., Scott, D. B., and Mergenhagen, S. E.: Mineralization of bacteria, Science **135**:439, 1962.

Rizzo, A. A., and Mergenhagen, S. E.: Local Schwartzman reaction in rabbit oral mucosa with endotoxin from oral bacteria, Proc. Soc. Exp. Biol. Med. **104**:579, 1960.

Rovin, S., Costich, E. R., and Gordon, H. A.: The influence of bacteria and irritation in the initiation of periodontal disease in germfree and conventional rats, J. Periodont. Res. **1**:193, 1966.

Rowles, S. L.: Biophysical studies on dental calculus in relation to periodontal disease, Dent. Pract. **15**:2, 1964.

Russell, A. L.: World epidemiology and oral health. In Environmental variables in oral disease, Washington, D. C., 1966, American Association for the Advancement of Science.

Schultz-Haudt, S. D.: Biochemical aspects of periodontal disease, Int. Dent. J. **14**:399, 1964.

Sharawy, A. M., Sabharwal, K., Socransky, S. S., and Lobene, R. R.: A quantitative study of plaque and calculus formation in normal and periodontally involved mouths, J. Periodont. **37:** 495, 1966.

Sicher, H.: Orban's oral histology and embryology, ed. 5, St. Louis, 1962, The C. V. Mosby Co.

Smith, D. T.: Oral spirochetes and related organisms in fuso-spirochetal disease, Baltimore, 1932, The Williams & Wilkins Co.

Socransky, S. S., Gibbons, R. J., Dale, A. C., Bortnick, L., Rosenthal, E., and Macdonald, J. B.: The microbiota of the gingival crevice of man. I. Total microscopic and viable counts and counts of specific organisms, Arch. Oral Biol. **8:**275, 1963.

Takazoe, I.: Microbial calcification in dental calculus formation, Parodontologie **20:**22, 1966.

Theilade, J., and Schroeder, H. E.: Recent results in dental calculus research, Int. Dent. J. **16:**205, 1966.

Weinstein, E., and Mandel, I. D.: The present status of anti-calculus agents, J. Oral Ther. **1:** 327, 1964.

Zander, H. A.: The attachment of calculus to root surfaces, J. Periodont. **24:**16, 1953.

Zander, H. A., Hazen, S. P., and Scott, D. B.: Mineralization of dental calculus, Proc. Soc. Exp. Biol. Med. **103:**257, 1960.

8 / Dental caries

Dental caries is a bacterial disease of the dental hard tissues and occurs in certain localized sites in the dentition. These sites are, in order of frequency of attack, the pits and fissures, particularly those on the occlusal surfaces of the teeth; the approximal contacting surfaces; and those labial, buccal, and lingual surfaces of the dentition adjacent to the gingivae. These sites, protected from the cleansing action of saliva, the tongue, and the oral musculature, are the regions where food is retained and where bacteria, salivary protein, and other oral debris readily collect. The tenaciously adhering and loose deposits of bacteria and proteins in these non–self-cleansing regions are commonly referred to as the *dental plaque*,[12] without which the caries process cannot occur (Figs. 8-1 and 8-2).

THEORIES OF CARIES FORMATION

The theory for dental caries formation now accepted by most investigators is the one usually referred to as the *acid decalcification theory*,[51] first proposed toward the end of the nineteenth century. In its original form it stated that the bacterial breakdown of dietary carbohydrate retained in the non–self-cleansing regions of the dentition produced acid which then dissolved the underlying tooth enamel, thus initiating the caries lesion.

At the time, and for a period after the acid decalcification theory was first formu-lated, enamel was thought to be inorganic in composition and not to contain an organic component. Consequently, it was believed that only acid decalcification applied to enamel; whereas the mechanism of breakdown of dentin, known to contain an organic matrix, was believed to be acid decalcification followed by the proteolytic breakdown of the organic matrix.

When it was discovered histologically that enamel contains a small amount of organic material,[6] the well-established acid decalcification theory was challenged by a new theory. This theory, called the *proteolytic theory*, proposed that the first step in the caries process was the proteolytic breakdown of the organic matrix of the enamel by the oral bacteria[26]; and that, once the organic matrix of the enamel was destroyed, the mineral portion crumbled, much like the bricks of a building when the mortar is removed. Subsequently, the proteolytic theory was modified to indicate that proteolysis of the enamel protein released either sulfate[53] or glutamic and aspartic acids,[1] which dissolved the inorganic portion of the enamel. Then a second modification was made which suggested that the end products of proteolysis acted as chelating agents and that these substances facilitated the solubilization of calcium.[56] With this second modification, the theory has been termed the *proteolysis-chelation theory*.

Because of the overwhelming amount

of evidence in support of the acid decalcification theory and the absence of comparable data to support the proteolytic theories, the latter now receive very little attention from most investigators. Support for the acid decalcification theory was not so one-sided when it was observed histologically that the organic portion of the enamel loses structural detail ahead of the invading microorganisms. However, when it was shown that the enamel matrix contained proteins soluble in acid,[60] a major

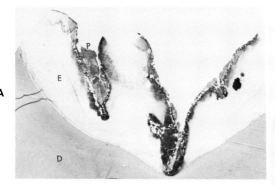

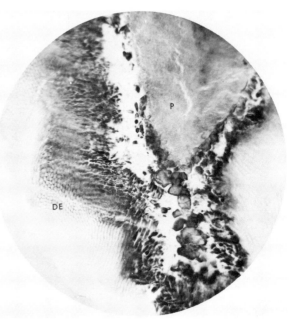

Fig. 8-1. A, Bacterial plaques in carious occlusal pits (12 ×). *P,* Bacterial plaque; *E,* Enamel; *D,* dentin. **B,** Left occlusal pit in **A** (465 ×). *P,* Plaque microorganisms demineralized enamel, *DE.* (Courtesy Dr. S. S. Arnim, Houston, Tex.)

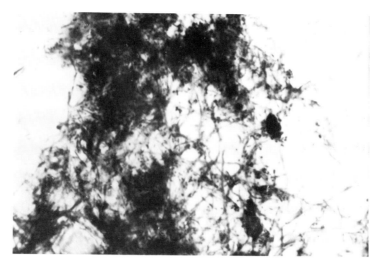

Fig. 8-2. Photomicrograph of stained smear of teased dental plaque showing the variation in its bacterial composition.

objection to the acid decalcification theory, namely that acid decalcification precedes proteolysis, was removed.

It has been shown recently[44] that at a pH of 5.6 hydrolysis of enamel phosphoprotein by phosphoprotein phosphatase accelerates solubilization of the enamel mineral by acid. This suggests a regulatory role for the organic portion of the enamel in the decalcification process, one of altering by its presence (and removal) the rate and severity of enamel destruction by the acid. Deposits of organic material derived from the bacteria and proteins of the plaque during and after periods of decalcification may play a similar role (Fig. 8-3).

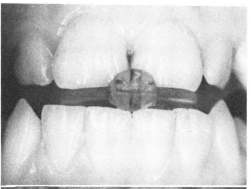

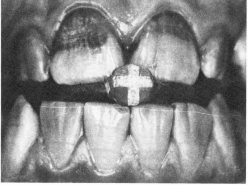

Fig. 8-3. Protein impregnated enamel demineralized by caries. Following rubber cup prophylaxis, teeth were photographed under visible (top) and under ultraviolet light (bottom). Demineralized enamel enables plaque remnants and excess pellicle (more easily seen under ultraviolet illumination) to accumulate.

Bacterial breakdown and invasion of the dental hard tissues

As the enamel is destroyed, microorganisms are able to penetrate the interior of the individual enamel rods and the inter-rod matrix of the enamel.[21] Penetration is usually more extensive in the region of the enamel core than in the region of the inter-rod matrix. In areas of deeper penetration the microorganisms are few in number compared to areas closer to the enamel surface. The microorganisms at the leading edge of the caries lesion are spheroidal and gram-positive, while the structure of those in the remaining portion of the lesion is heterogeneous. The spheroidal microorganisms are replaced by gram-positive and gram-negative threadlike forms as destruction of enamel continues.

Initial invasion of the dentin occurs through the odontoblast fibrils, following which decalcification and softening of the tubules take place. With further invasion and production of acid, decalcification of the intertubular dentin results.

The deepest layers of the active lesion in the dentin are nearly always sterile, and not until a very late stage in the development of the caries lesion do the bacteria enter the dental pulp.

Localization of acid and fall in pH in dental plaque

For caries to occur, the acid formed during the breakdown of carbohydrate by bacteria in the dental plaque must be capable of dissolving the enamel of the tooth before the continuously flowing saliva can wash away the acid. Two properties of plaque enable this to take place: (1) the plaque contains a high concentration of bacteria, which permits the production of large quantities of acid in a short period of time[62, 63]; and (2) the diffusion of materials through the plaque matrix is comparatively slow so that acids formed in the plaque require a comparatively long period to diffuse outward into the saliva. Because

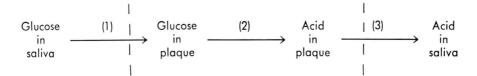

the rate of acid formation is faster than the rate at which the acid can diffuse from the plaque (step 2) into the saliva (step 3), acid accumulates in the plaque.[63] The sequence of metabolic and diffusion steps shown above illustrates this point.

When acid accumulates in plaque, the plaque pH falls and can be measured with relative ease with either antimony[34, 61, 63] or glass[10] pH microelectrodes. When the mouth is rinsed with a 10% glucose solution and the pH is measured before, during, and for approximately one hour after the rinsing, a pH curve with the general characteristics of that shown in Fig. 8-4 will result.[61] A curve of this type is commonly referred to as a Stephan curve.

During the 10% glucose rinsing some of the glucose enters the plaque, while the remainder is diluted and cleared from the mouth by saliva. The glucose entering the plaque is transient, and, since its rate of conversion to acid is faster than the rate of acid removal, the acid concentration in the plaque undergoes a rapid rise. Once the plaque glucose is used up, the concentration of the acid slowly falls.[34]

However, if the amount of glucose available to the plaque is increased, by an increase in either the glucose concentration or the time that glucose is available to the plaque bacteria, a Stephen curve with a larger area between the curve and the base line is produced. A further increase in the amount of glucose will result in the pH remaining at a minimal level for a longer period (Fig. 8-5).

Experiments such as these have clearly shown that the availability of glucose or dietary carbohydrate to the plaque bacteria determines the extent and duration of the plaque pH response.[39] Availability is defined as the amount of carbohydrate available per unit of time and is the product of the concentration and duration of exposure. A soluble carbohydrate such as ordinary sugar usually results in a high concentration and an exposure of short duration. On the other hand, a poorly soluble carbohydrate, such as the starchy foodstuffs, results in a low concentration and an exposure of long duration. When the availability of carbohydrate is unlimited, and, therefore, in excess, the pH falls to a minimum value and remains at this minimum as long as there is carbohydrate still available. Once the carbohydrate is used up by the plaque bacteria or washed away by the saliva, or both, the pH rises. If the exposure to glucose or dietary carbohydrate is repeated, then a second Stephan curve results. Thus, increase in the frequency of ingestion of dietary carbohydrate increases the frequency of acid response; the longer dietary carbohydrate remains in the mouth following ingestion, the longer it takes for the pH to return to starting levels.

The more frequently acid forms and the longer the acid remains on the surface of a tooth, the more frequently and the longer the enamel is subjected to acid attack. Whether dissolution of the enamel results is dependent upon the solubility conditions for calcium phosphate prevailing within the plaque and on the tooth surface.

Calcium phosphate, the salt making up nearly all of the inorganic portion of enamel and dentin, has a very low solubility at neutral and slightly acidic pH but becomes increasingly more soluble as the pH is lowered, particularly below pH 5.0.[19]

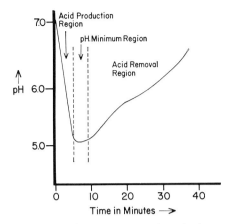

Fig. 8-4. Typical pH curve in dental plaque in response to rinsing the mouth with a strong sugar solution for a few minutes. This curve is commonly called the Stephan curve. The pH falls when the rate of acid formation exceeds the rate of acid removal; the pH remains at the minimum when these are in balance and rises when acid removal exceeds acid formation. Acid can be "removed" by (1) acid's diffusing out of the plaque into the saliva; (2) acid's being neutralized by salivary and plaque buffers and by ammonia and amines formed in the plaque; and (3) stronger acids' (such as lactic) being converted to weaker ones (such as acetic and propionic).

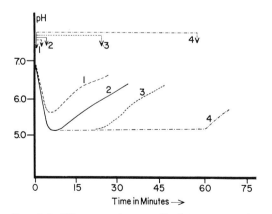

Fig. 8-5. Effect on plaque pH of increasing the availability of glucose to the plaque bacteria. Curves *1, 2, 3,* and *4* are typical of those obtained when a glucose solution of a particular concentration is made available for progressively longer periods of time.

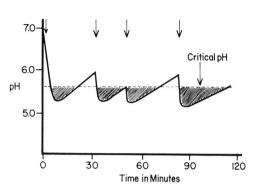

Fig. 8-6. Effect of the frequent ingestion of carbohydrate (arrows) on the pH of plaque and the relation of the plaque pH to the critical pH. Shaded areas indicate the period during which, and approximately the extent to which, the plaque is unsaturated with respect to calcium phosphate.

When there is no plaque on the surface of a tooth and tooth enamel is in continuous contact with saliva, no dissolution of the mineral portion of the enamel occurs since there is more than enough calcium and phosphate in the saliva to keep the tooth from dissolving. As long as the saliva remains "supersaturated" with calcium phosphate, the enamel is protected, and the formation of a certain amount of acid can be tolerated before the tooth will dissolve. The pH at which the saliva (and any calcium and phosphorus in the plaque) fails to protect the enamel from acid dissolution is called the *critical pH* (Fig. 8-6). This pH is rarely reached in the absence of plaque.

ORGANISMS INVOLVED IN THE CARIES PROCESS

Our present-day knowledge of the specific microorganisms involved in the caries process has come from studies of human beings and of laboratory animals that include the hamster, rat, monkey, and miniature pig. Although for a long time there seemed to be little doubt from studies of human beings that bacteria were essential for dental caries to occur, it was not until research with animals had been done that proof was definitely established. However, the unanswered question still remaining even after many years of research is whether the disease is infectious and, if so, which microorganisms of those found in the complex oral microflora are the ones responsible for the disease. The microorganisms most intensively studied have been the streptococci and the lactobacilli, although to a much lesser extent other organisms such as yeast and *Veillonella* have also been examined.

At least twenty-seven varieties of microorganisms have been isolated from mature dental plaque,[27, 28] which, in addition to bacteria, also contains epithelial cells and leukocytes. The microscopic count is approximately 2.5×10^{11} bacteria per gram, while the total cultivable count performed anaerobically and aerobically is approximately 7.1×10^{10} microorganisms per gram,[25] suggesting that a large proportion of the microorganisms in plaque are dead or, if viable, are not able to grow on the media.

The predominant cultivable forms of microorganisms found in plaque removed from the enamel surface were as follows[25]: facultative streptococci, 27%; facultative diphtheroids, 23%; anaerobic diphtheroids, 18%; peptostreptococci, 13%; *Veillonella*, 6%; *Bacteroides*, 4%; fusobacteria, 4%; *Neisseria*, 3%; and vibrios, 2%. Since the lactobacilli were present at a level of less than 0.01% it is evident that they, unlike the streptococci, represent only a minor proportion of the plaque microflora. However, agar replicas of the mouth have demonstrated that the incidence of lactobacilli is much more localized and is highest within fissures, at interproximal embrasures, and at the gingival margins—the areas where caries tends to occur.[2] In the individual with rampant caries, the location of the lactobacilli becomes more widespread and can be detected even on more easily cleansed areas such as the palate.

Because streptococci are present in the mouth in large numbers and are capable of rapidly converting carbohydrate to acid, most investigators have concluded that streptococci must play a dominant role in the formation of the caries lesion. However, streptococci are abundant in both caries-active and caries-inactive individuals, and attempts to relate total streptococcal counts to caries activity have demonstrated only a slight positive correlation. Also, the streptococci are more widespread and not as localized as the lactobacilli to those regions of the dentition where caries occurs. For these reasons, investigators have turned their attention to differences in the streptococci in the respective floras, particularly in relation to their ability to form acid, intracellular and extracellular polysaccharide, and plaque.

High numbers of streptococci and a poor correlation with caries activity in contrast to low numbers of lactobacilli with a high correlation to caries activity are relationships that have been demonstrated and appear to be paradoxical. However, a close examination of the studies related to this seeming paradox indicates that these two relationships may not be mutually exclusive. There is the possibility that the streptococci provide much of the acid responsible for the fall in pH in plaque, gingivae, and other sites in the mouth such as the tongue; and that in some locations, particularly the poorly accessible surfaces of the teeth, this acid is sufficient for lactobacilli to become established and, once established, to favor an increase in the total acid produced when dietary carbohydrate is ingested.

Lactobacilli

In the caries-free mouth, lactobacilli are usually absent. Attempts to introduce this organism into the mouth of a caries-free individual by inoculation have usually not been successful, indicating that in these individuals conditions favoring the establishment of this microorganism are absent.

When the carbohydrate content of the diet of groups of individuals having high incidence of caries and high *Lactobacillus* counts is moderately restricted as in a Becks[4] diet, the counts rapidly fall and then rise when the carbohydrate content is returned to its original level.

When dietary carbohydrate is severely restricted as in the Jay[31] diet, some individuals who show a decrease in *Lactobacillus* counts to zero or to very low levels do not show a return to high counts for periods as long as six months. This may be because those individuals whose counts remain low continue to avoid carbohydrate in their diets or because in their mouths conditions develop that do not favor the reestablishment of this organism. There is the possibility, although it is not probable, that exposure to and reinfection with lactobacilli has not occurred.

If conditions in the mouth are altered so that the retention of ingested carbohydrate is increased, then without any alteration in the diet *Lactobacillus* counts will increase. For example, in the edentulous mouth, retention sites are virtually absent, and the *Lactobacillus* counts are either extremely low or zero. Once teeth erupt, as in the infant, or once artificial dentures are inserted, as in the edentulous adult, presence of teeth provides retention sites for dietary carbohydrate, and the *Lactobacillus* counts rise sharply.

In mouths containing open caries lesions, the lesions provide retention sites for dietary carbohydrate, and accordingly the number of lactobacilli is usually high. However, once these retention sites are eliminated by restorative dentistry the *Lactobacillus* count rapidly falls. The *Lactobacillus* counts observed in individuals living in low-fluoride areas are higher than in those living in areas where the fluoride content is optimal; the higher counts have usually been attributed to the presence of more cavities and, therefore, of more retention sites.

Perhaps the most dramatic demonstration of the effect of increased retention sites on the *Lactobacillus* count was shown in a study in which palatal prostheses were inserted into the mouths of individuals initially showing low *Lactobacillus* counts.[51] The counts immediately rose and just as rapidly fell to the original levels once the appliances were removed. These changes parallel those commonly observed clinically where the caries activity on those surfaces of the teeth previously free from caries increases markedly when the teeth come into contact with newly placed prosthetic or orthodontic appliances.

From these studies it is obvious that the presence of teeth in the mouth, alterations of the form of teeth by caries, and the insertion of appliances can all provide conditions favoring the retention of dietary carbohydrate that enable the *Lactobacillus* organism to become established or, if already present, to increase in number. Because these microorganisms are aciduric, that is, a low pH (usually pH 5.0) favors their growth, then only those locations in the mouth where the pH can remain low for long periods of time would favor their establishment. This is possible only in areas of the dentition that have the poorest saliva access. Since these sites constitute only a small percentage of the total area upon which bacteria can grow, one can see why these organisms constitute such a small percentage of the total oral flora. Since these are also the sites where the mouth is most acid and where caries occurs, it is easy to see why past investigators believed that lactobacilli were the cause of the caries, rather than that their presence was indicative of those conditions favoring both an aciduric flora and in turn dental caries. Even if the additional acid supplied by the lactobacilli were necessary in a particular site to exceed the critical pH because most of the acid comes from the more numerous streptococci, it would not be correct to assume that lactobacilli are the "cause" of dental caries.

The *Lactobacillus* count seems to be related to the age of the individual.[7] In children up to 8 years of age, these organisms are present in approximately 35% of mouths; in young people from 8 to 20 years of age, they are present in from 85% to 95% of mouths; and in people older than 20 years, the frequency is approximately 50%. This variation with age seems to correspond to the caries incidence of the respective age groups.

Culturing of scrapings obtained from whitened areas of enamel (suggestive of initial active caries and commonly found in the cervical regions of the teeth) or from beginning and deep cavities, shows the presence of lactobacilli in a high percentage of cases.[8] On the other hand, in a high percentage of individuals giving no evidence of caries, positive *Lactobacillus* cultures are rarely obtained.

Although the presence of a high or low *Lactobacillus* count is generally indicative of caries activity or inactivity, respectively, there are cases in which no relationship appears to exist. One probable reason for this lack of relationship is that there is considerable difficulty in correlating the presence of lactobacilli with caries activity when the caries activity is determined by measuring the increase in the number or size of caries lesions over a period of time. Since at least a few months are needed for such changes to become clinically evident, the *Lactobacillus* count, which responds rapidly to alterations in the dietary carbohydrate, has an opportunity to fluctuate between zero and several millions many times during the same period.

Streptococci

Of the streptococci in the mouth, the aciduric streptococci, like the lactobacilli, grow in an acidic environment and represent only a minor portion of the total flora; they include the hemolytic, lactic, and enterococcal groups.[43] Of the remaining streptococcal organisms, S. mitis, S. salivarius, and more recently S. sanguis and S. mutans have received the most attention in the role of the streptococci in the caries process.

S. salivarius appears to be the predominant streptococcus on the tongue and other oral soft tissues, yet in dental plaque its incidence is generally low.[23] S. mitis, on the other hand, generally shows a reverse pattern and is found in much greater numbers in the dental plaque than S. salivarius.

Increasing retention sites by the placing of orthodontic appliances has demonstrated that, like lactobacilli, S. mitis and S. salivarius in plaque both increase.[3] Prior to insertion of the appliances the numbers of S. salivarius and S. mitis are comparable; but with increase in carbohydrate availability, resulting from the presence of an appliance, S. mitis increases more sharply (Fig. 8-7). This suggests that a much higher incidence of S. mitis than S. salivarius occurs in the plaque when conditions that favor carbohydrate retention are present.

S. salivarius can produce carieslike lesions in vitro and there is some evidence that a relationship exists between the incidence of this organism and dental caries. S. mitis has been shown to be predominant among those microorganisms in the plaque capable of storing polysaccharide (Fig. 8-7), a property that enables the plaque to continue acid formation once dietary carbohydrate is no longer available as substrate.[24, 55]

As mentioned earlier, total streptococcal counts in saliva obtained by chewing paraffin wax are slightly but not significantly higher in caries-active individuals than in those who are caries-inactive. However, the number of streptococci present only in plaque is significantly higher in the caries-active group.[43] The reason that a significant correlation between caries activity and total streptococcal counts in a saliva sample has not been demonstrated is obvious when one also considers that a major proportion of the streptococci in saliva comes from the tongue and the surfaces of the other oral soft tissues. That a slight correlation exists between S. salivarius and caries activity can be attributed to the fact that conditions in the mouth favoring acidogenic microorganisms in dental plaque also favor the existence of a higher number of acidogenic organisms such as S. salivarius on the tongue and oral soft tissues.

In addition to having more streptococci

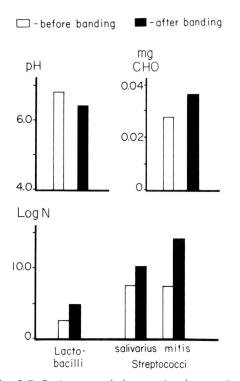

Fig. 8-7. Environmental changes in plaque stimulated by the presence of orthodontic appliances. Note the drop in pH and increase in the carbohydrate, streptococci, and lactobacilli that occurs in plaque following orthodontic banding. (Adapted from Balenseifen, J. W., and Madonia, J. V.: J. Dent. Res. **49:**320, 1970.)

per milligram of plaque, caries-active individuals also have a higher incidence of *Candida* in both plaque and saliva, and there is also some suggestion of a higher incidence of *Veillonella*.[43] All of these factors indicate that conditions in the mouths of caries-active individuals favor the presence of a larger number of acidogenic microorganisms.[22]

The net effect is a lower plaque pH in response to dietary carbohydrate in the caries-active individual.

Animal studies to determine the bacteria involved in the caries process

That dental caries does not occur without bacteria can be demonstrated by a technique in which small laboratory animals are reared in a bacteria-free environment.[52] Rats raised by this germ-free procedure show rates of growth, development, and general metabolism comparable to those of rats raised conventionally. When germ-free and conventional rats are fed a cariogenic diet, the germ-free rats show complete absence of dental caries, even at the microscopic level. On the other hand, the conventional animals develop numerous caries lesions. When the germ-free animals are deliberately inoculated with specific strains of bacteria cultured from caries lesions in conventional rats, some of the bacteria produce caries, but most do not.

Infection resulting in caries formation in germ-free animals has been most successfully accomplished with several strains of streptococci taken from caries-active human beings. Caries formation has also been accomplished in the germ-free animal with an enterococcus[52] and with lactobacilli.[17] The streptococci capable of causing caries were strongly acidogenic and produced lactic acid as their only end product when incubated with sugars in vitro.

In addition to being acidogenic, the streptococci were capable, particularly in the presence of sucrose, of adhering firmly to the surfaces of teeth and to a number of inert materials.[47] This adherence has been attributed to the large amounts of extracellular carbohydrate formed by these streptococcal strains, since those streptococci unable to produce caries produce only small amounts of such extracellular carbohydrate.

In addition to the germ-free technique a less arduous method has also been used to test the cariogenicity of specific microorganisms in laboratory animals.[32] The normal oral flora in a caries-active pregnant female is suppressed with an antibiotic. The offspring and animals of subsequent generations show the same depressed flora and can be used as experimental animals to test the cariogenicity of specific microorganisms by reinfection.

Hamsters treated with antibiotics in this way and their offspring remain caries-free on a cariogenic diet that would ordinarily produce rapid and rampant dental caries.

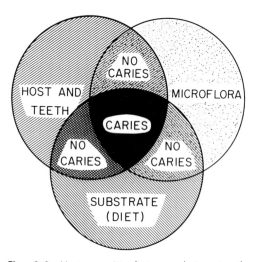

Fig. 8-8. Host-parasitic-dietary relation to the initiation of dental caries. Caries occurs when there is a critical combination of the three variables shown. Prevention consists of modifying these factorial areas so that the critical combination does not occur. (From Keyes, P. H.: Int. Dent. J. **12**:443, 1962.)

Should these animals be placed in contact with caries-active animals, caries lesions will develop, clearly showing that the animals treated with antibiotics do not harbor a cariogenic microflora. Such experiments have demonstrated that dental caries can be transmitted and that infection can be induced with specific strains of streptococci and other pure strains of microorganisms isolated from the oral cavity.

It is important, however, in relating the animal studies to the human condition, that one keeps in mind that most human beings harbor many of the microorganisms found to be cariogenic in animals. One must therefore consider human beings generally to be infected and host-dietary factors to be primarily responsible for caries absence in man (Fig. 8-8). Since saliva and carbohydrate availability have marked effects on the flora, caries in man can be considered to be more of a shift in the composition of the flora and its associated acid-base metabolism (see following section) rather than infection as in the animal studies. Should antibiotics be used in the human mouth and lead to the disappearance of the cariogenic organisms from the microflora, then, as in the animal studies, their reintroduction would be true infection. For this reason, methods successful against the classic infectious diseases may be unsuitable for preventing or controlling dental caries.

BASE PRODUCTION IN PLAQUE

Microorganisms in the plaque are capable of rapidly producing ammonia from nitrogenous substrates. Urea, an end product of protein metabolism in the body, is secreted in the saliva and its breakdown causes the pH of the plaque to rapidly rise.[35] Interestingly, catabolism of urea by the plaque bacteria is even more rapid than catabolism of glucose.[33] Amino acids and protein from saliva and from the oral soft tissues can also serve as substrates for

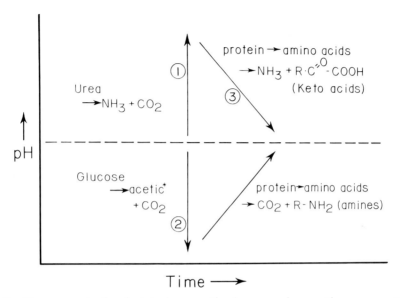

Fig. 8-9. pH response in the dental plaque with glucose and urea. The response in each case consists of a pH displacement (1 and 2) and a pH return component (3 and 4). The pH-rise from a minimum with glucose and the pH-fall from a maximum with urea comprise both the acidic and basic return components of the acid-base homeostatic processes of the mixed microbial flora in salivary sediment and in dental plaque. *Acetic acid is the acid formed at low glucose levels. Lactic acid and propionic acids appear when the glucose level rises and, as a result, acid formation increases. (From Kleinberg, I.: Int. Dent. J. **20**:451, 1970.)

Fig. 8-10. Oxygen uptake, glucose utilization, and lactic and pyruvic acid formation during incubation of mixed salivas of caries-active and caries-resistant individuals. Glucose concentration in these experiments was 250 mg. per 100 ml. and the experiments were carried out for 30 minutes at 37° C. Rate of oxygen consumption is expressed in cubic millimeters per milliliter of salivary mixture per hour, and the glucose and acid concentrations are in milligrams per 100 ml. Mean and standard errors for eight subjects in each group are shown. (Data taken from Eggers-Lura, H.: Deutsch. Zahn Mund Kieferheilk. **21**:97, 1954; reprinted from Kleinberg, I.: J. Dent. Res. **49**:1300, 1970.)

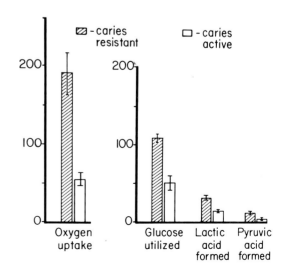

the formation of ammonia, but their breakdown by the microorganisms in the plaque is slower than that of urea and their degradation does not lead to a high pH as with urea[38] (Fig. 8-9).

Because the diet to a large extent provides the substrate for the microorganisms in plaque that produce acid, whereas the saliva is mainly responsible for providing the substrate for the microorganisms that produce base, a delicate balance exists between the availability of substrate from these two sources. Alteration of this balance would favor accordingly acid or base production and the pH in the plaque. The same plaque can, as a result, be responsible for a low pH and enamel dissolution or for a high pH and the deposition of calcium and phosphorus from the saliva and its accumulation in the plaque to form calculus.[33]

The microflora in the saliva of caries-free individuals paradoxically uses glucose and forms acid at a more rapid rate than that of caries-active persons.[16, 37] This could be taken as evidence against the acid decalcification theory for dental caries. However, along with an accelerated rate of acid formation, saliva of caries-free persons appears capable of also producing more base. Thus, fermentable carbohydrate would be used more rapidly and cleared from the mouths of caries-free subjects (Fig. 8-10) with less injurious fall in pH than in caries-active individuals. It has been suggested that caries and a cariogenic flora may actually arise from a deficiency in the base-forming capability of the plaque microflora rather than from an increase in its acid-forming potential.[5]

pH of plaque in various dentition locations and its relation to caries activity

The lowest pH reached during a Stephan curve, the pH minimum, is generally lower in plaques of caries-active individuals than of those showing low caries activity (Fig. 8-11). In addition, plaques

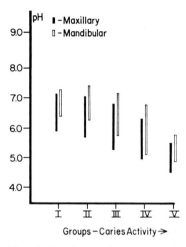

Fig. 8-11. pH levels in plaques on the labial gingival surfaces of the anterior maxillary and mandibular teeth of individuals with varying caries activity. The top of each bar is the pH before rinsing with 10% glucose; the bottom is the minimum pH reached during the rinse. (Adapted from Stephan, R. M.: J. Dent. Res. **23:**257, 1944.)

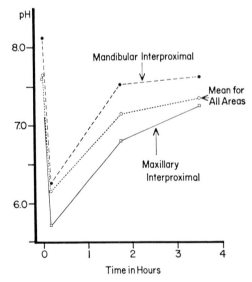

Fig. 8-12. Relationship between pH of plaque and time of eating. Fasting plaque pH levels are above that for resting saliva (mean pH, approximately 6.7); pH minima are below. (Adapted from Kleinberg, I., and Jenkins, G. N.: Arch. Oral Biol. **9:**493, 1964.)

on the labial surfaces of the maxillary anterior teeth show lower pH minima than do plaques on corresponding surfaces of the teeth in the mandible, a relationship which is consistent with the relative caries susceptibilities of these areas.[42]

The pH in carious lesions is approximately 0.7 pH unit lower than in plaques on noncarious surfaces. If the opening into a carious lesion is a narrow one, the pH in the cavity will be lower than if the opening to the cavity is wide and accessible to the saliva.[14]

Extensive studies of subjects before and after they have eaten[42] have shown that plaques located in different areas of the dentition (Fig. 8-12) (embrasure areas and those surfaces adjacent to the gingivae) all show a pH curve of approximately the same shape as a typical Stephan curve,

except that the curve extends over a longer time period.

The pH of plaque is highest before breakfast and is almost invariably higher than that of the saliva continually washing it. At this time, base production in the plaque overshadows acid production and is greatest in plaques on the anteriors of the mandible and least on corresponding plaques in the maxilla. Plaques in those areas of the mouth readily washed by saliva show the highest pH levels and the largest pH difference from that of the saliva.

As soon as food is eaten, the pH falls in plaques located in all areas of the mouth and reaches a minimum that is lowest in those areas that showed the lowest starting pH. Also, all levels are lower than the pH of the saliva.

The difference between the fasting pH and pH minimum, usually referred to as the plaque pH range, is larger for interproximal than for labial and buccal plaques since plaque is thicker in interproximal regions. The reason given for this is that a thick plaque contains more organisms than a thin one, thus enabling it to produce not only more base and a higher fasting pH but also more acid and a lower minimum pH. Plaques located on the labial and interproximal surfaces of the maxillary and mandibular anteriors show the largest differences (Fig. 8-13). This parallels the wide difference in caries incidence in these two regions of the dentition.[13]

Bacterial factors responsible for shape and minimum pH of the Stephan curve

In an attempt to determine the bacterial factors responsible for the shape of the Stephan pH curve and to account for the different pH minima in plaques located in different areas of the same mouth and in corresponding areas of different mouths, experiments have been carried out in which pure cultures of microorganisms isolated from dental plaque have been incubated

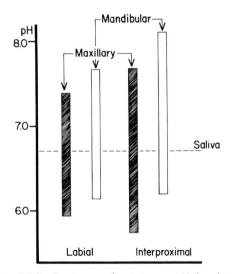

Fig. 8-13. Fasting and minimum pH levels in plaques on labial and interproximal surfaces of the maxillary and mandibular anterior teeth. The top of each bar is the fasting pH level, the bottom is the minimum pH. Note that the pH in maxillary plaques is lower than in mandibular plaques. Also the pH range is greater for interproximal than for labial plaques. (Adapted from Kleinberg, I., and Jenkins, G. N.: Arch. Oral Biol. **9:**493, 1964.)

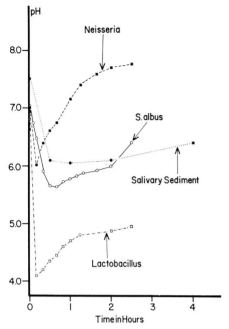

Fig. 8-14. pH curves with three pure cultures of microorganisms isolated from dental plaque and salivary sediment. Cell and sediment concentrations were each 33.3% (V/V). The glucose concentration was 0.18% with the three pure cultures and 0.1% with the sediment. Salivary sediment is the cell-containing portion of wax-stimulated whole saliva and is obtained by centrifuging the saliva. (Adapted from Stephan, R.M., and Hemmens, E. S.: J. Dent. Res. **26:**15, 1947, and Kleinberg, I.: Arch. Oral Biol. **12:** 1457, 1967.)

alone and in combination in an artificial buffer medium designed to simulate the ionic and buffering properties of saliva.[62]

When the microorganisms were present in high concentration and glucose was added in low concentration, the pH rapidly fell and then slowly rose, thus showing pH curves similar to the Stephan curve in Fig. 8-4. Most, but not all, of the microorganisms showed Stephan curves that were shaped differently (Figs. 8-14 and 8-15, *A*). Those microorganisms not showing such curves showed either no curve at all or one in which the pH fell to an

asymptote and did not subsequently rise. With higher glucose levels and the substrate therefore in excess, the pH fell and remained low for the duration of the experimental period, a situation much like that seen in plaque in situ when carbohydrate was in excess.

When microorganisms were combined, the pH curves reflected the acid-producing and acid-removing properties of each of the microorganisms involved in the combination. For example, streptococci prevented lactobacilli from reaching as low a pH as that reached by lactobacilli when present alone (cf. Fig. 8-15, *B* with Fig. 8-15, *A*). Other experiments have shown that the lactic acid produced by streptococci can be either utilized once glucose in the mixture has been used up[29] or rapidly converted by microorganisms such as *Veillonella* to the weaker propionic and acetic acids.[30] On the basis of experiments such as these, it is reasonable to suggest that a microorganism that is cariogenic alone, as in the germ-free animal experiments, will more than likely not behave in the same way when combined with the mixture of microorganisms that constitute the microflora of a dental plaque.

Under conditions of limited substrate, more likely to occur where there is an excess of saliva as on the smooth surfaces of the teeth, only those organisms capable of rapidly forming and maintaining low plaque pH levels would be capable of producing caries.[62] Such a situation could lead to the view that specific bacteria are required for the initiation of the disease. On the other hand, under conditions favoring the availability of substrate for long periods of time as in fissures and on proximal surfaces of the dentition, many of the microorganisms in the mouth could be cariogenic and moreover could supplement one another in the formation of the acid required to reach the critical pH for enamel dissolution. Thus, conditions favoring the increased availability of fermentable carbo-

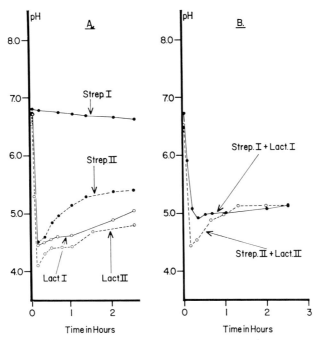

Fig. 8-15. pH curves with two strains of streptococci and lactobacilli individually, **A,** and combined, **B.** Cell concentrations are 33.3% (V/V); glucose concentration is 0.18% (W/V). Note in **A** that *Streptococcus* I does not show the characteristics of a Stephan curve. Note in **B** that the combined curves are very similar except near the pH minimum region. (Adapted from Stephan, R. M., and Hemmens, E. S.: J. Dent. Res. **26:**15, 1947.)

hydrate would decrease the possibility of specific microorganisms being responsible for the disease.

Factors favoring prolongation of low plaque pH levels

The rate of salivary flow, the form of the teeth, and those properties of a carbohydrate foodstuff (for example, stickiness) that favor its intra-oral retention are factors that can, alone or in combination, affect the length of time that dietary carbohydrate remains in the mouth after its ingestion. If the time is increased, then the time that acid is produced by the plaque bacteria will also be increased.

When fermentable carbohydrate is ingested, the plaque cells respond by producing acid, while the salivary glands respond by producing an increased flow of saliva.[41] The increased rate of salivary flow accelerates the clearance of carbohydrate from the mouth and the removal of acid from the plaque; by providing fresh saliva at a more rapid rate, it accelerates the diffusion of acid out of the plaque and, most important, by providing buffers, the neutralization of acid within the plaque. Removing acid from the plaque by either or both of these processes favors both a reduction in the plaque pH fall and an increase in the rate at which the pH returns to its starting level. Conversely, a slow salivary flow rate favors low pH levels and the pH remaining low for longer periods of time.

Should the form of the teeth or the physical properties of the ingested carbohydrate prolong the time that substrate is available to the plaque bacteria, duration of a low plaque pH will also be prolonged. For example, when a piece of bread is retained on the teeth, the pH falls to a minimum and remains at the minimum so long as bread remains in the retention site. Once the bread is gone, the pH slowly rises. Sugars, on the other hand, because of their much greater solubility, can be cleared more rapidly from saliva than can starchy foodstuffs. But, also because of their greater solubility, they raise the sugar level in saliva to a very high level with the result that it takes almost as long for the sugar to be cleared from the mouth as it takes for bread.[45]

The plaque microorganisms can also prolong the time that the plaque pH is below its base-line level by synthesizing cellular polysaccharide while dietary carbohydrate is present in the mouth. Subsequently, acid is formed from this stored carbohydrate when dietary carbohydrate is no longer present. In the last few years there has been considerable interest in the synthesis of both intracellular and extracellular polysaccharide. Although several experimental systems have been used (pure cultures of microorganisms isolated from dental plaque; intact plaque in situ and in vitro; and the microorganisms harvested from the mouth by chewing wax, referred to as salivary sediment[36]), in each system the synthesis of carbohydrate reserves and the catabolism of these reserves to form acid have both been demonstrated.

Experiments with human beings have shown that the number of intracellular polysaccharide-storing microorganisms in the plaque microflora decreases markedly when carbohydrate in the diet is restricted and subsequently increases when this restriction is removed.[64]

Synthesis and degradation of extracellular carbohydrate by plaque responds similarly to variation in the dietary carbohydrate, the levels in plaque rising during availability and falling once ingestion is complete.[11] Extracellular carbohydrate, in addition to being involved in the maintenance of a low plaque pH by providing substrate for acid formation (probably at a reduced rate), may, by contributing to the intercellular matrix material of the plaque, interfere with diffusion of acid out of the plaque.

PLAQUE FORMATION

Some studies have shown that initial deposits of plaque contain few bacteria whereas in other studies microorganisms are seen adhering directly to the enamel surface.[20] Where an initial layer of salivary protein deposits on the surface of the tooth, microorganisms from the saliva become attached[48] and invasion of the film takes place from the attached bacteria and any organisms present in cracks and other defects in the enamel. Colonization of these bacteria and further deposition of bacteria and protein from the saliva then take place, resulting in an increase in both bulk and density of the plaque.

One of the earliest theories concerning formation of the initial plaque was that acid from the oral bacteria, presumably those present on the tongue and the oral soft tissues, favored the precipitation of mucin from the saliva, and that this precipitated mucin then underwent denaturation by bacterial enzymes, dehydration, or surface inactivation to form a firm initial layer.[15]

Another theory about the same process suggests that neuraminidase, an enzyme in saliva, splits the sialic acid portion from sialo-containing salivary protein, thus altering the solubility of the protein by raising its isoelectric point and favoring precipitation under mildly acidic or even neutral conditions.[46]

Other investigators have shown that proteins in saliva are in a metastable state and, being colloidal, precipitate slowly but spontaneously from the saliva.[40] This precipitation appears to be a function of pH and of time, occurring slowly at neutral or alkaline pH and more rapidly as the pH is lowered. Consequently, in the individual having a slow flow rate of resting saliva and a salivary pH therefore slightly acidic, precipitation may occur more easily than in the person with a more rapid salivary flow rate and a more alkaline saliva. Adsorption of salivary protein to hydroxyapatite and clumping of the plaque bacteria also occur more readily at acidic than at neutral or alkaline pH.[49, 58] Thus, an increase in acidogenic microorganisms would favor increased plaque acidity, which in turn would favor more plaque formation.

Such a sequence of events could explain why individuals whose mouths are highly caries-active seem to have both higher numbers of acidogenic organisms and also more plaque than individuals whose mouths are caries-free.[43] Formation of extracellular polysaccharide by the bacteria that may be involved in plaque formation might facilitate the adhesion of these bacteria either to the tooth surface or to an initial protein layer. Early plaque shows a high frequency of S. *sanguis* and S. *mutans*, both of which form abundant amounts of extracellular polysaccharide, particularly dextran, when exposed to sucrose.[9] For organisms such as these, extracellular polysaccharides may contribute significantly to interbacterial adhesion and bacterial adhesion to the tooth surface.

Changes in plaque microflora during plaque formation

The predominant groups of microorganisms that first appear during the formation of plaque are the micrococci and streptococci. Yeasts, *Nocardia,* and *Streptomyces* are also found, but none of these constitutes more than a very small proportion of the plaque. Fungal filaments are rare at this stage but occur later; lactobacilli are also quite rare.

Mature plaque, on the other hand, contains a small amount of cellular and organic debris and consists mainly of gram-positive filamentous microorganisms embedded in an amorphous matrix. The filaments are closely packed and parallel to one another, running perpendicularly to the enamel surface. Near the enamel surface the filaments are less regular and in some cases lie flat. Toward the plaque surface cocci, rods, and occasionally *Leptothrix* are observed. It has been suggested that some of the filamentous forms are really streptococci that have lost their capacity for cell division. Nocardial microorganisms are restricted to the most superficial portions of the plaque.

CARIES SUSCEPTIBILITY TESTS

Many attempts have been made to develop a suitable diagnostic test for the determination of the caries susceptibility of an individual. Most of these tests have been based upon differences in the type of bacteria present in the microflora of caries-active and caries-inactive individuals and whether these microfloras are capable of producing acid when incubated with sugar, usually glucose. The most widely used procedures have been: (1) *Lactobacillus acidophilus* counts in a sample of wax-stimulated saliva,[54] and (2) acid formation during a 24- to 72-hour interval in a diluted aliquot of saliva (Snyder test).[59] Tests of a shorter time interval have also been suggested[54] but have not been used too widely. One involves a determination of the amount of acid formed when glucose is added to undiluted saliva, and the other, the Fosdick[18] test, determines the amount of calcium dissolved when a glucose saliva mixture is incubated in the presence of calcium phosphate. All of these tests suffer from the difficulty of obtaining a reproducible and representative sample of the acidogenic oral microflora. Consequently, they are suitable for determining the caries susceptibility of large groups but unfortunately are of limited value for individuals.

CITED REFERENCES AND ADDITIONAL READINGS

1. Atkinson, H. F., and Matthews, E.: An investigation into the organic components of the human tooth, Brit. Dent. J. 86:167, 1949.
2. Bahn, A. N., and Quillman, P. D.: Localization of oral lactobacilli, Dent. Progress 3:94, 1963.
3. Balenseifen, J. W., and Madonia, J. V.: Study of dental plaque in orthodontic patients, J. Dent. Res. 49:320, 1970.
4. Becks, H., Jensen, A. L., and Millarr, C. B.: Rampant dental caries: Prevention and prognosis. A five year clinical survey, J. Amer. Dent. Assoc. 31:1189, 1944.
5. Biswas, S. D., and Kleinberg, I.: Effect of urea concentration on its utilization, on the pH and the formation of ammonia and carbon dioxide in a human salivary sediment system, Arch. Oral Biol. 16:759, 1971.
6. Bödecker, C. F.: A report of further investigations on the organic matrix in human enamel, J. Dent. Res. 6:117, 1924-1926.
7. Bunting, R. W., Crowley, M., Hard, D. G., and Keller, M.: The prevention of dental caries through the limitation of the growth of *Bacillus acidophilus* in the mouth, J. Amer. Dent. Assoc. 16:224, 1929.
8. Bunting, R. W., Nickerson, G., and Hard, D. G.: Further studies of *Bacillus acidophilus* in its relation to dental caries, J. Amer. Dent. Assoc. 14:416, 1927.
9. Carlsson, J.: Plaque formation and streptococcal colonization on teeth, Odont. Rev. 19: Suppl. 14, 1968.
10. Charlton, G.: A micro-glass electrode for hydrogen ion determinations, Aust. Dent. J. 1:174, 1956.
11. Critchley, P.: Effects of foods on bacterial metabolic processes, J. Dent. Res. 49:1283, 1970.
12. Dawes, C., Jenkins, G. N., and Tonge, C. H.: The nomenclature of the integuments of the enamel surface of teeth, Brit. Dent. J. 115: 65, 1963.
13. Day, C. D. M., and Sedwick, H. J.: Studies on the incidence of dental caries, Dent. Cosmos 77:442, 1935.
14. Dirksen, T. R., Little, M. F., Bibby, B. G., and Crump, S. L.: The pH of carious cavities. I. The effect of glucose and phosphate buffer on cavity pH, Arch. Oral Biol. 7:49, 1962.
15. Dobbs, E. C.: Local factors in dental caries, J. Dent. Res. 12:853, 1932.
16. Eggers-Lura, H.: Untersuchungen über den aeroben und anaeroben Abbau der Kohlehydrate im Speichel, Deutsch. Zahn Mund Kieferheilk, 21:97, 1954.
17. Fitzgerald, R. J., Jordan, H. V., and Archard, H. O.: Dental caries in gnotobiotic rats infected with a variety of *Lactobacillus acidophilus*, Arch. Oral Biol. 11:473, 1966.
18. Fosdick, L. S., Hansen, H. L., and Epple, C.: Enamel decalcification by mouth organisms and dental caries: A suggested test for caries susceptibility, J. Amer. Dent. Assoc. 24:1275, 1937.
19. Fosdick, L. S., and Starke, A. C., Jr.: Solubility of tooth enamel in saliva at various pH levels, J. Dent. Res. 18:417, 1939.
20. Frank, R. M., and Brendel, A.: Ultrastructure of the approximal dental plaque and the underlying normal and carious enamel, Arch. Oral Biol. 11:883, 1966.
21. Frisbie, H. E., Nuckolls, J., and Saunders, J. B.: Distribution of the organic matrix of the enamel in the human tooth and its relation to the histopathology of caries, J. Amer. Coll. Dent. 11:243, 1944.
22. Frostell, G.: Studies on the ammonia production and the ureolytic activity of dental plaque material, Acta Odont. Scand. 18:29, 1960.
23. Gibbons, R. J., Kapsimalis, B., and Socransky, S. S.: The source of salivary bacteria, Arch. Oral Biol. 9:101, 1964.
24. Gibbons, R. J., and Socransky, S. S.: Intracellular polysaccharide storage by organisms in dental plaques. Its relation to dental caries and microbial ecology of the oral cavity, Arch. Oral Biol. 7:73, 1962.
25. Gibbons, R. J., Socransky, S. S., de Araujo, W. C., and van Houte, J.: Studies of the predominant cultivable microbiota of dental plaque, Arch. Oral Biol. 9:365, 1964.
26. Gottleib, B., and Hinds, E.: Some new aspects in pathology of dental caries, J. Dent. Res. 21:317, 1942.
27. Hemmens, E. S., Blayney, J. R., Bradel, S. F., and Harrison, R. W.: The microbic flora of the dental plaque in relation to the beginning of caries, J. Dent. Res. 25:195, 1946.
28. Hoffman, H.: Oral microbiology. In Umbreit, W. W. (ed.): Advances in applied microbiology, New York, 1966, Academic Press Inc., vol. 8, p. 195.
29. Hu, G., and Sandham, H. J.: Lactic acid utilization by Streptococci, International Association for Dental Research, Forty-seventh General Meeting, 1969, Preprinted abstracts, Abstract 173.
30. Hungate, R. E.: Ecology of bacteria. In

Gunsalus, I. C., and Stanier, R. Y. (eds.): The bacteria: the physiology of growth, New York, 1962, Academic Press, Inc., vol. 4, p. 95.

31. Jay, P.: The reduction of oral *Lactobacillus acidophilus* counts by the periodic restriction of carbohydrate, Amer. J. Orthodont. Oral Surg. **33**:162, 1947.

32. Keyes, P. H.: Research in dental caries, J. Amer. Dent. Assoc. **76**:1357, 1968.

33. Kleinberg, I.: Biochemistry of the dental plaque. In Staple, P. H. (ed.): Advances in oral biology, New York, 1970, Academic Press Inc., vol. 4, p. 43.

34. Kleinberg, I.: The construction and evaluation of modified types of antimony micro-electrodes for intra-oral use, Brit. Dent. J. **104**:197, 1958.

35. Kleinberg, I.: Effect of urea concentration on human plaque pH levels in situ, Arch. Oral Biol. **12**:1475, 1967.

36. Kleinberg, I.: Effect of varying sediment and glucose concentrations on the pH and acid production in human salivary sediment mixtures, Arch. Oral Biol. **12**:1457, 1967.

37. Kleinberg, I.: Formation and accumulation of acid on the tooth surface, J. Dent. Res. **49**:1300, 1970.

38. Kleinberg, I.: Regulation of the acid-base metabolism of the dentogingival plaque and its relation to dental caries and periodontal disease, Int. Dent. J. **20**:451, 1970.

39. Kleinberg, I.: Studies on dental plaque. I. The effect of different concentrations of glucose on the pH of dental plaque in vivo, J. Dent. Res. **40**:1087, 1961.

40. Kleinberg, I., Chatterjee, R., Kaminsky, F. S., Cross, H. G., Goldenberg, D. J., and Kaufman, H. W.: Plaque formation and the effect of age, J. Periodont. **42**:497, 1971.

41. Kleinberg, I., and Jenkins, G. N.: Further studies on the effect of carbohydrate substrates on plaque pH in vivo, J. Dent. Res. **38**:704, 1959.

42. Kleinberg, I., and Jenkins, G. N.: The pH of dental plaques in the different areas of the mouth before and after meals and their relationship to the pH and rate of flow of resting saliva, Arch. Oral Biol. **9**:493, 1964.

43. Krasse, B.: The relationship between lactobacilli, candida, and streptococci and dental caries, Odont. Rev. **5**:241, 1954.

44. Kreitzman, S. N., Irving, S., Navia, J. M., and Harris, R. S.: Enzymatic release of phosphate from rat molar enamel by phosphoprotein phosphatase, Nature **233**:520, 1969.

45. Lanke, L. S.: Influence on salivary sugar of certain properties of foodstuffs and individual oral conditions, Acta Odont. Scand. **23** (suppl.):3, 1957.

46. Leach, S. A.: Release and breakdown of sialic acid from human salivary mucin and its role in the formation of dental plaque, Nature **199**:486, 1963.

47. McCabe, R. M., Keyes, P. H., and Howell, A., Jr.: An in vitro method for assessing the plaque forming ability of oral bacteria, Arch. Oral Biol. **12**:1653, 1967.

48. McDougall, W. A., Studies on the dental plaque. III. The effect of saliva on salivary mucoids and its relationship to the regrowth of plaques, Aust. Dent. J. **8**:463, 1963.

49. McGaughey, C., and Stowell, E. C.: The adsorption of human salivary proteins and porcine submaxillary mucin by hydroxyapatite, Arch. Oral Biol. **12**:815, 1967.

50. Miller, W. D.: The micro-organisms of the human mouth, Philadelphia, 1890, S. S. White Dental Mfg. Co.

51. Onisi, M., and Kondo, W.: Establishing an environment for growth of aciduric bacteria in the oral cavity, J. Dent. Res. **35**:596, 1956.

52. Orland, F. J., Blayney, J. R., Harrison, R. W., Reyniers, J. A., Trexler, P. C., Wagner, M., Gordon, H. A., and Luckey, T. D.: Use of the germfree animal technic in the study of experimental dental caries. I. Basic observations on rats reared free of all microorganisms, J. Dent. Res. **33**:147, 1954.

53. Pincus, P.: The study of caries: Attack on enamel without acids, Dent. Record **59**:615, 1939.

54. Rickles, N. H.: The estimation of dental caries activity by a new colorimetric laboratory test. A preliminary investigation, J. Dent. Res. **32**:3, 1953.

55. Sandham, H. J., and Kleinberg, I.: Utilization of glucose and lactic acid by salivary sediment, Arch. Oral Biol. **14**:597, 1969.

56. Schatz, A., and Martin, J. J.: Some perspectives of dental caries research: Microbiological and biochemical considerations. Ann. Dent. **17**:1, 1958.

57. Scherp, H. W.: Introduction: Why another conference? J. Dent. Res. **49**:1191, 1970.

58. Silverman, G., and Kleinberg, I.: Studies on factors affecting the aggregation of the microorganisms in human dental plaque, Arch. Oral Biol. **12**:1407, 1967.

59. Snyder, M. L., Suher, T., Porter, D. R., Claycomb, C. K., and Gardner, M. K.: Evaluation of laboratory tests for the estimation of caries activity, J. Dent. Res. **35**:332, 1956.

60. Stack, M. V.: The chemical nature of the

organic matrix of bone, dentin, and enamel, Ann. N. Y. Acad. Sci. **60**:585, 1955.

61. Stephan, R. M.: Changes in hydrogen-ion concentration on tooth surfaces and in carious lesions, J. Amer. Dent. Assoc. **27**:718, 1940.

62. Stephan, R. M., and Hemmens, E. S.: Studies of changes in pH produced by pure cultures of oral microorganisms, J. Dent. Res. **26**:15, 1947.

63. Strålfors, A.: Investigations into the bacterial chemistry of dental plaques, Odont. T. **58**:153, 1950.

64. Van Houte, J.: Relationship between carbohydrate intake and polysaccharide-storing microorganisms in dental plaque, Arch. Oral Biol. **9**:91, 1964.

9 / Infections of pulp and periapical tissues

Endodontia is that branch of dental science which seeks to conserve teeth when the pulps and their associated structures become involved in disease processes. In accomplishing this objective, the dentist applies the fundamental principles of surgical practice and by gentle, nontraumatic procedures establishes drainage, performs debridement, maintains asepsis, and obtains sterility. After these and other technical procedures have been accomplished, the prepared root canal is filled so that microorganisms and tissue fluids can no longer reenter and the tooth may be restored to its proper form and function (Fig. 9-1).

Microorganisms are of importance as frank incitants and significant contributors to inflammatory diseases of the pulp and periapical tissues. Their elimination during treatment procedures is essential to post-treatment repair and the successful outcome of the case.

THE PATHOGENESIS OF PULPAL AND PERIAPICAL INFECTION
Pathways to pulpal infection

The principle ways by which infection of the pulp occurs are by the extension of a carious lesion and by pulp exposure resulting from tooth fracture sequent to trauma or during a dental procedure; whenever dental tubules are cut by a bur, stone, or chisel or exposed by caries, erosion, or attrition, a path is opened to the pulp. Microbial elements may also enter the pulp from a periodontal pocket by direct invasion of lateral or accessory canals or apical foramina, by extension from a neighboring tooth, or by the localization or fixation of microorganisms from the bloodstream.

The term "anachoresis" was suggested[45] for the latter phenomenon, which probably occurs in a clinically insignificant number of cases as compared with the large number of cases resulting from dental caries. However, it has been shown that bloodborne bacteria may localize in areas of inflammation within 30 minutes of injury. While the presence of microorganisms in a normal pulp does not necessarily lead to disease, their presence in an inflamed pulp could conceivably compound the injury and lead to pulp necrosis. The course of events may be summarized as: (1) traumatic, operative, or postoperative irritation of the pulp with production of asymptomatic pulpitis; (2) subsequent development of a transient bacteremia; and (3) localization of bloodborne microorganisms in the inflamed pulp with resultant infective pulpitis.

There seems to be full agreement that bacteria do not appear in the dental pulp until a very late stage of caries. Changes in the dental tubules including the presence of PAS-positive material are evident pulpward to the bacterial penetration.

McKay[35] studied the advancing front

271

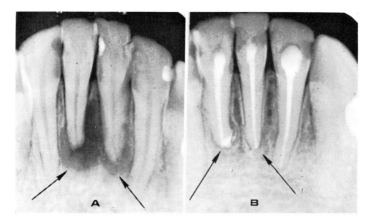

Fig. 9-1. Three mandibular incisors showing varying amounts of apical bone destruction prior to endodontic treatment, **A,** and the filling in of these lesions approximately 1 year after treatment, **B.**

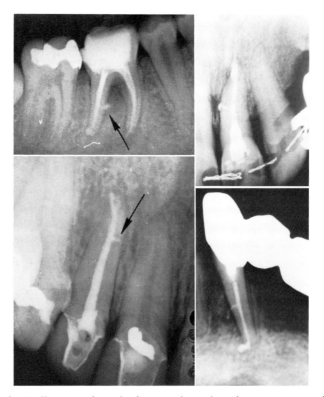

Fig. 9-2. Endodontically treated teeth showing lateral and accessory canals (arrows) at different anatomic positions.

of the carious lesion by culture. He dissected into the lesion from the pulp chamber and on several occasions stopped dissecting and culturing because the dentin was so soft that he assumed it must be infected. Yet in a number of instances he found the cultures were negative. The organisms in the primary wave of carious dentin were exclusively lactobacilli. Shovelton[47] found lactobacilli and streptococci, including anaerobic forms.

Shovelton[47] has shown that where the thickness of dentin remaining between the floor of the cavity and the pulp was greater than 0.8 mm. no signs of pulp inflammation were found and considerable pulp inflammation was observed when the thickness of the remaining dentin was less than 0.3 mm. Bacteria were found in the pulp only when the cavity floor was 0.2 mm. or less from the pulp.

Combined periodontal and pulpal involvement

The high incidence of periodontal disease and the surprisingly high incidence of accessory canals make combined periodontal-pulpal involvement a potentially important entity (Fig. 9-2).

The term "retrograde periodontitis" has been applied to cases in which a periodontally induced pulpitis exists and in which a feedback mechanism could serve to perpetuate both diseases. In deciduous molar teeth, for example, the earliest bone changes following pulpal inflammation are likely to be found at the crest of the interradicular bone. Since accessory canals leading to the interradicular aspect of the root of human deciduous molar teeth appeared to occur in approximately 25% of the teeth studied, these canals may serve as pathways for spread of the infectious process. Winter and Kramer[52] reported that they found in a high proportion of decidous molar teeth in kittens an accessory canal extending from the pulp chamber to the periodontium in the bifurcation region. Severe pulpal changes were followed by changes in the periodontium at the opening of the accessory canal, and in time destruction of the interradicular bone occurred.

Recovery of organisms from pulp

The pulp and periapical tissue of vital, sound teeth are invariably free of microorganisms. The high incidence of positive cultures reported by early investigators probably resulted from contamination of the tissues during the process of tooth extraction. Careful studies have shown that it is virtually impossible to remove a tooth aseptically. Henrici and Hartzel[28] obtained no growth from twenty-two teeth free from caries and periodontal disease. Dutton and Cameron[15] found only 2.7% of pulps from clinically normal teeth infected, Gunter and his co-workers[25] found none in forty-six normal pulps, and Burket[12] obtained growth from only three of fifty-four pulps examined in situ at autopsy.

It was previously suggested that irritation of the pulp from cavity preparation, placement of filling materials, use of chemical agents, and heat, cold, and other stimuli may be sufficient to inflame the pulp to the point of attracting and fixing microorganisms. Bacteria have been recovered from the pulp chambers of the majority of traumatically devitalized teeth, even though there was no direct communication between the pulps and the oral cavity. It is assumed that the source of these organisms, because they are chiefly indigenous oral strains, is the oral cavity and that the route of invasion is the gingival sulcus and periodontal lymphatics and blood vessels. The rare nonoral microbial species isolated, presumably localizes from the bloodstream during transient bacteremia. For example, examination of three hundred fifty-three noncarious pulp-involved teeth in lepers revealed that one hundred fifteen showed *Mycobacterium leprae* in the pulp tissue. Localization of

Brucella abortus was demonstrated at the apex of nonvital guinea pig teeth.[14] There is evidence from animal and human studies that anastomoses occur between the gingival, periodontal, and pulpal lymphatics; microorganisms may readily pass through the walls of these vessels that serve as a normal pathway for particulate matter. Organisms have been observed in the perivascular lymphatics of the pulp and the periodontal ligament.

Although it has been suggested that the exposure of dentin from any cause opens a pathway to the pulp and that this may serve as a possible explanation for persistent discomfort occasionally associated with restorative procedures, there is lack of unanimity among investigators on this point. The ability of microorganisms to invade devitalized pulp by way of the odontoblastic processes of nonvital dentin has been shown under in vitro conditions with cultures of *Serratia marcescens* and an oral alpha hemolytic streptococcus[13] (Fig. 9-3). Experimental evidence from studies of dogs and monkeys[3] when cultures of *Streptococcus faecalis* were used suggests that pressure, as exerted in taking impressions with inlay wax or modelling compound, frequently forces microorganisms through the dentinal tubules into the pulp. A streptomycin-resistant strain of *Streptococcus faecalis* introduced into aseptically exposed pulps could be recovered from the bloodstream in four of nineteen instances after the placement of prednisolone powder.[32] If root canal instrumentation was confined to the root canal, no transient bacteremias occurred; however, if instruments were passed beyond the apex, bacteremias occurred in 25% of the cases.[6] On the basis of these findings, it would seem advisable to avoid excessive reduction in full crown preparations, to modify techniques to avoid heat and pressure on deeply involved dentin, and to use a nonirritating antimicrobial agent on prepared teeth when force must be exerted in taking an impression. Because living pulp is capable of absorbing foreign proteins, sensitization to tissue breakdown products and microbial metabolites may, and probably does, occur. Anaphylactic shock has been produced in guinea pigs

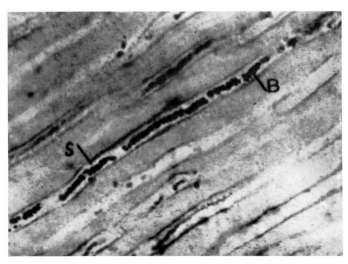

Fig. 9-3. Bacteria confined to the expected dimensions of the odontoblastic process. *B*, Bacteria; *S*, space occupied by calcific sheath in vivo (1,500 ×). (From Chirnside, I. M.: New Zeal. Dent. J. **54:**173, 1958.)

previously sensitized to horse serum by way of the pulp or by having had the biologic material placed in contact with freshly cut dentin.

Brown and Rudolph[9] obtained growth in 84% of samples from seventy nonvital, intact, traumatized teeth; Engström and Frostell (1957, 1961) showed growth in 58% of thirty-six cases; Chirnside,[13] in 54% of twenty-eight cases; and Macdonald and co-workers,[34] in 83% of forty-six cases. In many instances, microorganisms could be shown in stained smears from initial samples although no growth was obtained in culture (Engström and Frostell, 1957, 1961). With the aid of direct darkfield and phase contrast microscopic studies, Brown and Rudolph[9] found microorganisms in 90% of their samples versus 84% on cultivation. More organisms were seen than cultured, and often the predominant morphologic forms, fusiforms and vibrios, were not cultivable. A mixed infection was usually present.

Hampp[26] showed the presence of spirochetes in nonexposed, periodontally uninvolved, nonvital teeth and raised the important questions of their mode of entrance into the pulp chamber and their possible role. It was suggested that the spirochetes might have spread from the gingival sulcus by direct extension through the soft or hard tissues or both, or by lymphatic or blood channels. The results of a study on both dogs and monkeys[24] showed that in most instances *Serratia marcescens*, the indicator organism, was able to reach the pulp tissue or root canals of traumatized teeth from the gingival sulcus or damaged marginal gingiva. It is safe to conclude that almost all teeth rendered nonvital following impact injury become infected sooner or later.

Response of pulp to microorganisms

Pulps exposed to the oral environment in germ-free rats did not develop inflammatory changes or devitalization, and peri-apical changes did not occur.[31] Healing occurred in the presence of food impaction, while similarly treated animals under conventional conditions developed pulpal and periapical disease.

Once microorganisms have gained access to the pulp, this tissue reacts like other connective tissues of the body with an inflammatory response. Anatomic features at the site may play a significant role in determining the nature and course of the response. As a person ages, the apical foraminal area becomes increasingly constricted, allowing only the smallest possible lumen, sometimes to a point of obliteration. The fact that the pulp tissue is within a confined space precludes normal swelling, and the size of the apical foramen limits the possibility of collateral blood supply to the site of the injury.

The onset of the disease may be acute or chronic, and the extent of pulp involvement may be partial or total. In the early stages of acute pulpitis, relatively severe pain is elicited by thermal changes, particularly by cold drinks. The involved tooth may be extremely sensitive to percussion and palpation. As a greater portion of the pulp becomes involved, the pain becomes more continuous and severe, increasing in intensity when the person lies down. Heat may cause excruciating pain, especially when the opening to the oral cavity is obliterated and there is no opportunity for the inflammatory exudate to escape. Stained smears of this purulent material or pus will show large numbers of polymorphonuclear neutrophil leukocytes in various stages of maturation and disintegration, other leukocytic elements, occasional erythrocytes, connective tissue cells, fibrin strands, and the presence or absence of microorganisms.

Chronic pulpitis may arise from a previously acute stage that has quieted, but more frequently it occurs in a chronic form from its onset. The associated mild, dull pain is intermittent rather than continuous, and the response to thermal stimuli is barely perceptible. Chronic low grade pulpitis may be symptom-free. The pulp tissue is infiltrated by large numbers of small round cells, chiefly lymphocytes and plasma cells. There is evidence of fibroblastic activity and proliferating capillaries in the infected area, suggesting a walling off or containment. An excessive proliferation of chronically inflamed pulp tissue may occasionally occur in children; this results in the formation of a mass of tissue extending from the pulp chamber of the involved tooth and is characterized as chronic hyperplastic pulpitis. As a rule, untreated disease will culminate in necrosis of the entire pulp tissue.

Periapical disease

Except in the case of mechanical injury, periapical disease occurs by way of a descending pulpitis with concomitant pulp necrosis as just described. Periapical lesions are subject to essentially the same progressive and retrogressive changes that occur in the pulp. The inflammatory reaction may be acute or chronic and may involve apical cementum and dentin, the periodontal membrane, the lamina dura, and the cortical bone of the alveolar process. The rate at which the disease proceeds depends upon anatomic relationships, the resistance of the host, and the number and virulence of the invading parasites. The process may be arrested at any stage, with evidence of destruction and repair apparent simultaneously. As periapical disease progresses, resorption of the root can often be seen, and extension into the osseous support is depicted in a radiogram as loss of the bone pattern with rarefaction. Although the amount of tissue destroyed and the direction of spread of the disease are unpredictable, the disease always follows the path of least resistance (Fig. 9-4).

A common periapical pathosis arising from a low grade pulpitis is the granuloma. This walled lesion of granulomatous tissue is surrounded by a fibrous capsule that may break down and lead to an acute or chronic alveolar abscess. A fistulous tract or sinus may form, providing an egress for the suppurative material formed in the expanding lesion. The external manifestation of this condition is a tender buccal, labial, lingual, or palatal swelling that may draw intraorally and, on occasion, extraorally. Often the infectious material and its by-products will track through the soft tissues, causing a cellulitis with extensive swelling, redness, heat, pain, and impairment of function of the associated structures; they may track through the bone and bone marrow, causing an acute or chronic osteomyelitis.

One important feature of a chronic periapical granuloma is the presence of epithelium originating from the rests of Malassez. The inflammatory process may stimulate this epithelium to proliferate extensively, giving rise to an apical periodontal or radicular cyst filled with fluid.

Substances released as result of tissue destruction

Active substances, released as a result of tissue destruction and the inflammatory process, significantly alter that very process. The exudate changes from alkaline to acid. Neutrophils are active at alkaline or neutral pH and begin to disintegrate at an acid pH when the microphages become active. The autolyzing neutrophils release lysozyme and trypsinlike enzymes whose digestive products contribute to the semiliquid exudate called pus. Active agents present in alkaline exudates are *leukotaxine,* a polypeptide, which increases capillary permeability; *leukopenin,* which causes an initial leukopenia; *leukocytosis-promoting factor* (LPF), which stimulates pronounced leukocytosis and promotes phagocytosis; *granulocytic substance* (GS), which enhances diapedesis and an increase in temperature.

In acid exudates, comparable active sub-

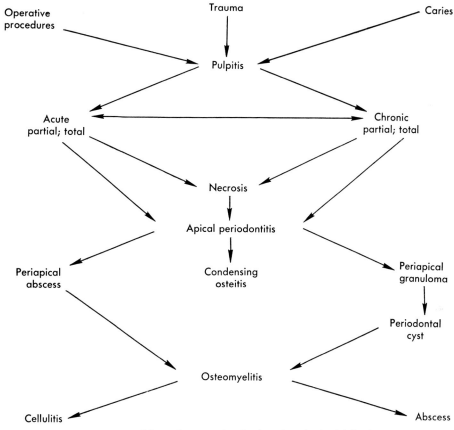

Fig. 9-4. Possible pathways of pulpal and periapical infections.

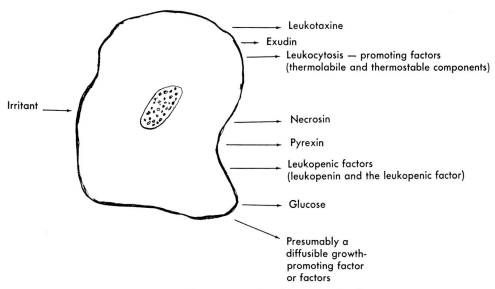

Fig. 9-5. Substances produced by injured cells.

Table 9-1. Changes in differential leukocytic count and pH inflammatory exudate with length of time the irritant is acting

Duration of action of irritant in hours	Differential white count in exudate			pH
	Polymorphonu- clear leukocytes	Lymphocytes	Monocytes	
19	78	2	20	7.45
43	78	1	21	7.23
67	87	1	12	7.23
93	31	3	66	6.97
115	26	2	72	6.95

stances are produced such as *exudin,* which continues the enhanced capillary permeability; a *leukopenic factor* of acid exudates; a *thermostabile leukocytosis factor; pyrexin; necrosin;* and a *diffusible growth-promoting factor,* which promotes growth of fibroblasts and capillary endothelium (Fig. 9-5).

Pain-producing substances

Other substances found in increased amounts in inflamed and autolyzing tissues provide some insight into the origin of the exquisite pain that often accompanies an acute pulpitis or apical periodontitis. Among these pain-producing metabolites are histamine from mast cells, 5-hydroxytryptamine (serotonin) from platelets, and plasma kinins. In higher concentrations these agents stimulate pain endings directly; in lower concentrations or after indirect stimulation they may produce hyperalgesia that may so enhance the effect of physical agents or stimuli that arterial pulsations may be painful and some trivial contact barely perceived under normal conditions can cause agonizing pain. Increased tissue tension, commonly regarded as the cause of pain in inflammation, is effective only because the sensitivity of the nerve endings is much increased. Important factors in host resistance are lysozyme and the antimicrobial basic proteins and polypeptides that are normally present in tissues (Fig. 9-6). Large amounts of acidic polysaccharides and nucleic acids, how-

ever, are released during inflammation; these may combine with the basic agents, largely minimizing their antibacterial effectiveness.

The early investigations of Rickert and Dixon[44] suggested that the irritants responsible for the apical response originate in the necrotic pulp and its diffusing decomposition products. They found that sterile root apices filled and implanted in rabbits were tolerated well. Sterile apices without fillings implanted in the same manner produced gross irritation of the surrounding tissues. Similarly, if hollow platinum tubes 1 cm. long were implanted in the rabbits' skin for several months, the central parts of the tube appeared compatible with the tissues; but a wide area of inflammatory response could be found around the open ends of the tubes. Implantation of porous materials such as soft wood caused large zones of irritation. The inability of Torneck[50] to support the findings of the earlier investigators may in part result from differences in the experimental methods employed and the type of materials used for implantation.

• • •

We have attempted so far to build a broad picture of the possible dynamics of the pulp-involved tooth. The accumulated metabolic products and cellular components of the microbial elements coupled with the autolytic products and debris of the cells and tissues of the pulp provide the

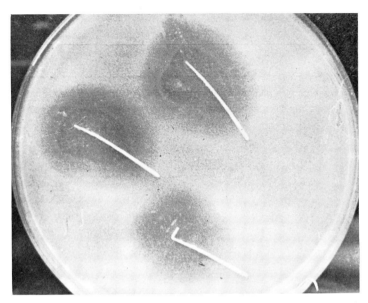

Fig. 9-6. Zone of inhibition is produced against *Micrococcus lysodeikticus* by lysozyme present in the purulent exudate on an absorbent point from pulp involved tooth.

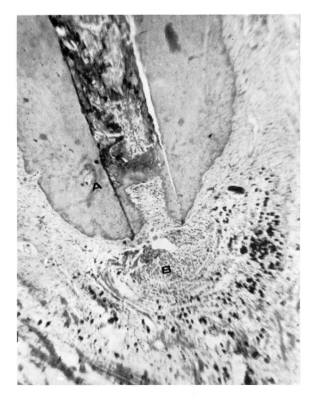

Fig. 9-7. Cementum bridge, *A*, in apical portion of root and granuloma, *B*, in periapical area of tooth. There is evidence of destruction and repair of apical tissues occurring simultaneously or sequentially.

irritant. The nature of the response must ultimately depend upon many factors related to the host. Among these are anatomic considerations including the diameter of the pulp canal, the size of the apical orifice, the presence of accessory canals and their location; and factors related to phagocytosis, bacteriostatic and bactericidal mechanisms of plasma and exudate fluid, and the changing chemical environment at the reaction site. The relative concentration of these components in the inflammatory exudate and the susceptibility of the pathogens to them determine, to a large degree, the course of the infectious process.

Since destruction and repair of tissue may occur simultaneously or sequentially, clinical manifestations are variable, often unpredictable (Fig. 9-7). The importance of systemic disease and nutritional and emotional stresses in modifying disease patterns has been discussed in earlier chapters, and their contribution to the course of pulpal and periapical disease is emphasized at this point.

In many cases the relatively enhanced role that microorganisms seem to play in the development of apical lesions depends to a great extent on the degree to which endodontic procedures upset the equilibrium between host and parasite. Various microorganisms with fairly great pathogenizing potential are isolated with some regularity from tooth pulps that do not show any demonstrable reaction to them; demonstration of the presence of microorganisms in cases of clinically obvious pulpitis with accompanying roentgenographic evidence of apical pathosis is not always possible. Acute symptoms may succeed the dentist's gaining access to clinically symptomless teeth, and, paradoxically, his simply obtaining access to a pulp canal is often sufficient treatment to eliminate acute distress. This apparent paradox can be explained only in terms of the subtle interplay of those determinant factors relating to host, to parasite, and to the interaction between them.

CULTURING FROM THE PULP-INVOLVED TOOTH
Asepsis in obtaining samples

Microorganisms may play an important role in the pathogenesis of pulpal and periapical disease; one of the more important objectives in endodontic practice is to eliminate them. At present the only available means of determining whether this objective has been attained is bacteriologic examination of the contents of the root canal.

Because the bacteriologic sampling of a root canal is performed under the most difficult of circumstances, a strict regimen of bacteriologic control and asepsis is required. The bacteriologic findings constitute the only objective evidence of microbiologic status of the pulp canal, and the significance assigned to a culture result must ultimately reside in the person who has taken the culture and his awareness of the circumstances under which it was taken.

Since the root canal culture is a test for sterility, preliminary sterilization of the endodontic field must be accomplished and maintained during the culturing procedure. Under no conditions may there be a breach of aseptic technique. Precleaning the pulp-involved tooth with prophylactic paste for 1½ minutes brings about a significant reduction in the number of contaminated samples.[39] A sterile rubber dam is then placed into position, and all the surfaces of the isolated tooth are painted with antiseptic solution. Tincture of iodine (2.5%), thimerosal, or benzalkonium chloride is satisfactory for this purpose. The antiseptic solution should be permitted to contact these surfaces for at least three minutes. Access to the pulp canal is obtained aseptically in the prescribed manner and the culture is taken with sterile paper points.

Later sampling is performed in a sterile field. The seal and the dressing are removed and the canal is flushed with approximately 1.0 ml. of sterile distilled water. The canal is then dried with sterile paper points until the last point comes out wet at the apex for a distance of approximately 1.0 mm. A sterile point is then placed in the canal as close to the apex as possible and allowed to remain in situ for from one to two minutes. This point is then transferred to suitable culture media.

Root canal cultures

Root canal cultures can be separated into types: the initial culture and the during-treatment or later culture. Even with the best of aseptic techniques, the chances of carrying organisms into the pulp canal chamber are great. This means that the number of positive cultures obtained from pulps that did not contain bacteria before preparation will be large; but the number of organisms per unit area will be small. Since many organisms reside in the deep carious lesion, it is likely that the initial root canal culture will yield a culture with a wide variety of microorganisms. Leakage from improper seals, carious dentin, and breaks in aseptic procedure provide gross sources of microbial contamination. The opportunity for chance contamination from the surrounding field of operation, from instruments, and from the hands of the dentist lessens as the case proceeds and as later cultures become available.

No predictions about the presence or absence of microorganisms can be made from looking at a roentgenogram, and the odor that occasionally emanates from a pulp-involved tooth does not necessarily indicate the presence of bacteria. It has been observed that the frequency of initial positive cultures is greater in areas with periapical rarefaction than in areas lacking such rarefaction. Diffuse areas are more likely to be associated with infection than circumscribed areas. A high proportion of

teeth having normal radiographic appearance yield positive cultures; the number of positive cultures obtained is higher from necrotic pulps than from vital pulps, but no large difference in flora seems to exist. An interesting finding is the negative correlation that appears to exist between the frequency of isolating micrococci and the skill of the operator.

Because many of the organisms that ultimately locate in the pulpal and apical tissues differ considerably in their metabolic needs, the isolation of all the members of this flora by means of a single culture medium has not been achieved. Conventional procedures yield limited data, and frequency tables depicting microorganisms isolated from pulp-involved teeth are incomplete. Morphologic forms that often predominate in smears cannot be cultivated. Several factors appear to modify the culturing procedure and result in absence of growth. Among these are carrying over antimicrobial medicament into the culture medium, or using too small an inoculum or excessive numbers of phagocytic cells in the sample.

An important diagnostic procedure of considerable value is a direct smear of the pulpal contents (Fig. 9-8). While the morphologic appearance and gram-staining reaction of the various microbial forms will provide presumptive diagnostic information and suggest culture procedures, the presence of increased numbers of phagocytic cells and their distribution will attest to the role that these microorganisms may be playing in the inflammatory process. Cocci usually predominate over rods and spiral forms, and their relationship becomes heavily weighted toward coccal forms in culture. In some instances the bacillary forms seen in smears fail to grow.

Suitable culture media. Meat or vegetable infusion broths with appropriate added enrichments such as 0.1% to 0.5% dextrose, soluble starch, or yeast extract; 5% to 10% serum, whole blood, or ascitic

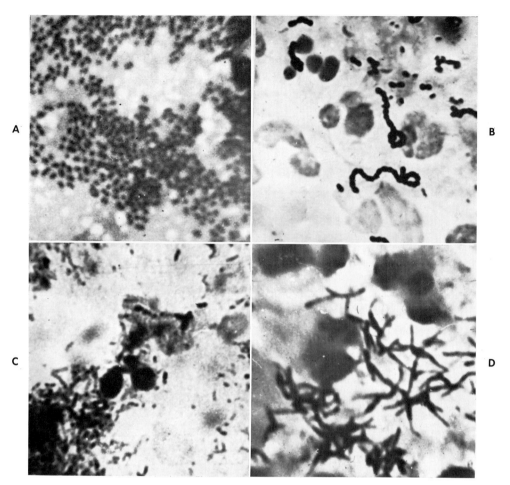

Fig. 9-8. Gram-stained smears of pulpal exudates. **A,** Staphylococci; **B,** streptococci; **C,** yeasts and other microbial forms; **D,** branched filaments.

fluid; and 0.1% to 0.2% agar are in common use (Figs. 9-9 and 9-10). Among the more widely used media are brain heart infusion broth or trypticase soy broth containing 0.1% agar, thioglycollate broth, cooked meat medium, and glucose ascites medium. Penicillinase may be added in concentration sufficient to inactivate any residual penicillin used in between-visit medication. No effective neutralizers are available for other antibiotics or for the many medicaments commonly used in endodontic practice. In most instances one has to depend primarily upon dilution to minimize the carry-over of antibacterial effects of such agents.

It is good practice, prior to use, to place the tube of root canal culture medium, with the exception of those containing heat coagulable protein, in a boiling water bath for five minutes to drive off dissolved air and then cool it to 45° C. before inoculating. Root canal cultures should be incubated at 37° C. for 48 hours before they are examined for growth and kept for at least one week if no growth has occurred. A number of small, inexpensive, thermostatically controlled incubators and pre-

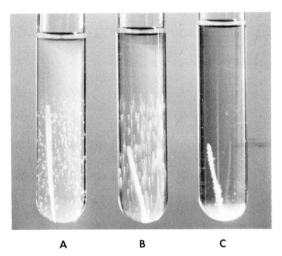

Fig. 9-9. **A,** 0.2% agar; **B,** 0.1% agar; **C,** 0% agar. Addition of small amounts of agar to a mixed culture of microorganisms in trypticase soy broth changes the character of growth.

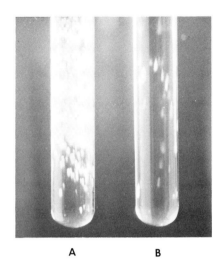

Fig. 9-10. **A,** Yeast extract added; **B,** no yeast extract added. Addition of yeast extract (2%) to brain heart infusion with starch (1%) and agar (0.2%) enhances growth of *Fusobacterium* species.

pared media in plastic capped tubes are readily available from several laboratory supply houses. Thermostatically controlled electric sterilizers using molten metal and extra-fine glass beads or salt maintained at a temperature of from 425° to 475° F. are used for the sterilization of root canal instruments during endodontic procedures. Effective sterilization requires that the instruments be immersed in the sterilizing medium for at least 10 seconds.

Positive versus negative cultures. The reversal rates following one negative culture and two negative cultures have been studied by several investigators. The wide disparity that exists among them may be explained by differences in sampling procedures and culturing techniques. Other factors are the length of time between treatments, leakage of temporary seal, and the presence of residual medicament. With proper techniques the probability of a positive culture after two negative cultures is low, 2% to 3% for experienced operators, 8% to 9% for students. It has been estimated that a single 48-hour nega-

tive culture as one criterion for obturation would be inaccurate 6% to 10% of the time[30] and 16% of the time if the case had been recultured prior to filling.[5] Bender and co-workers[5] compiled data after six months for more than 2,300 teeth and for 706 after a two-year follow-up and found no significant difference in success of repair, measured radiographically, between those teeth filled after a positive culture as compared with those filled after a negative culture.

This was not in agreement with the observations of Zeldow and Ingle[53] who concluded from their studies that successful results are significantly higher in cases of teeth filled after negative cultures and Engström and colleagues[20] who found that the frequency of failure was 24.1% when the bacteriologic sample taken at the time of root-filling had showed growth, and 10.7% when it had not. The period of observation in the latter study was from four to five years, and the difference between the groups was statistically significant.

The percentage of positive or negative

cultures obtained and reported in any one study will in large measure depend upon the proportion of teeth with vital and non-vital pulps, the status of the nonvital teeth selected, and the presence or absence of periradicular rarefaction. Engström,[17] for example, obtained 80% positive cultures from teeth with necrotic and gangrenous pulps with apical rarefaction and about 24% from previously root-filled teeth without rarefaction about the root apex. Table 9-2 summarizes the findings of several investigators correlating culture results with the clinical outcome of the pulp-involved tooth.

Between 14% and 40% of pulp-involved permanent teeth, vital and nonvital, have been reported as yielding no growth in initial cultures. These figures seem remarkably high in view of the fact that the chances of carrying microorganisms from a carious cavity into the pulp during perforation of the roof of a pulp chamber are great; chance contamination of the culture from the air, from instruments, or from the hands of the operator is also possible. Since chance contamination may be superimposed on the flora already present in an infected canal, it is not meaningful to associate microbial isolates from pulp-involved teeth with unusual pathog-

enizing ability based on histologic or clinical findings.

Microorganisms isolated from root canals

The organisms most frequently isolated from root canals are streptococci representing three of the four main divisions of the aerobic and facultative anaerobic species of the genus *Streptococcus*. Occasionally, obligate anaerobes of the genus *Peptostreptococcus* are also recovered. The predominant streptococci are clearly the viridans streptococci, followed by the nonhemolytic, gamma, or indifferent streptococci including enterococci; and small percentages of hemolytic—largely members of group H and K—and anaerobic streptococci. Tables 9-3 and 9-4 indicate the frequency of isolation of streptococci from

Table 9-2. Correlation of culture result with clinical outcome

Investigators	Percentage of clinical success	
	Positive cultures	Negative cultures
Ingle and Zeldow (1963)	83.3 (42)°	92.9 (14)°
Buchbinder (1941)	82.0 (94)	92.0 (151)
Rhein, Krasnow, and Geis (1926)	84.8 (152)	94.1 (340)
Oliet (1962)	55.1 (67)	83.8 (31)
Engström (1964)	69.3 (95)	82.8 (140)
Seltzer and Bender (1964)	82.2 (175)	81.9 (404)
Vanek (1968)	64.7 (17)	94.5 (72)

°Numbers in parentheses indicate actual number of cases reported on.

Table 9-3. Frequency of isolated organisms from 1,141 positive cultures from vital and necrotic pulps*

Organism	In pure culture	In mixed infection	Total
Streptococcus faecalis	240	45	285
Streptococcus mitis	153	130	283
Streptococcus salivarius	5	15	20
Streptococcus hemolyticus	33	22	55
Anaerobic streptococci	54	15	69
Indifferent streptococci	81	71	152
Other streptococci	11	17	28
Total streptococci	577	315	892
Micrococci	161	71	232
Lactobacilli	57	41	98
Diphtheroids	45	13	58
Gram-positive rods	10	11	21
Bacillus species	9	12	21
Actinomyces	17	3	20
Fusiformis	5	3	8
Sarcina	1	—	1
Neisseria	1	14	15
Gram-negative rods	5	23	28
Yeasts	15	8	23
Mixed infection	238		
Total positive cultures	1,141		1,417

°From Winkler, K. C., and van Amerongen, J.: Oral Surg. **12:**857, 1959.

pulp canals in pure and mixed cultures. Enterococci occur in approximately 15% of the positive root canal cultures, *Streptococcus faecalis* being the species most frequently isolated.

Mixed cultures are usually isolated from infected pulps, and a wide variety of microbial forms including *Mycoplasma* and yeasts and protozoa have been reported. The more than thirty categories, groups and species which have been isolated from pulp-involved teeth, principally represent the indigenous oral microbiota. It would seem reasonable to expect that every cultivable member of the indigenous oral flora might at one time or another be isolated from root canal cultures. While one cannot distinguish between the frank pathogen and the chance contaminant or secondary invader, those organisms that tend to persist in pulp canals after several treatments constitute the main threat as actual or potential pathogens. These appear to be mainly streptococci of the viridans and enterococcal varieties, staphylococci and *Pseudomonas* species.

Although pulpal microbial isolates in and of themselves are of a low order of intrinsic pathogenicity, it is likely that the metabolic products and physicochemical changes resulting from mixed cultures probably result in unpredictable, and often profound, tissue alterations. While pulpal isolates have been shown to produce a variety of virulence factors including hemolysins, toxins, and enzymes, no correlation appears to exist between the size or type of roentgenographic lesion and the number or kinds of substances produced by the microbial isolates from the involved teeth (Tables 9-5 and 9-6). Yet to be defined is the effect of sensitization of the apical and periapical tissues by microbial metabolic products and cellular components and the production of remittent and intermittent lesions of the allergic type or the Shwartzman variety or both.

Little attention has been given to defining the role of obligate anaerobes in the pathogenesis of pulpal and periapical disease, although several investigators have reported that anaerobic streptococci can be isolated from 15% to 20% of positive cultures if proper provisions are made for their cultivation. In infectious processes in other body tissues, these organisms produce fetid odors often accompanied by various degrees of tissue dissolution.

Presence of microorganisms in radicular dentin and surrounding tissue

Many methods have been used in the microbiology of the apical and periapical tissues of the pulp-involved tooth. Among the sampling and removal procedures used are aspiration techniques, intraboney trocars, apical curettage, apical sectioning to include the surrounding tissue, and tooth extraction. The high percentage of positive cultures reported must be considered in large measure the result of contamination, not infection.

Table 9-4. Prevalence of streptococci in root canal cultures

Number of positive cultures	Number of cultures containing streptococci			Number of cultures negative for streptococci
	Pure culture	Mixed culture	Total	
357[*]	191 (53%)	103 (29%)	294 (82%)	63 (18%)
256[†] vital	101 (39.4%)	107 (45.4%)	208 (86.3%)	48 (13.7%)
165 nonvital	52 (32.1%)	76 (46.0%)	129 (78.1%)	37 (22%)

[*]Sommer, R. F., Ostrander, F. D., and Crowley, M. C.: Clinical endodontics, Philadelphia, 1956, W. B. Saunders Co., p. 398.
[†]Author, unpublished data.

In many instances root canal infection extends from the pulpal tissue to include the radicular predentin and dentin. Chirnside,[13] Shovelton,[47] and Shovelton and Sidaway[48] demonstrated the presence of bacteria in selected tubules of the radicular dentin and Matsumiya and Kitamura,[37] in the accessory canals and in apical cemental lacunae. From a clinical point of view, these findings emphasize the need for careful debridement and mechanical preparation of the root canal and the desirability of using deeply penetrating antimicrobial agents to eliminate microorganisms (Figs. 9-11 and 9-12).

Hedman,[27] using an intracanal cannula-culture wire method, reported on eighty-two cases of pulp-involved anterior teeth

that had radiolucent areas (Fig. 9-13). Fifty-six cases or 68.5% had viable bacteria in both the pulp canal and periapical area, 8.5% had bacteria in the canal only, and 23% yielded no growth from either area. All of the patients having streptococci in the pulp canal also had them in the periapical tissue. Of clinical import is the finding that after two successive negative cultures were obtained from the root canal, no growth was obtained in cultures from the periapical area in any of the fifty-six patients evaluated.

Shovelton (1964) studied gram-stained sections of extracted, pulp-involved teeth and found that when a granuloma was associated with a root canal containing bacteria, organisms were rarely found within the granuloma. In longitudinal sections, the granulation tissue could generally be seen up to or just inside the apical foramen of the involved tooth, apparently forming an effective barrier preventing escape of organisms from the canal. Although the main part of the canal might have been heavily infected, no organisms were present in the granulation tissue at the foramen. As a rule, there was less bacterial invasion of dentin around a lateral root canal than around the main canal of the same tooth. In teeth with carious exposures of vital pulp tissue, even when heavy bacterial contamination was present at the surface of the pulp, very few orga-

Table 9-5. Production of various enzymes by strains of bacteria isolated from diseased pulp canals

Enzyme	Number of strains tested	Number of strains positive
Hemolysin	95	Alpha 15 Beta 36
Fibrinolysin	65	29
Coagulase	86	4
Hyaluronidase	95	25
Chondroitin sulfatase	71	0
Proteolytic enzyme (collagenase)	44	12

Table 9-6. Enzymes produced by organisms isolated from pulp canals of teeth showing various types of roentgenographic lesions

Roentgeno-graphic lesions	Alpha hemo-lytic strepto-cocci	Beta hemo-lytic strepto-cocci	Alpha and beta strepto-cocci	Anhemo-lytic strepto-cocci	Fibrino-lysin	Coagu-lase	Hyalu-ronidase	Chon-droitin sulfatase	Proteolytic enzymes (collagenase)
Defined	7/36*	14/36	1/36	14/36	12/20	1/32	11/36	0/25	8/16
Diffuse	4/18	10/18	0/18	4/18	8/15	2/15	12/18	0/14	2/9
Negative	1/9	2/9	2/9	4/9	5/7	1/9	1/9	0/7	2/4
Root re-sorption	2/12	5/12	0/12	5/12	6/7	1/10	5/12	0/8	2/6

*Number of cases positive over number of cases studied.

nisms could be seen in the deeper pulp tissue. Of academic and pragmatic interest is the finding of a "polar" distribution of organisms in transverse sections of pulp-involved teeth. In teeth with oral or flattened roots, there was a definite tendency toward invasion of dentin much more in the direction of the major axis of the root than in the minor axis. The uninvolved dentin appeared less tubular and was covered by a layer of amorphous material. In such teeth particular attention should be paid to the preparation and to the "poles" of the canal because pulp remnants will

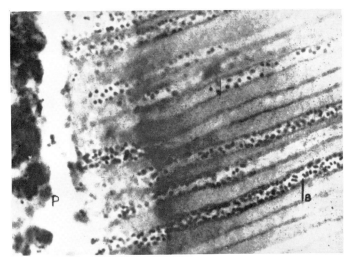

Fig. 9-11. Invasion of dentinal tubules in vitro by *Serratia marcescens*. P, Pulp canal; B, bacteria in dentinal tubules (1,500 x). (From Chirnside, I. M.: New Zeal. Dent. J. **54:**173, 1958.)

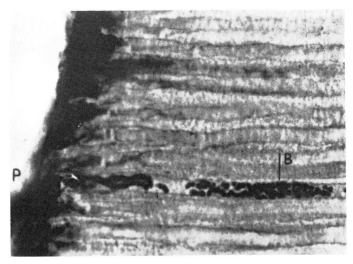

Fig. 9-12. Bacterial invasion of selected tubule. P, Pulp canal; B, bacteria in tubule (1,500 x). (From Chirnside, I. M.: New Zeal. Dent. J. **54:**173, 1958.)

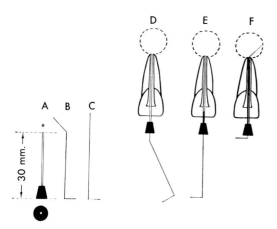

Fig. 9-13. *A, B,* and *C,* Cannula and culture wires; *D, E,* and *F,* method of inserting angular culture wires. (From Hedman, W. J.: Oral Surg. **4:**1173, 1951.)

tend to be left in these areas and dentin involvement by microbial elements will probably be greater there than at the sides of the canal.

INTRACANAL STERILIZATION PROCEDURES

Significant numbers of microorganisms and large masses of infected soft and hard tissues are removed during the processes of debridement, canal enlargement, and irrigation with antimicrobial agents of the halogen, surface-active, or oxidant types. However, it remains for antimicrobial adjuncts in the form of germicidal irrigants and between-visit medicaments to complete the destruction of microorganisms. Bacteriologic studies of the effect of mechanical preparation and irrigation of infected root canals suggest that a significant number of these canals can be rendered sterile by careful and effective procedures. It has been said that what you take out of a canal is at least as important as what you put into it.

Intracanal sterilization procedures no longer widely used include ionization, iontophoresis or electromedication, desic-

cation, and incineration. Among the many substances used for the between-visit sterilization or maintenance of the tooth under treatment are phenolics, volatile oils, halogens, sulfonamides, and antibiotics. Often mixtures of two or more antimicrobial agents are used together. Chapter 14 on chemotherapy in this book provides additional, detailed information.

On the basis of their in vitro studies on dentin permeability, Marshall and colleagues[36] concluded that the cervical and midroot dentin areas are very permeable, whereas the apical area is highly impermeable. While mechanical enlargement of the canal had relatively little effect, hydrogen peroxide and sodium hypochlorite used alternately produced a significant decrease in permeability.

The injudicious use of physical agents (files and reamers) and chemical agents (irrigants and medicaments) may be followed by a mild to severe apical periodontitis. Occasionally an acute and painful flare-up occurs. Sometimes merely gaining access to a pulp canal is sufficient to bring on acute symptoms. When generalized symptoms such as fever, malaise, localized swelling, tenderness, and lymphadenopathy appear, the systemic administration of chemotherapeutics is indicated. Access to the pulp canal is obtained to permit intraoral drainage, and the tooth is left open. If the fluctuant mass points, incision and drainage are established. Additionally, the pulp-involved tooth is taken out of occlusion by grinding whenever possible so as to reduce, even eliminate, premature and functional contacts. When the acute phase subsides, routine procedures are instituted. Continued flare-ups during treatment are often iatrogenic, resulting from overinstrumentation, excessive medication, or reinfection from leaky seals or resistant persisters.

In some cases periapical surgery is necessary because sterilization of the pulp canal cannot be accomplished, the apex

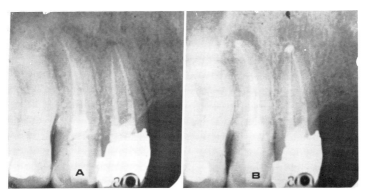

Fig. 9-14. Left maxillary first and second premolars. These teeth did not respond favorably to conservative endodontic treatment, **A,** and were retreated surgically and filled apically with amalgam, **B.**

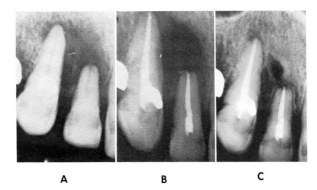

A   B   C

Fig. 9-15. Left maxillary lateral incisor and canine. **A,** Extent of the lesion; **B,** following surgical intervention and apical curettage; **C,** teeth approximately 3 years later.

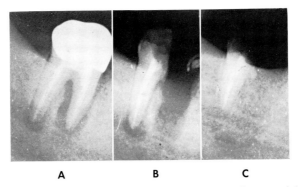

A   B   C

Fig. 9-16. Left maxillary first molar. **A,** There is evidence of successful endodontics on distal root and failure on mesial root. **B,** Hemisection of tooth and, **C,** retention of the distal root permit retention of the root as an abutment.

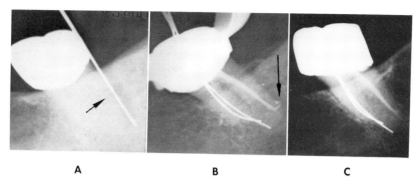

A	B	C

Fig. 9-17. Retrograde pulpitis presumably extended from distal infraboney periodontal pocket. **A,** Wire probe delineates the extent of the pocket depth; **B,** note lateral canal and extrusion of gutta-percha into the pocket. **C,** Infraboney lesion has largely disappeared 3 years after endodontic treatment.

Table 9-7. Medicaments suggested for endodontics

Designated as	*Composition*
PBSC (Grossman, 1951)	Penicillin, bacitracin, streptomycin, sodium caprylate (1958—nystatin)
PSCC (Bender and Seltzer, 1952)	Penicillin, streptomycin, chloramphenicol, sodium caprylate
DCP (Stewart, 1954)	Benzathine penicillin (Bicillin), chloramphenicol, (chloromycetin), antihistamine, (Perazil), propylene glycol, lidocaine (Xylocaine Ointment)
ACB (Sullivan and Jolly, 1955)	Aminacridine, alkyltrimethyl ammonium bromide, methyl, propylparabens
Nibacetin (Holst, 1956)	Neomycin, bacitracin
Oxpara (Cran, 1956)	7.6% phenol, formalin, creosote, thymol
Tact (Blitzen, 1956)	Oxytetracycline, hydrocortisone free alcohol (Cortril Acetate), tripelennamine (Pyribenzamine), tetracycline (with or without hyaluronidase)
PNB (Cran, 1957)	Polymyxin, neomycin, bacitracin, methyl, propylparabens
PBN (Ingle and Zeldow, 1958)	Polymyxin, bacitracin, neomycin, nystatin
PBSN (Ingle and Zeldow, 1958)	Penicillin, bacitracin, streptomycin, nystatin
ATF (Fubbo, Reich, and Dixson, 1958)	Neomycin, bacitracin, polymyxin, and 5-chloro-2-benzthiazole tartrate (fungicide) and 1:1000 noradrenalin
XP7 (Dietz, 1957)	Parachlorophenol, metacresylacetate, camphor
PATS (Gurney, 1959)	Para-aminotoluene sulfonamide (Benzylog)
Kanamycin-nifuroxime (Grossman, 1960)	Kanamycin sulfate, 5-nitro-2 furaldehyde oxime

cannot be negotiated, instruments have been broken, or the periapical lesion is of unusual size or type. The surgical procedures involve raising the flap over the root apex of the tooth, creating a window in the labial or buccal plate of bone and performing either periapical curettage or apical sectioning (apicoectomy) followed by curettage, and root end filling with gutta-percha or amalgam (Figs. 9-14 to 9-17).

INTRACANAL MEDICATIONS

In recent years antibiotic mixtures with or without added antifungal, anti-inflammatory, and antihistaminic agents among

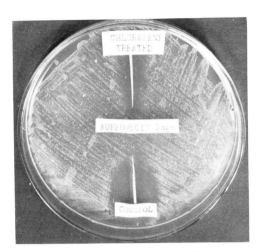

Fig. 9-18. Plate sensitivity testing. The presence of residual oxidizing agents such as peroxides or hypochlorites in teeth under treatment may significantly modify the antibacterial activity of antibiotics.

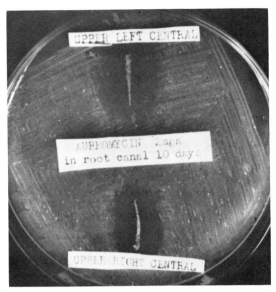

Fig. 9-19. Plate sensitivity testing. Absorbent point saturated with chlortetracycline, 2 mg. per milliliter, demonstrated antibacterial activity against a mixed culture of oral microorganisms after being sealed for 10 days in root canals of maxillary right and left central incisors.

other things have been recommended and used for intracanal medication. A list of some of these is given in Table 9-7.

Many leading endodontists continue to prefer using the classic medicaments: eugenol, formocresol, beechwood creosote, cresatin, paramonochlorophenol as such or in mixtures with other agents including antibiotics so as to obtain a broad spectrum of antimicrobial activity. Some clinicians have expressed concern that the use of antibiotic mixtures for endodontic treatment is attended by hypersensitization and the production of resistant strains of pulpal isolates. Although sensitization is a distinct possibility and allergic reactions to antibiotic mixtures used in root canals have been reported, it is very unlikely that resistant strains emerge.

Since solutions of some antibiotics are unstable and are rapidly inactivated by heavy metals and alkalis and oxidizing agents, the clinician should have a comprehensive knowledge of the properties and compatibilities of the agents he is using (Figs. 9-18 and 9-19). Plate sensitivity testing procedures provide a method for assessing the effect of antibiotic mixtures against known strains of microorganisms and provide a means for determining isolated strains' relative sensitivity or resistance to known concentrations of antibiotics and other pulp canal medicaments.

**CITED REFERENCES AND
ADDITIONAL READINGS**

1. Bartels, H. A., and Buchbinder, M.: Yeast-like microorganisms isolated from root canals, Oral Surg. 7:98, 1954.
2. Bartels, H. A., Naidorf, I. J., and Blechman, H.: A study of some factors associated with "flare-ups," Oral Surg. 25:255, 1968.
3. Bender, I. B., Seltzer, S., and Kaufman, I. J.: Infectibility of the dental pulp, by way of the dental tubules, J. Amer. Dent. Assoc. 59:466, 1959.

4. Bender, I. B., Seltzer, S., and Soltanoff, W.: Endodontic success-A reappraisal of criteria. Parts 1 and 2, Oral Surg. **22**:780, 1966.
5. Bender, I. B., Seltzer, S., and Turkenkopf, S.: To culture or not to culture? Oral Surg. **18**: 527, 1964.
6. Bender, I. B., Seltzer, S., and Yermish, M.: The incidence of bacteremia in endodontic manipulation, Oral Surg. **13**:353, 1960.
7. Birch, R. H., and Melville, T. H.: Preliminary sterilization of the endodontic field: Comparison of antisepsis, Brit. Dent. J. **111**:362, 1964.
8. Blechman, H.: Bacteriology in endodontic treatment, Dent. Clin. N. Amer. p. 845, Nov. 1957.
9. Brown, L. E., and Rudolph, C. E.: Isolation and identification of microorganisms from unexposed canals of pulp involved teeth, Oral Surg. **10**:1094, 1957.
10. Buchbinder, M.: A statistical comparison of cultured and non-cultured root canal cases, J. Dent. Res. **20**:93, 1941.
11. Buchbinder, M., and Bartels, H. A.: Criticism of the use of root canal cultures in evaluating antibiotic therapy, Oral Surg. **4**:886, 1951.
12. Burket, L. W.: Recent studies relating to periapical infection, including data obtained from human necropsy studies, J. Amer. Dent. Assoc. **25**:260, 1938.
13. Chirnside, I. M.: The bacteriological status of dentine around infected pulp canals, New Zeal. Dent. J. **54**:173, 1958.
14. Csernyei, J.: Anacoresis and anacoric effect of chronic periapical inflammations, J. Dent. Res. **18**:527, 1939.
15. Hatton, E. H.: Pulp abscesses and root resection, J. Amer. Dent. Assoc. **19**:742-746, 1932.
16. Engström, B.: The significance of enterococci in root canal treatment, Odont. Rev. **15**:87, 1964.
17. Engström, B.: Some factors influencing the frequency of growth in endodontia culturing, Odont. T. **72**:249, 1964.
18. Engström, B., and Frostell, G.: Experience of bacteriological root canal controls, Acta Odont. Scand. **22**:43, 1964.
19. Engström, B., and Lundberg, M.: The frequency and causes of reversal from negative to positive bacteriological tests in root canal therapy, Odont. T. **74**:189, 1966.
20. Engström, B., Segorstad, L. H., Ramstrom, G., and Grostell, G.: Correlation of positive cultures with the prognosis of root canal treatment, Odont. Rev. **15**:257, 1964.
21. Gier, R. E., and Mitchell, D. F.: Anachoretic effect of pulpitis, J. Dent. Res. **47**:564, 1968.
22. Grossman, L. I.: Bacteriological status of periapical tissue in 150 cases of infected pulpless teeth, J. Dent. Res. **38**:101, 1959.
23. Grossman, L. I.: Endodontic practice, ed. 6, Philadelphia, 1965, Lea & Febiger.
24. Grossman, L. I.: Origin of microorganisms in traumatized pulpless sound teeth, J. Dent. Res. **46**:551, 1967.
25. Gunter, J. H., Appleton, J. L. T., Strong, J., Reader, J. C., Zimmerman, E. A., and Brooks, J. J.: Bacteriology of dental pulp, J. Dent. Res. **16**:310, 1937.
26. Hampp, E. G.: Isolation and identification of spirochetes obtained from unexposed canals of pulp involved teeth, Oral Surg. **10**:1100, 1957.
27. Hedman, W. J.: An investigation into residual periapical infection after pulp canal therapy, Oral Surg. **4**:1173, 1951.
28. Henrici, A. T., and Hartzell, T. B.: The bacteriology of the vital pulps, J. Dent. Res. **1**:419, 1919.
29. Ingle, J. I.: Endodontics, Philadelphia, 1965, Lea & Febiger.
30. Ingle, J. I., and Zeldow, B. J.: An evaluation of mechanical instrumentation and the negative culture in endodontic therapy, J. Amer. Dent. Assoc. **57**:471, 1958.
31. Kakehashi, S., Stanley, H. R., and Fitzgerald, R.: The effects of surgical exposures of dental pulps in germ-free and conventional laboratory rats, Oral Surg. **20**:340, 1965.
32. Klotz, M. D., Gerstein, H., and Bohn, A. N.: Bacteremia after topical use of prednisolone in infected pulps, J. Amer. Dent. Assoc. **71**: 871, 1965.
33. Leavitt, J. M., Naidorf, I. J., and Shugaevsky, P.: Aerobes and anaerobes in endodontics. I. The undetected anaerobe in endodontics. II. A sensitive culture medium for the detection of both aerobes and anaerobes, New York Dent. J. **25**:377, 1955.
34. Macdonald, J. B., Hare, G. C., and Wood, A. W. S.: The bacteriologic status of the pulp chambers in intact teeth found to be nonvital following trauma, Oral Surg. **10**:318, 1957.
35. McKay, G. S.: The pattern of bacterial invasion of carious dentin, International Association for Dental Research, British Div., 1969, Abstract 10.
36. Marshall, F. J., Massler, M., and Dute, H. L.: Effects of endodontic treatments on permeability of root dentine, Oral Surg. **13**:208, 1960.
37. Matsumiya, S., and Kitamura, M.: Histopathological and histo-bacteriological studies of the relation between the condition of sterilization of the interior of the root canal and the healing process of periapical tissue experimentally infected and root canal treatment, Bull. Tokyo Dent. Coll. **1**:1, 1960.

38. Mazzarella, M. A., Hedman, W. J., and Brown, L. R.: Classification of microorganisms from the pulp canal of nonvital teeth, Res. Project N M 008-015-10. 01 U.S. Navy Dental School, Bethesda, Md., 1955.

39. Melville, T. H., and Birch, R. H.: Preliminary sterilization of the endodontic field, Brit. Dent. J. 110:313, 1961.

40. Melville, T. H., and Birch, R. H.: Root canal and periapical floras of infected teeth, Oral Surg. 23:93, 1967.

41. Melville, T. H., and Slack, G. L.: Bacteria isolated from root canals during endodontic treatments, Brit. Dent. J. 109:127, 1961.

42. Menkin, V.: Dynamics of inflammation, New York, 1940, The Macmillan Company.

43. Myers, J. W., Marshall, F. J., and Rosen, S.: The incidence and identity of microorganisms present in root canals at filling following culture reversals, Oral Surg. 28:889, 1969.

44. Rickert, U. G., and Dixon, C. M.: The controlling of root surgery, International Dental Congress (8), Trans. Sect. IIIa, 15, 1931 Fédération Dentaire Internationale.

45. Robinson, H. B. G., and Boling, L. R.: The anachoretic effect in pulpitis. I. Bacteriologic studies, J. Amer. Dent. Assoc. 28:268, 1941.

46. Seltzer, S., Bender, I. B., and Turkenkopf, S.: Factors affecting successful repair after root canal therapy, J. Amer. Dent. Assoc. 67:641, 1963.

47. Shovelton, D. S.: Bacterial invasion of dentine around infected root canals, Alabama Dent. Rev. 7:7, 1959.

48. Shovelton, D. S., and Sidaway, D. A.: Infection in root canals, Brit. Dent. J. 108:115, 1960.

49. Stewart, G. S.: A study of bacteria found in root canals of anterior teeth and the probable mode of ingress, J. Endont. 2:8, 1947.

50. Torneck, C. D.: Reaction of rat connective tissue to polyethylene tube implants, part I, Oral Surg. 21:379, 1966; part II, Oral Surg. 24:674, 1967.

51. Winkler, K. C., and vanAmerongen, J.: Bacteriologic results from 4000 root canals, Oral Surg. 12:857, 1959.

52. Winter, G. B., and Kramer, I. R. H.: Changes in periodontal membrane and bone following experimental pulpal injury in deciduous molar teeth in kittens, Arch. Oral Biol. 10:279, 1965.

53. Zeldow, B. J., and Ingle, J. I.: Correlation of the positive culture to the prognosis of endodontically treated teeth: A clinical study, J. Amer. Dent. Assoc. 66:9, 1963.

10 / Hypersensitivity and its clinical considerations

Untoward reactions in man to plants, foods, and drugs are recorded in the earliest medical writings. Bronchial asthma was described in the third century B.C., and hay fever was recognized in the sixteenth century. But it was not until the latter half of the nineteenth century that specific instances of experimental hypersensitivity were reported. In 1890 Koch described his observations of a guinea pig's allergic reaction to the tubercle bacillus; later Flexner (1894), von Behring (1895), Richet (1898), and Portier (1902) described a reaction opposite from prophylaxis, namely anaphylaxis (against protection). Local anaphylaxis was described by Arthus in 1903, and in the same year Hamburger and Moro discussed serum sickness. By 1906 von Pirquet had coined the term "allergie," and from then on a great interest in hypersensitivity developed.

Over the years allergy has become a focal point for the convergence of many basic disciplines such as endocrinology, pharmacology, microbiology, and immunology. With the development of appropriate materials for skin testing for local and systemic sensitization, clinical allergy has become a recognized specialized study in medicine; a wide variety of clinical entities including contact dermatitis, allergic rhinitis, bronchial asthma, drug and insect allergies, hypersensitivity to physical agents, and certain so-called autoimmune diseases of connective tissue and specific organs were identified as being basically related immunologic diseases.

Allergy is of interest to the dental practitioner for several reasons, among them the facts that the chemicals, drugs, and dental materials and procedures used may evoke reactions of hypersensitivity in himself or in his patient; and that allergic reactions may directly affect the oral cavity.

From 10% to 15% of the earth's population suffer from major allergic reactions, including rashes, hives, headaches, fevers, various wheezes, swellings, and palpitations. Among the inciting agents are such diverse entities as food proteins, metals, cosmetics, odors, cigars, drugs, denture powders, animal dander, light, heat, and cold. Many of these functionally and physically different materials have common or closely related chemical structures. It has been said that one man's meat is another man's poison. Although emotional and psychosomatic factors have been causally related to many cases of allergy, the mechanisms involved are poorly understood.

While the term "allergy" denotes an altered reactivity of tissues, in common usage it refers to hyperactivity or hypersensitivity. The paradox of increasing resistance and at the same time reducing

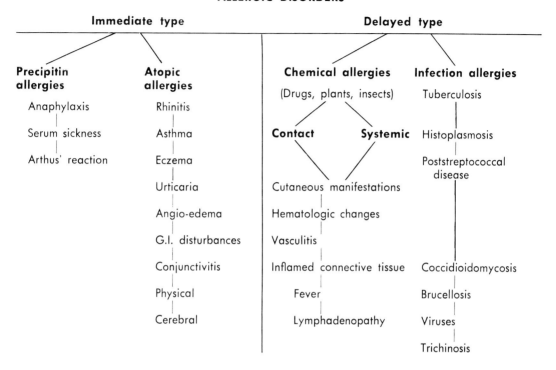

ALLERGIC DISORDERS

Immediate type		**Delayed type**	
Precipitin allergies	**Atopic allergies**	**Chemical allergies** (Drugs, plants, insects)	**Infection allergies**
Anaphylaxis	Rhinitis		Tuberculosis
Serum sickness	Asthma	**Contact Systemic**	Histoplasmosis
Arthus' reaction	Eczema		Poststreptococcal disease
	Urticaria	Cutaneous manifestations	
	Angio-edema	Hematologic changes	
	G.I. disturbances	Vasculitis	
	Conjunctivitis	Inflamed connective tissue	Coccidioidomycosis
	Physical	Fever	Brucellosis
	Cerebral	Lymphadenopathy	Viruses
			Trichinosis

Table 10-1. Characteristics differentiating immediate from delayed hypersensitivity

Characteristics	*Immediate type*	*Delayed type*
Time course	Begins within minutes and disappears within hours	Begins within hours and disappears within days
Gross reactions	Shock with respiratory and vascular symptoms; erythema, angioedema, eczema, hay fever, asthma; anemia, leukopenia, purpura	Necrosis, induration, slow healing; eczematous reaction of the skin
Mechanism	Release and participation of histamine, slow reacting substance (SRS-A), serotonin, bradykinin, and heparin	Mechanism of reaction unknown
Histologic and physiologic components	Dilation of capillaries and arterioles; shock-organs (smooth muscle), blood vessels, and collagen; polymorphonuclear platelet thrombi and vessel occlusion	Exudation and cellular proliferation and infiltration; early polymorphonuclears followed by mononuclear concentration around small venules; all tissues vulnerable
Circulating antibody	Present; frequently as precipitating antibody; sensitization by passive transfer	Absent; transfer by use of sensitized lymphocytes and macrophages
Treatment	Epinephrine, aminophylline, antihistamines, and corticosteroids	Corticosteroids

it depends upon the presence of "imperfect" immunologic mechanisms and the artificiality of the conditions under which sensitization occurs. In acquired resistance to an infectious agent or a toxic product, neutralizing antibodies are produced against the incitants which react with it and neutralize its infectivity and toxicity. In hypersensitivity, neutralization, if it occurs, is a side issue since the union of antigen (allergen) and antibody itself results in untoward bodily effects. The skin is often extremely sensitive to very minute amounts of allergen, and, accordingly, allergic diseases are often classified in terms of the type of skin reaction they produce. The diagram and Table 10-1 give a partial listing of allergic disorders according to duration of response, tissues chiefly involved, the nature of the incitant, and other differentiating characteristics.

IMMEDIATE HYPERSENSITIVITY

Allergic reactions that are mediated by circulating antibody and begin within seconds or hours of the union of antigen-antibody are labeled "immediate." An acute systemic reaction, occasionally terminating in death, following the injection of antigen intraperitoneally or intravenously into prepared animals is called *anaphylaxis;* local tissue necrosis resulting from intracutaneous application is known as *Arthus' reaction.* Although the time course in *serum sickness* is somewhat longer than that of the former two types of allergy, similar skin-sensitizing reagins and classic antibodies occur. Anaphylaxis, serum disease, and Arthus' reaction are primarily induced diseases, whereas the atopic diseases result from natural exposure to allergens.

Precipitin allergies
Anaphylaxis

The early investigators found that an anaphylactic state could be induced by nontoxic and nonpathogenic agents in most of the animal species, including man. The profound shock symptoms accompanying this condition of sensitization, occasionally resulting in death of the animal, could be produced by active immunization (sensitization) or by the administration of an antibody produced in another host (passive sensitization).

In *active anaphylaxis* the first injection is known as the sensitizing dose (0.1 mg. often suffices); and the second injection, from ten to one hundred times greater, given from 10 days to three weeks later, as the shocking dose. While sensitization may be induced by any route, including inhalation, shocking doses administered intravenously produce uniform results. Small doses produce mild shock; large doses result in death within 10 minutes. After receiving a sublethal dose of antigen, the animal may become temporarily or completely refractory to the antigen (desensitized).

Different animals show different symptoms. Within seconds of receiving the shocking dose the guinea pig becomes restless, his hair bristles, he sneezes, and his respiration increases. Later, the animal gasps for breath, urinates, defecates, undergoes tonic and clonic convulsions, and dies. Death results from asphyxia following an extreme spasm of the bronchioles and unsuccessful expiration. In the rabbit there is evidence of obstruction and constriction of pulmonary arterioles and right-sided heart failure. The dog shows extreme muscular weakness and engorgement and congestion of the liver and other organs. Human beings rarely develop anaphylaxis, but when it does occur it is characterized by circulatory collapse and labored respiration. Death may occur within a matter of minutes or hours.

In *passive anaphylaxis,* sensitizing antibody is usually administered intravenously or intraperitoneally, and an intravenous injection of antigen is given from 24 to 48 hours later. A *reversed passive anaphylaxis* can be induced by giving antigen first and then an intravenous injection of antibody one or two days later.

Regardless of the species of the recipient, the symptoms seen in anaphylaxis are caused by an increase in capillary permeability and the contraction of smooth muscle. Isolated strips of uterine or intestinal smooth muscle from sensitized animals contract when challenged with homologous antigen (Schultz-Dale reaction). The in vitro sensitization of strips from normal animals may also be accomplished. The union of antigen-antibody leading to the shock syndrome probably takes place not in the circulation but in the tissues. The union presumably results in the liberation of histamine, serotonin, and other physiologically active substances from damaged mast cells, other tissue cells, and platelets.

The term "anaphylactoid," or anaphylaxislike reaction, more appropriately applies to man. In such a reaction precipitating antibodies are not demonstrable. There is often no history of a primary or sensitizing dose; desensitization is difficult and passive transfer to animals unsuccessful. Skin-sensitizing antibodies (reagins) are found in the serum. In atopic individuals, anaphylaxislike symptoms may occur in response to challenges by pollens, fungi, stinging insects, and an assortment of drugs, chemicals, and even foods. Life-threatening symptoms are treated with epinephrine, antihistamines, oxygen, and even tracheotomy.

Serum sickness

Serum sickness is a type of hypersensitivity first observed in a number of individuals receiving antitoxins or antibacterial sera produced in animals. In recent years serum disease-like syndromes have been seen as a consequence of sulfonamide, arsenical, and penicillin therapy. Three types of clinical reactions can occur. *Primary serum sickness* manifests itself from 7 to 21 days after injection of serum and is characterized by fever; neutropenia; adenitis; erythematous or urticarial eruptions; edema at the site of injection and of the eyelids, face, and ankles; arthralgia; and hematuria. The symptoms may be mild and transitory, lasting from two to four days, or severe and lasting several weeks. *Accelerated serum sickness* occurs in individuals who have previously received an injection of horse serum and manifests itself from one to three days after injection (anamnestic reaction). The *atopic-type serum reaction* occurs in individuals with known allergic disorders and sensitivity to animal danders or sera. Persons who have serum sickness produce heterophilic, skin-sensitizing precipitin and anaphylactic antibodies. An initial injection of animal serum presumably results in the production of antibodies that react with the residue of serum still circulating in the blood.

Arthus' reaction

Arthus' reaction is characterized by edema, extensive cellular infiltration, hemorrhage, and secondary necrosis that results from the deposition of antigen and precipitating antibody complexes in blood vessels at the site of the lesion. It differs from anaphylaxis in that it is dependent upon cell-fixed antibody, it takes several hours to develop to its maximum, and it is associated with a striking granulocytic infiltration. The classic experiments on rabbits inoculated with horse serum in the same subcutaneous region are often cited: while the initial injections were without detectable effect, later injections in the same site resulted in an intense and persistent local reaction. Reactions of this type have been reported following the intramuscular injection of penicillin in an oil and beeswax vehicle. Arthus' reactivity can be passively transferred from the same or another species. Antihistamines have little or no effect on the reaction.

Atopic allergies

The atopic allergic diseases observed chiefly in man appear to have several characteristics in common. They show a familial distribution, and more than 10% of the population have allergies of this type. The clinical symptoms evoked are related to the site of contact and route of exposure. The antibodies are of the nonprecipitating, skin-sensitizing (reagin) variety. The most common allergens are grass and tree pollens; dander, feathers, hair, eggs, milk chocolate; house dust, bacteria, viruses, and fungi. The active antigenic components are usually protein in nature with some carbohydrate, having molecular weights between 3,000 and 4,000. Cross-sensitization frequently occurs between physically and functionally different materials because they have common or closely related chemical structures. Chlorogenic acid (3-caffeoylquinic acid), for example, has recently been shown to be a common allergenic determinant in green coffee beans, castor beans, and oranges.

Among the clinical diseases most frequently seen and described are hay fever, asthma, infantile eczema, atopic dermatitis, urticaria, and a host of drug and food idiosyncrasies. The allergen presumably combines with the reagin (univalent, nonprecipitating, sessile or attached antibody) in the tissues, the union resulting in the liberation of humoral agents that produce functional impairment of the tissues. In 1921 Prausnitz and Küstner in a study of passive sensitization described the cutaneous manifestations of atopic diseases. When a little serum from Küstner, who was fish-sensitive, was injected into the skin of a normal person and fish antigen was injected into the same site 24 hours later, a wheal and flare reaction was observed within from 20 to 30 minutes. It was found later that if the specific allergen is injected into some remote tissues or the bloodstream or ingested or inhaled, the same reaction will be elicited at the prepared site. These localized reactions appear and disappear quickly in contrast to the delayed and persistent reactions produced by microbial hypersensitivity.

The skin-sensitizing antibody (reagin) in sera of allergic individuals is much more labile than are the "immune" antibodies. Heating, storage, freezing and thawing, dialysis, fractionation procedures, and acidification lead to partial or total loss of activity. The homocytotropic (skin-sensitizing) antibody of atopic sera has been tentatively classified as γE immunoglobulins.

Skin testing for atopy may be performed by various scratch or intradermal techniques, and the procedure is frequently helpful in the diagnosis of seasonal rhinitis, asthma, and the many eczematous and urticarial rashes affecting infants and adults.

Emotional and psychogenic factors, weather, infectious diseases, and probably various other ill-defined factors of everyday living likely modify the allergic response by way of the autonomic nervous system.

Pharmacologically active mediators

The symptom complexes briefly described in the previous sections appear to be related mainly to the release of four recognized mediators: histamine, slow reacting substance (SRS), serotonin, and plasma kinin. No clearly defined role can be established for a given mediator in a given allergic disease. The following discussion presents a brief characterization of each of the pharmacologically active substances.

Histamine formed from L-histidine is associated chiefly with the granules of the mast cell, platelets, and basophilic leukocytes. Histamine increases capillary permeability and bronchiolar and other smooth muscle contraction and stimulates the exocrine glands. It appears to be the principal mediator of the systemic anaphylaxis in the guinea pig and the dog and an important contributor to the reaction in man. The *slow reacting substance* (SRS) refers to antigen-antibody released material that contracts smooth muscle more slowly than histamine and is presumably acidic and lipid in character. SRS probably arises from mast cells, and its exact role in clinical disease remains undefined. Although *serotonin* (5-hydroxytryptamine) is not present in the mast cells of many species, it can be identified in the platelets of most. It increases capillary permeability and constricts smooth muscle, and its action is inhibited by lysergic acid. The *plasma kinins*—kallidin I or bradykinin, a nonapeptide; and kallidin II, a decapeptide; and related polypeptides—are derived from kallikrein (glandular, pancreatic, or urinary) by the action of plasma aminopeptidases. Five pharmacologic activities have been demonstrated: smooth muscle constriction, vasodilation of cutaneous vessels, increase in capillary permeability, migration of leukocytes, and stimulation of pain fibers. Although *acetylcholine, heparin, leukotaxine,* and *anaphylatoxin* have been mentioned as contributory mediators, there are no firm data on the basis of which to assess the significance of their role.

PHYSICAL ALLERGIES

Hypersensitivity to light, heat, and trauma are common causes of cutaneous allergic manifestations. In all cases of light urticaria it must be assumed that the absorption of electromagnetic energy causes liberation or formation of a substance or substances in the skin which are capable of eliciting an urticarial response. Although the normal individual does not form antibodies to the metabolite, the allergic individual does. Studies with monochromatic light have shown that a person may react to several specific wave lengths. The eruptions that occur are characterized by pruritus at the site often within 30 seconds of exposure, followed by erythema and, in a few minutes, by urticarial edema; the lesions usually persist from one to four hours.

Topically applied benzoic acid derived preparations that absorb or reflect light afford partial protection. Photoallergic reactions that follow the ingestion, injection, or topical application of photosensitizing drugs may also cause eruptions on light-exposed areas. It has been postulated that the drug setting off the photoallergic reaction is converted in the skin into a new compound after it absorbs a specific wavelength of the light spectrum. It is this newly formed substance that acts as an antigen. Sulfanilamide, promethazine, and chlorothiazide have been shown to induce reactions of the type described. The photoallergic reaction must not be confused with the phototoxic reaction, a first exposure response which is nonimmunologic.

Both localized and generalized forms of heat urticaria are described. While temperatures of 118° F. for five minutes at a localized site produce only a mild erythema in normal control subjects, the allergic person will show urticarial eruptions. A diffuse form of heat urticaria, cholinergic urticaria, most conspicuous on the trunk but also present elsewhere on the body, may be produced following exposure to heat, exercise, or emotional stimuli. Cold urticaria occurs as a localized phenomenon appearing at the point of contact only, or as a localized urticaria followed by systemic manifestations. Familial and acquired varieties are recognized, the only inciting factor being a drop in temperature. Itching and edema characterize the lesions, which remain for only an hour or two. About one third of the cold allergic individuals have an atopic background and strong family history of allergy.

Cutaneous hypersensitivity reactions to mechanical stimuli appear as wheals (urticarial dermographism). The force required to elicit an urticarial response in a hypersensitive person is about one fifth of that required by a normal individual. Itching may accompany the trauma urticaria. Pressure urticaria is characterized by the appearance of wheals or edematous plaques

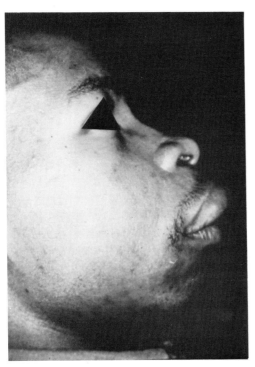

Fig. 10-1. Angioedema of upper lip.

following immediately or as long as eight hours or more after persistent pressure. These may persist for periods to 24 hours. Antihistamines diminish the reactions caused by light, heat and cold, and trauma. The dental practitioner should consider pressure urticaria in attempting to determine the cause of postoperative edema.

The *Sanarelli and Schwartzman phenomena,* which resemble Arthus' reaction in appearance and manner of development, should be differentiated from it because the phenomena do not depend upon an antigen-antibody mechanism. It is possible to prepare a skin site with one bacterial endotoxin or culture filtrates and to elicit a severe hemorrhagic and necrotic lesion by the intravenous injection from 8 to 32 hours later of unrelated culture filtrates or certain nonbacterial materials such as starch, glycogen, or agar. Localized reactions have been produced in the oral mucosa of rats by endotoxins from oral *Veillonella* and other members of the indigenous flora. Besides the localized, dermal Shwartzman reaction, a generalized phenomenon is described in which both the preparatory and shocking doses are given intravenously. The neutropenia and thrombocytopenia that follow the eliciting injection are associated with the development of leukocyte-platelet thrombi in the small veins of the kidney, resulting in bilateral renocortical necrosis.

DELAYED HYPERSENSITIVITY

In the delayed type of hypersensitivity neither demonstrable antibodies nor passive transfer can be successfully shown. The challenging dose is followed some 6 to 12 hours later by a faint redness at the site that reaches a peak within 24 to 72 hours and usually persists for several days. Hemorrhage and thrombosis, so frequently present in the antibody-specific Arthus' phenomenon and the nonspecific Shwartzman reaction, are conspicuously absent. This type of allergy, while antigenically specific, can be transferred with the leukocytes but not with serum. Many of the contact allergies (dermatitis venenata) caused by chemicals, drugs, plants, and insects and certain systemic drug reactions are of the delayed type. Additionally, many infectious diseases of bacterial, fungal, parasitic, and viral origin are characterized by hypersensitivity to various extractives or metabolites of the infectious agent. The injection of these into the skin results in cellular infiltration, hyperemia, and increasing induration. The classic Koch's phenomenon, in which tuberculous guinea pigs were found hyperreactive to superinfection with living cells or extracts from dead tubercle bacilli (O.T.), is typical of the allergy of infection and microbial hypersensitivity.

Four types of lesions—local, focal, ocular, and systemic—may be produced, depending upon the method of challenge with allergen. The cells mainly responsible for this reaction are probably small lymphocytes that are attracted to sites of antigen deposition. The occurrence of generalized tissue damage accompanying delayed hypersensitivity may result from the release of toxic substances from injured lymphocytes. Yet to be assessed is the relative importance of this type of hypersensitivity as a protective mechanism against neoplastic growths and certain infectious diseases such as tuberculosis, brucellosis, systemic mycosis, and viral infections.

Several factors influence the induction of delayed hypersensitivity. The intradermal and subcutaneous routes of administration rather than other parenteral routes favor development of hypersensitivity. The use of adjuvants such as oil or another emulsifying agent that delays absorption influences induction. A number of human diseases affect the delayed hypersensitivity state; these include Hodgkin's disease, leukemia, sarcoidosis, multiple myeloma, lymphoma, and agammaglobulinemia.

One investigator injected 0.3 ml. to 0.5 ml. of packed leukocytes obtained from human donors with intense delayed hypersensitivity to tuberculin into tuberculin-negative recipients. Typical tuberculin reactions were obtained in the formerly negative recipients. Similar transfers of hypersensitivity to streptococcal products, procaine, and other antigens have been demonstrated.

Allergic eczematous contact dermatitis is the clinical expression of delayed sensitivity to various water soluble and fat soluble natural products and defined chemical substances. The reaction time is from 12 to 48 hours, with a possible range of from 4 to 72 hours. Sensitization may take at least five days with the resultant lesions varying from macules, papules, and vesicles in the acute phase to encrusting, scaling, and thickening of the skin in the chronic variety. The location of the lesion is related to site of major exposure to the allergen (Fig. 10-2). Flare-ups and recurrences may follow systemic administration. The agents chiefly associated with this type of dermatitis are small molecular compounds, dyes, cosmetics, topical medicaments, plastics, metals, soaps, perfumes, and so forth. Not uncommon are allergic reactions to many antibiotics, sulfonamides, organic arsenicals, hormones, iodides, bromides, barbiturates, aspirin, local anesthetics, and antithyroid agents to name only a few. The eyelids, sides of the neck, and genitalia are highly reactive, while the scalp, palms, and soles are relatively resistant. A familial tendency has not been demonstrated; and since the allergens are chiefly haptens, it is presumed that these denature cutaneous proteins to form complete antigens. It has also been suggested that the type of protein with which the hapten links determines whether an immediate or a delayed type of hypersensitivity is induced. The fibrous proteins of the skin are involved with the delayed type, the globular proteins of the serum with the immediate type. Although the spontaneous loss of contact sensitivity has been reported, this condition, once established, persists for years. The discovery and elimination of the causative agent are the best approaches to therapy.

Allergic reactions to insects are mainly of the delayed type and result from inhalation of or contact with parts of the insect or from its sting or bite. The reactions are usually urticarial, followed occasionally by papular, vesicular, or eczematous lesions. Reactions of the immediate type caused by stings of honeybees, ants, wasps, hornets, and yellow jackets have been reported. An immediate reaction occurs in 98% of the cases and ranges from urticaria to anaphylaxis. The delayed reaction, on the other hand, appears some 24 hours to 10 days later and is similar to serum sickness. Bernton and Brown (1967) found that almost half of 170 asthmatic patients in New York City allergy clinics who did

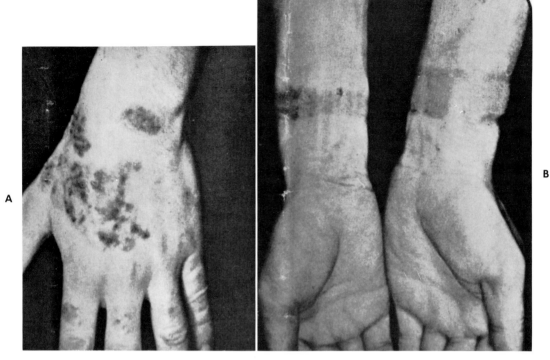

Fig. 10-2. Allergic eczema. Dermatitis was caused by **A,** chromic acid and **B,** wrist watch band dye.

not react to commonly used allergens did respond to extracts of cockroaches. Indeed, almost one quarter of 755 allergic patients screened were found hypersensitive to roaches.

It is generally accepted that the excitant in the common poison ivy plant is identical with that of poison oak and of poison sumac. Since these plants infest all parts of the country, the likelihood of an individual's being exposed to one of them is extremely great. About 60% of the population are susceptible to "poisoning" by poison ivy. Although insect parts play an important role as inhaled allergens, plant pollens are the principal offenders. Ragweed is a prolific producer of pollen, a potent antigen and the most common cause of hay fever. As atopic allergens the weeds are followed by the grass pollens and finally the relatively unimportant tree pollens. Molds, important sources of airborne

spores and allergic incitants, should not be overlooked. The desquamated skin epithelium and dander of domesticated animals also cause atopic rhinitis and eczema.

Allergy in microbial diseases

After the active disease state has subsided, many microbial diseases may be followed by manifestations of illness that can only be characterized as being the result of delayed hypersensitivity. The rather infrequent poststreptococcal diseases, rheumatic fever and glomerulonephritis, may result from the alteration of tissue proteins by the presence of the infectious microorganism and, hence, subsequent autosensitization. The latent period preceding the appearance of rheumatic fever suggests an allergic basis; rheumatic fever may follow any of the more than fifty types of beta hemolytic, group A, streptococcal diseases. Glomerulonephritis follows only a few types, particularly type 12. Allergy to streptococci has been well studied in laboratory animals. Delayed hypersensitivity to viridans streptococci has been shown in rabbits, producing cutaneous, ophthalmic, and systemic lesions after intracutaneous challenge.

In tuberculosis the response of the host to the proteins of the bacterial cell is best demonstrated. The use of old tuberculin (O.T.) or the purified protein derivative (P.P.D.) is followed by a delayed reaction in individuals sensitized to tubercle bacilli or their products; the intracutaneous test is read in 72 hours, the patch test in 48 hours. Similarly, sensitization to the arthrospores of the fungus *Coccidioides immitis* during the infective process may be detected by the administration of coccidioidin and indicates prior infection and a "relative" immunity.

In histoplasmosis, however, hypersensitivity per se seems to play a more important role in the development of the disease in later life than does the actual spread of the infectious microorganisms. This apparent paradox of an increasing and, at the same time, decreasing immunity requires further explanation. It would seem that while hypersensitization undoubtedly plays a large part in the localization of the disease and the destruction of many microorganisms by macrophages during the early stages of the disease, the reinfective and chronic varieties of these diseases are related to the acquired hypersensitivity. After *Brucella* strains invade the tissues, the organisms localize within monocytes, and granulomatous lesions evolve. Coincident with the appearance of the granuloma, *Brucella* agglutinins are found in the serum, and dermal *Brucella* hypersensitivity of the delayed type can be demonstrated. The contribution of this acquired hypersensitivity to the degree of illness has been studied in veterinarians and laboratory workers. It seems that the severity of the reaction was directly related to the presence or absence of sensitizing antibodies.

Animal parasites often take complex routes in the host before reaching their site of maturation. Usually, the greater the invasiveness and migration, the greater the host response. Helminths entering the host by the percutaneous route induce a dermatitis that, particularly on reinfection, appears to result from hypersensitivity. The visceral pathosis may also be linked to the same mechanism. The "swimmer's itch" or schistosome dermatitis is an example of the skin lesions referred to previously. One of the striking features of helminthic disease is the large number of eosinophils that appear in both the invaded tissue and the circulating blood.

Heated preparations of vaccinia, mumps, and lymphogranuloma introduced into the skin of sensitized individuals produce a delayed type of hypersensitivity. This type of reaction may develop following the injection of or infection with related viruses belonging to the herpesviruses; poxviruses; certain myxoviruses namely influenza; measles; and *Coxiella burnetii (Rickettsia diaporica)*, the causative agent of Q fever. The postinfection or postvaccination encephalomyelitis, which may appear as a complication in some virus diseases, is thought to have an underlying allergic basis. In general it may be said that in those virus diseases in which host resistance is of long duration, dermal hypersensitivity and resistance to infection show good correlation. The corollary is also true: where the resistance to reinfection tends to be of short duration, the correlation is poor.

Jones-Mote hypersensitivity

A mild type of reaction known as the *Jones-Mote type of delayed hypersensitivity* may occur if, for example, repeated doses of guinea pig serum are injected into the skin of man. Three to six days after the initial injection a small area of redness persisting for from 18 to 24 hours appears on the skin. With continuing injections there is an abrupt transition from the delayed to the immediate wheal and flare type of reaction. The appearance of the latter coincides with the appearance of precipitating serum antibodies.

DIAGNOSTIC METHODS

Diagnostic procedures for atopy include various skin tests for immediate reactivity utilizing extracts of pollens, mold spores, house dust, dander, and miscellaneous substances such as egg white, fish, seeds, nuts, feathers, wool, and so forth. These are administered by scratch and intradermal techniques inducing a wheal and flare reaction.

The more commonly used materials for skin testing in cases of allergy resulting from infections are tuberculin, histoplasmin, blastomycin, and coccidioidin. Proper doses of relatively pure preparations should be used for testing because serious focal, even systemic, reactions can occur in people who react positively. When both immediate and delayed responses arise, each should be evaluated independently. One must also remember that in advanced stages of all diseases the skin may fail to respond (anergy), and even positive reactions may be of limited practical value. A reaction to an extract of *Candida*, for example, might be expected in view of its ubiquity. Also, during intercurrent infections the host may temporarily cease to give skin reactions.

A carefully taken history, however, remains the basic and essential diagnostic procedure; indeed, a well-taken and well-studied history can often be all that is necessary. Most of the fatal reactions have occurred in persons having known histories of bronchial asthma, hay fever, or atopic eczema. One should ask about previous use of a drug and any reactions to it; and if one is still in doubt, a skin test should be used starting with 1 unit per milliliter and increasing to from 10 to 10,000 units per milliliter by intracutaneous methods. A positive reaction is of real value since it indicates an anaphylactic form of the allergy, the reaction at the end of a 15- or 20-minute period being a wheal and flare response. In any case, a bottle of epinephrine, 1:1,000, and a sterile syringe and needle should be available at all times in the dental operatory; from 0.5 ml. to 1.0 ml. should be administered intramuscularly, subcutaneously, or preferably intravenously if the signs of anaphylactic shock appear.

HOMOGRAFT REJECTION

The destruction of a homograft, a graft transplanted from one individual to another of the same species, by the host is not innate but rather immunologic in nature. At first the graft is accepted and thrives under the conditions of transplantation. After a few days, however, dramatic changes occur. First the tissue becomes swollen and infiltrated; afterward it shrinks and sloughs off. A second graft on the same or a different site in the same individual is rejected more rapidly. A convincing body of evidence is accumulating to support the view that homograft sensitivity and drug and bacterial delayed hypersensitivity are closely related. The death of the homograft may be caused by a local accumulation of mononuclear cells in proximal vessel walls and a direct cytopathogenic effect of these cells and sensitized lymphoid cells on the graft. Although grafts of bone and blood vessels may be destroyed, they remain useful as a supporting framework for host tissue repair. Corneal transplants, because they are not vascularized, appear to survive. In man homotransplants of skin, kidney, endocrine tissue, liver, lung, and spleen have functioned only temporarily.

A relative state of tolerance that may prolong the life of a homograft may be produced by whole body irradiation, treatment with corticosteroids, use of metabolic analogues and colloidal substances, neonatal thymectomy, and functional impairment of lymphoid tissues. Recent evidence suggests that chronic exposure to small doses of antigenic homograft cell preparations may confer tolerance to the recipient. A complication of inducing tolerance by the injection of tissue homogenates is a syndrome known as *runt disease,* homologous disease, or wasting disease. In young rodents it is marked by loss of weight and hair, eczema, diarrhea, and sometimes death. The main lesions appearing in the hematopoietic and lymphatic systems are initially hyperplastic and later atrophic.

MISCELLANEOUS DISEASE STATES AND ALLERGIC PHENOMENA

Endogenous antigens resulting from tissue damage or alteration may produce the serum sickness-like syndromes seen in the "collagen diseases," polyarteritis nodosa, lupus erythematosus, and rheumatoid arthritis. In the autoimmune diseases, by contrast, the lesions that appear are precisely in those tissues which served as antigenic stimuli. Experimental allergic encephalitis and chronic thyroiditis are the best studied examples. The idea of autosensitization in connection with acquired hemolytic disease has gained acceptance in recent years. The disease may be either of the "warm antibody" type, as seen primarily in the older age groups, especially postmenopausal women, and in chronic lymphocytic leukemia patients; or of the "cold active" autoantibody type, which is characterized by intermittent massive hemolysis following exposure to coldness and affecting all age groups. One of the better known acquired hemolytic diseases is *cold agglutinin disease,* which commonly follows Eaton agent pneumonia. The onset of purpura and severe bleeding following the destruction, abnormal functional activity, or decreased life span of

platelets may, in some cases, be explained on an autoimmune basis. The platelet is capable of binding a multitude of foreign materials including viruses, bacteria, endotoxins, and so forth, which may alter it and render it antigenic. Several clinical investigators have suggested that allergic phenomena may play a role in some forms of headache, namely the classic migraine, cluster headaches, and those associated with allergic rhinitis. Indeed there are some clinicians who suspect some cases of epilepsy and Meniere's disease of having an allergic origin.

Control of allergic diseases involves interrupting the reaction before, during, or after functional impairment of tissues has occurred. While roentgen rays and radiometric drugs like nitrogen mustard have been useful in controlling the rejection of homografts, they are of limited usefulness. Cortisone and related compounds inhibit antibody production, relax smooth muscle, and suppress inflammation. While rheumatic fever, some types of acquired hemolytic disease, and rheumatoid arthritis respond dramatically to corticosteroid therapy, the results of such therapy in systemic lupus erythematosus, polyarteritis, polymyositis and dermatomyositis, scleroderma, Sjögren's syndrome, and the demyelinating diseases have not been as impressive or as long-lasting. Antihistamine drugs effectively inhibit by prior administration the bronchoconstrictor effect of releases of histamine. Their action during the allergic response or after it has taken place is limited. The sympathomimetic drugs such as epinephrine, isoproterenol, aminophylline, and others reverse the bronchoconstriction and stimulate cardiac function. The use of mild sedation such as that provided by the barbiturates is often a valuable adjunct to therapy.

CLINICAL CONSIDERATIONS

The broad, often indiscriminate, use of chemical agents and drugs by individuals for cosmetic, prophylactic, and therapeutic purposes and the accompanying marked increase in the incidence of allergic reactions in persons to these and related substances have made it imperative that the modern dental practitioner be well informed on the subject of reactions to chemicals. He must be able to differentiate drug hypersensitivity from drug intolerance or idiosyncrasy and from drug toxicity.

The most common manifestations of allergy to drugs and simple chemicals are skin eruptions varying from transient rashes or hives to serious exfoliative dermatitis and fever. A drug applied to the skin is much more allergenic than the same drug taken into the gastrointestinal tract. The presence of adjuvants of an oily or lipid nature tends to evoke focal tissue reactions and contributes to the intensity of contact and the degree of sensitization. The so-called inert materials, fillers, dyes, antiseptics, and flavoring agents in dental fillings, prosthetic materials, medicaments, dentifrices, denture adhesives, soaps, creams, mouthwashes, and so forth, are often-overlooked sources of drug allergy. Although various systemic manifestations of drug sensitivity have already been mentioned in this chapter, little has been said about the isolated or accompanying facial and oral lesions that may arise. The intraoral lesions are usually multiple, ranging from erythematous raised papules through vesicles and coalescing ulcers. In "fixed drug" eruptions, the eruptions reappear at the same location whenever the causative drug is taken. The tongue is a common site. The use of penicillin in an allergic individual, for example, may be accompanied by an angioneurotic edema about the eyes, chin, lips, or tongue within 5 to 20 minutes that may persist for 24 hours or several days. The site may itch or burn before swelling. Additionally, diffuse fiery red stomatitis and cheilitis may be present and even glossitis with subsequent loss of filiform papillae.

When no obvious oral lesion can be found to explain a cellulitis, the dentist should consider angioneurotic edema, among other clinical entities, to account for the acute swelling.

Occupational allergies of dental practitioners

Available surveys indicate that at one time or another about 3% of all dentists suffer from occupational allergic eczematous dermatitis. This condition threatens to be disabling to somewhat less than 1% of those in the profession. In 1949 the Council on Dental Therapeutics of the American Dental Association reported on the incidence of occupational dermatitis in some 750 members of the dental profession. All of the respondents believed that their dermatitis was related to one or more of the following materials used in dental practice in order of frequency: local anesthetics of the procaine and benzocaine family, soap, acrylic, roentgenographic solutions, formaldehyde, rubber or latex, phenolics, and quaternary ammonium compounds, namely benzalkonium chloride. In a survey of some 1,200 dentists one investigator reported that more than 6% appeared to have occupational allergic eczema since the fingers were involved in most of the cases. In my experience with dental students, the chief allergens encountered have been developing solutions, formaldehyde, hexachlorophene, methyl methacrylate monomer, and benzalkonium chloride (Fig. 10-3).

Although the reaction of skin sensitivity to local anesthetics used topically is usually apparent within 2 days, it may not appear for as many as 45 days. The local response may appear only as redness or itching. Continued application results in gradual extension of the lesions, with swelling, vesiculation, oozing, encrusting, and often marked discomfort. Other studies have named mercurials, antibiotics (especially penicillin), and iodine as offenders. The

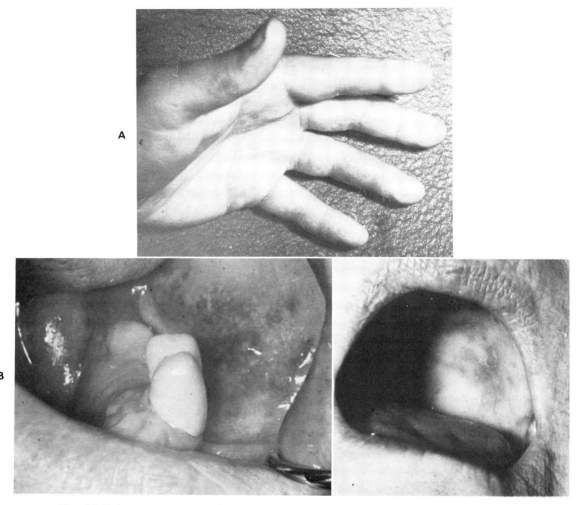

Fig. 10-3. In response to acrylic monomer, acute vesicular eruption and ulceration of **A,** palmar surface of fingers; **B,** buccal mucosa contacting temporary acrylic crowns; and **C,** palatal mucosa under relined denture.

use of skin tests, particularly patch tests and alternate exposure (avoidance and re-exposure), serves to prove the allergenic basis for the occupational dermatitis. Cross-sensitization to chemically related substances is common.

Hansen,[9] after studying more than 900 cases, stated that true hypersensitivity to soap does not exist. The few subjects in his study who seemed to be hypersensitive proved to react to the antiseptic, dye, filler, or perfume in the soap but not to

the soap itself. Other investigators concur with this conclusion.

In recent years a growing concern has been expressed by the dental profession about the health hazard that may result from the inhalation and fallout of the particulate matter, inanimate and viable, suspended in the aerosols generated by high speed drills. Aside from the frank infectious nature of the material and the possibility of respiratory, eye, and cutaneous infections, consideration should also be given to its potential irritant and antigenic properties. The increasing number of cases of rhinitis, coryza, and eczematous dermatitis among dentists and the circumstances leading to them can be explained only on the basis of hypersensitivity.

Since the likelihood of dermatitis increases with frequency and intensity of exposure, it becomes important to identify and avoid the responsible substance. If possible the dentist should use a drug with similar action but different chemical structure, for example lidocaine instead of procaine. He should also minimize contact with allergens by using rubber gloves or finger cots when possible and water-repellent "barrier" or "protective" creams.

Hypersensitivity in patients

Hypersensitive patients may develop a wide range of reactions, local and systemic, immediate and delayed, to dental procedures, materials, and medicaments.

Sensitivity to local anesthetics of the procaine and benzocaine group and related compounds is widespread. Kroll[14] described a patient who developed urticaria followed by pharyngeal edema 45 minutes after receiving an injection of procaine. Another patient died from anaphylactic shock after having used a lozenge containing benzocaine and tyrothricin. Although allergic reactions to lidocaine are rare, cases of anaphylactoid condition and even fatal anaphylaxis have been reported following the injection of 0.8 ml. of a 2% solution with 1 : 50,000 epinephrine. A magnificent example of cross-sensitization is described by Tzanck.[26] It seems that the patient applied picric acid to his shingles and developed a dermatitis. Some 15 years later he dyed his mustache and suffered from a dermatitis of his upper lip. He applied an ointment containing a local anesthetic to hemorrhoids and had a dermatitis of the anogenital region and thighs.

He applied an ointment containing a different anesthetic for epididymitis and developed a dermatitis of the scrotum. His dentist injected a local anesthetic before doing a dental procedure and the man suffered a dermatitis of the face. By patch test he was sensitive to picric acid, paraphenylenediamine, aniline, procaine, and a host of chemically related substances.

Pearson[20] reports six cases of allergic parotitis in which the swelling was caused by obstruction of the main duct. The six patients were all women of middle age or older, and the swellings had recurred for from 2 to 14 years. Each had a history of asthma or seasonal hay fever. The glandular swelling was bilateral and in half the cases the submaxillary glands were also affected. Swelling usually followed or accompanied the taking or smelling of food. It occurred daily for several years at a time and was accompanied by discomfort but no real pain. Inhalants were suspected in Pearson's cases and food sensitivity in three cases reported by Waldbott and Shea.[27]

Many allergists and dermatologists are concerned with the rising incidence of hypersensitivity to deodorants, detergents, and cosmetics. Nail lacquer, applied by half the women in the United States once or twice monthly, causes 36.6% of the observed cases of allergic manifestations in the cosmetic-dermatitis group. Permanent wave solutions cause 25.2%; hair dye and tint, 23.8%; and lipstick, 14.4% (Fig. 10-4). Four cases of allergic cheilitis associated with cigar smoking have been reported.

Karaya gum has been pinpointed as the offending allergen in some adhesive denture powders, ointments, and creams. Various constituents of dentures are reported to give rise to sensitization; rubber, acrylic, nickel, and cobalt are the major offenders. The so-called rubber sore mouth was attributable to the red and pink rubbers that contained vermilion (mercuric sulfide) as

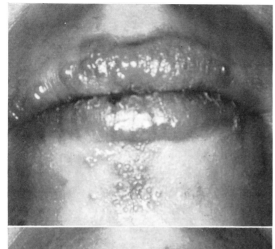

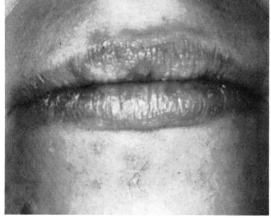

Fig. 10-4. **A,** Acute stage of contact allergy to lipstick. **B,** Ten days after acute vesicular eruption. (Courtesy Dr. Witkin, New York, N. Y.)

coloring matter; the use of carmine in place of vermilion overcame the problem. Miller[17] stressed the importance of taking a careful case history before making differential diagnosis between rubber sore mouth and other forms of stomatitis. In the cases reported by him, phenolphthalein was the offender in one instance, acetanilid in another, and uncontrolled diabetes in a third case. Most authorities agree that unpolymerized methyl methacrylate monomer is the chief offender in acrylic dentures, especially when self-curing materials are used (Figs. 10-5 to 10-7). This is a

very rare and unlikely problem, however, with the heat cured material. Since denture base materials can and do absorb and retain oral fluids and food residues, it is conceivable that these may act as irritants or allergens or both. It is the opinion of many investigators that the cure for inflamed denture-bearing tissues or burning sensations in the mouth is usually brought about by providing better fitting dentures and thus reducing trauma rather than by removing an allergen.

Untoward allergic responses to dentrifices are often attributed to the flavoring agent (usually an essential oil such as oil of anise), the antimicrobial agent, or an antienzyme. An investigator reported a case in which erythema, edema, and ulcerations of the buccal mucosa and tongue were induced by mint chewing gum. Although hypersensitivity to mercury is a relatively rare occurrence, the urticarial lesions can be relatively severe. In one case a boy 15 years old had six attacks of dermatitis affecting the mouth, eyelids, ears, and neck during a 12-month period.[23] He had used merbromin (Mercurochrome) or yellow oxide of mercury on each occasion. The seventh attack involved the hands, fingers, scrotum, and the face. The only clue to the problem was that he had had a tooth filled with amalgam before the last allergic episode. He gave positive skin reactions for merbromin, mercuric oxide, and fresh amalgam.

Another interesting case is that of a 32-year-old pregnant woman who suffered a severe eczematous skin reaction on the chin and neck following the insertion of two silver amalgam fillings.[4] The dermatitis increased and spread to the axillae and the inside of the arms a few days after additional fillings were inserted. It took from two to three weeks for the lesions to subside. Treatment was then postponed for 11 months at which point two fillings were inserted. A few hours later an eczematous reaction occurred, accompanied by oozing lesions and violent local itching. The patient responded positively to skin test of 0.1% mercuric chloride and the recently inserted two-week-old silver amalgam fillings. She took one of her children to the dentist and her eczema broke out again. Apparently there was enough mercury in the environment to elicit the allergic reaction. All of her amalgam fillings were subsequently removed and replaced with gold restorations. The possibility of an allergy to the local anesthetics and other materials used was excluded.

The influence of allergy on facial growth

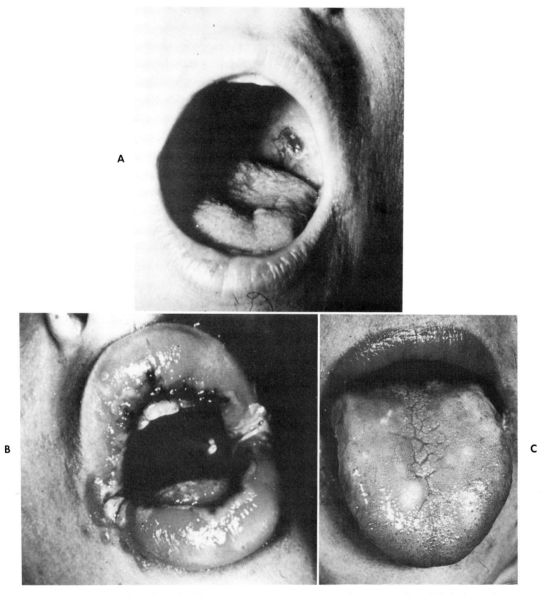

Fig. 10-5. Examples of oral allergic reactions to systemic drugs. **A,** Phenolphthalein; **B,** barbiturates; and **C,** gold salts.

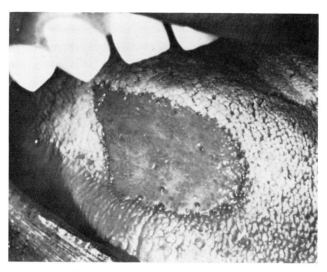

Fig. 10-6. Lingual glossitis from eugenol in a temporary filling. (Courtesy Dr. R. Moskow, New York. N. Y.)

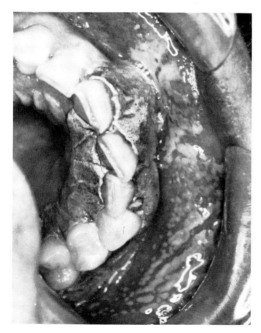

Fig. 10-7. Allergic patchy eruption of mucous membrane of upper lip in response to periodontal pack. (Courtesy Dr. R. Moskow, New York, N. Y.)

and development has received the attention of many investigators who agree that perennial nasal allergy interferes with the boney development of the nasal process of the maxilla, the anterior portion of the zygomatic arch, and the area over the antra. It also causes contraction of the anterior teeth. The phrases "mouth-breather," "adenoid face," and "allergic face" are often used to describe this condition. Hopkins[12] reported that a 12-year-old youngster developed a dermatitis from stainless steel orthodontic wire. Interestingly, the wire produced a skin reaction without any manifest oral mucosal reaction. Skin test reaction was positive to stainless steel.

Allergic reactions to drugs and antibiotics

The adverse response of patients to certain drugs and antibiotics deserves special attention. The oral lesions previously described that result from the ingestion or injection of drugs are collectively spoken

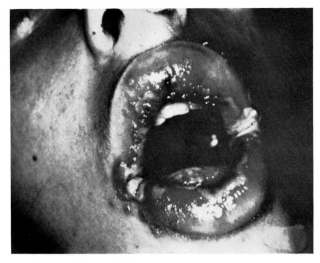

Fig. 10-8. Severe allergic stomatitis from barbiturate hypersensitivity. (Courtesy Dr. R. Moskow, New York, N. Y.)

of as *stomatitis venenata* (Fig. 10-8). Hypersensitivity to aspirin is well known; some 3% or 4% of individuals react to it and related compounds. In a series of 291 older asthmatic patients, 10% were aspirin-sensitive. Skin rashes are more commonly attributed to barbiturates than are respiratory manifestations. Edema of the tongue or epiglottis is a fairly frequent manifestation. Butler[2] recorded a case of hypersensitivity to meperidine in which urticaria and angioneurotic edema were followed by cyanosis and extreme hypotension; McDermott[16] cites the case of a patient who had a severe attack of asthma from meperidine. Photoallergic effects have been ascribed to several antihistamines which association results in the paradox of relieving and at the same time contributing to the occurrence of hypersensitivity. Anaphylaxis to chymotrypsin, a debriding agent widely used in oral surgery, has been reported, and oral eruptions of the fixed type have been reported following ingestion of meprobamate. It has been suggested that tic douloureux (trigeminal neuralgia) has an allergic basis and reported that antihistamine therapy and histamine desensitization brought permanent relief to 57% of the 183 patients studied.

Since the antibiotics, chiefly penicillin, are widely used in medical and dental practice and may be associated with a significant number of allergic responses, a detailed account of these will be presented. Since an anaphylactic reaction in some instances appears to be related to the inadvertent intravenous administration of the antibiotic, the practitioner must never fail to attempt aspiration before injection.

More than 500 tons of penicillin are produced annually, and more than one million injections are administered during a year. Some 6% to 8% of all individuals are allergic to penicillin, and between 90 and 125 people die each year from anaphylactic shock. Probably from five to ten times this number experience anaphylactoid shock. Penicillin is responsible for slightly more than 85% of the reactions attributed to antibiotics, mainly cases of angioneurotic edema and dermal lesions of the delayed type. Procaine penicillin G is involved in about 90% of all of the penicillin reactions, primarily because of its widespread use.

There are essentially five types of reactions to penicillin observed. The most common is the *delayed type* with an incubation period not shorter than 5 days and usually lasting from 7 to 14 days. The syndrome is serum sickness-like in nature with fever, urticaria, and arthralgia. The *immediate type,* far less common, occurs only in patients who have had penicillin some time previously. The reaction appears within seconds or perhaps a day or so and is characterized by pruritus, urticaria, angio-edema, dyspnea, asthma, or anaphylactic shock. The *hypoergic reaction* is a variety of the immediate type, showing more intense vascular and visceral involvement. The fourth type is the *erythematovesicular* or *"id-like" reaction* involving the hands, feet, and groin with an eczematous vesicular rash from one to three days after penicillin administration. The lesions represent an activation of sites previously sensitized by a dermatomycosis. *Contact dermatitis* occurs frequently in patients who are treated topically with the antibiotic and is an occupational hazard to persons who handle antibiotics. It has already been suggested that mild reactions may be treated with antihistamines, severe ones with epinephrine. Flare-up allergic reaction from the topical use of bacitracin and neomycin during endodontic treatment has been reported. The signs, which appeared in less than two hours, included a moderately severe eczema and an acute inflammation of the oral and pharyngeal mucosa. A similar reaction could be reproduced by giving neomycin orally to the same patient.

The dentist should be reminded that application of a finger rest during instrumentation or the mere act of retracting the lip before the administration of infiltration anesthesia may be sufficient to induce angioneurotic edema in a pressure-allergic individual.

Lastly, the contribution that hypersensitivity reactions and Shwartzman-like phenomena make to the pathogenesis of periodontal disease needs to be discussed. At present, evidence clearly identifying allergic phenomena as significant factors in the pathogenesis of gingival and periodontal pathosis is lacking. However, there are available some isolated observations and reasonable assumptions based upon an evaluation of the known interactive phenomena that appear to take place among the microbial populations of the periodontal pocket and between their metabolic products and the host. The erythema and edema associated with these tissues and the chronic inflammatory nature of the lesions and its infiltration with lymphocytic cells suggest an allergic response. Experimental animal studies indicate that the endotoxin of oral microorganisms is capable of inducing allergic sensitization and intermittent and remittent reactions of the Schwartzman type.

Patch tests

Several investigators have suggested that the oral mucous membranes are less reactive to allergic stimuli than is the skin, perhaps because of the diluting, absorbing, or neutralizing effect of the oral fluids. Whatever they may be, it is important to realize that many negative as well as false positive skin patch reactions can and do occur. The mucosal contact test, on the other hand, is carried out in the same environment in which the allergic reaction presumably has occurred and in which the dental material or appliance will be worn. If these tissues do not react to the test, it is unlikely that they will react to the constructed or placed material. Several methods have been proposed. Goldman and Goldman[6] suggest using a saucer-shaped rubber suction cup containing cotton moistened with the material in question; the cup is placed on the gingival tissues and attached to the adjacent teeth with dental floss. Farrington[3] described two modifications of that technique. One uses the cup attached to a denture appliance and in contract with the oral mucosa; the other, mainly for children, describes the use of a tightly rolled finger cot sutured with dental floss to a button and slipped between the teeth for retention. Jakobs[13] proposes painting soluble materials directly on the tissue and using heat softened plastic as a carrier for amalgam. Covering part of a denture for a period of time with a material impervious to contact with oral tissues, like tin foil, has been suggested by Nyquist.[19]

CITED REFERENCES AND ADDITIONAL READINGS

1. Billingham, R. E., and Silvers, W. K. (eds.): Transplantation of tissues and cells, Philadelphia, 1961, Wistar Institute Press.
2. Butler, L. B.: A case of hypersensitivity to pethidine in a woman in labor, Brit. Med. J. 2:715, 1951.
3. Farrington, J.: Modification of Goldman technique for contact testing of buccal mucosa, J. Invest. Derm. 8:59, 1947.
4. Fernstrom, A. I. B., Frykholm, K. O., and Huldt, S.: Mercury allergy with eczematous dermatitis due to silver-amalgam fillings, Brit. Dent. J. 55:204, 1962.
5. Freeman, S. O., and Fish, A. J.: The passive cellular transfer of delayed type hypersensitivity to intradermal procaine, J. Invest. Derm. 38:363, 1962.
6. Goldman, L., and Goldman, B.: Contact testing of buccal mucosa membrane for stomatitis venenata, Arch. Derm. 50:79, 1944.
7. Greenbaum, S. S.: Cheilitis venenata and allergy, Dent. Cosmos 75:768, 1933.
8. Hanes, W. J.: Clinical research on the etiology and treatment of tic douloureux on an allergic basis, Oral Surg. 23:728, 1967.
9. Hansen, P.: Einige Untersuchungen über die Einwirkung der Seife auf die Haut, Acta Dermatovener. 17:589, 1936.
10. Harkness, J. G.: Angular stomatitis and its association with artificial dentures, Brit. Med. J. 2:1,415, 1954.
11. Hesch, D. J.: Anaphylactic death from use of a throat lozenge, J.A.M.A. 172:12, 1960.
12. Hopkins, G. B.: A case of cutaneous sensitivity to stainless steel, Brit. Dent. J. 96:117, 1954.
13. Jakobs, F.: Über Epikutan- und Schleimhauttestungen, Derm. Wschr. 127:446, 1953.
14. Kroll, R. G.: Allergic reaction to local anesthetic, J. Oral Surg. 9:17, 1951.
15. Lawrence, H. S.: The cellular transfer of cutaneous hypersensitivity to tuberculin in man, Proc. Soc. Exp. Biol. Med. 71:516, 1949.
16. McDermott, T. F., and Papper, E. M.: Respiratory complications associated with demerol, New York J. Med. 50:1,721, 1950.
17. Miller, J. J.: The importance of case histories in making differential diagnosis between "rubber sore mouth" and other forms of stomatitis, Dent. Cosmos 75:357, 1933.
18. Mote, J. R., and Jones, T. D.: The development of foreign protein sensitization in human beings, J. Immun. 30:149, 1936.
19. Nyquist, G.: A study of denture sore mouth, Acta Odont. Scand. 9(suppl.):1-154, 1952.
20. Pearson, R. S. B.: Proceedings of First International Congress for Allergy, 1951, Basel, p. 868.
21. Pirila, V., and Rantanen, A. V.: Root canal treatment with bacitracin-neomycin as a cause of flare-up of allergic eczema, Oral Surg. 13:589, 1960.
22. Samter, M., and Alexander, H. L. (eds.): Immunological diseases, Boston, 1965, Little, Brown & Company.
23. Sedi, E., Casalis, F., and Longueville, L.: Dermatitis of face and scrotum due to dental amalgam fillings, Sem. Hop. Paris 30:1580, 1954.
24. Sugarman, M. M.: Contact allergy due to mint chewing gum, Oral Surg. 3:1145, 1950.
25. Turrell, A. J. W.: Allergy to denture-base materials—fallacy or reality, Brit. Dent. J. 120:415, 1966.
26. Tzanck, R. M.: Accidents cutanées pour sensibilisation à divers substances vontentant tautes une fonction amine premaire substituée en positionpara, Thèse no. 183, Paris, 1942, Librariea Louis Arnette.
27. Waldbott, G. L., and Shea, J. J.: Allergic parotitis, J. Allerg. 18:51, 1947.

11 / Focal infection

Infection refers to the ability of an organism to survive in a host for only a short period of time. If the organism can increase in number and produce sufficient quantities of toxic substances that affect the host in an abnormal way, a clinical change occurs and the condition is then referred to as disease. Infection may or may not result in disease, the outcome depending upon the resistance of the host and the virulence of the organism. The statement that man is sensitive to tuberculosis infection but resistant to the disease means that many people are infected with this organism but that their resistance is great and recognized disease does not develop. Infectious disease refers to those diseases caused by bacteria, fungi, viruses, PPLO forms, rickettsiae, and protozoa.

TYPES OF INFECTION

Various terms are used to describe types of infection. A *localized* infection is one in which the organism remains in or is confined to a particular area, as happens in pimples, abscesses, and boils. A *generalized* infection is one in which microorganisms invade the bloodstream and lymph circulation and spread through the body; examples are pyemia and miliary tuberculosis. A *mixed* infection involves more than one organism. For example, an individual may be infected with both the spirochete *Treponema pallidum* and the bacterium *Neisseria gonorrhoeae* simultaneously. Peri-

odontal disease may also be considered an example of a mixed infection because many different types of microorganisms appear to be involved.

An *acute* infection is one that runs a rapid course, is very serious, and generally terminates rather abruptly. Many of the common infectious diseases are of the acute type; typhoid fever is an example. In contrast, *chronic* infections are those that have a slow course. The symptoms are usually not severe, and the disease lasts for a long period of time. Tuberculosis in the adult is generally a chronic type of infection; periodontal disease might be considered a chronic infection also. Some infections are acute in the beginning but then change to a chronic nature, especially if not adequately treated.

Primary infection refers to the original infection; whereas *secondary* infection refers to one that follows and is generally caused by an opportunist. *Toxemia* refers to the presence of toxin in the bloodstream, as, for example, that condition resulting from infection with the diphtheria bacillus. *Latent* infection, such as brucellosis, is one in which the microorganism remains in a dormant state. *Subclinical* or *inapparent* infections usually occur naturally and are unrecognized; the symptoms may be so mild that the patient is not aware of having been infected. In such cases an individual develops antibodies to a disease which, to his knowledge, he has never had. The presence of antibodies to poliomyelitis in subjects who have never shown symptoms of polio infection is an example of subclinical infection. Superinfections are infections arising as the result of drug (broad-spectrum antibiotic) therapy. The drug may so greatly reduce the indigenous bacterial flora that nonsensitive organisms, such as *Candida albicans,* normally held in check by the bacterial flora, take over and cause serious infection difficult to treat. In other cases, antibiotic-resistant bacterial organisms such as *Proteus* in certain urinary infections might emerge as the result of broad-spectrum antibiotic therapy and might cause a superinfection. (See also Chapter 14.)

In general, *focal* infection refers to an infection localized in one part of the body, the focus, and disseminated elsewhere in the body. The term "focal infection" implies the metastasis or spread of microorganisms or their toxic products from chronic infected foci to other tissues where pathologic changes occur as the result of the toxin or the infecting organism. Other terms appearing in published materials that should be defined are bacteremia and septicemia. *Bacteremia* is the presence of bacteria in the circulating blood; *septicemia,* sometimes called blood poisoning, is a condition in which the organisms are actively multiplying in the bloodstream. Some authorities use the terms bacteremia and septicemia synonymously.

HISTORIC ASPECT OF STUDY OF INFECTION

The idea that infection may spread from the teeth and gums to other parts of the body was first presented in the United States by Benjamin Rush, a physician with the Continental Army. W. D. Miller, a dentist, in the 1890s stressed the important relationship of oral sepsis to diseases of other parts of the body. In the early 1900s the English physician William Hunter and the American physician F. Billings emphasized the apparent relationship between oral sepsis and bacterial endocarditis, osteomyelitis, nephritis, rheumatic fever, and other diseases. Oral sepsis includes dental decay, pyorrhea, and gingivitis. In addition to the teeth and gums, the tonsils were considered important foci of infection. Edward Rosenow's experimental work in the early 1920s emphasized the role of oral sepsis as the cause of diseases for which the physician had no explanation. Rosenow introduced the term "elective localization." His experiments led him to believe that streptococci acquired the trait of localizing in certain tissues. When streptococci isolated from root canals and apices of teeth of patients having nephritis, pains in the joints, appendicitis, and ulcers were cultured and injected into laboratory animals, the microorganisms colonized in similar organs in these animals. Rosenow's experimental work did much to incriminate the oral cavity as a focus of infection. During the next 20 to 30 years both physicians and dentists widely accepted the theory of focal infection. As a result, there were a great number of extractions of teeth and removals of appendices and tonsils, many of which were not infected but were thought to be the source of infection. With improvements in bacteriologic techniques, the work of Rosenow was questioned. He had frequently worked with mixed cultures and had injected large doses into the veins of animals. By comparison, it has been stated that the amount injected into animals would represent a pint of culture injected into man. Also, he had used cultures containing media that were probably responsible for some of the reactions he observed.[5]

Experiments in the 1940s demonstrated that when dyes or cultures of organisms are injected into the bloodstream of laboratory animals they localize in areas that have previously been injured, a phenomenon called anachoresis. The concept of focal infection was instrumental in helping to bring together the dentist and the physician in treating patients' conditions and in helping to elevate dentistry to the level of a scientific health service.

ORAL SOURCES OF BACTEREMIAS

Microorganisms may invade the bloodstream by several oral routes: (1) from carious lesions to the pulp and then to the blood, (2) by way of the periodontal pocket to the blood, (3) by surgical procedures such as the extraction of a tooth, and (4) by way of a fractured tooth. During the early part of the twentieth century it had not been common knowledge that microorganisms could invade the blood when a tooth was extracted.

Bacteremias are known now to follow almost all types of surgical procedures. Bacteremias of dental origin have been associated with rocking the tooth before extraction, periodontal scaling, gingivectomies, endodontic therapy, gingival massage, and administration of local anesthetics. The bacteremias are transitory in most instances; but there appears to be an association between the incidence of bacteremias and the degree of oral infection, especially periodontal disease. The importance of the microflora in the gingival crevice as a source of infection carried by the blood has been demonstrated by inoculating *Serratia marcescens* around the necks of teeth to be extracted. Recovery of this organism from the blood after tooth extraction shows that the gingival crevice is a source of bloodstream infection. The incidence of bacteremias following tooth extraction has been reported to vary between 50% and 85%. The organisms isolated most frequently are viridans streptococci. Transient bacteremias are of clinical importance because they may be the sources of bacterial growths in other tissues of the body through anachoresis. The relationship between oral infection and subacute bacterial endocarditis has thus been estab-

lished. Published reports cite cases that show a relationship between oral infection and chronic rheumatism and infection of the eyes, ears, and various tissues.

Bacteremias occurring after tooth extraction do not necessarily conform to the definition given for focus of infection. Nevertheless, the presence of microorganisms in the gingival crevice and the connection between these organisms and periodontal disease and periapical lesions constitute sepsis and appear to be a chronic infection. The highest incidence of bacteremias occurs following extraction of teeth from patients with periodontal disease. Brushing teeth is reported to yield positive blood cultures in approximately 24% of subjects having periodontal disease; chewing hard candy, in slightly more than 17%; and dental operations involving prophylactic treatment, 40%. Patients afflicted with periodontitis may show a positive bacteremia before prophylaxis is begun. As a result of subgingival scaling, positive blood cultures greatly increased. Finding a bacteremia before beginning any oral treatment indicates that periodontal disease may be involved in the sporadic spilling of microorganisms into the bloodstream. Therefore, this disease is instrumental in setting up bacteremias and may function as a focus of infection.

Technique for detecting bacteremias

The differences in percentages of positive blood cultures taken during various dental operations and during similar operations appear to be associated with the amount of blood drawn from the subject, the time interval between removing the blood and culturing it after the operation, the type of culture media used, and the conditions of anaerobiosis. If 45 ml. of blood is withdrawn from the subject and distributed among three rich culture media so that the ratio of blood to medium will greatly reduce the inhibitory action of the blood, a higher percentage of positive blood cultures should be obtained. With the use of this technique, postoperative positive blood cultures taken within five minutes were found in 82% of extraction cases and in 88% of periodontal patients after periodontal procedures were done. Of the organisms isolated from these two groups, 37% were identified as streptococci and 33% as diphtheroids.[12] Other microorganisms isolated are listed in Table 11-1.

A recent investigation supports the technique of using more than one type of culture medium in studying bacteremias.

Table 11-1. Approximate percentages of genera of bacteria isolated from blood following extractions and periodontal treatment*

Organisms	Periodontal cases	Extraction cases
Bacteroides	12	8
Gaffkya	8	6
Spirillum	4	4
Vibrio	2	2
Actinomyces	14	6
Micrococcus	2	2
Fusobacterium	14	0
Veillonella	10	0
Leptotrichia	2	0
Unidentified anaerobes	4	4

*Modified from Rogosa, M., Hampp, E. G., Nevin, T. A., Wagner, H. N., Jr., Driscol, E. J., and Baer, P. N.: J. Amer. Dent. Assoc. **60**:171, 1960.

The investigation shows that the addition of sodium polyanetholesulfonate to culture media inhibits the antibacterial activity of the blood and increases sensitivity. This material is an anticoagulant, it inactivates blood complement, and it has been reported to interfere with the phagocytic activity of leukocytes. Large volumes of blood, 16 ml. to 24 ml., cultured in aliquots of 4 ml. gave evidence of a greater number of bacteremias than did small volumes. Table 11-2 presents results of blood samples cultured in brain heart infusion broth, some taken immediately and others taken 10 minutes following extractions. The addition of the sodium polyanetholesulfonate increases the sensitivity of the blood culture media. Of the media, brain heart infusion broth with the antibacterial inhibitor appeared to be somewhat more sensitive than were trypticase or thioglycollate under conditions of this test (Table 11-3). Of the organisms cultured, viridans streptococci were recovered in the highest percentage of specimens.[2]

It is reported that bacteremias generally last for about 10 minutes. If blood samples are taken at times later than 10 minutes following certain types of dental operations and depending also upon the oral hygiene of the patient, the samples very well might be culturally negative, according to some investigators. The length of time cultures may remain positive will de-

Table 11-2. The effect of blood volume, Liquoid, and multiple aliquots on the number of positive blood cultures in forty-three cases detected with brain heart infusion broth*

Volume of blood (ml.)†	Number of aliquots	Percentage of positive		Volume of blood (ml.)†	Number of aliquots	Percentage of positive	
		Immediate	10 Minutes			Immediate	10 Minutes
4	Single	53.9‡	24.4‡	8 + L	Single	80.1	37.2
4 + L	Single	73.2‡	36.0‡	16 + L	Three	88.3	51.1
8	Two	67.4	34.9	24 + L	Five	88.3	58.1
8 + L	Two	81.4	48.8				

*From Bender, I. B., Seltzer, S., Meloff, G., and Pressman, R. S.: J. Dent. Res. **40**:951, 1961.
†L = Sodium polyanetholesulfonate (Liquoid)
‡Average for two 4-ml. samples

Table 11-3. Comparative incidence of bacteremia in multiple extractions following use of various media*

Study†	Media‡	Volume of blood (ml.)	Immediately after extraction			10 Minutes after extraction	
			Number of cases	Number of positive	Percentage positive	Number of positive	Percentage positive
1	B.H.I. + L.	8	50	40	80.0	15	30.0
1	Thio.	2	27	17	62.9	3	11.1
1	Thio. + L.	8	20	10	50.0	4	20.0
2	B.H.I. + L.	10	31	23	74.2	6	20.0§
2	Trypticase	10	29	11	37.9	2	7.1**
3	B.H.I. + L.	24	43	38	88.8	25	58.1
a	B.H.I. + L.	10	22	11	50.0	5	22.7
a	Trypticase	10	22	7	31.8	3	13.6

*From Bender, I. B., Seltzer, S., Meloff, G., and Pressman, R. S.: J. Dent. Res. **40**:951, 1961.
†a From another study in which single extractions were performed
‡B.H.I. = Brain heart infusion broth; Thio. = Thioglycollate; L = Liquoid (sodium polyanetholesulfonate)
§Based on thirty cases
**Based on twenty-eight cases

Table 11-4. Incidence of bacteremia following endodontic manipulation*

Procedure	Number of cases	Immediately after manipulation		10 Minutes after manipulation	
		Number positive	Percentage positive	Number positive	Percentage positive
Group A					
Within root canal	26	0	0.0	0	0.0
Group B					
Beyond root canal	24	6	25.0	0	0.0
Total	50	6	12.0	0	0.0

*From Bender, I. B., Seltzer, S., and Yermish, M.: Oral Surg. **13**:353, 1960.

Table 11-5. Comparative incidence of bacteremia following exodontic and endodontic procedures*

Procedure	Number of cases positive	Immediately after procedure		10 Minutes after procedure	
		Number positive	Percentage positive	Number positive	Percentage positive
Exodontic	93	79	84.9	41	44.1
Endodontic	50	6	12.0	0	0

*From Bender, I. B., Seltzer, S., and Yermish, M.: Oral Surg. **13**:353, 1960.

pend upon the numbers of organisms that spill into the blood, the efficiencies of the reticuloendothelial cells, and the immune reactions of the host.

Importance of bacteremias following dental procedures

In prophylaxis given periodontal patients there is no significant difference between the incidence of bacteremia produced by ultrasonics and that produced by hand instrumentation.[4] Reports concerning the incidence of bacteremia in endodontic manipulation indicate that if endodontic treatment is kept within the confines of the root canal no bacteremia is likely to develop; however, when those manipulations are performed beyond the apex of the root canal, positive blood cultures may be obtained immediately after the manipulation is done (Table 11-4). A comparison of the percentages of occurrences of bacteremia following endodontic and exodontic procedures shows that the extraction of teeth can result in a sevenfold increase in bacteremias over endodontic procedures. After 10 minutes, no bacteria were detected in the blood of endodontic subjects, although about 52% of the blood specimens were still positive for the exodontic subjects (Table 11-5). These results indicate that endodontic procedures are the safer and the treatment of choice for patients with valvular heart disease.[3] There are no case reports of subacute bacterial endocarditis following endodontic treatment.

Various studies concerning the causes of bacterial endocarditis have indicated that from 10% to approximately 50% of such cases are probably related to dental focus or previous dental extraction. It is now generally accepted as good medical practice to administer antibiotics prophylactically to patients with congenital or rheumatic valvular heart disease before performing extractions and other dental manipulations. Cases of bacterial endocarditis have been known to follow dental prophylaxis and tooth restoration. Close cooperation between the dentist, the patient, and the physician is important for prevention of bacterial endocarditis. Alpha streptococci have been associated with from 75% to 85% of cases of bacterial endocarditis. Of the streptococci isolated from the blood of patients with subacute bacterial endocarditis, it is reported that S. *mitis* was cultured from 23% of the subjects, S. *salivarius* from about 9%, and an organism identified as S. *sanguis* from 44%. *Streptococcus sanguis* is synonymous with *Streptococcus s.b.e.*[7, 14]

Unless there is a focus of infection, bacteremias traceable to alpha streptococci are unlikely to occur in an edentulous patient. It has been reported that poor fitting dentures can cause ulcers, which may become infected with alpha streptococci and act as a focus of infection. Case reports have shown that apical foci of upper lateral incisors have caused visual disturbances; restoration of vision has resulted when the infection was eliminated following root canal treatment. Published reports record cases in which gross dental sepsis appeared to be associated with arthritis of the hip. Clinical improvement was noted when the oral focus was removed.[13] Bacteremias have been reported to occur after extraction of teeth when either general or local anesthesia has been administered. Results of a study gave no evidence that subjects clinically free of inflammatory periodontal disease or having gingivitis or periodontitis suffered a bacteremia as a result of using an oral water irrigation device after brushing their teeth.[12]

Since bacteria present in the sulcus are considered the main source of bacteremias, the elimination or suppression of gingival sulcus bacteria should result in the reduction in bacteremias. Numerous studies have been carried out in an attempt to determine what measures may be effective in preventing bacteremias that follow dental procedures. Application of an iodine

Summary of chemoprophylaxis against bacterial endocarditis.*

Group I. *Standard chemoprophylaxis. Day of Procedure.* Procaine penicillin, 600,000 units crystalline penicillin, intramuscularly, 1 or 2 hours before procedure. If oral penicillin is to be employed, four doses (every 4 to 6 hours) of at least 0.25 gm. of alpha-phenoxymethyl penicillin (penicillin V), 0.25 gm. of alpha-phenoxyethyl penicillin (phenethicillin), or 500,000 units of buffered penicillin G should be given during the day of the procedure. In addition, an extra dose should be given 1 hour before the procedure.

For 2 days after procedure. Procaine penicillin, 600,000 units intramuscularly each day. In selected instances 0.25 gm. of alpha-phenoxymethyl penicillin (penicillin V), 0.25 gm. of alpha-phenoxyethyl penicillin (phenethicillin), or 500,000 units of buffered penicillin G four times daily by mouth may be prescribed for those patients in whom full cooperation is anticipated and ingestion is assured.

Group II. *Patients receiving small prophylactic doses of penicillin.*
A. With physician's consent, discontinue the penicillin for 48 hours; then treat as Group I.
B. Penicillin G, 2 million units, and streptomycin, 0.5 gm. 1 hour before procedure, followed by 2 million units of penicillin per day plus 0.5 gm. of streptomycin intramuscularly every 12 hours for 3 days.
C. 500 mg. cephaloridine (Loridine) intramuscularly 1 hour before procedure, followed in 6 hours by 250 mg. of erythromycin four times a day for 3 days.

Group III. *Patients sensitive to penicillin.* Initially, erythromycin estolate 500 mg. by oral administration 2 hours before the operation; followed in 6 hours by the oral administration of erythromycin estolate 250 mg. and continued thereafter at 6-hour intervals for 3 days.

Group IV. *Children.* The same dosage and duration of penicillin as recommended for adults. If erythromycin has to be used, a dose of 20 mg. per pound of body weight per day should be given, divided into three or four evenly spaced doses but not to exceed 1 gm. per day.

*Adapted from Myall, R. W. T., and Gregory, H. S.: Oral Surg. **28**:813, 1969.

lotion to the periodontal pocket five minutes before scaling was found to eliminate or greatly reduce the incidence of bacteremias. Treatment done before extraction, employing a phenolated antiseptic mouthwash for 30 seconds followed by gingival sulcus irrigation with the rinse, significantly reduced postoperative bacteremias. A 72.7% reduction in bacteremias was noted as compared to no reduction for the control goup, who had no oral rinse or sulcus irrigation. The use of saline as a rinse and sulcus irrigant was effective in bringing about a 29.5% reduction in bacteremias as compared to no reduction for the control group. As an added protection against transitory bacteremias, this preoperative treatment is recommended for all exodontic procedures.[6]

Patients whose history indicates that they are susceptible to subacute endocarditis, chiefly those with rheumatic and congenital heart disease, acquired heart valve abnormalities, or prosthetic cardiovascular appliances, should prophylactically be given antibiotics before and during

exodontic, periodontal, and traumatic endodontic treatment. Penicillin is the drug
of choice, but erythromycin is recommended for subjects who are sensitive to
penicillin.[8]

Some authorities believe that the administration of antibiotics for several days
before dental procedures are done could
create a resistant microbial flora that could
cause a form of bacterial endocarditis difficult to treat. Therefore, it is suggested
that the first dose of the antibiotic be
given at an interval before the dental procedure (such as extraction) is done in
order to create the highest blood level
of the antibiotic at the time of the procedure.

This procedure follows closely the antibiotic treatment schedule suggested by
the American Heart Association.[1]

Even though antibiotics are available,
there still remains a substantial mortality
of about 25%. When infection is thought
to be cured by early institution of therapy,
congestive cardiac failure, cerebral in-
farction, or renal insufficiency can cause
disability and shorten life.[8]

For the last 15 to 20 years, clinical experience coupled with better microbiologic
techniques have had a controlling effect
on the application of the focal infection
theory. When the presence of oral foci is
known for certain, especially in those subjects having a chronic systemic disease, the
foci should be removed. In one instance
removal of an impacted maxillary molar
resulted in the rapid recovery of a patient
with iritis. Physical examinations had
showed nothing significant; but roentgenograms of the mouth showed an area of infection around the upper right third impacted molar. A positive agglutination test
result for *Brucella abortus* was found. At
removal of the tooth, from a follicle of
gelatinous substance *B. abortus* was isolated. With the administration of streptomycin and sulfadiazine rapid recovery followed.[9]

The pathogenesis of focal infection is
not yet completely understood. It has been
suggested that the origin concerns infection allergy and autoimmunity. In the case
of dental foci, microorganisms per se and
tissue products resulting from their growth
may persist for a long time. This could
possibly sensitize the system with these
antigens and result in focal infection. Clinically, many investigators have demonstrated that the body can be sensitized
by products of dental foci, which result
in allergic response in the oral region.[10]

CITED REFERENCES

1. American Heart Association: Prevention of
   bacterial endocarditis, Circulation **31**:953,
   1965.
2. Bender, I. B., Seltzer, S., Meloff, G., and
   Pressman, R. S.: Conditions affecting sensitivity of techniques for detection of bacteremia, J. Dent. Res. **40**:951, 1961.
3. Bender, I. B., Seltzer, S., and Yermish, M.:
   The incidence of bacteremia in endodontic
   manipulation, Oral Surg. **13**:353, 1960.
4. Brandt, C. L., Korn, N. A., and Schaffer,
   E. M.: Bacteremias from ultrasonic and hand
   instrumentation, J. Periodont. **34**:214, 1964.
5. Grossman, L. I.: Focal infection. Are oral
   foci of infection related to systemic disease?
   Dent. Clin. N. Amer. 749, Nov. 1960.
6. Jones, J. C., Cutcher, J. L., Golbert, J. R.,
   and Lilly, G. E.: Control of bacteremia associated with extraction of teeth, Oral Surg.
   30:454, 1970.
7. Loewe, L., Plummers, N., Niven, C. F., Jr.,
   and Sherman, J. M.: Streptococcus s.b.e. in
   subacute bacterial endocarditis, J. A. M. A.
   130:257, 1946.
8. Myall, R. W. T., and Gregory, H. S.: Current
   trends in the prevention of bacterial endocarditis in susceptible patients receiving
   dental care, Oral Surg. **28**:813, 1969.
9. Newman, C. W.: Removal of impacted molar
   assists in diagnosis of brucellosis J. Amer.
   Dent. Assoc. **39**:754, 1949.
10. Okada, H., Aono, A., Yoshida, M., Mune-
    moto, K., Nishida, O., and Yokomizo, I.:
    Experimental study on focal injection in
    rabbits by prolonged sensitization through
    dental pulp canals, Arch. Oral Biol. **12**:1017,
    1967.
11. Rogosa, M., Hampp, E. G., Nevin, T. A.,
    Wagner, H. N., Jr., Driscol, E. J., and
    Baer, P. N.: Blood sampling and cultural

studies in the detection of postoperative bacteremias, J. Amer. Dent. Assoc. **60:**171, 1960.

12. Tamimi, H. A., Thomassen, P. R., and Moser, E. H., Jr.: Bacteremia study using a water irrigation device, J. Periodont.-Periodontics, **40:**424, 1969.
13. Weinstein, I., and Linz, A. M.: Infectious arthritis of the hip due to dental foci of infection, Oral Surg. **12:**83, 1959.
14. White, J. C., and Niven, C. F.: Streptococcus s.b.e. A streptococcus isolated with subacute bacterial endocarditis, J. Bact. **51:**717, 1946.

REFERENCES AND ADDITIONAL READINGS

Bartels, H. A.: The bacteriologist's view of focal infection, New York Dent. J. **19:**199, 1953.

Cobe, H. M.: Transitory bacteremia, Oral Surg. **7:**609, 1954.

Danielewicz, K., and Tarcynska, I.: Bacteremia after tooth extraction performed under general anesthesia and local anesthesia, Cesk. Stomat. **16:**147, 1963.

Dephilippe, J. L.: Diseases of the eyes caused by the upper lateral incisor, Med. Hyg. **20:**441, 1962.

Francis, L. E., deVries, J. A., Soomsawasdi, P., and Platonow, M.: Control of postextraction bacteremias with penicillin, J. Canad. Dent. Assoc. **28:**683, 1962.

Gutverg, M., and Haberman, S.: Studies on bacteremia following oral surgery: Some prophylactic approaches to bacteremia and the results of tissue examination of excised gingiva, J. Periodont. **33:**105, 1962.

Hampp, E. G.: Blood sampling and cultural studies in the detection of postoperative bacteremias, Proc. Inst. Med. Chicago **22:**314, 1959.

Harvey, W. P., and Capone, M. A.: Bacterial endocarditis related to cleaning and filling of teeth with particular reference to the inadequacy of present day knowledge and practice of antibiotic prophylaxis for all dental procedures, Amer. J. Cardiol. **7:**793, 1961.

Kassel, V.: Psychosomatic dentistry and medicine, Zahnaerztl. Rundsch. **71:**7, 1962.

Kraus, F. W., Casey, D. W., and Johnson, V.: The classification of nonhemolytic streptococci recovered from bacteremia of dental origin, J. Dent. Res. **32:**613, 1953.

Lazansky, J. P., Robinson, L., and Rodofsky, L.: Factors influencing the incidence of bacteremias following surgical procedures in the oral cavity, J. Dent. Res. **28:**533, 1949.

Leinback, R. C.: Bacterial endocarditis prophylaxis: Theory and practice, J. Dent. Med. **20:**66, 1965.

Losli, E. J., and Lindsey, R. H.: Fatal systemic diseases from dental sepsis—report of two cases, Oral Surg. **16:**366, 1963.

McGavic, J. S.: The relationship of oral infection to the eye, Dent. Clin. N. Amer. 527, July 1958.

Massaro, D., and Katz, S.: Subacute bacterial endocarditis in an edentulous man, New Eng. J. Med. **263:**911, 1960.

Müller, E. H.: Bacteremia after tooth extraction, Schweiz Mschr. Zahnheilk. **72:**283, 1962.

Robinson, H. B. G., and Boling, L. R.: The anachoretic effect in pulpitis. I. Bacteriologic studies, J. Amer. Dent. Assoc. **28:**268, 1941.

Schirger, A., Martin, W. J., Royer, R. Q., and Needham, G. M.: Bacterial invasion of blood following oral surgical procedures, Mayo Clinic. Proc. **35:**618, 1960.

Vargas, B., Collings, C. K., Palter, L., and Haberman, S.: Effects of certain factors on bacteremias resulting from gingival reaction, J. Periodont. **30:**196, 1959.

Winslow, M. B., and Kobernick, S. D.: Bacteremia after prophylaxis, J. Amer. Dent. Assoc. **61:**69, 1960.

Winslow, M. B., and Millstone, S. H.: Bacteremia after prophylaxis, J. Periodont. **36:**371, 1965.

12 / Microbial considerations in specialty areas of dental practice

In considering the role of microorganisms in specialty areas, we are concerned with their relation to diseases of the oral cavity and the general health of man. The specialties to be considered are: restorative dentistry, exodontics, prosthodontics, orthodontics, pedodontics, periodontics, preventive dental medicine, and endodontics.

This chapter should be of special interest to the dental student because it emphasizes the practical aspects of microbiology and shows why knowledge of this science is vital to modern dental practice. It should be of interest also to the practicing dentist because it should create in him a desire to refresh his knowledge of microbiology and make him more cognizant of the role that microorganisms play in his daily practice.

RESTORATIVE DENTISTRY
Microorganisms in the dentin of carious teeth

Carious dentin that has lost its structure and become soft contains many different types of microorganisms. It was reported in the early 1890s by W. D. Miller that microorganisms penetrate normal dentin beyond the area of decay. It has more recently been reported that a layer of partially decalcified dentin between carious and sound dentin is usually free of micro-

organisms and that in arrested caries this area is sterile. There is good evidence that microorganisms may penetrate at least to a depth of 1 mm. in sound dentin. Because of this fact it is questioned whether these microorganisms might not be instrumental in causing secondary decay in a tooth that has been restored. Whether the organisms in sound dentin tubules can continue to multiply under fillings would determine their role in secondary decay; also it would determine their importance in causing infection of the pulp. The size of dental tubules is such that the lumen at the dentin and enamel junction approximates 1 μ in diameter, and as the tubules approach the pulp they widen and reach a diameter of approximately 4 μ. From these dimensions, it can be concluded that microorganisms should be able to grow from the carious lesion through dental tubules to the pulp chamber.

In vitro tests showed that when *Serratia marcescens* and a strain of alpha streptococci were inoculated onto a section of freshly cut occlusal dental tubules, they could penetrate the tubules and could be isolated from the pulp chamber within several days.

Studies on the fate of bacteria sealed within dental tubules indicated that they do not multiply in a hermetically restored tooth. These organisms may remain viable in a latent state for periods longer than a year. It has been reported that when some decay was left in teeth covered with gutta-percha and sealed with zinc oxyphosphate cement, streptococci could be isolated from some teeth after 18 months.[6] Other reports show streptococci and lactobacilli to survive 26 months in carious dentin lined with a nonantiseptic base and sealed with amalgam.[1] When calcium hydroxide or zinc oxide and eugenol was used as a liner, organisms died quickly.[2, 25] This suggests that these lining materials create a better sealing of the cavity from mouth organisms than do filling materials and, in addition, may exhibit some degree of antimicrobial activity.[14] The condition in the restored tooth is such that there is free moisture and readily available nutrients sufficient only for microorganisms to metabolize slowly at a gradually decreasing rate until death. Although there is no evidence of increased growth, the role of organisms sealed under restorations in renewing caries activity and spreading to the pulp by way of the tubules must be considered.

CAVITY STERILIZING AGENTS

Should the prepared cavity be treated with a sterilizing agent as a routine procedure before being filled? Cavity sterilization is considered necessary and desirable by some workers, while others consider it an unnecessary step in tooth restoration. Chemical agents have been used to sterilize the dentin for more than 75 years. W. D. Miller observed that phenol required 45 minutes to sterilize a 1-mm. depth of dentin. Other workers have shown that a three-minute exposure with 95% liquid phenol was ineffective in destroying microorganisms in dentin. Aqueous silver nitrate solution was reported to sterilize carious dentin to a depth of 0.7 mm. within three minutes and 1.3 mm. within 10 minutes.[50] An evaluation of some of the common antiseptics used in cavity sterilization shows that they are ineffective in sterilizing dentin, to any depth, in three minutes. Such compounds as silver nitrate, iodine, chloramine-T, phenol, beechwood creosote, benzalkonium preparations (Zephiran), ethyl alcohol, benzethonium preparations (Phemerol), and 30% hydrogen peroxide were found to sterilize only the surface of the dentin. The failure to sterilize dentin beyond the surface is perhaps the result of adsorption, precipitation, and coagulation of the organic matter of the tooth. This would indicate that the sterilization of deep dentin is definitely not achieved.

The practice of cavity sterilization may lead the dentist to become less rigid in removing all discolored dentin. For deep cavities close to the pulp, he may rely on the germicide to kill the organisms that remained. In such cases the use of silver nitrate could result in irritation of the pulp and in pulp necrosis. The whole purpose of restoring the tooth and maintaining its viability would be defeated if this occurred. The idea that phenol and silver nitrate block dental tubules by coagulation of inorganic matter was refuted by studies using radioactive tracers. The results of these studies showed that phenol and silver nitrate diffuse rapidly through the tubules.

In discussing the presence of microorganisms in sound dentin and the effect that cavity sterilizing agents might have on these microorganisms, mention should be made as to the effect that dental filling materials might have. In vitro tests have shown that the various filling materials including silicous cement, zinc oxide and eugenol, copper amalgam, gold foils, zinc phosphate cement, copper cement, silver amalgams, and gold inlays all inhibit cultures of *Staphylococcus aureus, Escherichia coli, Candida albicans, Lactobacillus,* and others. Filling materials appear to have a bactericidal action only until they have set. The cements require several hours to set; silver amalgam may require several weeks. Copper amalgam has the

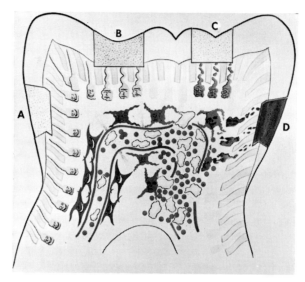

Fig. 12-1. Diagrammatic representation of the reaction of the pulp to filling materials. Material used in **A** was zinc oxide and eugenol; in **B**, crown and bridge cement; in **C**, silicate cement; and in **D**, copper cement. Injury of the pulp has been shown to lead to anachoretic pulpitis. (Courtesy Dr. S. S. Arnim, Houston, Tex.)

most powerful antibacterial activity. Silicous cement appears to have a residual antibacterial effect, probably because of its high fluoride content. This effect is noted by the lack of secondary caries about the margins of a tooth and the silicous restorative material. The fluoride is thought to react with adjoining enamel and dentin and thus reduce the enamel's solubility to acids. Zinc oxide and eugenol is the only filling material that has been shown to exhibit, in vitro, an inhibitory effect even after setting. Tests showed that zinc oxide and eugenol was effective in sterilizing completely infected slabs of dentin 1 mm. thick after contact for from 24 to 48 hours. Natural decay from extracted carious teeth was found resistant to the sterilizing effect of this material. Zinc oxide and eugenol was reported by some investigations to be bacteriostatic rather than bactericidal because of its hygroscopic property. Clinically its use in deep cavities suggests a sedative and bacteriostatic effect. (See Fig. 12-1.)

Marginal leakage

It is well known that there is marginal leakage between filling material and the tooth enamel. Radioisotope tracers have demonstrated the seepage of fluids between cavity walls and restorative material. This leakage may account for some of the postoperative sensitivity, marginal breakdown, and secondary caries which occur in teeth that have been filled.

Gold foil fillings and gold inlays appear clinically to be the most dependable restorations in the role of a sealing barrier and in the withstanding of the stress and strain of mastication. Amalgam restorations do not adhere well to tooth structure, and seepage of fluid between the restoration and the cavity preparation is considerable during the first few days after insertion.[37] The leakage, nevertheless, decreases markedly as the restoration ages. Very little or no leakage is observed for amalgam restorations after several months in the oral cavity. It is thought that the reduction in marginal leakage of amalgam restorations is associated with the accumulation of corrosive products, such as silver sulfite, that form at the interface of the restoration and the tooth. These products fill in this area and block the penetration of seepage fluids. Much of the clinical success in minimizing recurrent carries is possibly associated with this property of amalgam.

Clinical experience has shown that resin restorations have a very high thermal coefficient of expansion, do not prevent marginal leakage, and have no germicidal or anticariogenic effect. Gutta-percha has no antibacterial effect, does not form a good seal, and is not a good filling material. Calcium hydroxide has been shown to have a germicidal effect in in vitro tests. Calcium hydroxide or zinc oxide and eugenol, when used in the treatment of teeth by indirect capping, has been shown to bring about either sterility or a great reduction in the number of organisms in the residual carious dentin. Silver amalgam under the same conditions fails to produce sterility but does result in microbial reduction. Such restorations are considered clinically successful. Sodium or stannous fluoride incorporated into zinc oxide–eugenol reduces enamel solubility in vitro and may possess anticariogenic activity in vivo.[53]

Cavity varnishes

In order to help reduce or prevent the leakage around restorations such as silver amalgam, silicate, or foil, special types of varnishes have been applied to the walls and floor of the cavity preparation before insertion of the restorative material. Some studies using dyes and radioisotopes to determine leakage indicated that the application of cavity varnishes definitely reduced marginal leakage. The reduction in marginal leakage could therefore minimize postoperative sensitivity and also help in preventing recurrent caries. On the other hand, other results showed that the varnish might actually increase leakage under silver amalgam restorations. A recent study reported essentially no difference in preventing leakage to bacteria when cavity-lined silver amalgam restorations were compared with controls. Differences in the thermal coefficient of expansion of the amalgam restorative material, the varnish, and the tooth probably affect the adhesive quality of the varnish and explain this result.

Other investigations showed that varnishes decrease marginal penetration when the restoration is silicous cement. Silicous cement has a thermal expansion that is similar to that of the dentinal structure, whereas the thermal expansion of amalgam is given as nearly twice as great.

Restorative material plus antibiotics

The incorporation of antibiotics into certain dental materials has been investigated with specific reference to their use as cavity liners in deep carious lesions. The incorporation with zinc silicate cement of the antibiotics aureomycin, bacitracin, chloromycetin, streptomycin, and of combinations of penicillin, bacitracin, and streptomycin demonstrated increased bactericidal activity in vitro. The addition of a polyantibiotic consisting of dihydrostreptomycin, chloromycetin, aureomycin, and bacitracin to lithium cement used in restorations showed that the antibiotics inhibit growth in 93% of the restorations, whereas the lithium cement control showed inhibition in only 13%.

Antibiotics when incorporated into zinc oxide and eugenol and into zinc oxyphosphate cement show antibacterial effect (Fig. 12-2). A mixture of penicillin and camphorated parachlorophenol is effective in treating deep-seated cavities.

It has been observed that the incorporation of terramycin into zinc oxide and eugenol cement usually hastens the setting time and increases the crushing strength.

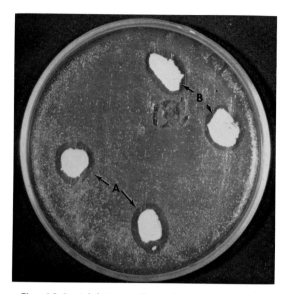

Fig. 12-2. Inhibitory effect of samples of zinc oxide and eugenol with and without penicillin. Zinc oxide and eugenol containing 250 units of penicillin were mixed to the proper consistency and held for 96 hours at room temperature. This material was tested in duplicates for antibacterial effect by the agar plate method. Samples *A* and *B* both showed inhibition zones for *Staphylococcus aureus.* Sample *A* containing penicillin showed a slightly wider zone than control sample *B.*

The incorporation of terramycin into silver amalgam, zinc oxyphosphate cement, and zinc oxide and eugenol appears to have no deleterious effect on the physical properties of these materials.

Antibiotic cements have been used for the past five years in pulp capping and no allergic reactions have been reported.

Resins plus bacteriostatic chemicals

A recent study showed that the cold cure acrylic resins—methyl methacrylate, polyethylene, styrol, nylon, cellulose acetate, polyvinylchloride, and other acrylic and phenolic resins—upon polymerization are bacteriostatically inert.

The incorporation of various bacteriostatic agents, including quinine hydrochloride, mercurous chloride, cadmium chloride,

silver chloride, proflavine, thymol iodine, silver proteninate, ethyl violet, and a mixture containing benzyl ammonium chlorides, propylene glycol, and boric acid, showed that the benzyl ammonium chlorides mixture in high dilution imparted a bacteriostatic property only to methyl methacrylate. Most of the bacteriostatic agents were found to be ineffective in inducing microbial inhibition when added to the acrylic resins.

In vitro tests show a fungistatic action for *Candida albicans* for the methyl methacrylate-benzyl ammonium chlorides mixture. This suggests its possible use in the denture base acrylic resin for preventing and for treating cases of denture sore mouth.

It was recently reported that an adhesive material applied to deciduous and permanent teeth and exposed to ultraviolet light, to induce hardening, resulted in 100% protection against cavities after one year.[7] After two years, 87% of the permanent teeth showed complete adhesive coverage and a 99% reduction in caries. For the same period, an 87% reduction in caries was noted for the deciduous teeth with only 50% tooth surface adhesive coverage. Use of the adhesive sealant makes available a simple procedure that appears promising in caries prevention.[8]

PREVENTIVE DENTISTRY
Oral hygiene

The relationship between material accumulated about the teeth and dental disease was recognized by early investigators. Preventive measures are concerned with the removal of this material by mechanical and chemical means. Various techniques involve the use of a brush, the use of floss, the rinsing effect of water, and the use of dentifrices and mouthwashes.

The function of the toothbrush is mainly to remove from the teeth both debris accumulation composed of microorganisms and beginning deposits of calculus. The brush also aids in the keratinization of the epithelium and stimulates the gingival tissue by creating a good blood supply. It has been shown that gingivitis can be produced at will by refraining from or inadequately brushing the teeth and that the gingiva can be restored to a normal healthy state by reinstituting good oral hygiene involving toothbrushing. Routine brushing of the teeth after each meal has been recommended as a means of preventing dental caries.

Automatic (electric) toothbrush vs. hand toothbrush

The automatic toothbrush was developed with the aim of doing a better job in removing materials from about the teeth than the conventional hand toothbrush, and accomplishing this within a shorter time. Since its develoment many investigations have been carried out to determine whether the electric toothbrush is more effective than the hand toothbrush. Clinical and nonclinical comparative studies using the electric and hand toothbrushes have been concerned with their ability to remove dental plaque and debris, and with their effect on trauma to the soft tissue, on gingivitis and bleeding of the gingiva, and on keratinization of the epithelium. Studies involving the assessment of these toothbrushes have been conducted on hospitalized patients, handicapped children and adults, mentally retarded children, normal children, patients with periodontal disease, edentulous patients, and others. There has been some disagreement as to which toothbrush is more effective.

A recent study concerning the effect of these two types of toothbrushes on dental plaque formation, gingivitis scores, and periodontal scores was made on a number of individuals over a period of four months. Results from this study indicated that there was no significant difference between the two toothbrushes. Both appeared to be equally effective in preventing and re-

moving plaque. There was no significant difference on the effect of the two types of brushes on gingivitis and periodontal scores.

A comparison between the electric and hand toothbrushes in cleaning the teeth of children indicates that the electric toothbrush appears to be superior. Studies with children showed that the automatic toothbrush may remove on an average of twice as much plaque as the conventional hand brush. These results possibly reflected the association of muscular coordination with more effective oral hygiene. The electric toothbrush is reported to require less time than the hand toothbrush as a cleaning instrument, and has definitely proven to be superior in cleaning the teeth of handicapped individuals who are unable to manipulate or control the hand toothbrush.

Floss and irrigating sprays

Effective oral hygiene is dependent upon removing subgingival as well as supragingival plaque from about the teeth. This is accomplished with the use of a toothbrush whether it be a hand toothbrush or an electric toothbrush and whether it have soft, medium, or hard bristles. Effective cleaning with minimal injury to the gingiva can be achieved with brushes containing medium or soft bristles. The interdental plaque that forms on the side of the teeth on approximal surfaces is difficult to remove. These surfaces are best cleaned with dental floss. The floss is gently passed between the teeth and underneath the edge of the gum. It is then held tightly against the proximal surface of the tooth and pulled over the surface toward the chewing edge. Dental floss is more effective in these areas than either the brush or the toothpick. The toothpick has been reported to be more effective than the ordinary toothbrush in removing plaque from the lingual interproximal surfaces of teeth.[19] Toothpaste and toothpowder may be employed as an aid to clean and polish the tooth surfaces. A very important step in oral hygiene is the use of the oral rinse. Irrigating sprays that hold reservoirs of water with or without mouthwash added or that may be attached directly to the water faucet are helpful in flushing between the teeth and gingival crevice. The water flushes away clumps of bacteria and food debris that are not removed by the brush or that are merely loosened by flossing. Irrigating sprays are also helpful in cleaning under bridges and braces and in flushing periodontal pockets.

Disclosing stains

To determine how effectively the teeth have been cleaned, disclosing stains may be used. These dye preparations may be applied to the teeth with a swab if they are liquid, such as merbromin. If they are in tablet form, such as the X-pose Disclosing Wafer,* which contains a harmless food color dye F.D.C. Red no. 3 known as erythrosine, the wafer is chewed, swished around the mouth for 30 seconds, and expectorated. With both techniques, bacterial plaque that adheres to the tooth will be stained by the dye. These accumulations can be seen with a mirror and special effort can be made to remove them. A disclosing wafer or solution may be used again to determine how effectively the hidden plaque has been removed. The patient now has a technique for evaluating the thoroughness of his tooth cleaning.[4]

The dye erythrosine in concentrations of 1.0% and 0.5% has been shown in vitro to inhibit various oral microorganisms, whereas another dye, fast green, in concentrations of 5.0% and 2.5% showed essentially no inhibitory effect. Erythrosine also appears to inhibit dextranase whereas fast green is reported to have no effect. If this inhibitory activity of erythrosine, demonstrated in vitro, is effective in vivo, its use

would have an added beneficial oral hygienic effect. Nevertheless, for the researcher who is quantitating dental plaque formation, fast green would be suggested in preference to erythrosine.[9]

Dentrifices

The use of a dentifrice merely as an abrasive compound to aid in removing microbial plaque from tooth surfaces has not proven satisfactory in preventing dental decay for the average person. A survey showed that approximately 30% of the people interviewed brushed their teeth immediately after each meal. It would appear desirable, therefore, to use a dentifrice that would have an inhibitory effect on plaque microorganisms.

Ammoniated dentifrices. In the late 1940s a concerted effort was made to introduce a new type of dentifrice that would be more effective in controlling dental caries. This type is known as the ammoniated dentifrice. Two basic types were introduced—one containing 5% dibasic ammonium phosphate plus 3% urea, and the other type containing 12% to 22% urea with or without 5% dibasic ammonium phosphate. Urea and dibasic ammonium phosphate were combined because they complement each other. The idea behind the use of the ammoniated dentifrices was to neutralize acids produced by the bacterial plaque. In so doing, the acids would not be allowed to accumulate to a high concentration and cause decalcification. Subjects using some of these dentifrices were instructed not to rinse their mouths after brushing. The dentifrice remaining in the mouth would then have a continued neutralizing effect because of ammonia production. Some of the dentifrices contained the enzyme urease to speed up ammonia production from the urea.

Dentifrices containing 5% dibasic ammonium phosphate plus 3% urea have not been shown to significantly reduce dental decay. Ammoniated dentifrices contain-

---

*Amurol Products Company, Naperville, Ill. 60540.

ing 13% urea and 5% dibasic ammonium phosphate have continuously been reported to reduce the incidence of new caries up to 25%. Dentifrices containing 22% urea have given even greater reductions.

No recent well-designed field tests have been reported concerning ammoniated dentifrices since 1957. These dentifrices were classified in 1951 as group C by the Council on Dental Therapeutics—meaning "needing further study." In a recent published report, ammoniated dentifrices have been considered of little importance in the current therapeutic dentifrice picture.[38]

Antienzyme dentifrices. After the ammoniated dentifrice, antienzyme dentifrices were introduced. These dentifrices contain enzyme inhibitors with the purpose of blocking bacterial enzyme systems and preventing the production of acids. The two compounds that have been incorporated into dentifrices as enzyme inhibitors are sodium N-lauroyl sarcosinate and sodium dehydroacetate. Only one study has been reported on use of a dentifrice containing sodium dehydroacetate, and it recorded a 55% reduction in caries.[52] Results from evaluation studies of sarcosinate use have proved somewhat conflicting and the true value of antienzyme dentifrices needs clarification, since reduction in tooth decay has varied from 0% to 50%. Muhler[35] made a clinical comparison of a sarcosinate dentifrice with a stannous fluoride dentifrice, reporting the fluoride dentifrice to be significantly superior in caries reduction. The sarcosinate dentifrice showed no reduction in caries and therefore no difference from the control.

Antibiotic dentifrices. Antibiotics, too, have found their way into dentifrices. Dentifrices containing penicillin have given results varying from 0% to 56% reduction in decay. There is always the question with the use of this type of dentifrice of the individual's becoming sensitized to the antibiotic, of antibiotic-resistant microbial

strains developing, and of overgrowth of nonsusceptible microorganisms. For these reasons dentifrices containing penicillin should not be recommended. Tyrothricin has also been incorporated into dentifrices and in clinical trials reduction in dental decay was noted. Further evaluation is required before this dentifrice is recommended.

Fluoride dentifrices. At the present time fluoride dentifrices have created great interest as caries-reducing agents. The exact mechanism by which they work is not known. It has been shown that the fluoride ion and the hydroxyl group of the hydroxyapatite in enamel react to form a less soluble fluorapatite. It is also believed that a remineralization effect may occur as the result of a tendency of calcium phosphate to precipitate from saturated solutions, such as saliva in the presence of fluoride, or that fluoride may work as an enzyme inhibitor. It has been reasonably established by many investigations that exposure of teeth to fluoride decreases its solubility in acids and thus increases resistance to dental decay.[20, 43, 45, 46] With stannous fluoride, the stannous ion is believed to react with the tooth to form stannous phosphate.

Evaluation studies have been conducted under nonsupervised and supervised conditions, and the percentage reduction of caries reported is somewhat difficult to evaluate. Some studies, in which the subjects were supervised, indicated a 57% reduction in dental decay at the end of one year and a 46% reduction at the end of the second year. Other studies indicated a much lower percentage of redution in dental decay. A number of studies, unsupervised as to brushing habits, reported negative results of use of a stannous fluoride dentifrice. Nevertheless, the incorporation of stannous fluoride into a dentifrice in well-supervised clinical tests has proved that stannous fluoride dentifrices have a caries-preventive action. Such dentifrices imparted more protection to teeth during eruption than to teeth after eruption.[21]

Although early tests with sodium fluoride dentifrices failed to demonstrate significant reduction in dental caries activity, Peterson and Williamson[39] demonstrated inhibition of caries using a sodium fluoride acid orthophosphate dentifrice.

In a clinical evaluation comparing stannous fluoride and a sodium monofluorophosphate dentifrice for a two-year period, both dentifrices demonstrated approximately a 21% reduction in cavities as compared to no reduction in the control.[15] In vitro evaluation of a prophylactic paste containing zirconium silicate plus 2% stannous fluoride was shown by Shannon[49] to reduce significantly enamel solubility. Recently, Muhler and co-workers[36] reported a one-year in vivo evaluation of a SnF_2-$ZrSiO_4$ paste, which showed a 41% reduction in new DMF teeth and a 64% reduction in new DMF surfaces in children. The incorporation of stannous fluoride, 0.4%, in a gel type of dentifrice has been demonstrated to significantly reduce enamel solubility in acid in laboratory tests.[48]

Organic fluorides have also been incorporated into dentifrices. A single clinical evaluation with an amine fluoride dentifrice demonstrated a 25% to 30% caries reduction. The organic fluorides appear promising but require further investigation.

Evaluation of the effect of fluoride on acid production in a saliva glucose mixture indicates that a concentration of 0.5 ppm. is required to produce a significant statistical depression in acid production. The maximum concentration of fluoride in saliva has been reported to be 0.35 ppm. This concentration is too small to cause any change in acid production or to have a direct effect on the oral flora itself.

Chlorophyll dentifrices. Chlorophyll has been incorporated as a therapeutic agent into dentifrices for its deodorizing property and for the inhibition of lactobacilli. Results do not show these dentifrices to be any more beneficial than those that do not contain chlorophyll.

Mouthwashes

Mouthwashes may be separated into two main types: (1) antibacterial, or those used to reduce the oral microflora and thus reduce mouth odor, aid in the prevention of caries and periodontal disease, and help reduce the hazards of oral aerosols created during dental operation; and (2) fluoride mouthwashes, or those that aid in the prevention of dental decay and help to reduce sensitivity at the necks of teeth.[47]

There appears to be a relationship between the amount of carbohydrate retained in the oral cavity and caries activity. Rinsing the mouth four or five times—the so-called swish and swallow technique—immediately after eating reduces appreciably the amount of sugar retained in the oral cavity. The use of sialogenous tablets stimulates salivary flow and is also reported to bring about a reduction in the caries incidence.

Results on the effectiveness of mouthwashes sold as oral antiseptics are quite confusing. By definition an antiseptic is a chemical agent that either inhibits or kills microorganisms. If the compound is a skin antiseptic, it has to demonstrate, by in vitro testing, the inhibition of microbial growth. On the other hand, if the compound is sold as an oral antiseptic it has to demonstrate, by in vitro testing, that it kills the test microorganism in a short time period. The mere rinsing of the mouth with tap water is reported to remove about 15% of the oral flora. Within a matter of 60 minutes or less the flora will regenerate to its normal pyramid level. If the microbial population is reduced 50% by a mouthwash, theoretically the remaining microorganisms would require 30 minutes to return to the original numbers. This is based upon a generation time of 30 minutes in the case of streptococci. If oral hygiene involving a mouthwash reduces the population 25%, the remaining microorganisms will require 60 minutes to reach the initial numbers. If the oral population is reduced to 0.1% of its original, those organisms that remain will require five hours to regenerate to the original population. The reduction to 0.1% means that 99.9% of the organisms were killed.[51] This, of course, cannot be achieved. The big problem in oral hygiene is the unaccessible areas that protect microorganisms from mechanical cleaning and from the antibacterial effect of oral antiseptics. The penetration of mouthwashes and dentifrices through dental plaque does reduce the number of organisms. Those organisms that survive regenerate quickly and the reduction is not effectively maintained.

In interpreting theoretic results based upon a constant generation time such as 30 minutes, one has to keep in mind that members of the oral cavity possess different generation times, some longer and some shorter than 30 minutes; also, that when one is working with masses of mixed organisms, as in plaque, the generation time of the respective organisms differs because of competition and is probably greatly extended. The effect of salivary flow, swallowing, movement of the tongue and cheek mucous membrane against the teeth removes oral organisms and also affects the theoretic calculation.

Another problem in evaluating the effectiveness of oral antiseptics involves variations in technique. Some techniques weigh plaque before and after the use of an oral mouthwash. Others determine the microbial population of paraffin-stimulated saliva before and at definite intervals of time after a mouthwash has been used. Other variations in technique have also been reported.

The results of well-planned experiments indicate that under practical conditions mouthwashes, depending upon how frequently they are used, can reduce the oral flora.[31] A recent study on the effect of the prolonged use of a specific mouthwash twice a day for more than a month showed

that there was initially a sharp drop in plate count, indicating reduction as the result of the mouthwash. Following this reduction there was a gradual increase in counts. This increase was interpreted as perhaps representing the adaptability of the normal flora to the mouthwash. When a second mouthwash was substituted, a sharp drop in plate count was also noted. It is recommended that when using a mouthwash, the subject alternate one type of mouthwash with another from time to time.[1]

Numerous reports[47, 48] give results indicating that fluoride mouthwashes offer a practical home care procedure for helping in the reduction of dental caries.

A clinical evaluation of the effect of dextranase mouthwash on the formation and dispersion of bacterial plaque on human teeth has presented somewhat conflicting results. Lobene[28] reported that dextranase mouthwash significantly reduced the dry weight of plaque but did not alter the area of plaque formation. The dextranase mouthwash had no observed adverse effect on oral soft or hard tissues.

These findings were more or less confirmed by Keys and co-workers,[24] who showed that the dextranase mouthwash resulted in less plaque deposit, and also reported no harmful effects on the subjects. In contrast, Caldwell and co-workers'[10] studies showed that dextranase mouthwash had no measurable effect on plaque scores or plaque weight.

In a series of experimental studies,[12, 29, 40, 42] it was reported that two daily rinses with a mouthwash containing 0.2% chlorhexidine prevented plaque formation whereas one daily rinse with this mouthwash did not completely inhibit plaque. A topical application of a 2% chlorhexidine gluconate solution once daily was as effective in plaque inhibition as the 0.2% mouthwash. The 0.2% chlorhexidine mouthwash also reduced the salivary microflora; whereas the topical application of the 2% solution showed no significant reduction of salivary flora. It was demonstrated that chlorhexidine is absorbed by hydroxyapatite, tooth surface, and salivary mucin. The absorption by tooth surface in vivo possibly acts as a reservoir from which this chemical is slowly released and inhibits bacterial colonization on tooth surfaces. The absorption by the oral mucosa is not lasting because the mucous flow causes a loss of inhibitory effect. The chlorhexidine mouthrinse appears to reduce the gingival microflora whereas the topical application of chlorhexidine to teeth appears to have little effect on the gingival flora.

Halitosis. Halitosis[32, 41, 54, 55, 56] means offensive or bad breath. The word is derived from the Latin *halitus*, which means breath, and the suffix *-osis*, which means disease. Breath odors can originate in the mouth, lungs, and nasal passage, the first of these being of main interest to the dentist. The chief sources of oral odors are stagnant saliva, tooth decay, periodontal disease, coated tongue, and necrotic lesions. Most people have a foul breath upon arising in the morning. This is normally because of local salivary stagnation. Morning breath, especially marked in the older age group, appears to be associated with a decreased nocturnal level of muscular and physiologic activity. In general, the saliva from mouths with periodontal disease decomposes more rapidly than saliva from a normal mouth. Mouth odors are attributed to the degradation of exogenous and endogenous sources of protein nutrients by the oral microflora.

Bert and Fosdick (1946) demonstrated that seventeen oral organisms could putrefy saliva. No single organism was capable of putrefying saliva as rapidly as the mixtures that are normally present in the mouth. Among the many products studied with reference to offensive breath are indole, skatole, sulfides, and cadaverine. Rizzo[41] demonstrated hydrogen sulfide in periodontal pockets from 2 to 6 mm. in depth. At least five genera of anaerobic oral microorganisms found in deep periodontal pockets can produce H_2S: spirochetes, fusiform bacilli, *Vibrio*, *Veillonella*, and some species of *Bacteroides*. Substrates for H_2S production, such as cysteine, cystine, methionine, glutathione, and thiocyanate, have been demonstrated to be present in saliva and serum. Isobutyric acid has been detected in fusiform filtrates, and putrescine in diphtheroid filtrates. The decomposition of food lodged between the teeth in cavities and between or under prosthetic appliances is a frequent source of foul breath. A positive correlation has been shown between coated tongue and mouth odor.

Bleeding and the accumulation of blood elements in various regions of the mouth and in the socket as the result of tooth extraction tend to be the source of undesirable odor.

The control of halitosis originating from the mouth involves treatment or removal of the possible cause. If the cause is associated with carious teeth, either restorations or extractions are indicated. If gingivitis or periodontal disease is the cause, specific treatment is initiated. In most cases, halitosis is associated with a dirty mouth, one that shows microbial plaque about the teeth and gingival margin, especially in stagnated areas, and a coated tongue. The rigid enforcement of good oral hygiene incorporating the mechanical removal of microbial debris by the use of a toothbrush, dentifrice, floss, and water irrigation under pressure will effectively aid in controlling offensive odors originating in the mouth. Swishing with a mouthwash will add to the effectiveness of the hygienic procedure.

Cleansing effect of chewing food and gum

The effect of eating apples on the dental health of children indicates that the chewing of crisp firm apples appears instrumental in creating a better gum condition. The efficacy of chewing fibrous food as a means of natural oral hygiene has been questioned. In one investigation,[3] chewing fresh sugar cane, unpeeled apple, celery, lettuce, and carrots resulted in comparatively little reduction in the area of plaque on tooth surface as shown by disclosing solutions (Fig. 12-3).

The effect of gum chewing on oral hygiene has been under investigation for many years. There is no evidence that chewing gum reduces dental decay. Chewing one piece of gum after meals has not been shown statistically to influence the caries incidence, but the excessive chewing of gum may create an environment favorable for dental decay. Certain enzymes that have been incorporated into some gums can retard the accumulations of soft accretions, stain, and calculus on teeth. Further investigation is needed to determine whether the added therapeutic agents, synthetic vitamin K, Nitrofuran, chlorophyll, and fluoride compounds, reduce tooth decay.

Most of the sugar from gum is released within the first 10 minutes of chewing; the increase in salivary flow may carry most of this sugar away. It has been suggested that sugar, such as that released when chewing gum, may furnish reserve energy to dental plaque organisms and result in an increase in oral acidity over extended periods of time. Present clinical evaluation does not support this idea. The incorporation of phosphate compounds into gum appears to be promising in preventing caries. Finn and Jamison[16] reported that under experimental conditions the chewing of five sticks of gum, each containing 225 mg. of dicalcium phosphate, daily, resulted in significant reduction in caries, a reduction not evident when sugar gum was chewed. Dicalcium phosphate gum and sugarless gum were comparable in their caries reduction capacity. Since there is no conclusive evidence that the chewing of gum removes debris from teeth, gum cannot be advocated as an oral cleansing agent for the teeth.

Smoking

It has been observed that swabs obtained from the mouth and throat of smokers show the presence of beta hemolytic streptococci about twice as frequently as swabs from nonsmokers or from past smokers. No

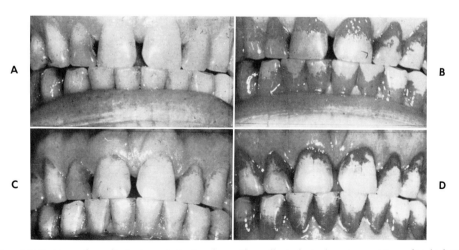

Fig. 12-3. Use of a disclosing stain to show the effect that chewing various foods has in removing plaque from the teeth. **A,** Initial plaque accumulations on unstained teeth. **B,** Initial plaque accumulations on teeth stained with basic fuchsin. **C,** Plaque accumulations on teeth not easily seen after celery, carrots, apple, and cane pulp had been chewed for 3 hours. **D,** Plaque accumulations made easily visible after teeth were restained following chewing. (From Arnim, S. S.: J. Tenn. Dent. Assoc. **39:**3, 1959.)

significant difference was noted in anti-streptolysin O titers of serum from either smokers or nonsmokers. Some reports show that there is a decrease in caries with increased smoking and an increase in severity of gingivitis.

ORTHODONTICS

The appliances used in orthodontics create a tremendous increase in sites about the teeth that favor the lodgement of foods and the accumulation of dental plaque. These conditions make keeping the teeth relatively free of the plaque by means of routine oral hygiene techniques more difficult. The orthodontist is particularly concerned about the effect of his treatment on caries susceptibility. It would be discouraging to create an appealing dentition through orthodontic treatment and then to have to restore or possibly extract some teeth because of decay resulting from lack of a good oral hygiene program.

Few articles concerning the relationship of oral microbial types to orthodontic appliances have been published. It has been reported that the *Lactobacillus* count increases with the placement of appliances and that the increase appears to be associated with the increase in the number of orthodontic bands. Upon placement of orthodontic appliances, the overall microflora increases numerically in staphylococci, streptococci, *Veillonella,* and yeast organisms, total aerobes and anaerobes, as well as lactobacilli. This increase in plaque microorganisms is associated with an increase in both extracellular and intracellular carbohydrate per milligram of plaque. Thus, the plaque is more cariogenic since there is an increase in numbers of acid-producing bacteria as shown by significantly lower pH levels in patients after banding as compared to before banding. The increase in extracellular carbohydrate makes the plaque more tenacious and reduces the neutralization of acids formed by the washing effect of saliva.[5]

A positive correlation was found between DMF teeth and the *Lactobacillus* count. It has been shown also that the caries incidence may increase with orthodontic treatment, and that the tooth surfaces affected are likely to be those covered by the bands from which cement has been washed away. By an agar replica technique, it was observed that *Lactobacillus* colonies developed on teeth along the band edge and along the gingival margin. With the removal of the bands, the salivary *Lactobacillus* count dropped and the lactobacilli disappeared from the sites on the tooth's surface that had previously shown their presence by the replica agar technique. Colonizing lactobacilli could be found only where areas had become carious.

It is recommended that topical application of fluoride be made before fitting fixed orthodontic appliances. Other preventive measures concerning the orthodontic patient require, in addition to a good oral hygiene, regular periodic check-ups by the patient's general practitioner. In the orthodontic patient, it is reported that an oral hygiene procedure that combined the use of an oral irrigating device with brushing is significantly more effective in reducing lactobacilli and other oral organisms than plain rinsing with brushing.[23] Dietary control involving the reduction of consumable refined carbohydrate food may also be necessary for certain patients.

EXODONTICS

It has been demonstrated that microorganisms invade the bloodstream following the extraction of teeth and may be carried to other parts of the body. In one study microorganisms were removed from the peripheral blood following tooth extraction in from 50% to 85% of specimens. The microorganisms recovered were similar to those present in the oral cavity.

The effect of a complete extraction of the dentition on the numbers of lactobacilli, yeasts, *Streptococcus salivarius,* and staphylococci has been that, following extraction and during the edentulous period, no lactobacilli or yeasts can be detected in the saliva. At the same time, streptococci appear to increase for the first several weeks after the dentures are placed and worn. With the placement of dentures, the lactobacilli reappear. Within a five-week period after the dentures are worn, the lactobacilli and yeast increase to the preextraction level and the streptococci show a decrease. Staphylococci remain essentially unchanged throughout the entire period. The return of acidogenic organisms with the wearing of dentures suggests that individuals with partial or full dentures be advised to follow a rigid oral hygiene procedure. The purpose is to reduce the acidogenic microorganisms to low levels and thus help prevent recurring decay in the partial denture patient and denture sore mouth in the complete denture patient.

Certain research work suggests that there may be a relationship between the extraction of teeth and the incidence of poliomyelitis. This correlation has not been substantiated in surveys. Therefore it might be concluded that the recommendation to postpone dental extractions during the polio season is without scientific basis.

Candidal fungemia has been reported to have followed dental extractions. The probable source of the candida organism is the oral cavity itself. Other infections associated with exodontia are discussed in Chapter 11.

The dry socket

The term "dry socket" is actually a misnomer. The so-called dry socket is the result of tooth extraction, particularly extraction in the molar area, and occurs in from 1% to 4% of extractions. The loss of the blood clot that forms originally in the socket results in necrosis of the denuded alveolar bone. A putrid odor is present and

there is generally a severe throbbing pain. Clinically the dry socket develops within two to four days from extraction. Its exact origin is not known. Some theories are that it represents a preexistent infection in the lamina dura from a root infection, others that it is the result of secondary infection after extraction, and others that it is the result of trauma to the bone during extraction. Prevention involves the local use of antimicrobial drugs such as sulfa cones and antibiotics, as well as the administration of systemic antibiotics. Treatment involves the alleviation of the pain, the irrigation of the socket with warm saline solution to clean out the foreign necrotic material, and the application of gauze containing an antimicrobial agent such as iodoform. Antibiotics are also administered.

Various organisms have been isolated from dry sockets, including *Actinomyces bovis, Corynebacterium diphtheriae, Neisseria meningitidis, Diplococcus pneumoniae, Haemophilus influenzae, Klebsiella, Pseudomonas aeruginosa,* and members of the coliform group.

ENDODONTICS
Evaluation of some culture media

The importance of microbiology in the practice of endodontics has been emphasized in Chapter 9. The information presented here pertains only to culture media.

To detect the presence of microorganisms in the root canal during treatment it is necessary that the practitioner use a culture medium rich in nutrients. The medium should support the growth of a variety of microorganisms and still be sensitive enough for the detection of the various types when they are present in small numbers. Fig. 12-4, *A,* presents the results of an evaluation of four media for growth-supporting of and sensitivity for a strain each of a fusiform bacillus, a lactobacillus, a viridans streptococcus, an actinomyces, and the yeast *Candida albicans.* These microorganisms are members of the oral

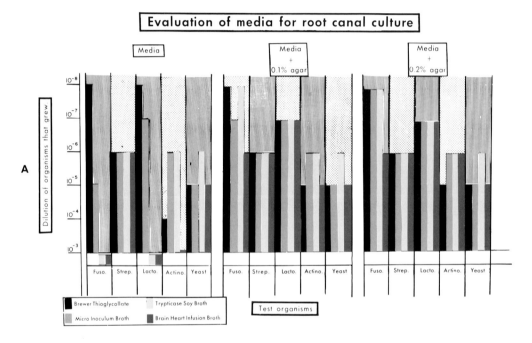

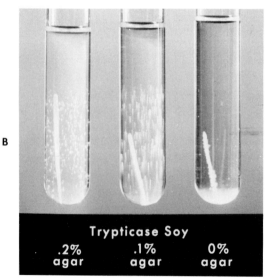

Fig. 12-4. Evaluation of media for root canal cultures. **A,** Sensitivity of media for root canal cultures of five different microorganisms indigenous to the oral cavity. **B,** Influence of agar added to culture media in the development of isolated colonies from contaminated paper points.

flora and represent some types that are quite fastidious in their nutrient and oxygen requirements. These media with or without 0.1% or 0.2% agar were found to be equally sensitive for the viridans streptococcus and the yeast. The addition of agar to Brewer thioglycollate, trypticase soy, brain heart infusion, and Micro Inoculum broths broadened their spectra and in some instances increased the sensitivity of these media for certain of the organisms tested. Of the media, trypticase soy plus agar was the most sensitive. The addition of agar appears to favor the development of isolated colonies throughout the medium in the tube. The amount of infected material picked up on the paper point from the canal, therefore, should give some idea of the numbers of microorganisms (Fig. 12-4, *B*). One might expect also to obtain some idea of the different microbial types involved in the infection by removing colonies with a Pasteur pipet, making smears, and observing under the microscope. The addition of 0.2% agar appears to favor better separation of colonies throughout the tubed media than does 0.1% agar.

PREVENTION OF CROSS-INFECTION

The patient goes to the dentist generally for relief of oral pain that is in most instances the result of infection. The dentist alleviates the pain and restores the oral cavity of the patient to a healthful state. During dental operations, microorganisms from the patient's mouth contaminate the dentist's instruments and fingers and are disseminated into the air by splatter and aerosols. In operational procedures, the dentist should use all possible measures to prevent the introduction of new infectious material into the patient's mouth. He should use methods to prevent cross-infection between himself and the patient and between patients. He should endeavor to maintain a chain of asepsis. This involves the sterilization of

dental instruments and other equipment that is used on the patient and the disinfection of office appurtenances with which the patient comes in contact.

Sterilization procedures of dental instruments have been discussed in other chapters and will not be considered here. Rather, other equipment that might be important as a possible source of cross-infection in the handling of patients will be considered—for example, the dental chair head rest. The patient entraps many different types of microorganisms in his hair and these may be transferred to the head rest of the chair. The operator's hands and his assistant's hands come in contact with the head rest and can transfer microorganisms from the head rest to the oral cavity of patients. Covering the head rest with a small plastic bag and changing the bag between patients eliminates this source of contamination. The handle of the head rest also becomes contaminated and may be disinfected by wiping with a germicide. Seventy percent alcohol or a solution of 0.5% chlorhexidine in 70% alcohol is reported to be effective. In decontaminating, the disinfectants mentioned or an aqueous solution of benzalkonium chloride can be used in wiping the bracket table, light handle, water spray, air syringe, call buttons, knobs, pens, and so forth. Water spray reservoirs used for cooling handpiece burs can be disinfected by the addition of chlorhexidine in concentrations of 1:5,000.

It has been shown that during various dental operations on tubercular patients, the washings from their oral cavities may contain *Mycobacterium tuberculosis*. Swabs taken from the throat and the anterior part of the mouth of these patients and glass slides held 3 inches from their lips while coughing all show the tubercular organism in a high percentage of samples. These findings indicate that when working on a tubercular patient the dentist, dental hygienist, and dental assistant, as well as their instruments, become contaminated with *Mycobacterium tuberculosis*. If the patient coughs, the atmosphere surrounding the dentist is likely to contain tubercular organisms, which are inhaled. Droplet nuclei containing tuberculosis bacilli were not demonstrated during oral prophylaxis when an ultrasonic scaler was used on patients with active pulmonary tuberculosis.[13]

High speed cutting instruments create an aerosol in the environment surrounding the dental chair. With the use of high speed dental drills (200,000 to 300,000 rpm) considerable heat is generated, which may cause injury to the tooth pulp. To prevent this, water spray is employed as a coolant and a lubricant. As a result, microbial aerosols are generated from the patient's mouth during dental operations which are comparable in bacterial concentrations to those produced during coughing and sneezing. It is possible to greatly reduce the bacterial aerosols generated by the effective use of high velocity suction during dental procedures. The suction apparatus should be placed as close as possible to the area of operation. The aerosol removed by this apparatus should be discharged so as to not contaminate the operatory.[33] It has been demonstrated that a preoperative rinse with distilled water may result in a 35% reduction in colony count when high speed handpieces are used for 60 seconds; whereas a rinse with a commercial mouthwash containing cetylpyridinium chloride resulted in a 76% reduction.[34]

Thus, use of a cetylpyridinium chloride mouthwash before and during dental high speed drill operations reduced the number of organisms in the air taken at a distance between the operator and patient by 89.3%. However, use of a sterile water rinse as required during the drilling procedure, or a sterile water rinse used preoperatively and as required during the procedure, gave results that were not significantly different from each other.[27]

Prosthetic material and appliances become contaminated with tubercular bacilli in the construction of dentures for tubercular patients. The various impression materials may be effectively sterilized by immersion in a 10% solution of formaldehyde for 30 minutes, followed by a rinse in cold running water. The formaldehyde appears to have no deleterious effect on black base plate, green Kerr modeling compound, and Kerr permlastic rubber impression materials. An antiseptic detergent containing sodium octy-phenoxyethoxyethyl ether sulfonate and hexachlorophene has been reported effective in sterilizing denture materials contaminated with tubercular bacilli. The contaminated material should be soaked for five minutes in a solution of this detergent and then rinsed.

Face masks, rubber gloves, eye glasses, and plastic covering gowns are some of the items that the dentist may use in order to reduce the hazards of infection. In an evaluation of the protective effect of surgical masks,[18] it was shown that the filtering efficiency varied between 15% and 99%. The types of masks tested included gauze of various weaves, paper, plastic foam, nonwoven synthetic fiber, and masks incorporating fine fiber mats. The plastic foam, paper, and cloth masks were found to be the least adequate filters for bacterial aerosols. Masks of glass or synthetic fiber demonstrated great filtering efficiency. Almost all the particles that penetrate the efficient filtered mask are 5 mμ or less in diameter. Particles of this size may be hazardous if they penetrate the alveoli of the human lungs. Bacterial aerosols do remain airborne for many hours after certain dental procedures have been used unless they are removed by an efficient ventilation system.

When working on a carious lesion, the dentist can reduce the numbers of organisms in the aerosol by removing as much of the soft decayed material as possible with hand instruments before using the high speed handpiece.

The effectiveness of hexachlorophene soaps, detergent creams, and germicidal rinses in reducing the microflora of the skin to low levels is presented in Chapter 13. The application of a 0.5% chlorhexidine digluconate in 70% alcohol for two minutes following a germicidal soaping was shown to reduce the skin microflora 99.98%. To protect himself and his patients against the spread of tubercular organisms, the dentist should have a yearly chest x-ray. In some countries it is suggested also that if his results from a Mantoux test are negative, he should be vaccinated with BCG vaccine.

The dentist's hands are exposed to infections that result not only in discomfort, embarrassment, and loss of income, but more important, infection on the dentist's hands may be instrumental in the spread of infection to his patients. The most common infections of the dentist's hands are acute cellulitis, chronic infectious eczema, yeast infections, and fungus infections. Prompt diagnosis and effective treatment are essential.

It has been demonstrated that if an injection is made into the oral mucous membrane before the site of injection is swabbed with a skin germicide, the needle will become contaminated with microorganisms of the indigenous oral flora. Viridans streptococci have been the most frequent contaminants. Other contaminants isolated have been *Neisseria catarrhalis, Micrococcus tetragenus, Staphylococcus pyogenes,* diphtheroids, beta hemolytic streptococci, and nonhemolytic streptococci. When the mucus is dried before injection, the number of organisms on the mucous membrane is greatly reduced, but although reduced, there is still contamination of the syringe needle. For this reason it is recommended that some germicide be swabbed over the mucous membrane before intra-oral injection. If infection does follow injections, the dentist may be accused of neglect and be subjected to legal action. The use of sterile disposable needles eliminates the needle as a source of cross-infection. Once used, the disposable needle should be thrown away and not resterilized for reuse. There is no safe way to thoroughly clean small-gauge needles, and such needles can possibly be responsible for cross-infection.

CITED REFERENCES

1. Alderman, E. J., and Scallon, V. L.: An in vivo study of the effect of prolonged use of a specific mouthwash on the oral flora, Chron. Omaha Dent. Soc. **28:**284, 1964.
2. Aponte, A. J., Hartsook, J. T., and Crowely, M. C.: Indirect pulp capping success verified, J. Dent. Child. **33:**164, 1966.
3. Arnim, S. S.: Microcosms of the human mouth, J. Tenn. Dent. Assoc. **39:**3, 1959.
4. Arnim, S. S., Diercks, C. C., and Pearson, E. A., Jr.: What you need to know and do to prevent dental caries and periodontal disease, J. N. Carolina Dent. Soc. **46:**296, 1963.
5. Balenseifen, J. W., and Madonia, J. V.: Study of dental plaque in orthodontic patients, J. Dent. Res. **49:**320, 1970.
6. Besic, F. C.: The fate of bacteria sealed in dental cavities, J. Dent. Res. **22:**349, 1943.
7. Buonocore, M. G.: Adhesive sealing of pits and fissures for caries prevention with use of ultraviolet light, J. Amer. Dent. Assoc. **80:**324, 1970.
8. Buonocore, M. G.: Caries prevention in pits and fissures sealed with an adhesive resin polymerized by ultraviolet light: A two year study of a single adhesive application, J. Amer. Dent. Assoc. **82:**1090, 1971.
9. Caldwell, R. C., and Hunt, D. E.: A comparison of the antimicrobial activity of disclosing agents, J. Dent. Res. **48:**913, 1969.
10. Caldwell, R. C., Sandham, H. J., Mann, W. V., Jr., Finn, S. B., and Formicola, A. J.: The effect of a dextranase mouthwash on dental plaque in young adults and children, J. Amer. Dent. Assoc. **82:**124, 1971.
11. Council on Dental Therapeutics: Council classifies Colgate with MFP (sodium monofluorophosphate) in group A, J. Amer. Dent. Assoc. **79:**937, 1969.
12. Davies, R. M., Jensen, S. B., Rindom Schiott, C., and Loe, H.: The effect of topical application of chlorhexidine on the bacterial colonization of the teeth and gingiva, J. Periodont. Res. **5:**96, 1970.
13. Duell, R. C., and Madden, R. M.: Droplet nuclei produced during dental treatment of tubercular patients, Oral Surg. **30:**711, 1970.
14. Eidelmann, E., Finn, S. B., and Koulourides, T.: Remineralization of carious dentine treated

with calcium hydroxide, J. Dent. Child. **32:** 218, 1965.

15. Fanning, E. A., Gotjamanos, T., and Vowles, N. J.: The use of fluoride dentrifices in the control of dental caries. Methodology and results of a clinical trial, Aust. Dent. J. **13:** 201, 1968.

16. Finn, S. B., and Jamison, H. C.: The role of a dicalcium phosphate chewing gum in the control of human dental caries—30 months result, J. Amer. Dent. Assoc. **74:**987, 1967.

17. Fisher, F. J.: The viability of microorganisms incarious dentine beneath amalgam restorations, Brit. Dent. J. **126:**355, 1969.

18. Ford, C. R., and Peterson, D. E.: The efficiency of surgical face masks, Amer. J. Surg. **106:**954, 1963.

19. Gjermo, P., and Flotra, L.: Plaque removal effects of dental floss and toothpicks in group comparative studies, J. Periodont. Res. **4:**170, 1969.

20. Gordon, G. E., and Shannon, I. L.: Treatment of root surfaces with stannous fluoride, N. Zeal. Soc. Periodont. Bull., no. 29, p. 24, 1970.

21. Heifetz, S. B., and Horowitz, H. S.: An appraisal of therapeutic dentifrices, J. Public Health Dent. **30:**206, 1970.

22. Hoover, D. R., and Lefkowits, W.: Reduction of gingivitis by toothbrushing, J. Periodont. **36:**193, 1965.

23. Hurst, J. E., and Madonia, J. V.: The effect of an oral irrigating device on the oral hygiene of orthodontic patients, J. Amer. Dent. Assoc. **81:**678, 1970.

24. Keyes, P. H., Hicks, M. A., Goldman, B. M., McCabe, R. M., and Fitzgerald, R. J.: Dispersion of dextranous bacterial plaques on human teeth with dextranase, J. Amer. Dent. Assoc. **82:**136, 1971.

25. King, J. B., Crawford, J. J., and Lindahl, R. L.: Indirect capping: A bacteriologic study of deep carious dentine in human teeth, Oral Surg. **20:**663, 1965.

26. Law, D. B., Berg, M., and Fosdick, L. S.: Chemical studies on periodontal disease, J. Dent. Res. **22:**373, 1943.

27. Litsky, B. Y., Mascis, J. D., and Litsky, W.: Use of an antimicrobial mouthwash to minimize the bacterial aerosol contamination generated by the high-speed drill, Oral Surg. **29:** 25, 1970.

28. Lobene, R. R.: A clinical study of the effect of dextranase on human dental plaque, J. Amer. Dent. Assoc. **82:**132, 1971.

29. Löe, H., and Rindom, Schiott, C.: The effect of mouthrinses and topical application of chlorhexidine on the development of dental

plaque and gingivitis in man, J. Periodont. **5:**79, 1970.

30. Löe, H., Theilade, E., and Jensen, S.: Experimental gingivitis in man, J. Periodont. **36:** 177, 1965.

31. McCormick, J.: A critical review of the literature on mouthwashes, Ann. N. Y. Acad. Sci. **53:**274, 1968.

32. Massler, M., Ernslie, R., and Bolden, T.: Fetor ex ore, Oral Surg. **4:**110, 1951.

33. Micik, R. E., Miller, R. L., Mazzarella, M. A., and Ryge, G.: Studies on dental aerobiology. 1. Bacterial aerosols generated during dental procedures, J. Dent. Res. **48:**49, 1969.

34. Mohammed, C. I., and Manhold, J. H.: Efficacy of preoperative oral rinsing to reduce air contamination during use of air turbine handpieces, J. Amer. Dent. Assoc. **69:**715, 1964.

35. Muhler, J.: A clinical comparison of fluoride and antienzyme dentrifrices, J. Dent. Child. **37:**59, 1970.

36. Muhler, J., Kelley, G., Stookey, G., Lindo, F., and Harris, N. O.: The clinical evaluation of a patient-administered SnF_2-$ZrSiO_4$ prophylactic paste in children. 1. Results after one year in the Virgin Islands, J. Amer. Dent. Assoc. **81:** 142, 1970.

37. Noonan, R. G.: Silver amalgam is not antibacterial, J. Dent. Child. **32:**147, 1965.

38. Peterson, J. K.: The current status of therapeutic dentifrices, Ann. N. Y. Acad. Sci. **153:** 334, 1968.

39. Peterson, J. K., and Williamson, L.: Three-year caries inhibition of sodium fluoride acid orthophosphate dentifrice compared with a stannous fluoride dentifrice and a non-fluoride dentifrice. International Association for Dental Research, Forty-sixth General Meeting, Program and abstracts. San Francisco, 1968, p. 254.

40. Rindom Schiott, C., Loe, H., Jensen, S. B., Kilian, M., Davies, R. M., and Glavind, K.: The effect of chlorhexidine mouthrinses on the human oral flora, J. Periodont. Res. **5:**84, 1970.

41. Rizzo, A. A.: The possible role of hydrogen sulfide in human periodontal disease. 1. Hydrogen sulfide production in periodontal pockets, Periodontics **5:**233, 1967.

42. Rolla, G., Loe, H., and Rindom Schiott, C.: the affinity of chlorhexidine for hydroxyapatite and salivary mucins, J. Periodont. **5:** 90, 1970.

43. Sandoval, E., and Shannon, I. L.: Stannous fluoride and dentin solubility, Texas Rep. Biol. Med. **27:**111, 1969.

44. Schouboe, T., and MacDonald, J. B.: Pro-

longed viability of organisms sealed in dental caries, Arch. Oral Biol. 7:525, 1962.

45. Shannon, I. L.: Dural application of fluorides, New Mexico Dent. J. 21:12, 1970.
46. Shannon, I. L.: Enamel solubility reduction by topical application of combinations of fluoride compounds, J. Oral Med. 25:12, 1970.
47. Shannon, I. L.: Evaluation of prophylaxis pastes and topical applications prepared with X-14 stannous fluoride solution, Techn. Docum. Rep. SAM-TDR 63-103. U. S. Air Force Electron. Syst. Div. 1-7.
48. Shannon, I. L.: Preventive dental services in the Veterans' Administration Hospital, J. Public Health Dent. 30:156, 1970.
49. Shannon, I. L.: A pumice-zirconium silicate prophylaxis paste containing 2% stannous fluoride in water-free solution, Pharm. Ther. Dent. 1:24, 1970.
50. Stephan, R. M., Muntz, M. S., and Dorfman, A.: In vitro studies on sterilization of carious dentin. III. Effective penetration of germicides into carious lesions, J. Amer. Dent. Assoc. 20: 1905, 1943.
51. Stralfors, A.: Disinfection of dental plaques in man, Odont. T. 70:183, 1962.
52. Sulser, G. G., Fosket, R. R., and Fosdick, L. S.: Use of sodium dehydroacetase sodium oxalate dentrifrice in the control of dental caries, J. Amer. Dent. Assoc. 56:368, 1958.
53. Swartz, M. L., Phillips, R. W., and Norman, R. D.: Effect of fluoride-containing zinc oxide-eugenol cements on solubility of enamel, J. Dent. Res. 49:576, 1970.
54. Tonzetich, J., Eigen, E., King, W. J., and Weiss, S.: Volatility as a factor in the inability of certain amines and indole to increase the odour of saliva, Arch. Oral Biol. 12:1167, 1967.
55. Tonzetich, J., and Kestenbaum, R. C.: Odour production by human salivary fractions and plaque, Arch. Oral Biol. 14:815, 1969.
56. Tonzetich, J., and Ritchter, V. J.: Evaluation of volatile odoriferous components of saliva, Arch. Oral Biol. 9:39, 1964.

REFERENCES AND ADDITIONAL READINGS

Abbott, J. N., Briney, A. T., and Denaro, S. A.: Recovery of tubercle bacilli from mouth washings of tuberculous dental patients, J. Amer. Dent. Assoc. 50:49, 1955.

Arnim, S. S.: How the dentist can help people learn to prevent and control dental disease, Northwest Dent. 45:3, 1966.

Arnim, S. S.: The use of disclosing agents for measuring tooth cleanliness, J. Periodont. 34: 227, 1963.

Bahn, A. N., and Michalsen, R. C.: Addition of bacteriostatic agents to acrylic resins, J. Prosth. Dent. 11:237, 1961.

Barber, D. B., and Massler, M.: Penetration of isotopes through liners and bases under silicate cement restorations, J. Amer. Dent. Assoc. 65: 786, 1962.

Bartels, H. A.: Cavity sterilization—a recommended procedure, Dent. Clin. N. Amer. 647, Nov., 1960.

Belting, C. M., Haberfelde, G. C., and Juhl, L. K.: Spread of organisms from dental air rotor, J. Amer. Dent. Assoc. 68:648, 1964.

Beube, F. E., Schwartz, M., and Thompson, R. II.: A comparison of effectiveness in plaque removal of an electric toothbrush and a conventional hand toothbrush, Periodontics 2:71, 1964.

Bloom, R. H., and Brown, L. R., Jr.: A study of the effects of orthodontic appliances on the oral microbial flora, Oral Surg. 17:658, 1964.

Briner, W. W., and Francis, M. D.: The effect of enamel fluoride on acid production by *Lactobacillus casei,* Arch. Biol. 7:541, 1962.

Brown, R. V.: Bacterial aerosols generated by ultra high speed cutting instruments, J. Dent. Child. 32:112, 1965.

Burdick, K. H.: Dermatitis involving the dentist's hands, J. Amer. Dent. Assoc. 63:643, 1961.

Colton, M. B., and Ehrlich, E.: Polyantibiotic dental cement as a cavity sterilant—in vitro and in vivo report, New York Dent. J. 23:23, 1957.

Conroy, C. W., and Melfi, R. C.: Comparison of automatic and hand toothbrushes cleaning effectiveness for children, J. Dent. Child. 33:219, 1966.

Coykendall, A. L.: "Swish and swallow" is effective, J. Dent. Child. 33:162, 1966.

Dikeman, T. L.: A study of acidogenic and aciduric microorganisms in orthodontic and non-orthodontic patients, Amer. J. Orthodont. 48:627, 1962.

Finn, S. B.: Cavity sterilization—an unnecessary step, Dent. Clin. N. Amer. 663, Nov. 1960.

Finn, S. B.: Chewing-gum studies, Ann. N. Y. Acad. Sci. 153:350, 1968.

Gardner, A. F., and Higel, R. W.: An evaluation of agents used in cavity sterilization, Aust. Dent. J. 7:53, 1962.

Gibbons, P.: Clinical and bacteriological findings in patients wearing silastic 390 soft liner, J. Mich. Dent. Assoc. 47:64, 1965.

Goldfarb, S. K.: The dental x-ray machine, a possible route of disease transmission, New York Dent. J. 34:391, 1964.

Harrison, L. M., Jr.: Cavity varnishes shown ineffective, J. Dent. Child. 33:174, 1966.

Hoffman, M. M.: Questionable relationship of exodontia to poliomyelitis, Fortn. Rev. Chicago Dent. Soc. **25**:27, 1953.

Horowitz, H. S., and Heifetz, S. B.: The current status of topical fluorides in preventive dentistry, J. Amer. Dent. Assoc. **81**:166, 1970.

Ingervall, B.: The influence of orthodontic appliances on caries frequency, Odont. Rev. **13**:17, 1962.

Kantorowicz, G. F.: A study of organisms associated with injections into the oral mucosa, Arch. Oral Biol. **1**:183, 1959.

King, J. B., Jr., Crawford, B. A., and Lindahl, R. L.: Indirect pulp capping: A bacteriologic study of deep carious dentine in human teeth, Oral Surg. **20**:663, 1965.

Kutscher, A. H.: Terramycin in dental filling materials: Preliminary report, New York Dent. J. **19**:77, 1953.

Levens, P.: Prevention of caries in the patient undergoing orthodontic treatment, J. Amer. Dent. Assoc. **65**:316, 1962.

Lucente, J.: Use of an electric toothbrush in severely retarded children, J. Dent. Child. **33**:25, 1966.

Mandel, I. D., and Cagan, R. S.: Pharmaceutical agents for preventing caries—a review, J. Oral Ther. **1**:218, 1964.

McCue, R. W., McDougal, F. G., and Shay, D. E.: The antibacterial properties of some dental restorative materials, Oral Surg. **4**:1180, 1951.

Newton, A. V.: Denture sore mouth: A possible aetiology, Brit. Dent. J. **112**:357, 1962.

Parikh, S. R., Massler, M., and Bahn, A.: Microorganisms in active and arrested carious lesions of dentin, New York Dent. J. **29**:347, 1963.

Phillips, R. W.: Some current observations on restorative materials, J. Dent. Assoc. S. Afr. **21**:11, 1966.

Pleasure, M. A., Duerr, E., and Goldman, M.: Eliminating a health hazard in prosthodontic treatment of patients with pulmonary tuberculosis, J. Prosth. Dent. **9**:818, 1959.

Ray, K. C., and Fuller, M. L.: Isolation of mycobacterium from dental impression material, J. Prosth. Dent. **14**:93, 1964.

Richardson, A. S., and Castaldi, C. R.: Current status of chewing gum in preventive dentistry, J. Canad. Dent. Assoc. **31**:713, 1965.

Rothenberg, F., and Landman, R.: A review of drug therapy for dry socket, J. Oral Ther. **2**:229, 1965.

Saslaw, M. S., and Streitfeld, M. M.: Relation between smoking habit and presence of streptococci, Bl. Zahnheilk. **22**:141, 1961.

Shklair, I. L., and Mazzarella, M. A.: Effects of full-mouth extraction on oral microbiota, D. Progress **1**:275, 1961.

Slack, G. L., and Martin, W. J.: Apples and dental health, Br. Dent. J. **105**:366, 1958.

Slanetz, L. W., and Brown, E. A.: Studies on the numbers of bacteria in the mouth and their reduction by use of oral antiseptics, J. Dent. Res. **28**:313, 1949.

Toto, P. D., Rapp, G. W., and Goljan, K. R.: The effect of manual and mechanical toothbrushing on oral hygiene, caries conduciveness and pH of the oral cavity, J. Oral Ther. **1**:612, 1965.

Turkheim, H. J.: Bacteriological investigations on dental filling materials, Br. Dent. J. **95**:1, 1953.

13 / Sterilization and disinfection

This chapter presents the general principles of sterilization and disinfection and relates how these processes are indispensable to the practice of dentistry. There is a distinct difference between sterilization and disinfection. Sterilization refers to those processes by which all forms of microbial life, vegetative and spores, are destroyed or killed whereas disinfection refers to those processes that result in the destruction of only the vegetative forms of microbial life, and not spores. The processes of sterilization primarily use moist and dry heat, and those of disinfection are often restricted to the use of chemicals. It is reported that a 1-ml. salivary sample from the mouth of an average healthy person contains about 750 million microorganisms. Since the dentist's hands and instruments are repeatedly contaminated in his operations on patients, he should be well informed of sterilization and disinfection procedures in order to prevent cross-infection between patients and to protect himself from this occupational source of infection.

Suits of malpractice filed against dentists have specified that the dentist in his operation had broken the chain of asepsis. A malpractice suit brought against a dentist stated that the chain of asepsis was broken by the dentist's hygienist who, while performing a prophylactic treatment, was repeatedly interrupted to answer the telephone and make appointments. She re-turned to the patient without washing her hands during the treatment. A week later the patient became ill with symptoms diagnosed as those of tetanus. With recovery following antiserum therapy, the patient sued the dentist, claiming that the hygienist was responsible for the transfer of the organism *Clostridium tetani* from the objects she had touched to the patient's mouth during the prophylaxis, thereby causing the infection. There have been cases of serum hepatitis reportedly associated with dental operations. Some of these have been traced to the injection of an anesthetic with syringes and needles not properly sterilized. As little as 0.0004 ml. of virus contaminated blood remaining in the lumen of a needle has been reported to result in infection. The hepatitis virus in blood dried on instruments employed in periodontal treatments or oral surgical procedures is also a means of spreading this infection to the patient. The hepatitis virus appears to be more resistant to chemical disinfectants and heat than are other viruses. It is obvious that the nature of the dentist's work lends itself to the transfer of infectious agents from one patient to another. He should know about those aseptic procedures that protect his patients, his ancillary help, and himself.

Microorganisms are found everywhere in man's environment. In order to control those that cause disease, man has employed both physical and chemical meth-

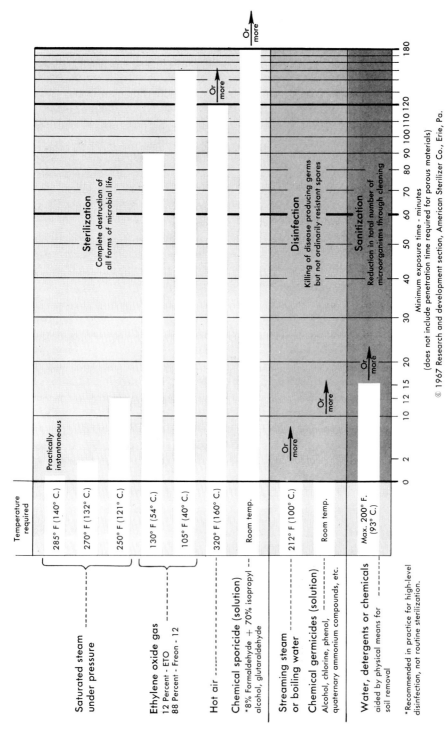

Fig. 13-1. Methods for controlling microbial life.

ods. Some of the most acceptable methods are presented in Fig. 13-1.

TERMINOLOGY

Besides understanding what is meant by sterilization and disinfection, the dentist should be familiar with other terms regarding the destruction or removal of microorganisms associated with infection. Some of the more common terms are presented here and are generally restricted to the use of chemical agents.

bactericide A chemical agent that kills bacteria, pathogenic and nonpathogenic, but not necessarily spores, when applied to either living tissues or inanimate objects.

germicide Same as bactericide; used especially with reference to killing pathogenic bacteria.

virucidal or *virucide* A chemical agent that inactivates or destroys viruses when applied to either living tissues or inanimate objects.

sporicide A chemical agent that kills bacterial and mold spores; refers usually to agents applied to inanimate objects.

fungicide A chemical agent that destroys pathogenic and nonpathogenic fungi. Such agents are used on living tissues and inanimate objects.

antiseptic A chemical agent that inhibits or destroys microorganisms. Such agents are applied to living tissues.

sanitization A term used in public health to indicate reduction of microorganisms to safe levels. Sanitization is not synonymous with sterilization or disinfection.

degermination Refers to the mechanical removal of microorganisms from tissue surfaces—such as hand washing.

DEATH RATE FOR BACTERIA

The exposure of bacteria to agents that have a killing effect does not result in instantaneous death to the entire population. The rate of death of a specific organism under uniform conditions appears to follow a certain pattern. Regardless of the initial size of the microbial population, the number of organisms is reduced by physical or chemical agents by the same percentage during each specific time period. For example, the percentage of microbial cells dying per unit

of time is constant. This is sometimes referred to as the logarithmic death rate. If the initial microbial population is one million microorganisms, at termination of the first unit of time 90% will have been killed, thus leaving 100,000 surviving. After the second unit of time, 90% of the 100,000 would die, thus leaving 10,000. After the third unit of time, 90% of the 10,000 would be killed, thus leaving 1,000 surviving. This pattern of death is followed until the entire microbial population has been killed. This observation of the logarithmic death rate shows that the number of microorganisms killed per unit of time is proportional to the numbers present. The unit of time may be expressed in minutes; as one minute would be the first unit of time, two minutes the second unit of time, etc. Some deviation from this logarithmic death rate pattern has been observed for certain organisms.

ANTIMICROBIAL PHYSICAL AGENTS
Heat

Practical methods of sterilization employ heat. These methods may be divided into dry heat and moist heat procedures.

Dry heat

Examples of dry heat sterilization are the open flame and the hot air oven. In the laboratory, the microbiologist uses the flame to sterilize Nichrome or platinum culture transfer wires. These instruments are held in the flame until they glow, thus incinerating all microorganisms, vegetative and spores, that contaminated the flamed portion. The dentist employs this method to a limited extent in taking cultures from specific isolated areas of the oral cavity using a transfer wire. The mere passage of dental instruments through a flame several times does not ensure sterilization. The dentist sometimes uses the flaming procedure for forceps previously sterilized by other methods. Here the forceps are generally dipped into 70% alcohol and ignited by passage through a flame. This procedure is used to ensure disinfection when such instruments are used several times as in the placing of a sterile paper point for a root canal culture. Flaming in alcohol cannot be relied upon to kill spores (Table 13-1).

The hot air oven is employed in the sterilization of microbiologic equipment such as glassware—Petri dishes, pipets, flasks. It is also used in the dentist's office for sterilizing certain instruments and materials. These ovens are generally heated electrically and have an outer jacket in

Table 13-1. Effect of simple sterilizing methods on *Bacillus subtilis* spores*

Method	Number of tests	Results		Efficiency percentages
		Growth	No growth	
Times flamed				
3	3	3	0	0
6	3	3	0	0
10	4	4	0	0
15	20	19	1	5
20	20	3	17	85
95% alcohol and flame	30	27	3	10
40% formalin (1 part), 95% alcohol (3 parts), and flame	25	2	23	92
Benzene, phenol, alcohol, boiling water (each 30 seconds)	26	22	4	15.4
Flaherty molten metal sterilizer	68	6	62	91.2

*From Bartels, H. A., and Rice, E.: J. Amer. Dent. Assoc. **29**:1398, 1942. Copyright by the American Dental Association. Reprinted by permission.

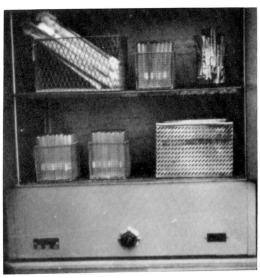

Fig. 13-2. Hot air sterilizer. This unit is electrically heated and contains an air blower for circulation of the heated air.

which the heated air is passed to the oven chamber by either normal air convection or convection currents forced by a fan (Fig. 13-2). Since air is a poor conductor of heat, a relatively high temperature is necessary for sterilization. A temperature of 160° C. (320° F.) for an exposure period of one hour is generally required. Only articles not deteriorated or destroyed by dry heat may be sterilized by this method. The dentist uses the hot air oven for sterilization of certain items and instruments that rust when exposed to moisture; for example, carbon steel cutting instruments, files, broaches, cotton pellets, and paper points that are used in endodontics.

It has been shown that pathogenic *Streptococcus pyogenes*, *Staphylococcus aureus*, and salivary oral microflora dried on dental instruments are destroyed in 20 minutes at 160° C. Therefore, 160° C. for 60 minutes should add a considerable safety factor, to ensure sterility of dental instruments that have been thoroughly cleaned of all debris and properly packaged before sterilization.

During endodontic dental procedures, the dentist uses hot air-sterilized broaches and reamers repeatedly in enlarging the root canal. He requires a quick method for resterilizing these instruments during the procedure so as to not reintroduce contamination into the canal. The molten metal sterilization introduced by Flaherty (Fig. 13-3) has been used for this purpose. The working end of the instrument is immersed in the molten metal, which is a mixture of lead-tin solder of equal parts. Since the molten metal has a tendency to adhere to the instruments and can be carried into the canal of the tooth, the metal has been replaced by salt crystals or small glass beads 1 mm. in diameter. The temperature and time required for this method of sterilization is 220° C. for 10 seconds. Paper points and cotton pellets contaminated with *Staphylococcus aureus* and spores of *Clostridium welchii* and *Cl.*

sporogenes were demonstrated to be sterilized by this method.

Hot oil baths represent another method of sterilization employed in dentistry. Mineral oil or certain silicone preparations are used to sterilize dental handpieces. The handpieces are first placed in a solvent cleaning solution to remove debris and then placed in the hot oil sterilizer (175° C.) for 10 minutes. The handpiece is removed from the sterilizer, the oil allowed to drain, and the outer sheath wiped with sterile gauze. If temperatures of around 150° C. are used, the hot oil cannot be relied upon to kill spores.

Moist heat

The most effective means of sterilization is the use of moist heat in the form of steam under pressure. Heat transfer is rapid when moisture is present. The autoclave uses steam under pressure. Hospitals

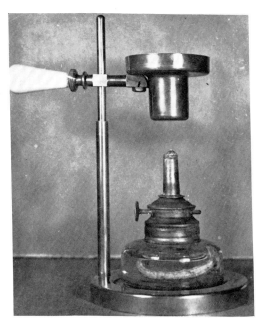

Fig. 13-3. Flaherty molten metal sterilizer. This original model in which the tin-lead solder is melted by heat from the alcohol lamp has been replaced by an electrically heated unit which may be attached to the dental unit.

and microbiologic laboratories' autoclaves (Figs. 13-4 and 13-5) are connected to a main steam line and by means of a reducing valve the pressure of the steam is controlled to 20 pounds of pressure per square inch upon entrance into the autoclave. Small autoclaves are especially designed for use in the dental office and generate steam from a water reservoir by means of gas or electricity (Fig. 13-6). In operation of the autoclave, the chamber is loaded and the door closed and bolted because the pressure generated by the steam on the inside will reach 15 pounds

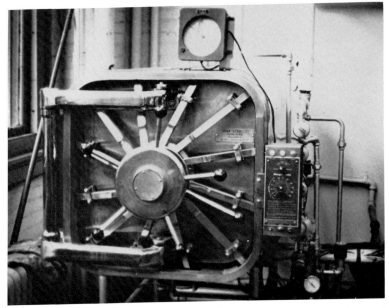

Fig. 13-4. Large autoclave using steam under pressure. Chamber may be packed with gowns, towels, rubber gloves, and instruments in individual packets as well as various media in flasks or tubes or contaminated glassware.

Fig. 13-5. Longitudinal cross section of an autoclave. The body of the sterilizer is made up of a cylindrical sterilizing chamber surrounded by a steam jacket. The outside of the steam jacket is insulated and covered. The chamber is loaded with supplies to be sterilized through a door which closes the front end of the sterilizing chamber. This is a safety steam-locked door made tight against a flexible heat resistant gasket. Pressure is first generated in the steam jacket; then steam is admitted to the sterilizing chamber, and the load (materials to be sterilized) is heated to the temperature of the steam in the chamber. A constant pressure within the steam jacket is maintained during the sterilizing procedure to keep the walls of the sterilizing chamber heated and dry. The moisture which condenses on the door or back part of the sterilizing chamber drains downward from behind a steam deflector plate to the bottom of the chamber and is then discharged. When the pressure of the chamber is suddenly exhausted, the heat initially transferred to the load helps to dry the load. This residual heat effects vaporization of the moisture in the load; if this vapor is allowed to escape freely, the load will be satisfactorily dried within a brief period of time. (From Smith, A. L.: Principles of microbiology, ed. 5, St. Louis, 1965, The C. V. Mosby Co.)

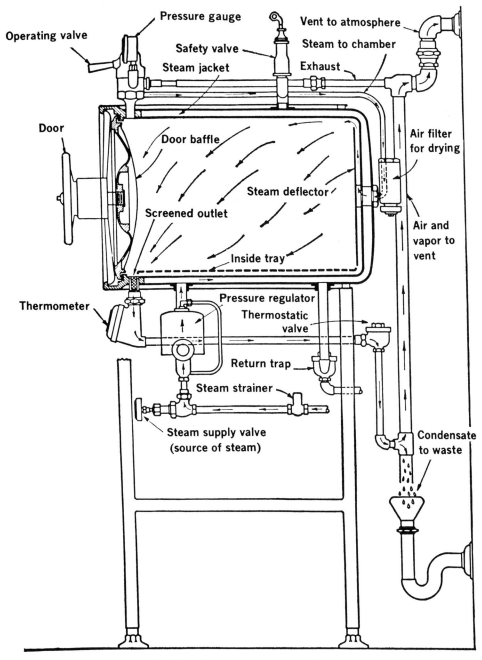

Fig. 13-5. For legend see opposite page.

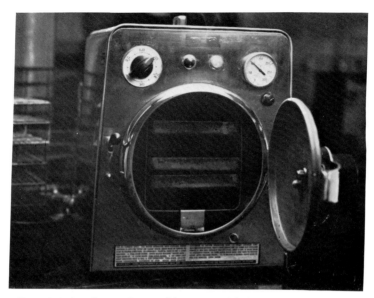

Fig. 13-6. Small autoclave (table top model) for dental office use.

or slightly more per square inch. The outer jacket surrounding the autoclave chamber is freed of air, which is replaced with steam to a recording gauge pressure of 15 pounds. A valve is then opened and steam enters the sterilizing chamber, forcing the air out until a pressure of 15 pounds is reached. When this pressure is reached, the recording thermometer attached to the steam escape drainage pipe should read 121° C. At this point, the period of sterilization is recorded. Depending upon the type of material and amount of load in the autoclave, the time period for sterilization varies. Generally the minimum time is 15 minutes and the maximum 30 minutes. When steam condenses on the surface of an object, latent heat of condensation raises the temperature of the object to that of the steam under pressure. At 10 pounds pressure per square inch, the temperature of steam would be 116° C.; at 15 pounds, 121° C.; and at 30 pounds, 136° C. No microorganism, including spores, can survive 10 minutes of direct exposure to steam at 121° C. Articles that can be sterilized in the autoclave

include most culture media; saline and other solutions not broken down by the high temperature; syringes, needles, dressings, sponges, gowns, rubber gloves, tubing and aprons and certain instruments. By the use of negative pressure, which is created by the rapid exhaust of pressure through a gauge control, articles such as gowns, instruments, and the like can be dried. For culture media and solutions, the release of pressure from the chamber has to be slow to avoid blowing out the stoppers and causing bubbling and overflow of these liquids from the flasks and tubes in which they were sterilized.

Also available for use in the dental office are small autoclaves that utilize chemical vapors instead of steam and operate according to the standard procedures. The chemical solution consists of various alcohols, acetone, formaldehyde, and 5% distilled water. Under pressure of 15 pounds, the temperature exceeds 121° C. It has been shown that these vapor sterilizers will destroy spores within 15 minutes, and that the vapor is less corrosive to instruments than steam under pressure.

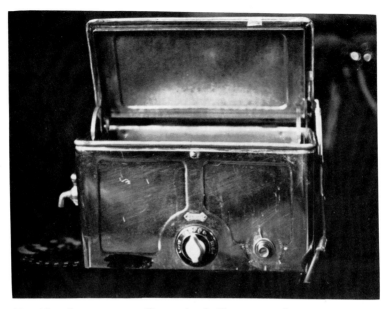

Fig. 13-7. Instrument sterilizer using boiling water plus antirust tablet.

Indicator controls to ensure sterilization. To ensure that the autoclave is operating effectively, controls should be run periodically. Among the various types available are pressure-temperature-sensitive tapes that change color when the proper temperature is reached. Other types are spore suspensions of *Bacillus stearothermophilus* or some similar spore-resistant bacillus. In the case of *Bacillus stearothermophilus*, a thermophile, the spore suspension is prepared in an indicator broth in a sealed vial. Some preparations consist of spore suspensions fixed to paper strips by drying. In either case, the controls are placed in the autoclave in wrapped articles and after the sterilizing process is completed they are cultured. If no growth occurs, the autoclave is operating effectively; if growth occurs on culture, the autoclave cannot be relied upon to ensure sterility and should be checked by an authorized autoclave mechanic.

Boiling water. The apparatus most commonly employed in many dental and medical offices for sterilization is the boiling water sterilizer (Fig. 13-7). Many instru-ments, syringes, needles, sutures, and other items are sterilized by exposure to boiling water for at least 30 minutes. In the strictest sense, boiling water (100° C.) will not kill spores; therefore, this is a *disinfection* process and *not a sterilization* process. Boiling water will kill vegetative bacterial cells within five minutes or less. *Mycobacterium tuberculosis* is killed at 58° C. within 30 minutes, and at 65° C. within 2 minutes. A period of 30 minutes at 100° C. is recommended in order to destroy the virus of hepatitis, which may contaminate instruments through dental operations on carriers of this virus or patients with unrecognized cases. Boiling water destroys microorganisms by coagulating protein. Water corrodes carbon steel instruments. When boiling water is used, the addition of sodium carbonate, trisodium phosphate, or 0.2% nitrate to the water should help prevent corrosion. The addition of a 2% oil (AC 10) and 2% sodium carbonate decahydrate to boiling water forms an emulsion. This procedure has been recommended for use in (sterilizing) disinfecting dental handpieces and carbon dental

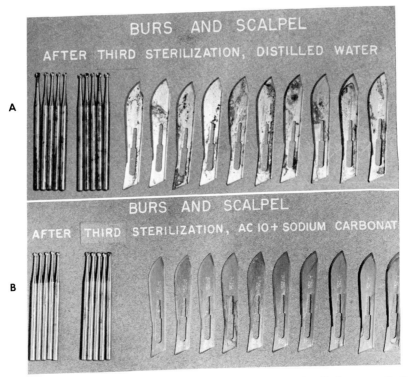

Fig. 13-8. A, Burs and scalpels after third sterilization in distilled water. **B,** Burs and scalpels after third sterilization in A.C. 10 and sodium carbonate. Corrosion occurred only in the distilled water. (From Nolte, W. A., and Arnim, S. S.: J.A.D.A. **50:**133, 1955. Copyright by the American Dental Association. Reprinted by permission.)

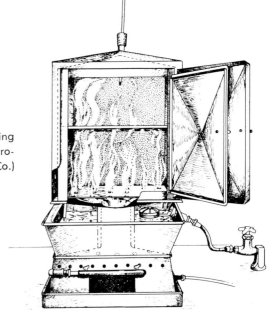

Fig. 13-9. Arnold sterilizer using free-flowing steam. (From Swatek, F. E.: Textbook of microbiology, St. Louis, 1967, The C. V. Mosby Co.)

Table 13-2. Effect of three boiling media on dental instruments inoculated with microbial cultures*

Cultures used in inoculating instruments	Sterilization media† exposure 5 minutes	Number of instruments used for each culture						
		40 scalpels	40 burs	8 straight handpieces			8 contra-angles	
				Outside spindle	Inside spindle	Chuck plunger	Gear head	About gear
Serratia marcescens	A	−	−	−	−	−	−	−
	B	−	−	−	−	−	−	−
	C	−	−	−	−	−	−	−
Staphylococcus pyrogenes var. aureus	A	−	−	−	−	−	−	−
	B	−	−	−	−	−	−	−
	C	−	−	−	−	−	−	−
Streptococcus hemolyticus	A	−	−	−	−	−	−	−
	B	−	−	−	−	−	−	−
	C	−	−	−	−	−	−	−
Candida albicans	A	−	−	−	−	−	−	−
	B	−	−	−	−	−	−	−
	C	−	−	−	−	−	−	−
Bacillus subtilis	A	+	+	+	+	+	+	+
	B	+	+	+	+	+	+	+
	C	+	+	+	+	+	+	+
Human saliva	A	−	−	−	−	−	−	−
	B	−	−	−	−	−	−	−
	C	−	−	−	−	−	−	−

*From Nolte, W. A., and Arnim, S. S.: J. Amer. Dent. Assoc. **50:**133, 1955. Copyright by the American Dental Association. Reprinted by permission.
†A, A.C. 10 soda emulsion; B, distilled water plus 2% W/V sodium carbonate (decahydrate); C. distilled water
+ Denotes growth
− Denotes no growth

instruments since it prevents corrosion (Fig. 13-8). It does not kill spores (Table 13-2).

Intermittent sterilization. Another method of using steam is known as intermittent sterilization, tyndallization, or Arnold sterilization. This method is applied in the microbiologic laboratory to sterilization of those media and solutions that are adversely affected by the high temperatures of the autoclave. The method utilizes free flowing steam of a temperature of 100° C. The instrument employed, the Arnold sterilizer, has a steam generator (Fig. 13-9). The steam generated rises, enters the sterilizing chamber, and escapes about the sides of the door and through a vent. Media and solutions to be sterilized are exposed to the free flowing steam for 30 minutes, which process kills vegetative bacteria but not spores. These materials are then removed and incubated overnight at either room temperature or 37° C. During this time, most spores if present will germinate into vegetative cells. A second 30-minute sterilization exposure followed by incubation as before is carried out. Then there is a third exposure to the steam and incubation. This procedure should result in the sterilization of the materials.

Moist heat versus dry heat

It was early demonstrated by Koch that moist heat is more effective than dry heat as a medium for sterilization. By placing maximum and minimum recording ther-

Table 13-3. Physical sterilization of reusable instruments and supplies*

Method	Administration		Application
	Temperature	*Time*	
Autoclave	121° to 123° C. (250° to 254° F.), 15 to 17 lbs. pressure†	30 minutes	Gloves, drapes, towels, gauze pads, instruments, glassware, and metalware
Dry heat	170° C. (340° F.)	1 hour	Glassware, metalware, and dull instruments (any temperature)
	160° C.	2 hours	Small quantities powders, petrolatum (Vaseline), oils, and petrolatum (Vaseline) gauze
	150° C. or lower	3 hours	Sharp instruments and metal-tip syringes
	121° C. (250° F.)	6 hours or longer	
Boiling	100° C. (212° F.)†	30 minutes	Method not recommended when dry heat and autoclave sterilization available

*From Smith, A. L.: Principles of microbiology, ed. 5, St. Louis, 1965, The C. V. Mosby Co.
†Atmosphere pressure, sea level.

mometers within various thicknesses of linen, Koch found that after their exposure to hot air at 130° C. for four hours, the temperatures recorded by thermometers wrapped in 20, 40, or 100 thicknesses of linen were 86°, 72°, and 70° C., respectively. On their exposure to moist heat (free flowing steam from 90° to 100° C.) for three hours, the temperature reached was 101° C. This observation indicates that moist heat has penetration superior to that of dry heat. Spores of the anthrax bacillus were reportedly killed by exposure to free flowing steam within 10 minutes; whereas dry heat required three hours at 140° C. Table 13-3 compares various methods of using heat for the destruction of microorganisms.

When heat is used, the time of exposure and the temperature of the heat are most important. The term "thermal death point" (T.D.P.) refers to the lowest temperature that will kill a bacterial culture in 10 minutes. The term "thermal death time" (T.D.T.) refers to the shortest period of time required to kill a bacterial culture at a specific temperature. The relationship between time and temperature required to kill microorganisms varies for different microorganisms and is influenced

by many factors, such as type of heat (moist or dry), kind and number of microorganisms, presence of spores, and the nature of the material to be sterilized.

Pasteurization

Pasteurization is not a method of sterilization; it is a process used principally in the food industries for the preservation of milk and other dairy products, fruit juices, beer, and wine. This process consists of exposing the product to a temperature of 62.8° C. for 30 minutes and then cooling it immediately. Vegetative microbial forms such as the tubercule bacillus, beta hemolytic streptococci, and *Brucella* organisms, other pathogens, nonpathogens, and most viruses are killed. Pasteurization does not kill thermophiles or spore formers.

Cold

Cold temperatures are employed to retard microbial growth in foods and to preserve many biologic materials. Regarding their temperature requirements for growth, bacteria have been classified as follows: (1) The psychrophilic organisms are those that grow best at low temperatures, the optimum being around 15° C. These organisms are found in the soil and in the sea. (2) The mesophilic bacteria are the pathogens of man and animals and grow best around 37° C. (3) The thermophilic organisms, which grow best around 55° C., are found in the soil and hot springs. The household refrigerator with a temperature of around 4° C. (39.2° F.) is especially unfavorable for the growth of thermophiles and most mesophiles. Psychrophilic and some mesophilic bacteria grow only at a slow rate. Temperatures around 0° C. have a greater growth inhibitory effect on bacteria than subzero temperatures of around –20° C. Low temperatures of from –20° to –76° C. are used to preserve cultures of certain microorganisms. Viruses that are used in research are best preserved at –76° C. Cold affects the bacterial cell in several ways: (1) It increases the viscosity of the proteins, thus slowing the streaming action of the protoplasm, and affects its colloidal state; (2) it impedes the diffusion of toxic products from the cell; (3) it causes a decrease in enzyme activity; and (4) it results in the formation of ice crystals within the outside of the bacterial cell, which mechanically ruptures the cell. At extremely low temperatures many microbial cells are destroyed, but a sufficient number of cells survive to permit the propagation of the culture.

Lyophilization

Lyophilization is a freeze-drying procedure used to maintain viable organisms for long periods of time. An 18- to 24-hour pure culture of the organism is suspended in a medium such as sterile milk or serum. A small amount of the suspension (0.1 ml. or less) is aseptically transferred to several ampules. The ampules are placed in dry ice (–76° C.) and the suspension mixture is frozen instantaneously. Immediately the ampules are attached to a high vacuum system. The water in the suspending medium is rapidly withdrawn so that it passes from the solid to the vapor state without going through the liquid phase.

When all water is removed, the ampules are hermetically sealed by an oxygenated needle flame. Most organisms processed by this method retain their viability for years.

Radiation

Ultraviolet light, x-rays, and gamma rays are examples of different types of radiation. Radiant energy emanates from the sun in the form of waves that reach the earth in approximately eight minutes. The lethal effect to man of some of these waves is prevented by the blocking effect of the earth's atmosphere. Some of these rays can be produced artificially by man.

Waves of the electromagnetic spectrum have different lengths. Their size is measured in the Angström unit, which is equivalent to $\frac{1}{10}$ of a millimicron or $\frac{1}{10,000,000}$ of a millimeter.

The cosmic rays are the shortest in length (0.1 A). X-rays and cathode and gamma rays range between 0.01 and 0.06 A in length. The ultraviolet rays cover the spectrum between 1,000 and 3,000 A in length. The visible light and its color components are found in the spectrum range of from 4,000 A (violet) to 8,000 A (red). Infrared or heat waves are longer waves and are in the range of from 8,000 to 40,000,000 A. Radio waves extend to 2 $\times 10^{12}$ A.

Cosmic rays, x-rays, and cathode and gamma rays are of small wave size, are powerful and penetrating, and are deadly to life. Use of these rays in the preservation of foods through their lethal action on microorganisms has been studied intensively. Of these, gamma rays obtained from isotopes are used most frequently. The rays penetrate cans, paper boxes, and plastic bags and destroy the microorganisms in foods that are irradiated. The concentration of gamma rays necessary for bactericidal activity depends on the organism; that is, whether it is the vegetative or spore form. The spore form requires longer and more concentrated exposure. The unit of exposure, called the rad (radiation absorbed dose), is equivalent to 100 ergs of energy absorbed by 1 gm. of exposed material. A megarad is equivalent to 1 million rads. Doses of more than several megarads may be necessary to destroy spores. A study has shown that bacon contaminated with from 600,000 to 2 million *Clostridium botulinum* spores and packed in cans was rendered free of viable spores after exposure to gamma rays of from 2.5 to 3.0 megarads. Sterilization of foods by this procedure appears to result in characteristic changes in flavor and odor. Radiation does not result in the denaturation of protein. It appears to induce ionization of vital cell units, particularly the deoxyribonucleic acid of the nucleus.

Ultraviolet radiation

The ultraviolet rays of sunlight filter through the earth's atmosphere and have been shown to possess bactericidal or bacteriostatic properties. The maximum killing effect is at 2,600 A units of the spectrum. Ultraviolet lamps called "sterilamps" have been recommended to reduce the microflora of the air in operating rooms, communicable disease wards, schoolrooms, nurseries, bacteriologic laboratories, and food processing plants such as bakeries and meat packing plants. The exposure of microorganisms to ultraviolet light causes an excitation rather than ionization of the molecules in vital cell units, particularly nucleic acids.

The effect of ultraviolet light on microorganisms may be reversed if after being exposed to ultraviolet light the microorganisms are exposed to normal light and placed in fresh culture medium. This regeneration is called photoreactivation. Sublethal doses of ultraviolet rays are mutagenic and this is one method used in producing mutant strains in the laboratory. The energy required to destroy most vegetative forms of bacteria is approximately

40,000 ergs per centimeter. This energy may be obtained within several minutes from a low pressure mercury vapor lamp (30 watts) placed at a distance of several feet and emitting ultraviolet rays in the 2,500 to 2,600 A region of the spectrum.

Ultraviolet germicidal lamps placed in a cabinet have been found effective for the storage and maintenance of previously sterilized materials and instruments in the dental office. These lamps are not effective in sterilizing gauze, cotton, and dental handpieces because the rays have poor penetrating power and cannot reach all contaminated surfaces. An ultraviolet lamp with a quartz pencil-shaped extension has little therapeutic value in the treatment of Vincent's infection. Recently use has been made of ultraviolet light's ability to induce hardening of an adhesive material that is applied to teeth to protect against cavities.

Ultrasonic vibrations

The human ear can detect sound wave frequencies less than 9,000 cycles per second. Supersonic vibrations are considered to be between 9,000 and 200,000 cycles per second, and ultrasonic waves are at higher frequencies, more than 200,000 cycles per second. The effect of sound waves depends more on their amplitude than on their frequency. Waves of low frequency but high intensity are more effective than high frequency waves of low intensity. Because of their small size, bacteria are more resistant to the effects of sonic vibrations than the cells of higher plants. When microorganisms are in liquid suspension and exposed to sonic vibrations of appropriate rate and intensity generated electrically by a sonifier, microbubbles are formed about the cell walls of the microorganisms. The bubbles cause disruption of the cell, a process known as cavitation. Also during sonification, a temperature of 50° or 80° C. is reached and effects destruction of organisms. At lower temperatures, 20° C.

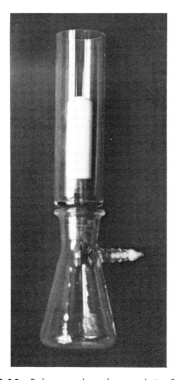

Fig. 13-10. Selas unglazed porcelain filter assembled in glass mantle and connected by bored rubber stopper with mouth of Erlenmeyer flask. Side neck of flask is connected with vacuum pump.

and lower, some organisms survive sonification as demonstrated by growth on culture. Bacteria differ greatly in their susceptibility to the effects of sonification. Spores are extremely resistant. Sonification cannot be relied upon to sterilize, especially viscous materials such as human saliva.

Sonation tanks have been recommended for the cleaning of dental and surgical instruments, but not for sterilizing them. Sonic operated handpieces may be used in dental prophylaxis. A commercially available sonic denture cleaning bath has been shown to destroy oral microorganisms dried in saliva on glass rods.

Filtration

Microorganisms can be removed from solutions and fluids by filtration. These solutions are then sterile. This method is used for solutions and fluids that cannot be exposed to heat or chemicals without being chemically changed. Microorganisms are not killed by filtration but are physically separated from the fluid as it passes through the filter. Filters with a pore size

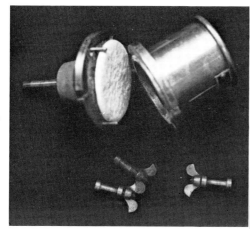

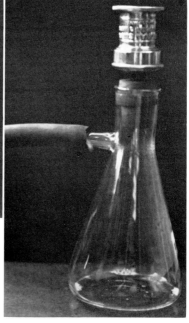

Fig. 13-11. A, Seitz asbestos fiber pad filter with metal assembly. **B,** Seitz asbestos fiber pad filter assembled and attached to Erlenmeyer flask.

of 0.2 μ in diameter will remove bacteria and microorganisms other than viruses. Filters of porosity of 10 mμ are recommended for the removal of viruses. Filtration is used to remove microorganisms from biologic fluids such as normal sera, antisera, microbial toxins, enzyme-containing solutions, various sugar solutions, and other materials that are put in solution that cannot be sterilized by other methods. Microbiologic filters are made of unglazed porcelain, diatomaceous earth, asbestos, sintered glass, collodion, and cellulose acetate.

The Berkefeld and Mandler filters are made of diatomaceous earth and are available in three different porosities, coarse, normal, and fine. The Chamberland filter is an unglazed porcelain one made of mixtures of kaolin and sand that are oven fired to a specific temperature. These filters are made in different porosities, designated L1, L2, and L3; the porosity of L3 is given as 0.2 μ in diameter. These filters are shaped like a hollow candle and the base is attached to glazed porcelain or metallic nipples that can be fitted to flasks for the collection of filtrates (Fig. 13-10).

The Seitz filter is shown in Fig. 13-11. This filter consists of a metallic holder for an asbestos pad. Pads of different porosities are available. Fresh pads are used for each filtration. This filter does not require special methods of cleaning as do the Berkefeld, Mandler, Chamberland, and sintered glass types. This latter type is made of pulverized glass that is placed in molds and heated to just less than its fusion temperature, thus leaving the glass porous. The discs are then fused into spiral-designed glass funnels. These filters can be obtained in three pore sizes: coarse, medium, and fine.

Membrane filters are very popular today because of the simplicity of the filtering apparatus available. The filter membranes, made of cellulose esters, are available in porosities of from 10 mμ to 5 μ (Fig. 13-12). These membranes can be obtained in various size diameters for use with syringes with large funnel filters. Membrane

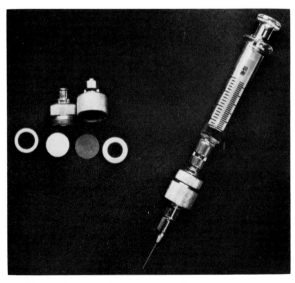

Fig. 13-12. Swinny filter. The metal parts are attached to syringe and needle. When assembled, the metal parts contain a cellulose acetate filter which rests upon a perforated metal disk; both are supported by an inner and an outer gasket to prevent leakage.

filters have replaced to a great extent all other filters.

The Chamberland, Berkefeld, Mandler, and sintered glass filters have to be thoroughly cleaned by special methods before they can be sterilized for reuse. This requires time and, therefore, use of these filters has decreased in popularity. The membrane filter apparatus after use is disassembled, the old filter discarded, the apparatus thoroughly washed, and a new filter fitted and the assembly sterilized. Today, there are available special disposable plastic filter units with membrane filters. After use, the entire assembly is discarded.

The use of filtration is important to the microbiologist to sterilize solutions and fluids. Some solutions that the dentist uses are sterilized by this method by the manufacturer.

ANTIMICROBIAL CHEMICAL AGENTS

The use of chemical agents as a means of preventing infection was first introduced in the medical field. In 1847, Semmelweis, a physician, noted that mortality caused by puerperal fever was extremely high in certain clinics. He believed that the physician and the medical student were responsible for transferring infectious material from one patient to another. He enforced the use of chlorinated lime soak after a thorough washing of the hands between examinations of patients on his wards. Through this measure, he was instrumental in significantly reducing the death rate caused by childbed fever.

Lister, the father of aseptic surgery, in 1867 introduced the use of aqueous solutions of phenol as wet dressings in the treatment of fracture wounds. He also introduced the use of phenol as a soak for instruments and used a phenolic solution in washing the skin before operating. In 1870, Lister employed a phenolic acid spray in the environment in which he was operating, believing that it would kill the germs in the air before they came in contact with the wound. As a result, a drop of 35% in mortality followed the use of phenol in surgical procedures.

In addition to these measures, aseptic surgery soon included the sterilization of all instruments, gowns, drapes, and dressings before use.

Disinfectant spectrum

The exposure of microorganisms to low, intermediate, and high concentrations of a germicidal agent produces various effects ranging from stimulatory to killing. This variation in the activity of germicidal agents on microorganisms has been referred to as the disinfectant spectrum. This disinfectant spectrum may be separated somewhat into different zones regarding the effect of the germicide. In extremely low concentrations, the germicidal agent may have no effect on the microorganisms; this is referred to as the ineffective zone. With slightly increased concentrations of the germicide, a stimulation of growth of the organisms may occur; this is referred to as the stimulatory zone. Increased concentration of the germicide produces an inhibition or static effect; this range of concentration is referred to as the inhibitory zone. In higher concentrations, a lethal effect is known and this is referred to as the germicidal zone. Higher than the germicidal zone are concentrations of the chemical agent that are not practical to use because of their insolubility or toxicity to tissues. The zones referred to as a disinfectant spectrum blend into one another and are not sharply separated.

Bacteriostat versus bactericide

A bacterial cell is considered to be dead when it is unable to multiply in an ideal environment. When organisms are exposed to certain chemical agents, such as organic mercurials, for short time periods, they can be revived by being subcultured in a medium containing free sulfhydryl groups.

The effect of the mercury compound is reversed by the –SH groups. The action of the mercurials under this condition is known as bacteriostasis, for if the organism were subcultured to a medium not containing sulfhydryl groups, it would fail to grow. A bacteriostatic agent is one that inhibits microbial reproduction. A bactericidal agent is one that has an irreversible action and results in death of the microbial cell. Germicides and disinfectants act as bactericidal agents when used in the concentrations recommended; whereas antiseptics may be either bactericidal or bacteriostatic in their action. The basic difference between these types of action is largely determined by the concentration of the agent and the time of exposure. To determine whether a chemical agent is bactericidal, the evaluation test must be designed to exclude bacteriostatic inhibition. As was discussed with the disinfectant spectrum, many germicides in high dilutions are bacteriostatic. If after the exposure period minimal amounts of the agent are transferred along with the test organism to subculture medium, bacteriostasis may continue. The absence of growth on subculture would lead to a false assumption of a bactericidal action of the agent. To nullify this misinterpretation, certain substances are added to the subculture medium to inactivate traces of the agent carried over. For example, sodium thioglycollate 0.05% is added to neutralize mercury compounds; 1% sodium thiosulfate to inactivate chlorine and iodine; 1% Tween 80 to inactivate phenol and phenol compounds as hexachlorophene; and 1% Lubrol and 0.5% lecithin to inactivate quaternary ammonium compounds.

Factors affecting germicidal activity

Effective concentration of agent. The chemical agent should be used in the concentration recommended by the manufacturers and prepared according to the directions. Some agents are readily soluble in water; others are not and require special preparation in order to obtain an effective germicidal concentration.

The cresols are only moderately soluble in water but, when properly saponified, can be diluted with water to an effective germicidal concentration. On the other hand, phenol is readily soluble in water in an effective germicidal concentration.

Time of exposure. All microorganisms are not killed instantly when in contact with a germicidal agent. The death rate follows a logarithmic pattern related to time of exposure. There is a relationship of time to temperature, kind and number of organisms, type of material to be disinfected, and the presence of organic matter. *Mycobacterium tuberculosis* and spores are quite resistant to chemical germicides, and pneumococci are very susceptible.

Temperatures. An increase in temperature results in increased lethal activity of germicides. For each 10° C. rise in temperature, the disinfectant velocity of a germicidal agent increases. A threefold increase is noted for silver nitrate; the lethal effect of carbolic acid is reported to increase twofold to fourfold for each 10° C. rise in temperature.

pH. Some chemical agents have a greater germicidal effect in an acid reaction, and others are more active in an alkaline medium. Cationic detergents (quaternary compounds) demonstrate their maximum antibacterial or inhibitory activity in an alkaline pH range whereas the anionic detergents (lauryl sulfate type) are more active germicidally in the acid range.

Presence of contaminants. Some chemical germicidal agents combine with organic matter such as blood, pus, or saliva, and as the result the germicidal efficiency of the chemical is greatly reduced. The chemical agent may coagulate proteinaceous material and thus form films about the microorganisms that protect the microbe from the germicidal activity of the agent. Whenever chemical agents are used to disinfect instruments or other items, it is essential that the instruments be thoroughly cleaned of all debris before being placed in the disinfectant.

Methods of evaluating chemical agents for antimicrobial activity

The evaluation of chemical agents for their antiseptic or disinfection activity and their toxicity toward man and animals is made according to standard methods designed by the Federal Food and Drug Administration.

The official method, presented in *The Association of Official Agricultural Chemists—Method for Testing Disinfectants,** is known as the A.O.A.C. phenol coefficient method. Methods other than the phenol coefficient are used also in the evaluation of chemical agents for germicidal activity.

Phenol coefficient. The phenol coefficient method is based on testing dilutions of chemical agents soluble in water for antimicrobial activity and comparing their activity with that of phenol under standard conditions.

*Ed. 10, 1965.

The test compound is diluted in a series of decreasing concentrations. To 10 ml. of each dilution, a specific amount (0.5 ml.) of the test microorganism grown from 22 to 26 hours at 37° C. in a standard broth is added, mixed, and held at 20° C. At specific time intervals of 5, 10, and 15 minutes, a sample (one standard wire transfer loop, 4 mm. inside diameter) of the mixture is aseptically removed from each dilution, transferred to respective tubes of standard nutrient medium, and incubated at 37° C. for 48 hours. The phenol standard is tested in 1:80, 1:90, and 1:100 dilutions following the same technique. No growth on subculture indicates that the organism has been killed. The highest dilution of the unknown chemical agent that kills in 10 minutes and not in 5 minutes is divided by the highest dilution of phenol that kills in the same time period. This ratio is the *phenol coefficient.* The test organisms used in the phenol coefficient are *Salmonella typhosa* (Hopkins strain) and a strain of *Staphylococcus aureus* number 209. The following is a sample test:

Disinfectant dilution	5 minutes	Exposure time 10 minutes	15 minutes
Phenol			
1:80	−	−	−
1:90	+	−	−
1:100	+	+	+
Test germicide			
1:10	−	−	−
1:100	−	−	−
1:200	−	−	−
1:300	+	−	−
1:400	+	+	−
1:500	+	+	+

+ indicates growth; − indicates no growth

$$\text{Phenol coefficient} = \frac{\text{Highest dilution germicide kills in 10 minutes}}{\text{Highest dilution phenol kills in 10 minutes}} = \frac{300}{90} = 3.3$$

This test is highly standardized as to the specific brands of basic nutrients used in making media for growing and subculturing the test organism, the pH of the media, age of the test culture, amount of culture used in tests, temperature at which the tests are carried out, and other factors. Under these conditions the test organisms remain sufficiently constant in their resistance to phenol. *Salmonella typhosa* is resistant to exposure of 1:90 dilution of phenol for 5 minutes but is killed by this dilution within 10 minutes. *Staphylococcus aureus* is resistant to 1:80 dilution of phenol for 5 minutes but is killed by this dilution within 10 minutes. The phenol used must meet the requirements of the United States Pharmacopoeia and should congeal at 40° C. or above. The stock, a 5% phenol solution, is standardized by a specific A.O.A.C. method and is held in an amber stoppered bottle in a relatively cool place.

If the antimicrobial agent is recommended for external use, the evaluation is carried out at 20° C.; if the agent is to be used in the body cavity, such as a mouthwash, the evaluation is carried out at 37° C. It is frequently desirable to test substances in the presence of organic matter, and such tests are conducted using 10% sterile blood serum.

The phenol coefficient method has its limitations in that it is an in vitro test, is adapted to the testing of substances that are miscible in water, and is especially favorable for testing substances similar to phenol. It has been suggested that other tests be made to supplement the information obtained from phenol coefficient results. Such tests should furnish information regarding tissue toxicity, the effect of inactivation on the bactericidal activity of the chemical agent, and the effect of the agent on other organisms, including spores.

Use-dilution test. The use-dilution test confirms the phenol coefficient results and indicates the maximum dilutions of the agent effective for practical disinfection. Specially prepared sterile small steel cylinders are inoculated by immersion into a broth culture of the test microorganism. The inoculated cylinders are dried for one hour at 37° C. in an incubator. The dilutions prepared of the disinfectant are approximately twenty times that determined in the phenol coefficient, or 20 × 3.3 of the sample test which equals 1:60 to 1:70 dilutions. The inoculated cylinders are then placed in respective dilutions of the disinfectant for 10 minutes, removed aseptically, rinsed in a tube of sterile broth, and then placed in a second tube of broth. This procedure is followed to remove adherent disinfectants that may act as a bacteriostat. The broth tubes are incubated at 37° C. for 48 hours and observed for growth. This test gives information as to the dilution found germicidal. Organic matter such as blood, serum, saliva, or milk may be added to the dilutions of the disinfectant to furnish information regarding the effect of organic matter on germicidal efficiency.

Infection-prevention test (Nungester and Kempf). The infection-prevention test is an in vivo test for evaluating germicides. The tips of the tails of anesthetized mice are contaminated by being swabbed with a broth culture of either type I pneumococcus or a beta hemolytic streptococcus. The tails are then dipped into the germicide and allowed to remain for two minutes. The tips of the tails (½ inch long) are severed and inserted into the peritoneal cavity of the mice through a previously prepared incision; the incisions are then sutured. The mice are observed daily for from 7 to 10 days. If the mice die, heart blood is cultured and the organism identified. If the mice survive, the germicide was effective in killing the organism and preventing infection. This test is limited to use of those microorganisms that are pathogenic for mice and does not provide for toxicity evaluation.

Toxicity tests. Numerous methods are used to determine toxicity of germicidal chemical agents. The agent may be added to the drinking water of laboratory animals, and the animals observed for a period of weeks or months for symptoms of toxicity. Upon death, the animals are autopsied and sections of the various organs are examined histopathologically. Antiseptic agents may be tested by being applied to the forearm of volunteers each day who are observed for skin sensitivity. Also, germicidal and antiseptic agents may be tested in the presence of leukocytes to determine whether phagocytosis will be inhibited, or tested in the presence of tissue cultures to determine their effect on cell multiplication.

Halogens

Chlorine and iodine are the most widely used halogens. These chemicals are used in the food industry, water purification and sewage disposal plants, swimming pools, home use, hospitals and clinics, and dentists' and physicians' offices.

Chlorine. Chlorine in gaseous form is widely used in water purification and in sewage disposal plants. A final concentration of about 0.1 to 0.2 part per million of residual chlorine in water used for drinking purposes should render it free of pathogenic vegetative microorganisms and therefore safe.

Other forms of chlorine in common use are sodium and calcium hypochlorite. Household chlorine compounds are used generally in the form of sodium hypochlorite in a concentration of from 5% to 12% available chlorine. Hypochlorite compounds of from 50% to 70% available chlorine are used in the food and dairy industries to disinfect equipment.

The antibacterial effect of chlorine and chlorine compounds is dependent upon the formation of hypochlorous acid (HCLO) with water. The release of nascent oxygen from hypochlorous acid probably also involves the destruction of microorganisms. Chlorine compounds are most effective as germicides in an acid environment, around pH 5.0. The antibacterial activity of chlorine compounds is greatly reduced by the presence and amount of organic matter.

Chloramines. Chloramines are organic chlorine compounds that are relatively stable and liberate chlorine slowly. They may be used for wound dressing because they are less irritating than other forms of chlorine. Their application today is mainly as disinfectants and sanitizing agents.

Dakin's solution was introduced during World War I for treating wounds. This solution is a compound of calcium hypochlorite, boric acid, and sodium carbonate and contains about 0.5% available chlorine. It is somewhat irritating to tissue and delays wound healing.

Of these compounds, many dentists use sodium hypochlorite with hydrogen peroxide in the irrigation of root canals for antimicrobial effect and removal of debrided material.

Iodine. Probably the most widely used skin disinfectant is iodine. It is an effective germicide against a wide variety of microorganisms, including *Mycobacterium tuberculosis,* viruses, fungi, and even spores on long exposure of one hour or more.

The germicidal activity of iodine is thought to be attributable to direct iodination of protein of the microorganisms. Iodine used as a disinfectant is prepared as a tincture. Formerly, a 7% (alcohol) solution was recommended, but this concentration proved too caustic and irritating for local skin application, and therefore the preparation in common use today is a 2% alcoholic tincture. This solution contains 2% iodine plus 2.4% sodium iodide in dilute (approximately 50%) alcohol. Vegetative microorganisms are killed within one or two minutes when exposed to tincture of iodine. Iodine is also prepared in a 2% aqueous concentration and is used by some dentists for disinfection of oral mucosa before injection of an anesthetic.

Iodophors. Iodophors are compounds that possess germicidal power and are nonstaining and nonirritating. They are made by combining iodine with a solubilizing agent, which results in a complex that liberates free iodine slowly when diluted with water. The carriers are generally a surface-active agent of nonionic type; but cationic detergents may be used. The surface-acting agent increases permeability so that the iodine is more readily absorbed.

PVP-iodine or povidone-iodine complex is an iodophor in which iodine is complexed with polyvinylpyrrolidone. Such compounds may contain 25% iodine, but 20% is unavailable in the complex. PVP-iodine is reported to be more effective and less toxic than tinctures or aqueous solutions of iodine. Several preparations (Isodine and Betadine) are available as antiseptics for external use by man. These preparations are used on the skin and oral mucosa as presurgical antiseptics. They have also attained wide acceptance as a topical antiseptic for home use.

Commercial preparations are available for general disinfection of equipment in hospitals, dental operatories, and clinics. Iodophors used as general disinfectants in dilutions of from 25 to 75 parts per million in water are bactericidal for vegetative microorganisms within 10 minutes or less. The iodophor (Wescodyne, a polyethoxy polypropoxy ethanol-iodine complex) is reported to be tuberculocidal in 10 minutes at a concentration of 450 parts per million. This preparation is recommended for general disinfection of walls, floors, tables, and similar objects.

Oxidizers

Hydrogen peroxide, zinc peroxide, potassium permanganate, and sodium perborate are oxidizers that decompose and liberate nascent oxygen (O). In general, these compounds have very limited use. Potassium permanganate in 1:5,000 dilution was used as an irrigant for treating wounds and gonorrheal infections before the discovery of the sulfa drugs and antibiotics. Hydrogen peroxide (3%) is not widely used as a skin germicide because more effective preparations are available. In addition to being used in the office for treatment, hydrogen peroxide is frequently recommended by the dentist as a mouthwash for home use in cases of Vincent's infection and periodontal disease. This peroxide decomposes by the enzyme catalase, which is present in aerobic microorganisms, blood and epithelial cells, and saliva. The nascent oxygen liberated is toxic for anaerobic bacteria, which are associated with these oral infections.

Zinc peroxide is incorporated into a gingival pack in office treatment of periodontal disease. This peroxide liberates nascent oxygen slowly and therefore has a more lasting effect than that obtained from hydrogen peroxide from which the oxygen is dissipated quickly.

Sodium perborate is incorporated into a dentifrice and has been recommended for home treatment of Vincent's infection. Its daily use is not recommended because the alkaline reaction often results in irritation of the mucous membrane.

Heavy metal compounds

Certain heavy metal compounds, such as silver, mercury, copper, arsenic and zinc, have antimicrobial activity. The inhibition of microbial growth by the metals is attributed to ionization and is referred to as oligodynamic effect. Perhaps the first drug containing a heavy metal was arsphenamine specifically synthesized in the laboratories by compounding arsenic with an organic group and used for the treatment of syphilis.

Heavy metals exert their antimicrobial

effect by coagulating proteins and reacting with $\sqrt{SH}$ groups, and, in the case of enzymes, inactivating them. Mercury compounds in particular react with $\sqrt{SH}$ radicals. In the testing of mercury compounds for germicidal efficiency, if the medium used contains $\sqrt{SH}$ radicals, as found in compounds such as glutathione, or thioglycollate, the substance containing $\sqrt{SH}$ will combine with the mercury and render it innocuous to the test organism.

Bichloride of mercury in concentrations of 1:1000 may be used as a general disinfectant. It is, however, very toxic to tissue and corrosive to metal instruments. When mercury is combined with an organic substance, the antibacterial properties are enhanced and the compound is less toxic to tissue. Organic forms of mercury are commonly available as Mercurochrome, Merthiolate, and Metaphen. These compounds are widely used as antiseptics for the skin and mucous membrane and are added to biologicals to maintain sterility. Mercury compounds are essentially biostatic.

Silver nitrate in a 1% solution is routinely instilled in the conjunctiva sacs of eyes of newborn infants as a preventive measure against gonococcal ophthalmia. Penicillin has replaced silver nitrate to a great extent for this purpose. Ammoniated silver nitrate at one time was widely used in dentistry to arrest the carious process in cavity preparations before the placing of the restoration. It has been shown to cause pulp irritation and also causes the tooth to take on a grayish appearance. Ammoniated mercury ointments are effective in treating external infections, especially impetigo.

Organic colloidal preparations of silver known as Argyrol or Protargol are non-irritating and are available for treating eye infections of adults, although ophthalmic antibiotic ointments have in general replaced them. Many ophthalmic solutions contain phenylmercuric nitrate as a preservative.

Alcohol

The two alcohols that are most frequently used for disinfection, ethyl and isopropyl alcohol, are miscible in water and are effective germicides in concentrations ranging from 50% to 70%. Alcohols higher than 70% and lower than 50% lose effective germicidal activity. These alcohols are active against vegetative forms of bacteria, including *Mycobacterium tuberculosis*, but not against spores. Ethyl alcohol on standing becomes oxidized to acetic acid and acetaldehyde, which are corrosive to metal instruments, and thus its use for instrument sterilization is limited. Isopropyl alcohol on the other hand is only slowly oxidized and therefore is less corrosive. It is used to some extent to disinfect instruments. Both of these alcohols are widely used to sponge the skin to reduce the skin microflora before an injection is given.

Isopropyl is reported to be a more effective germicide than ethyl alcohol. Ethyl alcohol in 70% concentration required five minutes to kill smears of the oral microflora, whereas isopropyl alcohol in 70% required only two minutes and in a 50% concentration required only one minute.

The antimicrobial effect of alcohol is associated with the denaturation of the protein of microorganisms and the reduction of surface tension. It also is a lipid solvent.

Phenols and phenolic compounds

Phenol (carbolic acid) was introduced as a surgical antiseptic by Lister in the mid-nineteenth century. Because of its caustic and irritating effect on tissues and its toxic vapors, it has limited use today. It is employed as a standard for evaluating chemical agents for germicidal effect. An 0.8% to 1% phenol solution kills vegetative bacteria in from 10 to 15 minutes;

spores and viruses are resistant and fungi are susceptible.

Phenol is germicidal because of its ability to injure the cell's membrane and to denature protein. Hexylresorcinol, a phenolic derivative, is employed as a topical antiseptic and is also incorporated into a mouthwash and cough drops.

Cresols, which are alkyl derivatives of phenol, are more effective germicides; they are no more toxic and are less expensive than phenol. Many cresol preparations are widely used as general, industrial, and laboratory disinfectants. A cresol solution (Lysol) used by many as a disinfectant is four times more effective as a germicide than phenol. Some oral mouthwashes contain cresol for their antiseptic effect.

Bis-phenols. Bis-phenols are substances containing two phenolic groups. The incorporation of chlorine results in compounds that possess high antimicrobial activity. A widely used bis-phenol is hexachlorophene, also known as G-11. The formula for hexachlorophene is as follows:

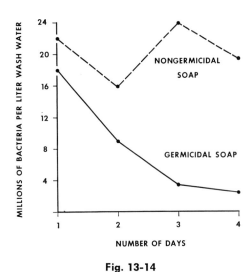

Although insoluble in water, G-11 retains its activity when mixed in oils, soaps, and similar agents. Soap containing hexachlorophene has been shown to reduce the microflora of the skin. Soap and similar hand washing preparations containing hexachlorophene (of 2% to 3% concentration) are used in the surgical scrub and have greatly replaced tincture of green soap.

To be effective in maintaining a low microbial count of the hands, hexachlorophene soap should be used exclusively in order to build up and maintain an effective antimicrobial concentration (Figs. 13-13 and 13-14; Table 13-4).

Although some workers report that the use of hexachlorophene soap obviates use

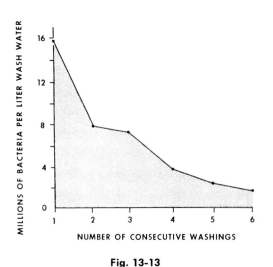

Fig. 13-13   **Fig. 13-14**

Fig. 13-13. Effectiveness of washing with nongermicidal soap in reducing bacterial flora of the hands.

Fig. 13-14. Comparison of a germicidal soap and a nongermicidal soap in reducing the bacterial flora of the hands.

of the brush in the surgical scrub, other workers do not agree.

Chlorhexidine is another bis-phenol with high germicidal activity. It is used as a wound irrigant in concentrations of 1: 1,000 and higher and is also incorporated with other agents as a general disinfectant. Experimentally, it has been incorporated into a mouthwash and has been shown to effectively reduce dental plaque formation.

A chlorophenol preparation in a mixture with camphor (ratio 1 part chlorophenol to 2 parts camphor) is known as camphorated p-monochlorophenol. This preparation is widely used as an antiseptic in root canal treatment, having replaced beechwood creosote because of its lower toxicity to tissue.

Surface tension depressors

Soaps. Soaps are potassium or sodium esters of fatty acids. They do have some antimicrobial activity against the spirochete of syphilis, pneumococci, and several other types of pathogenic microorganisms. In general they show weak antibacterial activity. Soaps possess surface tension-reducing power and therefore are effective in removing microorganisms and debris from the skin and instruments in the emulsion formed in the washing process.

Detergents. There are substances referred to as nonionic, anionic, and cationic detergents or surfactants. The nonionic surfactants (no electric change) are relatively nontoxic to microorganisms. One type, Tween 80, is favorable for the growth of certain bacteria as *Mycobacterium tuberculosis* and lactobacilli. Examples of the anionic type are soaps and synthetic detergents such as triethanolamine lauryl sulfate, known as Drene. The anionic detergents yield negatively charged ions, are most active at acid pH, and are effective against gram-positive microorganisms.

Cationic substances carry a positive electric charge and are germicidal for both gram-positive and gram-negative bacteria. Perhaps the most important and useful of the cationic detergents are those known as the quaternary ammonium compounds, the so-called quats. These agents are most active at an alkaline pH. The first was discovered by Domagk (1936), who reported on benzalkonium chloride, among whose trade names are Zephiran Chloride and Roccal, which has this formula:

The quat benzalkonium chloride possibly acts by lowering the surface tension, thus increasing the permeability of the bacterial cell membrane and allowing for the leak-

Table 13-4. Effectiveness of liquid soaps in reducing bacterial flora of hands

Number of subjects	Number of washings	Soap used*	Average number of bacteria per liter wash water		Percentage reduction
			Initial wash	Wash after 2 days	
15	27	T	11,309,000	120,800	98.9
21	37	S	12,150,000	3,950,000	67.5
4	6	A	4,711,000	811,000	82.8
17	34	Y	6,759,000	7,378,000	none

*Letters T, S, and A refer to three different liquid soaps containing hexachlorophene; Y refers to a cocoanut oil soap.

age of nitrogen and phosphorous components and other substances. With this increased permeability, the quat agent may enter the cell and cause denaturation of cellular protein and enzyme inhibition. This agent is somewhat more active against gram-positive than gram-negative bacteria. It is reported ineffective against *Mycobacterium tuberculosis, Pseudomonas aeruginosa,* spores, and viruses. Virucidal activity has been shown for the influenza virus. The presence of blood, serum, saliva, or pus reduces its antimicrobial activity. As a mucous membrane and skin antiseptic, it is used in concentrations of from 1: 100 to 1:1,000 in either aqueous solutions or alcoholic tinctures. As a disinfectant for instruments, an aqueous 1:750 solution is recommended. To reduce corrosion, 0.3% sodium nitrate is added. Soaps and anionic detergents inactivate benzalkonium chloride. Therefore, after being washed with a soap the hands should be thoroughly rinsed with water, then rinsed with alcohol, and finally immersed in the solution of benzalkonium chloride. When it is used to disinfect instruments, the instruments should be thoroughly scrubbed with soap and water to mechanically remove the debris, rinsed thoroughly to remove all soap, and then immersed in the "quats" for at least 30 minutes.

These agents are referred to as cold sterilizing solutions, a misnomer. At best they are effective disinfectants only if used in the proper concentrations (1:750) and if the exposure time is at least 30 minutes.

Besides being used in the dental and medical fields, quaternary compounds are employed as sanitizers in food processing plants, dairies, and restaurants.

Aldehydes

Formaldehyde. Formaldehyde is a gas. Aqueous solutions of from 3% to 8% formaldehyde called formalin are germicidal even in the presence of organic matter. These solutions are irritating and toxic

and are not used as general disinfectants.

The antimicrobial effect of formalin is attributed to direct alkylation of the microbial cells' protein. Formalin solution in 5% concentration is reported to kill *Bacillus anthracis* spores within 90 minutes at 37° C. Formalin in concentrations of from 0.2% to 0.4% are used in the preparation of viral vaccines as an inactivator of the virus.

Isopropyl alcohol solutions of formaldehyde have been used for instrument disinfection. These solutions are objectionable mainly because of their irritating effect, fumes, and their tendency to produce dermatologic conditions.

Glutaraldehyde. Glutaraldehyde is a dialdehyde having a formula $CHO–CH_2–CH_2–CH_2–CHO$ and possessing strong germicidal power in alkaline aqueous solution. It is tuberculocidal and sporicidal, as well as fungicidal and active against viruses, polio and *H. influenzae*. A 2% glutaraldehyde aqueous solution is buffered with 0.3% $NaHCO_3$ to pH 7.5 to activate it. This solution is moderately toxic and irritating to the skin and eyes. It is used for chemical disinfection of instruments, rubber tubing, and similar items. Instruments disinfected with glutaraldehyde should be rinsed with sterile water before being used, to remove this chemical.

Vegetative forms of bacteria, *Staphylococcus aureus, Escherichia coli, Pseudomonas* organisms, *Candida albicans,* and *Mycobacterium tuberculosis* are reportedly killed by this solution in five minutes. Spores require a three-hour exposure. The disinfectant exposure time to this germicide, recommended for non–spore-formers, is 20 minutes. The solution should not be used after two weeks because of its instability.

Chemical aerosols and gases
Aerosols

Certain chemicals when sprayed into the air have germicidal activity. Chemical substances that can be dispersed into the air in particle size of from 1 to 2 μ and remain suspended for some time are referred to as aerosols.

Several chemical agents, phenolic compounds, quaternary, hypochlorite, and glycols have been used for air sanitization. Of these, the glycols appears to be ideal. Ethylene, propylene, and triethylene glycols have proved, when in aerosols, to be effective in reducing airborne organisms. Propylene glycol in a concentration of 1 part in from 2 to 4 million parts of air will destroy airborne vegetative microorganisms, when the humidity is around 45% and the temperature between 50° and 70° F.

Glycols have a lethal effect on vegetative microbial forms because the glycol vapors are absorbed in water droplets that surround the airborne bacteria and result in dehydration. Triethylene glycol is the most effective of the glycols. It is reported to be lethal for the *H. influenzae* virus. These aerosols are relatively ineffective against surface bacteria that are protected by particulate matter.

Aerosols have been used to reduce respiratory infections in hospital wards, business offices, barracks, and public schools. One of the difficulties encountered with their use is maintaining the proper concentration of glycol and controlling the humidity in the air.

Sterilizing gases

The use of chemicals in a gaseous state for disinfection or sterilization offers many advantages: (1) it affords a method of disinfection for materials damaged by heat and moisture, (2) it enhances penetration, and (3) it affords a method of rapid distribution throughout an enclosed space.

Formaldehyde. Formaldehyde gas (CH_2O) was introduced in the mid-1800s for fumigating sickrooms. This gas was generated by heating paraformaldehyde or concentrated 37% solutions of formaldehyde. The gas is irritating and forms a paraldehyde film over exposed objects and therefore has had limited use. It is most effective as an antimicrobial agent in a relative humidity of 70% and at a temperature of 20° C. It has poor penetrating power.

Ethylene oxide. Ethylene oxide (CH_2–O–CH_2) has been used since 1936 as an antimicrobial agent. It is liquid at temperatures less than 10.8° C. and in the pure form is toxic, irritating and explosive. A nonflammable preparation is obtained when ethylene oxide is mixed with carbon dioxide in a ratio of 1:9, called carboxide. A combination of 20% ethylene oxide with 80% carbon dioxide is sold under the name Oxyfume; and a mixture of 11% ethylene oxide plus 89% halogenated hydrocarbons is known as Cryoxide.

Ethylene oxide is germicidal, virucidal, and sporicidal. It is a sterilizing gas when used according to prescribed methods. Its germicidal activity results from its alkylating action on proteins, and also possibly from its reaction with DNA and RNA.

A special closed chamber such as the autoclave is used when ethylene oxide is employed to sterilize, because humidity and temperature can be controlled. Ethylene oxide is selective for sterilization because it penetrates well and dissipates quickly from the exposed material.

Concentrations that sterilize are expressed in milligrams of ethylene oxide per liter of space at specific temperatures and humidity. Ethylene oxide will sterilize in from three to six hours at a concentration of from 500 to 1,000 mg. per liter at 30% humidity. After the sterilization period, the residual gas is removed from the autoclave by vacuum and fresh sterile air is admitted to the chamber by aeration.

This gas is used to sterilize wrapped surgical materials such as sponges, rubber goods, plastics, instruments, syringes, and many materials that cannot be sterilized by steam autoclaving or dry heat.

Beta propiolactone (CH_2)$_2$ CO, is liquid

at 20° C. and is nonexplosive. In aqueous solutions it is unstable. It requires the use of a closed chamber in which the temperature and humidity can be controlled. From 2 to 4 mg. of the lactone per liter of air at 25° C. in 70% to 80% humidity will sterilize items within two or three hours. Because it does not penetrate as well as ethylene oxide and has been stated to be carcinogenic, it has not come into routine use but is used to decontaminate rooms and buildings.

Dyes

Dyes are organic compounds originally introduced in microbiology to stain microorganisms so they might be seen more clearly under the microscope. They are also used to demonstrate differential characteristics of the microbial cell. Selective staining techniques such as the gram stain, the acid-fast stain, nuclear stain, the spore and capsule stain aid in classification of microorganisms. Many of these dyes possess bacteriostatic and bactericidal properties.

Ehrlich (1911) recommended acriflavine as a trypanocide. This dye possesses bacteriostatic effects for most bacteria at a 1:50,000 dilution. The dye probably interferes with the synthesis of nucleic acids.

Crystal violet, brilliant green, and methyl violet are dyes that demonstrate a greater inhibitory effect for gram-positive than gram-negative organisms. Some of these dyes are incorporated into culture media in concentrations to selectively inhibit certain groups of microorganisms and thus favor the growth of the insensitive types. Brilliant green bile agar contains both the dyes brilliant green and basic fuchsin in concentrations that favor the growth of coliform organisms and is employed to determine the density of coliforms in water samples.

Of the dyes, crystal violet is used to treat gram-positive bacterial infection and also certain fungal infections. Oral infec-

tions caused by *Candida* organisms respond favorably to topical applications of 0.5% aqueous solution of the dye.

• • •

Various measures to prevent cross-infection in the dental office are presented in Chapter 12. Procedures that apply to sterilization and disinfection of dental instruments and other materials have been interwoven throughout this chapter in order to include the practical application along with the general principles. Each dental school selects those methods that are particularly adapted to the design of its dental clinic.

The practicing dentist who understands the basic principles of sterilization and disinfection is better able to select wisely those methods that protect his patients as well as himself against oral infection.

REFERENCES AND ADDITIONAL READINGS

Anellis, A., Greez, N., Haber, D. A., Berkowitz, D., Schneider, M. D., and Simon, M.: Radiation sterilization of bacon for military feeding, Appl. Microbiol. 13:37, 1965.

Bartels, H. A.: Cavity sterilization, Dent. Clin. N. Amer. 647, Nov. 1960.

Bartels, H. A.: Consultant symposium: Our empiric cavity sterilization, New York Dent. J. 17: 3, 1951.

Burton, W. E.: Changing requirements for sterilization, J. Prosth. Dent. 14:127, 1964.

Ehrlen, I. R.: Advances in sterilization techniques, Pharm. Weekbl. 99:1430, 1964.

Ewen, S. J.: Ultrasound and periodontics, J. Periodont. 31:101, 1960.

Gillings, R. D., Dodd, C., and Martin, N. D.; An ultra violet sterile storage cabinet for medical and dental use, Aust. Dent. J. 10:444, 1965.

Green, G. H., and Sanderson, A. D.: Ultrasonics and periodontal therapy—a review of clinical and biologic effects, J. Periodont. 36:232, 1965.

Grogan, J. B.: New skin germicide, Antimicrob. Agents Chemother. 4:545, 1964.

Haberman, S.: Some comparative studies between a chemical vapor sterilizer and a conventional steam autoclave on various bacteria and viruses, J. S. Calif. Dent. Assoc. 30:163, 1962.

Hedgecock, L. W.: Anti-microbial agents, Philadelphia, 1967, Lea & Febiger.

Hildick-Smith, G.: Disinfection of the hands, Pediat. Clin. N. Amer. 12:137, 1965.

Kelsey, J. C.: Use of gaseous antimicrobial agents with special reference to ethylene oxide, J. Appl. Bact. 30:92, 1967.

Knighton, H. T.: Viral hepatitis in relation to dentistry, J. Amer. Dent. Assoc. 63:21, 1961.

Maibach, H. I. (ed.): Skin bacteria and their role in infection, New York, 1965, McGraw-Hill Book Company.

Maurice, C. G.: A critical survey of the methods of instrument disinfection and sterilization, J. Amer. Dent. Assoc. 55:527, 1957.

Monash, S.: Composition of sunlight and of ultraviolet lamps, Arch. Derm. 91:495, 1965.

Morton, H. E.: The relationship of concentration and germicidal efficiency of ethyl alcohol, Ann. N. Y. Acad. Sci. 53:191, 1950.

Nolte, W. A., and Arnim, S. S.: Sterilization, lubrication and rust-proofing of dental instruments and handpieces with a water-oil emulsion: Laboratory and clinical study. J. Amer. Dent. Assoc. 50:133, 1955.

Nungester, W. J., and Kempf, A. H.: An infection-prevention test for the evaluation of skin disinfectants, J. Infect. Dis. 71:174, 1942.

O'Brien, H. A., Mitchell, J. D., Haberman, S., Rowan, D. F., Winford, T. E., and Pellet, J.: The use of activated glutaraldehyde as a cold sterilizing agent for urological instruments, J. Urol. 95:429, 1966.

Perkulis, B., Engelhard, W. E., and Kramer, W. S.: Ultrasonics and benzalkonium chloride as a method of sterilizing dental instruments, J. Dis. Child. 37:69, 1970.

Radomski, J. L., Deichmann, W. B., Austin, B. S., and MacDonald, W. E.: Chronic toxicity studies on irradiated beef stew and evaporated milk, Toxic. Appl. Pharmacol. 7:113, 1965.

Reddish, G. F.: Antiseptics, distinfectants, fungicides and physical sterilization, ed. 2, Philadelphia, 1957, Lea & Febiger.

Rubbo, S. D.: Asepsis and antisepsis in dentistry, Aust. Dent. J. 5:61, 1960.

Rubbo, S. D.: Calculated risks in sterilization in dentistry, Aust. Dent. J. 56:1, 1952.

Rubbo, S. D., and Gardner, J. F.: A view of sterilization and disinfection, London, 1965, Lloyd-Luke (Medial Books) Ltd.

Spaulding, E. M.: Studies on the chemical sterilization of surgical instruments, Surg. Gynec. Obstet. 69:738, 1939.

Sykes, G.: Disinfection and sterilization, Princeton, 1958, Van Nostrand Co., Inc.

Sykes, G.: The problems of sterility, Practitioner 190:52, 1963.

Tinsley, I. J., Bone, J. F., and Bull, E. C.: The growth, reproduction, longevity and histopathology of rats fed gamma-irradiated flour, Toxic. Appl. Pharmacol. 7:71, 1965.

U. S. Naval Dental School: Sterilization and disinfection of dental handpieces, U. S. Navy Medical News Letter, 32(12):25-27, 1958.

Walter, C. W.: The aseptic treatment of wounds, New York, 1948, The Macmillan Company.

Walter, C. W.: Disinfection of the hands, Amer. J. Surg. 109:691, 1965.

Williams, R. E. O., Blowers, R., Garrod, L. P., and Shooter, R. A.: Hospital infection, ed. 2, Chicago, 1966, Year Book Medical Publishers, Inc.

14 / Chemotherapy

Chemotherapy is the chemical treatment of disease, especially disease caused by microorganisms. Its history may be traced to the oldest available records, but by the end of the nineteenth century only two agents were known that had specific antimicrobial activity effective enough to be useful for treatment without being overly toxic.[4] One of these was quinine, which may still be used in the treatment of cerebral malaria, and the other was ipecac, which was once used in the treatment of amebic dysentery.

The modern science of chemotherapy, however, dates from Paul Ehrlich's systematic investigations early in the twentieth century for a synthesized agent to cure trypanosomiasis. Ehrlich followed this effort with a search for an agent active against syphilis, synthesizing a large series of organic arsenicals. The six hundred and sixth of these proved active against the treponema and become widely known as salvarsan, the first drug highly effective against this very serious infection.

For about 25 years progress practically stopped, until Domagk in Germany uncovered the action of sulfonamides against the streptococci.[7] Since then, scientific advances in chemotherapy have developed in two directions: the synthesis of compounds related to essential metabolites and the isolation of antibiotic substances formed by microorganisms. The great success of these efforts is indicated by the estimate that for the 15-year period from 1938 to 1952 there would have been 1.5 million more deaths from certain infectious diseases in the United States if the trend of mortality from 1922 to 1937 had prevailed after 1937.[17] The chemotherapeutic agents must have been largely responsible for this impressive reduction.

SYNTHESIZED CHEMOTHERAPEUTIC AGENTS

Sulfonamides

The first line of development had its greatest modern triumph at its very inception in the discovery by Domagk in 1935 that Prontosil (sulphonamido-crysoidin) would cure otherwise fatal hemolytic streptococcal infections in mice. The subsequently developed sulfonamide drugs were widely used for more than a decade to treat a large number of bacterial infections. Unfortunately, these drugs have an inherent toxicity and today have been almost entirely replaced with the antibiotics in medical practice—except for urinary infections—and have been entirely dropped from the drugs used in dentistry.

Nevertheless, the sulfonamides represented an important advance, for they saved many lives; and they were the first group of chemotherapeutic agents for which the mechanism of action was unraveled, proving to be an antimetabolite. Sulfonamide compounds, it is now known, are bacteriostatic agents that compete with and block the use of para-aminobenzoic acid, necessary for folic acid production in the bacterial cell. Unfortunately, so little is yet known of the metabolism of both host and invaders that the development of a logical chemotherapy based upon the principle of interference with specific and critical points in cell metabolism has been a failure compared to the results obtained from the other line of chemotherapeutic development, an empiric search for useful agents.

Nitrofurans

This class of antimicrobial agents, the nitrofurans, is derived from the nitration of furfural (2-furaldehyde), a vegetable by-product. First reported in 1944, these drugs have since proved useful as bacteriostatic agents active against both gram-positive and gram-negative bacilli. Nitrofurantoin is useful for *Escherichia coli* infections of the urinary tract, and nitrofurazone is used as a topical antibacterial agent. Several attempts have been made to find a place for nitrofurans among drugs used by the dentist, but no outstanding usefulness has been demonstrated in comparison to older drugs or the standard antibiotics.

ANTIBIOTICS AND SYNTHESIZED DERIVATIVES

The term "antibiotic" is used to designate any chemical substance produced by a microorganism that in low concentration inhibits the growth of or kills other microorganisms. The scattered and unexploited observations concerning antibiotic effects by bacteria and fungi that were made during the latter part of the nineteenth century and early part of the twentieth failed to lead to any significant advances. It was not until September, 1928, when Alexander Fleming made his observations on the lysis of staphylococcal colonies by a mold contaminant, that the modern era of antibiotics can be said to have properly begun. Fleming's report in 1929 failed to

engender its eventual electrifying effects, however, until July, 1939, when Florey, Chain, and their associates became interested in isolating the active agent, penicillin.

Working at Oxford University under the limitations imposed by World War II, these investigators made such encouraging progress that by 1941 they were able to interest the National Research Council in Washington to take up the problem of large scale production. Intensive American efforts succeeded so well that large supplies of penicillin were available for the Armed Forces before the end of the war. Penicillin's effectiveness in combatting infections by gram-positive bacteria promptly earned it the appellation of "miracle drug." Infectious diseases that had resisted the sulfonamides or had been treated only with difficulty—syphilis and gonorrhea, for example—now came under therapeutic control.

Nevertheless, it gradually became apparent that there was only a limited range of microorganisms susceptible to penicillin and, moreover, that there were severe untoward reactions that might occur during penicillin therapy. These limitations have led to an intensive search for other antibiotics. There is now available, consequently, a large number of these agents, and many of them have been found useful in the fight against microbial diseases.

Mode of action

Both microbial and biochemical investigations have led to the suggestion that the antibiotics may be differentiated as being either bacteriostatic or bactericidal agents.[16] Bactericidal drugs actively kill bacteria, and these dead cells are then removed by the body defenses. Among the bactericidal antibiotics are ampicillin, penicillin, kanamycin, polymyxin, and streptomycin. Bacteriostatic drugs merely prevent the growth of the microorganisms, their final elimination depending more strongly

upon the killing effects of the body defenses. If the body defenses are ineffective
or if use of the drug is stopped too early,
the bacteria may begin to grow again and
the patient then may suffer relapse. Antibiotics in this group include chloramphenicol, erythromycin, novobiocin, and the tetracyclines. There is no strict demarcation
between the two groups since erythromycin, for example, is bacteriostatic at low
concentrations but bactericidal at high.

In general, bactericidal antibiotics act
in one of three ways: Either they affect
the bacterial cell wall so as to interfere
with the cells' osmotic balance, causing it
to absorb water and burst; or they affect
the cell membrane and so probably cause
loss of vital metabolites; or they inhibit
protein synthesis (streptomycin and kanamycin). In most instances, bacteriostatic
drugs interfere with protein synthesis, preventing the growth and multiplication of
the bacteria without actually destroying
them.

Among the bactericidal drugs, penicillins, cephalosporins, and cycloserine affect
bacterial cell wall synthesis. The first two
antibiotics prevent the cross-linking by
transpeptidization of the glycopeptide backbone of the cell wall. Penicillin is most
effective on actively growing bacteria
where a continuous biosynthesis of cell
wall is occurring. Cycloserine is an ana-
logue of D-alanine, one of the amino acids
that forms a substrate for the formation of
the penta-peptide side chain of the cell
wall backbone. The close resemblance allows cycloserine to be mistaken for D-ala-
mine and, in being accepted by the cell,
it disrupts the cell wall building process
by competitively inhibiting the enzymes
involved.

Antifungal antibiotics that kill, such as
amphotericin B and nystatin, bind to a
sterol in the cell membrane and so interfere with its osmotic barrier activity. Polymyxin B and colistin have the same effect
by acting as cationic detergents with an
affinity for phosphate radicals in the case
of gram-negative bacteria.

The mode of action of the bactericidal
antibiotics such as kanamycin and streptomycin is not clearly established, but it is
known that these agents interfere with
protein synthesis by causing a distortion
of the 30S portion of the ribosomes in the
bacterial cytoplasm. This results in a mis-
reading of the instructions from messenger RNA and in consequence causes the
manufacture of false proteins. Protein synthesis may also be completely blocked by
streptomycin forming aberrant complexes
to portions of ribosomes (30S particles).

In the case of bacteriostatic antibiotics,
such drugs as the tetracyclines and erythromycin interfere with the attachment
of the amino acid-transfer RNA complex
to the ribosome. Chloramphenicol interferes with the attachment of messenger
RNA to the ribosome so that the coding
instructions from the nuclear DNA fail
to reach the ribosome and the relevant
protein is not manufactured. Nalidixic
acid, griseofulvin, and novobiocin affect
the DNA replication of the chromosome.

CAUSES OF CHEMOTHERAPEUTIC FAILURE

The failure to obtain an adequate response to chemotherapy[16] or the need to
withhold or withdraw use of the antibiotic
are complex problems involving any of a
number of possible causes. Among the factors that must be considered are: (1) microbial drug resistance, (2) bacterial "persistence," (3) host defense responses, (4)
poor drug absorption, (5) drug inactivation
by the host's protein or flora, and (6)
poor penetration of the drug into tissues or
cells.

Drug resistance

Drug resistance conveniently divides into
three major groups: (1) natural drug resistance, occurring in organisms that have
not been exposed to the drug, at least in
that particular patient; (2) acquired drug

resistance, which results from exposure of the organism to the drug and which may occur during the treatment of an individual patient; and (3) transferred drug resistance, by which genetic material conferring resistance may be transferred from a resistant to a sensitive species or strain.

Natural drug resistance

Natural drug resistance may occur either as a part of the make-up of the entire species or as restricted to particular strains of a species. It may result from (1) lack of the metabolic process affected by the specific agent; (2) a structural characteristic, such as absence of cell wall in mycoplasmata, which renders them resistant to penicillin; or (3) the production of enzymes that destroy the agent, such as penicillinase produced by staphylococci.

Acquired drug resistance

Acquired drug resistance is the condition in which a strain of microorganism infecting a patient that was originally sensitive to a particular chemotherapeutic agent has become resistant to that agent during treatment. This change occurs by virtue of a genetically determined capacity for adaptation by the infecting microorganism.

Chemotherapeutic agents may be separated into the following two groups in regard to this phenomenon: (1) resistance is acquired to the agent very rapidly, such as in the case of streptomycin, used for the treatment of infections with *Mycobacterium tuberculosis;* and (2) resistance is acquired slowly, such as resistance to tetracycline or chloramphenicol after treatment of infections with sensitive bacteria (staphylococci, others).

Rapidly acquired resistance. Great resistance may be obtained upon even the first subculture when microorganisms in this group are grown in vitro. This behavior is probably caused by mutations occurring in powerfully acting genes that confer a considerable degree of resistance.

In the case of streptomycin, for example, high degrees of resistance may be controlled by a single gene locus.

Slowly acquired resistance. Slowly acquired resistance, rare in clinical cases, is also demonstrable in the laboratory. If microorganisms are repeatedly cultured in increasing concentrations of a chemotherapeutic agent, subcultured on each occasion from the tube containing the greatest concentration in which growth has occurred, the degree of resistance may be slowly increased. This small-step increase is probably caused by mutations occurring in a number of genes, each of which is responsible for a slight increase in resistance. Some microorganisms such as the pneumococci may lose their pathogenicity in the course of slowly acquiring resistance to penicillin, but this does not occur with all species. The patient is able to throw off these resistant organisms more readily because of the loss in pathogenicity.

Clinical significance of acquired resistance. In chemotherapy for infections other than tuberculosis, the commonly used antibiotics may be classified as follows in regard to *risk of acquired resistance* by the infecting bacteria:

High risk
  Streptomycin
  Erythromycin
  Novobiocin
  Lincomycin

Low risk
  Penicillin
  Tetracyclines
  Chloramphenicol
  Colistin
  Polymyxin B
  Gentamycin
  Cycloserine

Resistance is rapidly acquired to almost all antituberculotic drugs if used alone, with the possible exception of cycloserine, which, however, suffers the disadvantage of giving rise to a high incidence of unpleasant toxic effects mainly involving the central nervous system. Rapidly acquired drug resistance is of such great importance and is such a complex problem in tuberculosis that therapy must be based upon use of a combination of drugs such as isoniazid (INH), streptomycin, and para-aminosalicylic acid (PAS). The PAS is only a weak antituberculotic drug that is not bactericidal for the organism. It is important, however, because it prevents or delays development of resistance to INH and streptomycin. It is never given alone.

Genetic mechanisms for transfer of drug resistance

Genetic material conferring drug resistance may be transferred from a strain or species resistant to a particular drug to another strain previously sensitive. Since such a transfer can occur within the intestine of man, there are grounds for apprehension concerning its role in human infections. Such a possibility exists not only in the intestine but in the upper respiratory tract and perhaps within the hospital environment.

There are three main mechanisms by which genetic material conferring resistance may be transferred from a resistant to a sensitive strain: (1) transformation, (2) conjugation, and (3) transduction.

Transformation. In transformation, genes are released from one cell into the medium containing the microorganisms and they then pass into another cell where they recombine with the DNA of the chromosome. This phenomenon occurs only under optimal laboratory conditions and probably is of little clinical significance.

Conjugation. Conjugation[42] depends on a "male" type of bacterial cell that can produce a pilus, a tubelike surface structure that allows conjugation with a "female" or receptor cell. There are two principal forms of conjugation known, the Hfr (high frequency) type and the R (resistance) factor type. In the Hfr type the male cells may transfer portions of the chromosome, perhaps including a gene for resistance, to a female cell that may incorporate the gene for resistance into its own chromosome, a phenomenon referred to as "recombination." In the R factor type a cytoplasmic episome, or R factor, which consists of cytoplasmic DNA responsible for multiple drug resistance, replicates itself within the cytoplasm and also induces the formation of a pilus that allows transfer of an R factor to a previously sensitive female type of cell upon direct cell-to-cell contact.[67] This transfer makes the recipient cell resistant and also induces the formation of a pilus in this cell, rendering it male in its turn. This cycle continues, but only for a limited period until an inhibitory process develops that prevents the formation of further pili. Nevertheless, when a small number of cells carrying R factor are mixed with a large number of drug-sensitive recipient cells and then incubated, there is a rapid acquisition of the R factor by a majority of the recipient cells. Antibiotic resistance mediated by the R factor includes the penicillins, cephalosporins, streptomycin, kanamycin, neomycin, chloramphenicol, the tetracyclines, and the sulfonamides.[15] It should be noted that resistance to the polymyxins and to chemotherapeutic drugs other than sulfonamides is not associated with R factors.

Transduction. Transduction consists of the transfer of genetic material for resistance from a resistant to a sensitive strain by means of bacteriophage. Staphylococci, particularly, have been shown to exhibit this mechanism. The bacteriophage may infect a coccus containing a cytoplasmic plasmid with a gene that carries the genetic determinants for penicillinase formation. During the replication of the phage in the coccus it may happen to incorporate the genetic material of the plasmid. The replicated phages are finally released, and a plasmid-bearing individual phage may infect a previously penicillin-sensitive coccus. The DNA of the plasmid will then induce the newly infected coccus to manufacture penicillinase.

Cross-resistance between antibiotics

The term "cross-resistance" refers to the condition where if a strain is resistant to one agent it is also resistant to another. Therefore, if use of a particular drug is unsuccessful in treatment, there is usually little point of changing to another to which there may be cross-resistance. The tetracyclines constitute such a group of drugs that exhibit cross-resistance. If there is cross-resistance in a group of drugs useful for particularly dangerous organisms, then this group should be reserved only for infections caused by these organisms to minimize possible development of resistant strains. Such a reserve group of drugs includes lincomycin and vancomycin. Oxacillin and cephalosporin, which originally were regarded as reserve drugs, are now primary agents in the treatment of staphylococcal infections because of the widespread appearance of penicillin-resistant strains. It should be remembered that there is little point of combining two drugs liable to cross-resistance, since each may be ineffective against the mutants in the population resistant to the other.

Problems of microbial resistance to antibiotics in dentistry

Several attempts have been made to find whether antibiotic therapy induces the appearance of resistant bacteria in the oral cavity and the upper respiratory tract. This question has been of particular concern for patients who have rheumatic heart disease, or congenital heart defects.

It has been shown that the bacteria occurring in the blood during postextraction bacteremias generally are quite sensitive to the commonly used antibiotics (Table 14-1).[34] In regard to patients who are on long-term antibiotic therapy for the prevention of recurrent rheumatic fever, relatively small doses of penicillin are taken daily by mouth for a long time. The salivary bacteria develop only a low level of penicillin resistance (first-step mutants) under these circumstances, and upon discontinuance of use of the drug, the antibiotic resistance tends to return to the original levels.[28] Penicillin-resistant viridans streptococci are rarely found in normal peoples' mouths.[59] The development of penicillin-resistant viridans streptococci in the oropharynx of patients receiving penicillin orally for prophylaxis or therapy, however, is being increasingly recog-

Table 14-1. Sensitivity of 133 postextraction bacteremia strains to eleven chemotherapeutic agents*

Antibacterial agent	Number of strains tested	Number of resistant strains	Percentage of sensitive strains
Erythromycin	128	0	100.0
Ampicillin	132	1	99.2
Chloramphenicol	132	1	99.2
Penicillin	130	1	99.2
Cephalosporin	132	3	97.7
Tetracycline	132	6	95.5
Lincomycin	43	4	90.7
Streptomycin	133	40	70.0
Sulfonamide	133	55	59.0
Neomycin	132	100	24.0
Kanamycin	131	118	9.0

*From Jokinen, M. A.: Suom. Hammaslaak. Toim. **66:**69, 1970.

nized,[56] but such resistant strains are rare in patients receiving the penicillin parenterally.

Local therapy in the oral cavity seems most likely to lead to the appearance of resistant strains. Placement of a periodontal pack containing oxytetracycline leads to the appearance of resistant bacteria in the mouth that persist for as long as two or three months after removal of the pack,[27] replacing the original sensitive flora. Several studies have been concerned with the development of bacterial resistance following endodontic therapy with locally applied antibiotics.[24, 53] Although the results are not entirely in agreement, their general trend is that resistance occurs following use of penicillin, streptomycin, tetracycline, oleandomycin, and neomycin. One study of resistance by bacterial isolates from root canals, to bacitracin, erythromycin, penicillin, polymyxin, chloramphenicol, chlortetracycline, and oxytetracycline, showed the most effective antibiotics were chloramphenicol, chlortetracycline, and oxytetracycline; for only from 5% to 6% of more than 1,000 microorganisms tested (predominantly streptococci) were resistant. The least effective antibiotic was polymyxin, for 77% of 873 bacteria were resistant to it. The study found that there had been a great increase in the number of penicillin-resistant streptococci, lactobacilli, and *Neisseria* organisms compared to three years earlier.[53]

Multiple-resistant *Staphylococcus aureus* infection may occur in the operative wound following surgery in the oral cavity. In one reported case[40] a pathogenic staphylococcus was isolated from an infected iliac bone graft in the mandible although the patient was receiving penicillin, streptomycin, and aureomycin. Sensitivity testing indicated the staphylococcus was resistant to both penicillin and streptomycin. When chloramphenicol was substituted for these two drugs, the infection promptly subsided. Multi-resistant staphylococci

have been a serious cause of hospital infections, the control of which has only recently been well established by improved hospital practice of sanitation and by the use of more effective antibiotics.[32]

The problem of resistance developing in fungi subjected to antimycotic therapy appears to be much less serious than for bacteria. Resistance is inducible in laboratory experiments if the fungus is repeatedly spread upon a substrate to which minimal inhibiting or gradually increasing concentrations of the antimycotic have been added. By means of these special procedures there can be demonstrated a one hundred fiftyfold increase in resistance to candidin. The increased resistance appears to result from mutational changes.[29]

Clinical reports, however, indicate that resistance to nystatin and amphotericin B is not likely to occur, especially in the case of *Candida albicans*,[13] unless treatment extends for a prolonged period of time. A slow and moderate increase in vitro has been shown when *Actinomyces bovis* is exposed to oxytetracycline, tetracycline, chloramphenicol, or dihydrostreptomycin, but not when exposed to erythromycin, carbomycin, or penicillin.[58]

The rare occurrence of resistance by fungi to high levels of the polyene agents, such as nystatin, is clear if it is remembered that their mode of action consists of combining with membrane sterol.[36] This results in membrane changes that allow leaking of essential constituents; apparently, mutational changes cannot adequately reduce the risk the membrane runs of complexing with a polyene antibiotic.

Synergism and antagonism between antibiotics

In general there is virtually never a synergistic effect between bacteriostatic antibiotics.[16] On the other hand, if two bactericidal agents are used together in concentrations that for each alone would be only marginally effective, the bactericidal effect is greatly increased. This effect, however, is demonstrable only with certain organisms. It may be because of a double action on two metabolic processes, but perhaps also because of the elimination of L-form persisters.

In most infections use of a single antibiotic is quite successful, provided the microorganism is sensitive to it. In those infections difficult to eliminate the combination of two bactericidal antibiotics may be particularly useful. An important example of this is the superiority of penicillin combined with streptomycin in the treatment of enterococcal bacterial endocarditis. However, so-called fixed-dose preparations, antibiotic combinations prepared by drug houses on the basis of in vitro studies, should not be used because they prevent selection of the proper dosage for each drug in the combination and they fix the ratios between the drugs at what may not be the most effective levels.

Antagonism between antibiotics has no practical clinical importance, although this phenomenon has some theoretic interest. The lack of clinical importance arises from the fact that antagonistic effects develop only when the drugs are present in marginal doses, whereas under clinical conditions they are given in large doses.

Bacterial persistence

Bacterial persistence[39] refers to the survival of fully sensitive bacteria in the presence of a concentration of antibiotic that kills the great majority of the bacterial population. Persisters usually form only a very small proportion of a bacterial population exposed to a drug; nevertheless they have great clinical significance since they may be responsible for a relapse. They occur particularly in old bacterial populations or in the presence of pus, poor drainage, or a foreign body. They are less likely to occur if an infection is treated early and with adequate doses of a bactericidal drug. The faster the rate of killing, the smaller the chance of persisters arising. It is probable that persisters are bacterial cells that happen to be relatively dormant and so are only very slowly metabolizing at the time of exposure to the drug. Therefore, they are less readily eliminated.

Some persisters may be L-forms that have lost their cell walls and thereby ceased to be sensitive to drugs acting on cell walls. Such persisters might be eliminated by other drugs, according to in vitro studies, but in most cases they are eventually eliminated from the patient's body by the natural defense mechanisms. If the host defenses are poor, such as in patients with a congenital lack of immunoglobulins, the problem of eliminating persisters becomes correspondingly more difficult. *Treponema pallidum* is well established as a microbial persister, with the ability to break into overt infection again in treated cases that had seemingly been completely cured. Bacterial endocarditis is also an example of persistence, and chronic bronchitis and chronic genitourinary infections possibly are other examples.

Host responses; iatrogenic diseases from antibiotics

A very important complex of factors having to do with the success of chemotherapy is the host response to the drugs in the presence of infection.[8] The host, in fact, is probably the most important determinant of the outcome of therapy. These innate factors condition the kind of antibiotic used, the optimal and safest dose, the final effectiveness of treatment, and the risk of various reactions. Among these host factors are included age, sex, pregnancy, genetic background, immunologic defenses, renal and hepatic function, electrolyte balance, transport mechanisms, noninfectious disorders such as pernicious anemia or diabetes, and central nervous system disease. Only some of these are discussed here, by way of illustration.

In regard to age, renal function varies significantly in the excretion of certain antibiotics, thus requiring suitable adjustments in dosage; this problem is discussed in the next section in greater detail. Another aspect, of special interest to the dentist, is that the calcifying bone and dental tissues of young babies and children, as well as in the fetus of pregnant women, may be affected by therapy with the tetracycline antibiotics. One of the most apparent and long-lasting effects is the staining of the teeth. Initially, with tetracycline therapy, the tooth color is yellow, but with increasing age after therapy it becomes brownish or even grayish in some instances. The pigmentation first appears at the gingival margin and has been observed after only three days of therapy. The deciduous dentition is stained if the drug is administered to the mother during the last trimester of pregnancy or during the first nine months of the infant's life; at 10 months of age or later, the permanent dentition alone becomes discolored. Some investigators claim that hypoplastic areas of the enamel also may occur, but this point is disputed. When the pigmented structures are subjected to ultraviolet illumination, they show yellow fluorescence, the dentin reacting more strongly than the enamel. None of the dental changes are reversible.

All of the tetracyclines produce a yellowish fluorescence in bone. This effect may be observed in newborn infants whose mothers have been treated with a tetracycline during pregnancy or in premature infants given a tetracycline during the first four or five weeks of life. Given in large doses for a period of from 9 to 12 days, the tetracyclines cause a transient inhibition of bone growth of approximately 40%. However, there is no convincing evidence that this effect has resulted in congenital bone malformations in human beings. Tetracyclines deposited in the calcifying areas of bone may persist for at least several years.[19]

Several genetic factors influence the outcome of the chemotherapy on infection. Among these, one may note especially that of glucose-6-phosphate dehydrogenase (G-6-PD) deficiency. G-6-PD deficiency is present in from 10% to 15% of American Negro males and in from 1% to 2% of Negro females. The highest incidence occurs in Kurdish Jews; but the disease is also frequent in Sephardic Jews and in some African tribes, especially the Bantus. Among the antimicrobial compounds that may produce hemolysis and anemia in patients lacking or deficient in G-6-PD are a number of the sulfonamide drugs and chloramphenicol.[65]

The normal immunologic response to an infection may be aborted by antibiotic treatment in some cases if the infection is controlled before enough microbial antigen has been produced. With long-term tetracycline treatment of animals, however, it has been shown that there is suppression of antibody production. Penicillin seems to have a similar effect.

Absorption, protein binding, excretion, and destruction of antibiotics

Among many other factors, the effectiveness of an antibiotic in the body also depends upon its concentration in the immediate neighborhood of the bacteria in the lesion. This in turn is influenced by several factors. The tissue concentration of an antibiotic first of all depends upon its concentration in the free form in the blood, unbound to protein. Protein binding in the blood may be considerable, but it is relatively unimportant in the tissues. Some of this free circulating antibiotic, in the case of certain drugs, is destroyed in the liver and elsewhere by metabolic processes, and some is excreted by the kidneys.

Renal excretion of antibiotics varies according to the character of the antibiotic and the age of the patient. Penicillin, especially, has been very thoroughly investigated[12] and presents features of special interest. This drug is rapidly excreted in the urine, but the rate varies significantly according to patient's age. Babies in the first month of life need much less penicillin than older children because at this early period of life renal tubular function is relatively poor and the excretion of penicillin is impaired. Children older than this, on the other hand, have highly efficient kidney tubules and excrete penicillin very rapidly. With increasing age, tubular excretory capacity lessens, so that older people require much less penicillin than young children, even though they are much larger. A failure to keep these differences in mind may result in one's using too little for young children and too much for old adults.

The importance of the salivary route of drug excretion has not been fully assessed, but there are beginning to appear indications that this route may be of special significance for certain diseases. It has now been shown[31] that salivary excretion of antibiotic may well be useful for the prediction of antibiotic effectiveness in ridding nasopharyngeal carriers of *Neisseria meningitidis*. This observation indicates that the mucous glands of the nasopharynx perhaps handle antibiotics in exactly the same manner as the salivary glands.

It has been well established that antibiotics are excreted in varying patterns in the saliva. In the earlier studies, salivary excretion of penicillin following systemic administration either could not be demonstrated or was found to occur only at a very low level.[48] It has since been found that the oral flora produces a penicillin-inactivating factor that is not penicillinase.[3] It has been suggested that penicillinase from oral microorganisms may also have a role in the inactivation of salivary penicillin. However, since penicillin given intramuscularly will suppress dental caries in rats following surgical removal of the sublingual and submaxillary glands and ligation of severed parotid gland ducts, it appears that significant quantities of penicillin may reach the oral cavity without participation of the major salivary glands.[49]

In relation to total body excretion of penicillin during therapy, only an insignificant amount is lost through the saliva, whereas urinary excretion accounts for by far the greatest part of the loss.

Chlortetracycline given intravenously appears in the saliva within 15 minutes of being injected and reaches its peak in the saliva at the end of one hour.[10] Chloramphenicol given intravenously is secreted into the saliva and persists there almost as long as it does in the blood.[9]

In the rabbit, studies have found that antifungal drugs absorbed from the intestinal tract, such as nystatin, appear in inhibitory concentrations when pilocarpine is given to promote salivary flow.[2]

The concentrations of parenterally adminstered antibiotics in the various tissues forming the oral cavity are less thoroughly studied than those in the saliva. With a single intravenous dose of penicillin in dogs, concentrations of the drug in each preceding organ are greater than in the succeeding, in this sequence: kidney—small intestine—lung—buccal mucosa—bile—skin—liver—adrenal—voluntary muscle.[57] The dental pulp and periodontal membrane attain high concentrations of penicillin upon intravenous administration of the drug.[61] Penicillin is also able to pass from the blood into the fluid contents of the dentinal tubules, although its concentration there is much lower than in the blood serum. Lincomycin given intramuscularly to the laboratory rat produces higher concentrations than penicillin in the mandibular bone,[23] while human alveolar bone attains good therapeutic levels after three 600-mg. doses of lincomycin have been given intramuscularly.[18] Parenterally administered tetracycline appears in the dental pulp[6] and is deposited in the calcifying dentin and enamel of developing teeth.[11] Absorption of penicillin into the blood from the mouth, through the oral mucosa, has been shown to occur.

The tissue concentration of parenterally given antibiotic drops sharply with the distance from the blood vessel unless serum levels can be maintained for long periods, giving time for equilibrium to occur. This may be important in relatively avascular lesions, such as thick-walled abscesses. The drainage of an abscess will maintain tissue flow and thus assist diffusion.

Certain membrane barriers may act to prevent the entrance of antibiotic into an organ. The best known case of this type is the blood-brain barrier, which allows only a relatively small amount of penicillin to penetrate into the cerebrospinal fluid of normal people. More penicillin may pass the barrier in cases of meningitis, and since the cerebrospinal fluid has a low content of protein for binding, most of the penicillin is free and effectively active. Other drugs, such as isoniazid, penetrate the blood-brain barrier well.

Intracellular bacteria, resulting from phagocytosis, are protected from antibiotic action by the cell wall and membrane barriers, the cytoplasm, and the wall of the pinocytic vacuole, and even the fluid of the vacuole itself. Infections in which such barriers as these may be significant include brucellosis, salmonella infections, leprosy, and tuberculosis. Necrosis and abscess formation result in the release locally of a large variety of intracellular components and breakdown products of tissues that very probably contribute to the failure of drugs to act in established lesions. The larger the abscess, the less effective the therapy because the less free is the contact between the antibiotic and the lesion.

Inactivation of antibiotics by host flora

It is theoretically possible that an antibiotic such as penicillin might be inactivated by penicillinase produced by bacteria other than those causing the illness. This is not a frequent phenomenon, however. A possible instance of such a case may be the patient who is receiving peni-

cillin in the prophylaxis of rheumatic fever and in whom the presence of penicillinase-producing staphylococci in the throat might prevent the elimination of hemolytic streptococci.

Allergic reactions

Allergic reactions[55] are among the iatrogenic, or treatment-induced, diseases developing from the use of antibiotics. These reactions seriously complicate the antibiotic treatment of infectious diseases. Patients with a history of penicillin allergy should not be given penicillin. If a life-threatening infection such as bacterial endocarditis is present, however, and the most effective drug available is penicillin, then the risk may not outweigh the possible benefit. In such cases, preparations should be made for emergency treatment of anaphylactic shock, including the use of epinephrine and supportive measures, if the decision is made to proceed with use of the penicillin.

Effects on the intestinal flora

Antibiotic therapy has profound and, in a sense, undiscriminating effects upon the normal microbial populations of the various body surfaces. Only a few of these are here described.

Prolonged medication with penicillin suppresses or eliminates gram-positive bacteria and directly or indirectly stimulates the multiplication of gram-negative bacilli. On the other hand, prolonged therapy with relatively large doses of streptomycin may suppress the gram-negative bacilli and stimulate the growth of gram-positive cocci, although this effect is not as constant as the reverse one induced by penicillin. Coliform bacteria disappear from the intestinal tract within 72 hours after a total of 3 gm. of oxytetracycline has been given. A combination of oxytetracycline and neomycin is extremely effective in eliminating culturable aerobic and anaerobic microorganisms from the feces.

Such profound effects by these and other antibiotics are the basis for antibiotic preparation of the lower part of the intestinal tract for major surgery in conjunction with mechanical cleansing.[60] A rich mixture of microorganisms is present in the colon, consisting predominantly of bacteroides[33] but also including coliform bacteria, clostridia, *Staphylococcus aureus*, lactobacilli, *Proteus vulgaris*, *Pseudomonas aeruginosa*, streptococci, and *Candida albicans*. Complete sterilization of the lower-intestinal tract lumen before surgery of the intestinal tract, in the face of such a large and complex mixture of microorganisms, is not possible or even desirable. Among the antibiotics used for bowel sterilization, kanamycin[14] has been among the most successful. At the present time, however, the effort to attain so-called intestinal antisepsis for surgery is still controversial and remains under investigation.[21]

Effects on the oral flora

There are relatively few studies on the specific effects of antibiotic therapy on the oral flora, particularly upon long-term drug administration. Penicillin either given orally or injected systemically greatly reduces, in a short time, the number of penicillin-sensitive gram-positive bacteria.[37] Following this initial phase there is an invasion by gram-negative bacilli, which disappear when use of the antibiotic is discontinued. The total salivary count, once the gram-negative bacilli appeared during antibiotic therapy, rapidly returns to the level present before the antibiotic therapy was begun. Most of the gram-negative bacilli are of nonfecal type and probably are derived from food or water. Neither penicillin nor chlortetracycline ingested for seven weeks was able to change *Lactobacillus* counts in the mouths of young male adults.[38] A mouthwash containing 0.1% vancomycin used as a rinse for one week produces a significant decrease in the relative percentage of gram-positive micro-

organisms as seen from swabs of the dento-gingival region, but no significant change is produced in the occurrence of yeasts or staphylococci.[63]

Superinfection

The changes in the normal resident flora following upon antibiotic therapy may not lead to any untoward effects, but in some cases they may lead to superinfection. By superinfection, it is meant that the organisms colonizing upon administration of the antibiotic are clearly associated with a prolongation or exacerbation of the signs of infection or are associated with clinical evidence of a new infection.

Superinfection usually occurs from three to six days after the start of therapy and affects about 2% of the cases under treatment. In hospitals a significant proportion of the infections acquired during the hospital stay are superinfections, contracted while the patient is receiving broad-spectrum antibiotic.[44] Many microorganisms, ordinarily practically nonpathogenic, may result in fatal superinfections upon antibiotic therapy. Two organisms, however, have been the most commonly involved—staphylococcus and *Candida*.

Superinfections appear most frequently in children less than three years of age who have been administered broad-spectrum antibiotics. Typical of this class of infections is the development of a severe diarrhea. As a result of the effects upon the flora of the gastrointestinal tract, upon administration of an oral antibiotic preparation, a *Staphylococcus aureus* strain resistant to the antibiotic being used may multiply in the intestinal tract and elaborate enterotoxin. A severe and sometimes fatal enteritis is produced by the toxin and is characterized by a copious outpouring of voluminous liquid stool, a shocklike state, and frequently a high fever. Smears of the rectal discharge will show the staphylococci in large numbers and in almost pure culture. Gram-negative organisms, however, are also frequently found in superinfections.

The most thoroughly studied form of superinfection following antibiotic suppression of the normal flora is that of candidiasis of the oral and other mucous membranes of the body.[51] This occurs especially after tetracycline is administered orally but also, although less commonly, with other antibiotics. In most persons with normal host resistance, the proliferation of *Candida* organisms during antibiotic therapy may cause certain unpleasant side effects such as anal or vulval itching, or diarrhea, but it is not a serious consideration. In those patients who have a lowered resistance or are on corticosteroid therapy, however, candidiasis may result in serious or even fatal infection.

Problems with superinfection may arise in the course of dental treatment. In one series of 120 patients given oxytetracycline therapy for various dental problems, including periodontitis, pericoronitis, Vincent's infection, periostitis, and jaw fracture, nine of the patients (7.5%) had untoward side reactions, including four with diarrhea.

Prevention of candidal or bacterial superinfection can be aided by adding an antifungal drug to the therapeutic regime, particularly nystatin[68]; avoiding antibiotic combinations other than with nystatin; avoiding broad-spectrum antibiotics unless they are specifically indicated; and not using antimicrobial drugs prophylactically without there being a specific indication, particularly in hospitalized patients.[52]

Effects on nutrition

Prolonged use of antibiotics has resulted in serious deficiencies of vitamins K and B-complex in patients,[41] but the mechanisms involved are not known with certainty. These deficiencies perhaps result from: (1) elimination of intestinal bacteria that normally synthesize the vitamins;

(2) the diarrhea and vomiting that occurs with use of some antibiotics; or (3) the anorexia and subsequently diminished food intake that can result from the infection itself or from the antibiotic therapy.

Glossitis as an occasional side effect of antibiotic therapy remains unexplained, but it is possibly related to vitamin B-complex deficiency. Use of vitamin supplements has therefore been recommended for these patients by some clinicians, especially when a tetracycline is given for more than 10 days consecutively.

Direct toxicity

Toxicity is the property of a drug to cause damage to the body by virtue of the chemical properties of the drug. It always affects everyone sufficiently exposed to the drug.

The systemic toxicity[26] of the most commonly used antimicrobial drugs is quite low. Penicillin has been injected parenterally for several weeks into patients at daily doses of 60 gm. without causing any unpleasant side effects; but the appearance of peripheral neuritis in some cases has been attributed to use of the penicillin. Injection of penicillin into a nerve trunk may result in permanent destruction of nerve fibers.[64] Aqueous injection is often painful, but with procaine it is relatively free from causing local reactions.

The tetracyclines have unpleasant, but not serious, irritative effects upon the gastrointestinal tract such as nausea, vomiting, and diarrhea. They have these effects, however, only in a small proportion of the cases. Chloramphenicol results in aplastic anemia, in some cases only if very large doses (6 to 12 gm. daily) are given for an appreciable period of time (12 to 35 days); but in a small percentage of the population even relatively small doses can produce this effect.

Streptomycin damage to the eighth cranial nerve occurs primarily with long-term therapy. Neomycin also has toxic effects on the eighth cranial nerve, as well as irritating effects upon the kidneys. Kanamycin has a greater cochlear toxicity than dihydrostreptomycin, but less than neomycin.[25] Toxic manifestations have not been seen when polymyxin B is given orally, but parenteral administration may result in neurotoxic or nephrotoxic effects. Erythromycin in large oral doses may cause nausea, vomiting, abdominal pain, and diarrhea, but the intestinal flora is not suppressed to the same extent as with the tetracyclines. Lincomycin has been relatively free of serious side effects, but diarrhea occurs in from 10% to 15% of patients treated by the oral route.[46]

The antifungal drug amphotericin B induces nausea, vomiting, chills, fever, and myalgia in almost every patient taking it. Altered renal function occurs during treatment, but it does not generally lead to permanent kidney damage.[62] The toxic effects of griseofulvin include headache, drowsiness, skin rashes, and gastrointestinal disturbances.[33]

PRINCIPLES OF CHEMOTHERAPY IN DENTISTRY

Dental infections are probably just as frequent today as in the days before antibiotics, but the duration, severity, and complications have decreased greatly. Surgical intervention today is rarely needed. This is primarily a consequence of modern chemotherapy,[50] but the usefulness of antibiotics may be gravely compromised unless they are restricted to cases where one has first resorted to the conventional surgical, hygienic, and antiseptic measures. The failure to use these basic principles cannot and must not be covered over by routine use of antibiotic therapy. Similarly, the use of antibiotics for minor localized infections of the oral mucosa cannot be justified. Moreover, local or topical use of antibiotics in the form of ointments, troches, and pastes should be avoided because of the greater risk of sensitizing the

patient than when the drug is given systemically.

Systemic use of antibiotics in acute infections arising from the teeth or their supporting structures is instituted[66] with the following aims: (1) prevention of spreading of infection following tooth extraction, (2) control of acute infection in preparation for endodontic therapy, (3) resolution of oral infections, and (4) localization of infection in preparation for early local or surgical intervention.

Other dental indications for the systemic use of antibiotics include the following: (1) prevention or control of infections following extensive oral surgery, (2) prevention of infection in the oral cavity following accidental trauma, (3) prevention of infection after minor oral surgery when host defense mechanisms are impaired, (4) control of bacteremias in patients undergoing dental treatment who have a history of rheumatic fever heart valve damage or congenital heart disease.

In spite of the thoroughly established need to institute chemotherapy for the control of bacteremias in dental patients with rheumatic heart damage or congenital cardiac defects, cases of subacute bacterial endocarditis and subsequent death are still occurring because prophylactic antibiotic medication was not instituted. The recently recommended treatment[43] is presented in Chapter 11.

Selection of most effective antibiotic

A wide range of antibiotics is now available (Table 14-2) that have significant differences in their antimicrobial effects. Whenever it is possible, in one's dealing with specific infections, antibiotics should be selected as precisely as possible on the basis of the isolation and identification of the infecting organisms and determination of their antibiotic sensitivities. Some bacteria, such as *Haemophilus influenzae*, pneumococci, and group A streptococci, have predictable sensitivity patterns and

Table 14-2. Antibiotics commonly used for therapy for infectious diseases

Source	Antibiotic	Spectrum	Therapeutic use
I. Molds		**Antibacterial antibiotics**	
Penicillium notatum and other *Penicillium* species	Penicillin	Gram-positive cocci and bacilli; gram-negative cocci; *Treponema pallidum*	Diseases caused by streptococci and sensitive staphylococci; gonorrhea and syphilis
Cephalosporium strains	Cephalosporin	Broad spectrum	Penicillin-resistant staphylococci, some coliform organisms
II. Streptomyces			
Streptomyces griseus	Streptomycin	Gram-positive cocci and bacilli; some gram-negative bacilli; tubercle bacillus	Tuberculosis and *Pasteurella* diseases; other bacterial diseases
Streptomyces venezuelae	Chloramphenicol	Broad spectrum; gram-positive and -negative cocci and bacilli, some rickettsiae, and some of larger viruses	Enteric diseases, psittacosis-ornithosis-lymphogranuloma venereum viruses
Streptomyces aureofaciens	Tetracycline	Broad spectrum	Gram-negative bacilli, *Brucella, Haemophilus, Klebsiella, Bacteroides, Rickettsia,* and the large viruses
Streptomyces rimosus		Broad spectrum	
Streptomyces erythreus	Erythromycin	Similar to penicillin	Similar to penicillin, also against penicillin resistant staphylococci
Streptomyces lincolnensis	Lincomycin	Similar to penicillin	Similar to penicillin, also against penicillin-resistant staphylococci
Streptomyces niveus	Novobiocin	Narrow spectrum	*Proteus* strains and penicillin-resistant staphylococci
III. Bacteria			
Bacillus polymyxa	Polymyxin B	Narrow spectrum: gram-negative bacilli	*Pseudomonas* and *Escherichia coli*
Bacillus subtilis	Bacitracin	Similar to penicillin	Penicillin resistant stains; best used topically because of toxicity
		Antifungal antibiotics	
Streptomyces noursei	Nystatin	*Candida*	Candidiasis (superficial lesions)
Streptomyces nodosus	Amphotericin B	Yeasts and yeastlike organisms	Candidiasis, histoplasmosis, blastomycosis cryptococcosis, and coccidioidomycosis
Penicillium griseofulvum	Griseofulvin	Dermatophytes (molds)	Ringworm and athlete's foot

are not routinely tested. Bacterial species such as *Proteus* organisms, coagulase-positive staphylococci, and enterococci, which have a significant percentage of resistant strains, should be tested, however. These latter microorganisms are frequently implicated in dental infections.

Determination of antibiotic sensitivities

Results of sensitivity tests[45] in the laboratory will indicate which drug is most likely to be useful against the infecting strain or which second-choice drug can be given if the first is not effective clinically or is not well tolerated.

The usual laboratory technique is the disc method (Fig. 14-1). The surface of the agar plate is entirely inoculated with the bacterium to be tested. Individual filter paper discs, each with a different antibiotic, are placed equally spaced around the plate. Following overnight incubation the zones of clear medium around the disc are measured. The size of the inhibited growth zone, however, does not neces-

sarily imply that similar activity will occur in vivo since quite different factors are operating on the plate—rate of diffusion of the antibiotic through the agar medium, temperature of incubation, character of the agar enrichment, molecular weight of the antibiotic.

As a general rule, however, an organism is considered sensitive if it is inhibited by considerably less than the average blood level attained with ordinary dosage. It is rare for an antibiotic to be effective in treatment if the infecting bacterium can grow in a high concentration of the drug in vitro, but good clinical responses are sometimes found with antibiotics that would seem of little value on the basis of in vitro studies. Occasionally, an infection may be refractory to treatment even though the microorganism involved is found to be sensitive. In some cases this may be because of inadequate dosages of the drug. Certain areas of the body present a barrier to the entrance of antibiotics. In some cases there is a poor correlation be-

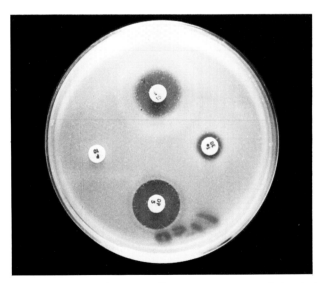

Fig. 14-1. Disc sensitivity test of a penicillin-resistant strain of *Staphylococcus aureus.* Clockwise from top disc are *E,* erythromycin; *T,* tetracycline; *DP,* methicillin; and *P,* penicillin. (Courtesy Dr. Sami Schaefler, Bureau of Laboratories, Department of Health, City of New York.)

tween in vitro tests and the results of treatment, such as in the instance of *Salmonella* carriers.

In many situations a decision must be made concerning a chemotherapeutic regime without laboratory sensitivity test results being available. In these instances an educated guess, aided by examination of gram-stained smears from the lesion, must be resorted to. When possible, cultures should be made to aid in the choice of the drug.

A much less frequently utilized technique for testing bacterial sensitivities to drugs is that of the broth tube dilution method (Fig. 14-2). In this procedure a standard inoculum of bacteria is seeded into tubes of broth containing decreasing concentrations of antibiotic. After an incubation period of from 18 to 24 hours, the endpoint (minimum inhibitory concentration) of the antibiotic is read as the lowest concentration inhibiting the development of visible growth. This procedure is used when minimal dosage must be determined when an infecting resistant bacterium is involved for which unusually high dosage is being considered, or for testing slow-growing organisms such as those of *Actinomyces* or some *Neisseria*.

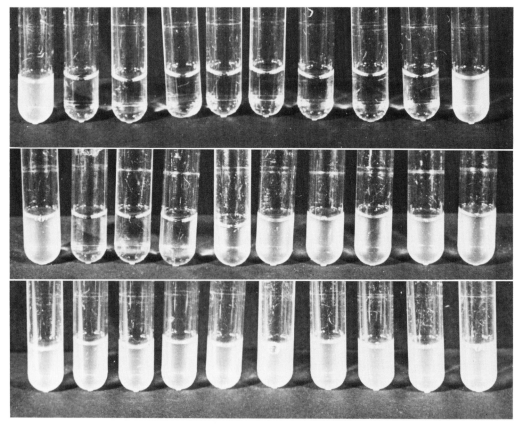

Fig. 14-2. Serial tube dilution test for the antibiotic sensitivities of a penicillin-resistant strain of *Staphylococcus aureus*. Top series, oxacillin (highly sensitive); middle series, tetracycline (medium resistance); bottom series, penicillin (highly resistant). (Courtesy Dr. Sami Schaefler, Bureau of Laboratories, Department of Health, City of New York.)

Therapeutic characteristics of some useful antibiotics

The term "antimicrobial spectrum" of a particular antibiotic refers to the range of microorganisms against which it is active.[5, 54] Narrow-spectrum antibiotics are effective against only a limited number of species. Penicillin, the most commonly used in this group, acts against gram-positive cocci and bacilli, the gram-negative *Neisseria*, and *Treponema pallidum*. Bacitracin has a similar narrow spectrum.

Broad-spectrum antibiotics include the tetracyclines and chloramphenicol. They act against gram-positive and gram-negative cocci and bacilli, the rickettsiae, and the intracellular parasites of the psittacosis group.

The agents referred to as reserve antibiotics are extremely useful because of their broad spectrum but are not prescribed routinely because of their toxicity or their ready propensity to evoke resistant mutants. The tetracyclines, chloramphenicol, erythromycin, and cephaloridine are among those included in this group.

Penicillins

Penicillin[30] today is produced from large scale culture of *Penicillium chrysogenum*. The penicillins are organic acids with a basic structure of a fused thiazolidine and beta-lactam ring. A number of acids are produced by the mold culture itself, differing from each other only in the side chain attached to the beta-lactam ring. Further variant forms are obtained by adding various chemicals to the culture medium. These variants are designed for specific properties such as gastric acid resistance, penicillinase resistance, and activity against gram-negative bacteria.

Benzylpenicillin (penicillin G) is the common drug meant by the term "penicillin." It is susceptible to penicillinase and is inactivated by gastric juice. It is active against gram-positive and gram-negative cocci and some gram-positive bacilli, but gram-negative bacilli are generally resistant to it. *Leptospira* and *Treponema* are also sensitive. *Staphylococcus aureus* readily becomes resistant. Intramuscular injection of procaine penicillin G in aluminum monostearate gives effective blood concentrations for from 48 to 72 hours. Penicillin G may be administered orally, but it must be taken on an empty stomach at least 30 minutes before meals and in a concentration from three to five times greater than penicillin in aqueous solution given parenterally.

Methicillin (dimethoxyphenylpenicillin) has the important quality of being highly resistant to penicillinase, especially that from *Staphylococcus aureus*. Since it is inactivated by gastric acid, it must be given parenterally. Its major use is in the treatment of infections caused by penicillinase-producing *S. aureus* not responding to penicillin G.

Oxacillin has the great advantage over methicillin that it is stable in gastric acid and is also resistant to penicillinase. It has greater activity than methicillin against other susceptible gram-positive organisms, such as pneumococci and group A streptococci. It is the antibiotic of choice in the treatment of serious staphylococcal infections.

Ampicillin (6 alpha-aminobenzyl penicillin) is acid-stable but not penicillinase-resistant. It is an important penicillin congener because of its wide antibacterial activity against gram-negative bacteria, including *Haemophilus influenzae*, alpha hemolytic streptococci, *Proteus mirabilis*, *Escherichia coli*, and *Salmonella* and *Shigella* species. It is not effective against penicillinase-producing staphylococci. It is acid-resistant and may be given orally.

Cephalosporins

Cephalosporins[1] are a family of antibiotics (7-aminocephalosporanic acid nucleus) produced by the fungus *Cephalo-*

sporium. They are effective against almost all the gram-positive cocci and many gram-negative bacilli, giving them a wider spectrum of antimicrobial activity than penicillin. Moreover, they are resistant to staphylococcal penicillinase, a property which makes them useful in penicillin-resistant infections. There is no cross-hypersensitivity with penicillin and very low toxicity, but it requires intramuscular injection. They are rapidly excreted by the kidney. Cephaloridine and cephalothin are included in this group.

Erythromycin

Erythromycin is effective against a wide range of bacteria, but not against the coliforms. It is also effective against many rickettsial infections. It has been frequently used in dentistry because it may be given by the oral route and is especially useful in cases of penicillin allergy. It may, however, present problems in clinical infections because resistant mutants may emerge and become dominant if the infection is not controlled within a few days.

Lincomycin

Lincomycin (Fig. 14-3), produced by *Streptomyces lincolnensis,* is an antibiotic of low toxicity that is chemically distinct from the other clinically available antibiotics, being a derivative of the amino acid trans-L-4-n-propylhygrinic acid. It is effective in vitro against gram-positive

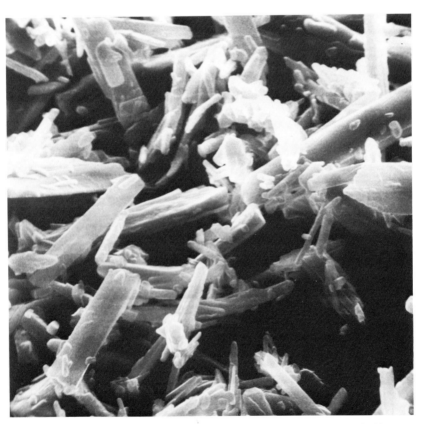

Fig. 14-3. Lincomycin hydrochloride, scanning electron microscopy (3,000 ×). (Courtesy The Upjohn Company, Kalamazoo, Mich. All rights reserved.)

cocci including staphylococci, *Strepto-coccus viridans*, *Streptococcus pneumoniae*, and beta hemolytic streptococci. Clinical studies have indicated its usefulness for oral infections[35] as well as for various others. Clinimycin (7-chloro-7-deoxy lin-comycin) is a chemical modification of lincomycin that is better absorbed after oral administration, has fewer gastrointes-tinal side effects than the parent com-pound, and is more active than lincomycin against gram-positive cocci.[47]

Tetracyclines

The tetracyclines,[23] a group of broad-spectrum antibiotics, are useful in the treat-ment of infections caused by rickettsia, the psittacosis-lymphogranuloma venereum group, mycoplasma, *Brucella*, *Pasteurella*, *Entamoeba histolytica*, *Shigella*, *Lepto-spira*, *Clostridium*, *Treponema*, and *Neisseria*. They also are active against *Staphylococcus* and *Streptococcus* infec-tions, but the problem of resistant strains makes use of another antibiotic preferable. They are absorbed rapidly from the gastro-intestinal tract and are usually adminis-tered by mouth. This group includes chlor-tetracycline, oxytetracycline, and tetracy-cline.

Chloramphenicol

Chloramphenicol[23] is a broad-spectrum antibiotic isolated first in 1947 from *Strep-tomyces venezuelae*. Its chemical structure is relatively simple, so that it is made synthetically. Its antibiotic spectrum is similar to that of the tetracyclines, but it is notably effective against *Salmonella ty-phosa*. This drug is completely and rapidly absorbed from the intestinal tract after oral administration, degraded by the liver, and excreted by the kidney. It rarely may cause aplastic anemia or fatal granulocy-topenia, so that the drug is now used with considerable caution. It is the drug of choice for treating the typhoid-paratyphoid infections and may also be used in other

infections that do not respond to safer antibiotics.

Antifungal antibiotics

These agents have no activity against bacteria but have powerful effects upon pathogenic fungi.

Nystatin is produced by a *Streptomyces noursei* strain isolated from a Virginia soil sample. It is a polyene antibiotic that retains its activity for several months when stored at 4° C. as a powder. It is used locally in the treatment of *Candida albi-cans* infections especially. It is also useful for gastrointestinal, vaginal, and cutaneous candidiasis; but poor absorption from the intestinal tract requires large doses by mouth for systemic candidiasis.

Amphotericin B is formed by *Strepto-myces nodosus* and is chemically a hep-tane. It is active in low concentration against both yeastlike and filamentous pathogenic fungi. Since it is not easily absorbed from the gastrointestinal tract, it has to be given intravenously for a sys-temic effect. It is highly toxic, having nu-merous side effects, among which are fever, nausea, renal damage, anemia, and leu-kopenia. It is indicated for histoplasmosis, coccidioidomycosis, North American blasto-mycosis, and cryptococcosis. Because of the severe side effects, the drug is used only when the diagnosis is established and the infection severe and widespread.

Griseofulvin is produced by a number of *Penicillium* molds, but especially by *Penicillium griseofulvum*. It was first dis-covered in 1938, then rediscovered in 1947, and introduced into clinical practice in 1958. Given orally, this antifungal agent is absorbed and then deposited in keratin as it is laid down. Fungi, and especially dermatophytes, do not grow in its pres-ence. It is not active against yeasts and bacteria. Its greatest value is in the treat-ment of ringworm infections of the scalp. Treatment consists of daily doses of from 0.2 to 1 gm. and may require six weeks or more. Ringworm of the nails does not respond as well and may require six months of treatment. Athlete's foot from *Trichophyton mentagrophytes* responds poorly to this drug, but most other fungus infections of the skin will respond.

CITED REFERENCES

1. Abraham, E. P., and Newton, G. G. F.: The cephalosporins, Advances Chemother. **2**:23, 1965.
2. Adler-Hradecky, C., and Kelentey, B.: Der Gehalt des Speichels an antifungalen Antibiotics nach Darreichung per os, Stoma **15**:83, 1962.
3. Adler-Hradecky, C., Kelentey, B., and Adler, P.: Inactivation of penicillin by saliva, Acta Med. Acad. Sci. Hung. **22**:81, 1966.
4. Albert, A.: Selective toxicity, ed. 3, London, 1965, Methuen & Co. Ltd., p. 68.
5. Alstead, S., Macarthur, J. G., and Thomson, T. J.: Clinical pharmacology (Dilling), ed. 22, London, 1969, Baillière Tindall & Cassell, p. 454.
6. Antalovská, Z., Lonská, V., and Pruchová, I.: Participation of vital dental pulp in the distribution of tetracycline in dental tissues, J. Dent. Res. **47**:806, 1968.
7. Baldry, P. E.: The battle against bacteria, a history of the development of antibacterial drugs for the general reader, New York, 1965, Cambridge University Press.
8. Beaty, H. N., and Petersdorf, R. G.: Iatrogenic factors in infectious disease, Ann. Intern. Med. **65**:641, 1966.
9. Bender, I. B., Pressman, R. S., and Tashman, S. G.: Studies on excretion of antibiotics in human saliva. II. Chloramphenicol, J. Dent. Res. **32**:287, 1953.
10. Bender, I. B., Pressman, R. S., and Tashman, S. G.: Studies on excretion of antibiotics in human saliva. III. Aureomycin, J. Dent. Res. **32**:435, 1953.
11. Bennett, I. C.: Measurement of tetracycline incorporated in enamel and dentin, J. Oral Ther. **3**:232, 1966.
12. Beyer, K. H.: Pharmacological basis of penicillin therapy, Springfield, Ill., 1950, Charles C Thomas, Publisher.
13. Bodenhoff, J.: Resistance studies of *Candida albicans*, with special reference to two patients subjected to prolonged antimycotic treatment, Odont. T. **76**:279, 1964.
14. Cohen, I., Jr.: Kanamycin for bowel sterilization, Ann. N. Y. Acad. Sci. **76**:212, 1958.
15. Cohen, S.: Ecologic consequences of resistance-transfer factors, Amer. J. Clin. Nutr. **23**:1480, 1970.
16. Crofton, J.: Some principles in the chemotherapy of bacterial infections, Brit. Med. J. **2**:137, 1969.
17. Dauer, C. C.: A demographic analysis of recent changes in mortality, morbidity, and age group distribution in our population. In Galdston, I. (ed.): The impact of the antibiotics on medicine and society, New York, 1958, International Universities Press, p. 99.
18. Davis, W. McL., Jr., and Balcom, J. H., III: Lincomycin studies of drug absorption and efficacy, Oral Surg. **27**:688, 1969.
19. Demers, P., Fraser, D., Goldbloom, R. B., Haworth, J. C., La Rochelle, J., MacLean, R., and Murray, T. K.: Effects of tetracyclines on skeletal growth and dentition, Canad. Med. Assoc. J. **99**:849, 1968.
20. Devine, L. F., Knowles, R. C., Pierce, W. E., Peckinpaugh, R. O., Hagerman, C. R., and Lytle, R. I.: Proposed model for screening antimicrobial agents for potential use in eliminating meningococci from the nasopharynx of healthy carriers, Antimicrob. Agents Chemother.—1968, p. 307, 1969.
21. Evaskus, D. S., Laskin, D. M., and Kroeger, A. V.: Penetration of lincomycin, penicillin, and tetracycline into serum and bone, Proc. Soc. Exp. Biol. Med. **130**:89, 1969.
22. Finegold, S. M.: Interaction of antimicrobial therapy and intestinal flora, Amer. J. Clin. Nutr. **23**:1466, 1970.
23. Florey, M. E.: The clinical application of antibiotics. Chloramphenicol and the tetracyclines, vol. 2, London, 1957, Oxford University Press.
24. Fox, J., and Isenberg, H. D.: Antibiotic resistance of microorganisms isolated from root canals, Oral Surg. **23**:230, 1967.
25. Frost, J. O., Daly, J. F., and Hawkins, J. E., Jr.: The ototoxicity of kanamycin in man, Antibiot. Ann. 1958-1959, p. 700, 1959.
26. Guthe, T., Idsöe, O., and Willcox, R. R.: Untoward penicillin reactions, Bull. W.H.O. **19**:427, 1958.
27. Handelman, S. L., Garnick, J., and Slusar, R. J.: Effect of oxytetracycline in a periodontal pack on sensitivity and number of tongue flora, J. Periodont. **40**:480, 1969.
28. Handelman, S. L., and Hawes, R. R.: The effect of long term antibiotic therapy on the antibiotic resistance of the salivary flora, J. Oral Ther. **1**:23, 1964.
29. Hebeka, E. K., and Solotorovsky, M.: Development of strains of *Candida albicans* resistant to candidin, J. Bact. **84**:237, 1962.

30. Hoeprich, P. D.: The penicillins, old and new: Review and perspectives, Calif. Med. **109**:301, 1968.

31. Hoeprich, P. D.: Prediction of antimeningococcic chemoprophylactic efficacy, J. Infect. Dis. **123**:125, 1971.

32. Jawetz, E.: Antimicrobial chemotherapy, Ann. Rev. Microbiol. **10**:85, 1956.

33. Jawetz, E., Melnick, J. L., and Adelberg, E. A.: Review of medical microbiology, ed. 9, Los Altos, Calif., 1970, Lange Medical Publications.

34. Jokinen, M. A.: Bacteremia following dental extraction and its prophylaxis, Suom. Hammaslaak. Toim. **66**:69, 1970.

35. Khosla, V. M.: Lincomycin in oral surgery, Oral Surg. **29**:485, 1970.

36. Lampen, J. O.: Interference by polyenic antifungal antibiotics (especially nystatin and filipin) with specific membrane functions, Symp. Soc. Gen. Microbiol., no. 16, p. 111, 1966.

37. Long, D. A.: Effect of penicillin on bacterial flora of the mouth, Brit. Med. J. **2**:819, 1947.

38. Ludwick, W. E., Bass, K., and Jay, P.: Evaluation of antibiotic agents in the control of lactobacillus counts, J. Amer. Dent. Assoc. **46**:174, 1953.

39. McDermott, W.: Microbial persistance, Yale J. Biol. Med. **30**:257, 1958.

40. McManis, T. F., Dehne, E., and Bingham, C. B.: Specific antibiotic therapy for an iliac bone graft in the mandible, Oral Surg. **6**:1396, 1953.

41. Milberg, M. B., and Michael, M., Jr.: Antibiotics and nutrition in infections, Ann. N. Y. Acad. Sci. **63**:252, 1955.

42. Mitsuhashi, S.: Review: The R factors, J. Infect. Dis. **119**:89, 1969.

43. Myall, R. W. T., and Gregory, H. S.: Current trends in the prevention of bacterial endocarditis in susceptible patients receiving dental care, Oral Surg. **28**:813, 1969.

44. Ogilvie, R. I., and Ruedy, J.: Adverse reactions during hospitalization, Canad. Med. Assoc. J. **97**:1445, 1967.

45. Petersdorf, R. G., and Sherris, J. C.: Methods and significance of in vitro testing of bacterial sensitivity to drugs, Amer. J. Med. **39**:766, 1965.

46. Price, D. J. E., O'Grady, F. W., Shutter, R. A., and others: Trial of phenoxymethyl penicillin, pheneticillin, and lincomycin in treatment of staphylococcal sepsis in a casualty department, Brit. Med. J. **3**:407, 1968.

47. Quintiliani, R., and McGreevy, M. J.: Clinda-

48. Rammelkamp, C. H., and Keefer, C. S.: The absorption, excretion, and distribution of penicillin, J. Clin. Invest. **22**:425, 1943.

49. Rosen, S., and Carpenter, L.: Effect of dietary and intramuscular administration of penicillin on dental caries in intact rats and in rats after sialoadenectomy, Antimicrob. Agents Chemother.—1965, p. 445, 1966.

50. Rubbo, S. D.: Chemotherapy and chemical sterilization in dentistry, Aust. Dent. J. **60**: 204, 1956.

51. Seelig, M. S.: Mechanisms by which antibiotics increase the incidence and severity of candidiasis and alter the immunological defenses, Bact. Rev. **30**:442, 1966.

52. Seelig, M. S.: The rationale for preventing antibacterial-induced fungal overgrowth, Med. Times **96**:689, 1968.

53. Slack, G. L.: The resistance to antibiotics of micro-organisms isolated from root canals, Brit. Dent. J. **102**:493, 1957.

54. Smith, J. W. (ed.): Manual of medical therapeutics, ed. 19, Boston, 1969, Little, Brown and Company, p. 181.

55. Smith, L. W., and Walker, A. D.: Penicillin decade, 1941-1951: Sensitizations and toxicities, Washington, D. C., 1951, Arundel Press Inc.

56. Sprunt, K., Redman, W. W., and Leidy, G.: Oral antibiotics in patients with heart disease, Pediatrics **43**:608, 1969.

57. Struble, G. C., and Bellows, J. G.: Studies on the distribution of penicillin in the eye, and its clinical application, J. A. M. A. **125**:685, 1944.

58. Suter, L. S.: In vitro development of resistance of *Actinomyces bovis* to antibiotics, Antibiot. Chemother. **7**:285, 1957.

59. Tozer, R. A., Boutflower, S., and Gillespie, W. A.: Antibiotics for prevention of bacterial endocarditis during dental treatment, Lancet **1**:686, 1966.

60. Turell, R., and Landau, S. J.: Antibiotics in the preoperative preparation of the colon: Evaluation of the present status, J. Int. Coll. Surg. **31**:215, 1959.

61. Ullberg, S.: Autoradiografiska undersökningar över penicillinets distribution i kroppen, Svensk Tandlak. T. **48**:141, 1955.

62. Utz, J. P., Treger, A., McCullough, N. B., and Emmons, C. W.: Amphotericin B: Intravenous use in 21 patients with systemic fungal disease, Antibiot. Ann. 1958-1959, p. 628, 1959.

63. Volpe, A. R., Kupczak, L. J., Brant, J. H.,

mycin (Cleocin®) in bacterial pneumonia, Curr. Ther. Res. **12**:701, 1970.

King, W. J., Kestenbaum, R. C., and Schlissel, H. J.: Antimicrobial control of bacterial plaque and calculus and the effects of these agents on oral flora, J. Dent. Res. **48:**832, 1969.

64. Walker, A. E., and Johnson, H. C.: Penicillin in neurology, Springfield, Ill., 1946, Charles C Thomas, Publisher.

65. Weinstein, L.: The present status of antimicrobial therapy, Resident Physician **15:** 63, 106, 110, 1969.

66. Weisberger, D.: Systemic therapy with antibiotics, Dent. Clin. N. Amer., March 1958, p. 109.

67. Wolstenholme, G. E. W., and O'Connor, M. (eds.): CIBA Foundation Symposium on bacterial episomes and plasmids, Boston, 1969, Little, Brown and Company.

68. Younger, D., Epifano, L. D., DiPillo, F., Hoffman, I., Thaler, E., and Yarvis, M.: A clinical comparison of the side effects of tetracycline-nystatin and tetracycline, Antibiot. Chemother. 6:216, 1959.

GENERAL REFERENCES AND ADDITIONAL READINGS

Anderson, E. S.: The ecology of transferable drug resistance in the enterobacteria, Ann. Rev. Microbiol. 22:131, 1968.

Hare, R.: The birth of penicillin and the disarming of microbes, London, 1970, George Allen and Unwin Ltd.

Herrell, W. E.: Lincomycin, Chicago, 1969, Modern Scientific Publications, Inc.

Jukes, T. H.: Antibiotics in nutrition, Antibiotics Monographs 4, New York, 1955, Medical Encyclopedia, Inc.

Mann, C. H. (ed.): Kanamycin: Appraisal after eight years of clinical application, Ann. N. Y. Acad. Sci. 132:771, 1966.

Resistance of bacteria to the penicillins, CIBA Foundation study group, No. 13, London, 1962, J. & A. Churchill Ltd.

Rosenblum, A. H.: Penicillin allergy, J. Allerg. 42:309, 1968.

Welch, H., and Finland, M. (eds.): Antibiotic therapy for staphylococcal diseases, New York, 1959, Medical Encyclopedia, Inc.

15 / Laboratory animals and their contribution to oral microbiology

Those engaged in the scientific pursuit of knowledge to alleviate human suffering eventually find it necessary to use human subjects in their experimentation. However, before any experiment can be performed on a human being, it must be deemed relatively safe to his health. In order to determine relative safety, it is necessary to perform appropriate experiments on a suitable animal.

Suitability of laboratory animals depends, in part, upon the premise of uniformity in nature: that is, what is true about one species may also be true about another. For example, both human beings and guinea pigs are susceptible to tuberculosis. The same microorganism, *Mycobacterium tuberculosis*, produces the same disease in both species. The guinea pig proved its worth in the laboratory when Koch was able to demonstrate that a particular organism caused tuberculosis without even exposing a human being to the etiologic agent.

In addition to showing that a particular microorganism causes a specific disease, laboratory animals can be used in various other ways. A drug or a procedure for the treatment of a disease is always tested on animals before it is used in human beings. The toxicity of a drug is determined by testing it on animals. Much of the basic knowledge in genetics, biochemistry, physiology, pharmacology, microbiology, immunology, and psychology has been obtained through the use of animals. New surgical techniques must first be tested on animals; animals preceded human beings into outer space, and animals have been used for the production of vaccines and antisera. Thus animals have contributed enormously to our body of biologic knowledge and have also contributed to man's welfare by increasing his lifespan and his comfort.

BASELINE STUDIES

There is little information about the composition of the normal oral flora of experimental animals, although many researchers have noted the need for such studies. Studies of this nature have numerous complications, which lead to highly variable data. Time and method of sampling, diet, and the age, sex, and strain of animal are among the important considerations in attempting to define oral flora.

The methods of sampling oral flora of experimental animals include brushing the oral cavity with a cotton swab, removing and grinding the teeth, removing a measured amount of saliva with a capillary pipet, and even macerating the entire head. Many types of diets are used in experimental studies. Undoubtedly the composition of the diet influences the numbers and types of microorganisms in the oral cavity. In human beings it has been shown that severe restriction of carbohydrates results in diminished numbers of salivary oral lactobacilli.

There exist several reports of the indigenous oral flora of experimental animals.

A summary of the indigenous oral flora of man and of certain laboratory animals is given in Table 15-1. The two groups of microorganisms common to all species are the lactobacilli and the streptococci. These particular microorganisms are able to cause dental caries in animals and presumably in human beings.

Table 15-1. Comparative distribution of oral microorganisms in man and certain animals

Genus or group	Human	Monkey	Rice rat	Albino rat	Cotton rat	Hamster
Actinobacillus			+			
Actinomyces	+		+			
Bacillus	±		+			
Bacterionema (Leptotrichia)	++		+			
Bacteroides	+	+	+			
Clostridium	0		+			
Coliform	±	+	++	++		
Corynebacterium and diphtheroids	+	+	++			
Diplococcus	±					
Fusobacterium	++	+	+			++
Hemophilus	±					
Lactobacillus	+	+	+	+	+	++
Mycobacterium	0					
Neisseria	±	+				
Pleuropneumonia-like organisms	+					
Paracolon bacillus			++			
Proteus	±					
Protozoa	±					
Pseudomonas	±					
Spirochaeta	++	+	0			+
Staphylococcus	+	++	++	+		+
Streptococcus	++	++	++	++	++	++
alpha	++	++		++		
beta	+	0		+		
gamma	+	++		++		
enterococci	±		++		++	
Peptostreptococcus	++					
Veillonella	++	+				
Vibrio	++	+				
Viruses	±					
Yeasts	+	+		±		+
Candida		+		±		
Other types		+				

++ Constitutes a significant percentage of the oral flora

 + Found less frequently or in smaller numbers than previous group

 ± Rarely occurring types; may appear as transients

 0 Sought but not discovered

Blank space signifies data not available.

DENTAL CARIES

In the area of oral microbiology, laboratory animals have been used to study diseases of the oral cavity, of which dental caries has been studied more extensively than all of the others. Dental caries may be characterized as a localized, progressive, molecular disintegration of tooth structure. Although the anatomic structure of human and rodent teeth differs in certain respects (Fig. 15-1, A), the appearance of a carious lesion in a human being (Fig. 15-1, B) is similar to that in a rat (Fig. 15-1, C).

Experimental animals

The albino rat has four teeth in each quadrant: an incisor and three molars. The incisor teeth are rarely affected by caries, since they are in constant eruption and have a smooth surface. The molars have narrow, deep fissures lined by enamel that does not continue over the entire occlusal surface (Fig. 15-1, A). The molars of certain strains of rats are susceptible to dental caries (Fig. 15-2).

The hamster dentition is similar to that of a rat in that it has one incisor and three molars per quadrant. The shapes of

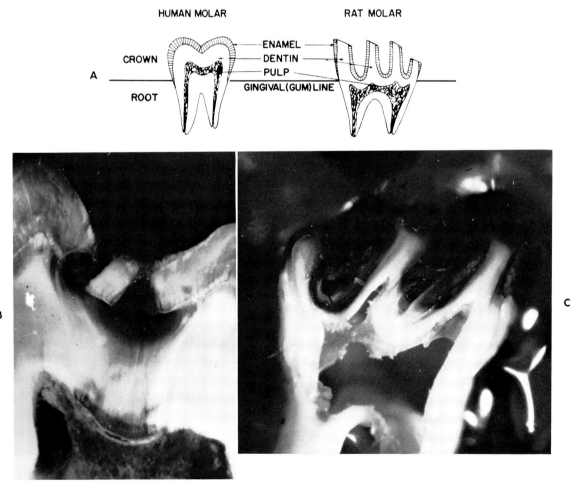

Fig. 15-1. A, Anatomic structure of human and rat molars. **B,** Dental caries in human tooth. **C,** Dental caries in rat molar.

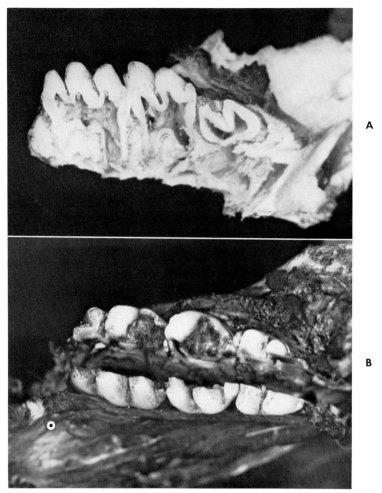

Fig. 15-2. A, Hemisection of noncarious rat molars. The third molar has barely erupted. **B,** Extensive carious lesions in first and second molars of a rat. The teeth have been hemisectioned to permit observation of the depth of caries penetration.

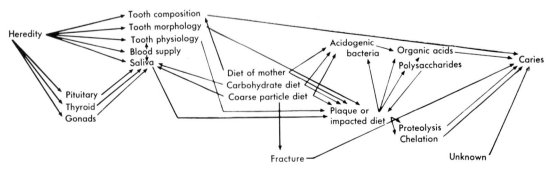

Fig. 15-3. Interrelation of certain etiologic factors of dental caries.

the teeth are different from those of a rat, but the teeth are also susceptible to caries.

Experimental dental caries has also been produced in the gerbil, the cotton rat, and the monkey.

Multifactorial origin

Dental caries undoubtedly has a multifactorial origin. The interrelation of certain but not all theoretic and known etiologic factors is given in Fig. 15-3. In the diagram each arrow represents a cause-and-effect situation and points from a cause to an effect. For example, acidogenic bacteria produce organic acids, which decalcify enamel, thus producing the initial or incipient carious lesion. Many of the causal arrows are justified by experimental studies, but some are hypothetical, particularly those originating at heredity. Certain relationships are better established than others. For example, the evidence for acidogenic bacteria's initiating dental caries is more extensive than is the evidence for the role of proteolysis in caries initiation. Some of the relations indicated are based on experiments with albino Norway rats, whereas others are based on observations of human beings or hamsters.

Heredity

The role of heredity in the incidence of dental caries has been elucidated by studies of rats. Caries-resistant and caries-susceptible lines of rats have been established by selection, inbreeding, and progeny testing (Fig. 15-4). The reversion from resistance to susceptibility when the stress of selection is relaxed indicates that these are not purebred lines. Nevertheless, the marked difference between these two lines suggests that potent heritable factors contribute to resistance or susceptibility to dental caries.

Microbiology

The laboratory animal has been particularly valuable in elucidating the microbial origin of dental caries. Until recently it was not known whether specific microorganisms caused caries. As a result of numerous studies performed on

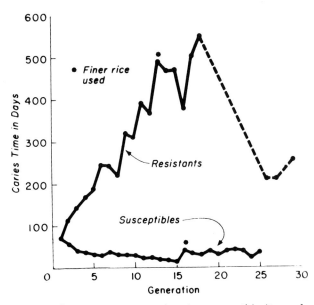

Fig. 15-4. Development of caries resistant and caries susceptible lines of rats. The decline in resistance was the result of relaxation of the stress of selection.

human beings and on animals, it was believed that the etiologic organisms be-
longed to the genus *Lactobacillus*. This
conclusion was based on the evidence that
lactobacilli were recovered more frequently
and in greater numbers from subjects with
caries than from those without caries.
However, all that was shown was an association of lactobacilli with caries; there
was no evidence that lactobacilli caused
caries. Since no other organism or particular group of organisms was found to
be associated with dental caries, by de-
fault the lactobacilli were believed by
some researchers to be etiologic organisms.
Others believed that any microorganisms
that were associated with the dental plaque
and that could produce acid from carbohydrates were capable of causing caries.

Two approaches have been used to differentiate cariogenic from noncariogenic
bacteria. One approach has used the germ-
free rat; the other, the conventional hamster or rat under conditions of relative
gnotobiosis. The germ-free technique was
developed by Reyniers at the University

of Notre Dame, Notre Dame, Indiana. At
first the housing chambers for germ-free
animals were constructed of stainless steel,
but today investigators are using a less
expensive chamber fabricated of a durable
flexible plastic (Fig. 15-5). These chambers are called "isolators" since they effectively house animals that are germ-free
or that bear one known microorganism or
more.

The term "gnotobiotic" has been used
to designate an animal bearing a known
microbial flora. "Gnotobiotic" may also be
used to include the germ-free animal, but
common usage has restricted this term to
animals bearing one or more known and
no unknown microorganisms. For animals
that have been born and reared in the
usual animal quarters, the term "conventional" has been used.

Gnotobiotic techniques have been applied to the study of dental caries. In
1954 it was shown that dental caries
would not develop in rats reared free of
all microorganisms, although the diet used
in this study was capable of producing

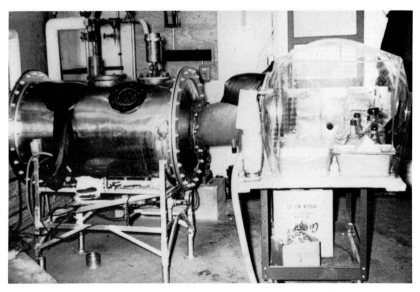

Fig. 15-5. At left, a stainless steel isolator which has been converted into a vacuum autoclave. At right, a flexible plastic isolator.

caries in the same strain of rat reared in a conventional environment. In the following year caries was produced in germ-free rats that were inoculated with either an enterococcus and a proteolytic bacillus or with the same enterococcus and a pleomorphic bacterium. In 1959 it was reported that this enterococcus could produce caries when maintained as a pure culture in the isolator.

Confirmation of the etiologic role of streptococci (Fig. 15-6) in dental caries has been obtained in numerous studies using experimental animals (Table 15-2). The species of streptococci listed as cariogenic include: *faecalis, liquefaciens, mitis, salivarius, sanguis,* and *mutans. Streptococcus mutans,* a recently recognized species, refers to a large spectrum of cariogenic streptococci that produce dextran and ferment sorbitol and mannitol. Two species of *Lactobacillus, acidophilus* and *casei,* have been listed as cariogenic (Fig. 15-7 and Table 15-2). These organisms are homofermentative, as are all streptococci, in that they produce primarily lactic acid as the end product of glucose metabolism. Two strains of *Actinomyces, viscosus* and *naeslundii,* have been found to cause root caries only. Certain strains of microorganisms that were tested for cariogenicity in gnotobiotic rats were shown to be noncariogenic (Table 15-2). This does not mean that these organisms are absolutely noncariogenic; under different conditions they may prove to be cariogenic. Testing an organism with a different strain of rat or using the hamster model system instead of the rat, using a different diet, or merely repeating the experiment may show that an organism once found noncariogenic is actually cariogenic.

In addition to the germ-free rat, the conventional hamster has been used to demonstrate the etiologic role of streptococci in caries (Table 15-2). Caries-inactive hamsters can be made caries-active by being caged with caries-active hamsters. This may be demonstrated by transferring the caries-inactive weanling albino hamster to a cage housing a caries-active hamster and maintaining the caries-inactive animal on a diet containing 56%

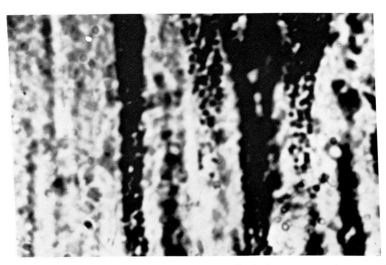

Fig. 15-6. Penetration of streptococci into the dentinal tubules in a gnotobiotic rat (1,000 ×).

sucrose. A study such as this displays the infectious and transmissible nature of dental caries. Also, specific microorganisms may be used to inoculate a freshly weaned hamster with a particular microorganism. From these studies it has been found that certain streptococci are capable of causing caries in the conventional hamster, whereas other microorganisms, including other streptococci, lactobacilli, and diphtheroids, are unable to produce caries (Table 15-2).

A similar procedure has been used to determine the cause of caries in the conventional rat. This is generally done by suppressing the gram-positive flora by feeding young rats (newborn to 35 days old) high concentrations of an antibiotic, for example, penicillin, for about one week. A test organism is then implanted usually by way of the drinking water. This technique, known as relative gnotobiosis, has reinforced previous knowledge that organisms of the *Streptococcus mutans* type cause caries. In addition, organisms of the *Strep-*

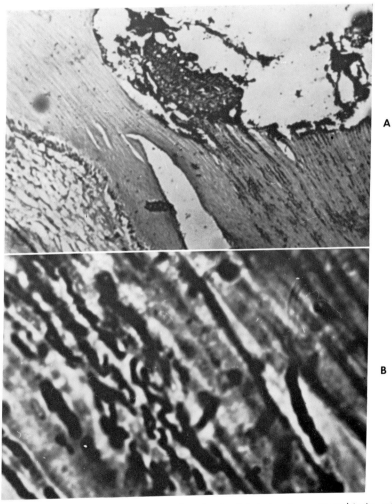

A

B

Fig. 15-7. Penetration of lactobacilli into the dentinal tubules in a gnotobiotic rat: **A,** 400 ×; **B,** 1,000 ×. (From Rosen, S., Lenney, W. S., and O'Malley, J. E.: J. Dent. Res. **47:** 358, 1968.)

Table 15-2. Cariogenic and noncariogenic strains of bacteria in gnotobiotic or relatively gnotobiotic rats and conventional hamsters

Genus and species	Cariogenicity	Reference*
Streptococcus		
faecalis	+	16
liquefaciens	+	16
mitis	+	8
salivarius	+	8, 11, 12, 15, 17, 20
sanguis	+	11, 12
mutans	+	1, 2, 3, 6, 7, 9, 10, 11, 12
		14, 15, 20, 21, 22
strain CHT	−	22
strain 112 R (*salivarius*)	−	4, 12
strain 4M4 (*uberis*)	−	12
strain JR8SM (*lactis*)	−	4
strain 2M2 (*bovis*)	−	12
strain OMZ 44 (*sanguis*)	−	11, 12
strain GS 15 (*mitis*)	−	9, 12
strain Bing 3-R (*faecalis*)	−	4
Lactobacillus		
acidophilus	+	5
casei	+	17, 18
strain HO 50X	−	7
Actinomyces (Odontomyces)		
viscosus	+	13
naeslundii	+	19

*References to Table 15-2:
1. Carlsson, J.: Arch. Oral Biol. **12**:1657, 1967.
2. Edwardsson, S.: Arch. Oral Biol. **13**:637, 1968.
3. Fitzgerald, D. B., and Fitzgerald, R. J.: Arch. Oral Biol. **11**:139, 1965.
4. Fitzgerald, R. J.: Caries Res. **2**:139, 1968.
5. Fitzgerald, R. J., Jordan, H. V., and Archard, H. O.: Arch. Oral Biol. **11**:473, 1966.
6. Fitzgerald, R. J., Jordan, H. V., and Stanley, H. R.: J. Dent Res. **39**:923, 1960.
7. Fitzgerald, R. J., and Keyes, P. H.: J. Amer. Dent. Assoc. **61**:9, 1960.
8. Gibbons, R. J., and Banghart, S.: Arch. Oral Biol. **13**:297, 1968.
9. Gibbons, R. J., Berman, K. S., Knoettner, P., and Kapsimalis, B.: Arch. Oral Biol. **11**:549, 1966.
10. Gibbons, R. J., and Loesche, W. J.: Arch. Oral Biol. **12**:1013, 1967.
11. Guggenheim, B.: Caries Res. **2**:147, 1968.
12. Houte, J. van, de Moor, C. E., and Jansen, H. M.: Arch. Oral Biol. **15**:263, 1970.
13. Keyes, P. H., and Jordan, H. V.: Arch. Oral Biol. **9**:377, 1964.
14. Krasse, B.: Arch. Oral Biol. **11**:429, 1966.
15. Krasse, B., and Carlsson, J.: Arch. Oral Biol. **15**:25, 1970.
16. Orland, F. J., Blayney, J. R., Harrison, R. W., Reyniers, J. A., Trexler, P. C., Ervin, R. F., Gordon, H. A., and Wagner, M.: J. Amer. Dent. Assoc. **50**:259, 1955.
17. Rosen, S.: Arch. Oral Biol. **15**:445, 1969.
18. Rosen, S., Lenney, W. S., and O'Malley, J. E.: J. Dent. Res. **47**:358, 1968.
19. Socransky, S. S., Hubersak, C., and Propas, D.: Arch. Oral Biol. **15**:993, 1970.
20. Zinner, D. D., and Jablon, J. M.: Arch. Oral Biol. **14**:1429, 1969.
21. Zinner, D. D., Jablon, J. M., Aran, A. P., and Saslaw, M. S.: Proc. Soc. Exp. Biol. Med. **118**:766, 1965.
22. Zinner, D. D., Jablon, J. M., Aran, A. P., Saslaw, M. S., and Fitzgerald, R. J.: Arch. Oral Biol. **11**: 1419, 1966.

tococcus sanguis type have been shown to be cariogenic by this technique. Although S. *sanguis* produces dextran, it does not ferment sorbitol or mannitol.

Why only certain organisms within a particular genus are able to cause caries in germ-free rats and in hamsters has been a subject of recent intensive investigation. The reason or reasons that these particular organisms cause caries should provide greater insight into the cause of dental caries. Apparently the acidogenic property of a microorganism, per se, is not a suitable explanation for its cariogenic potential because certain acidogenic bacteria, namely streptococci or lactobacilli, have not been able to cause caries (Table 15-2).

The colonial structures of cariogenic and noncariogenic streptococci can be distinguished when they are grown on *mitis-salivarius* agar, a differential medium con-

taining nutrients, dyes, inhibitory agents, and 5% sucrose. There are four morphologically characteristic groups (Fig. 15-8): Group 1 colonies are black, raised, rough, and of a crumblike appearance; they are surrounded by an emanation, or puddle, with a clear, gelatinous consistency. Examples of these colonies are AHT and HS-6. Group 2 colonies resemble group 1 colonies except these colonies do not show a gelatinous puddlelike emanation and have a rubbery consistency that makes it difficult to take a colony from the agar plate; these colonies are represented by FA-1 and BHT. The colonies in group 3 are large, heaped up, mucoid, and gummy and are represented by *Streptococcus salivarius* and HHT. Group 4 colonies are flat, gray, and smooth with no gelatinous emanations; these are represented by CHT. Although group 4 colonies are generally

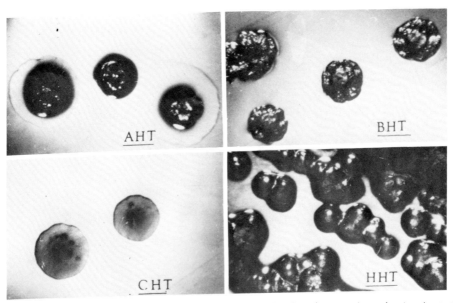

Fig. 15-8. Colonial structure of human cariogenic and related noncariogenic streptococci. AHT, human cariogenic strain similar to hamster strain (HS) of Fitzgerald; BHT, human cariogenic strain similar to rat strain (FA-1) of Fitzgerald; CHT, human noncariogenic strain with some antigens in common with the cariogenic strains; HHT, human strain, S. *salivarius* group, slightly cariogenic for hamsters. (From Zinner, D. D., and Jablon, J. M.: Human streptococcal strains in experimental caries. In Harris, R. S. [ed.]: Art and science of dental caries research, New York, 1968, Academic Press, Inc.)

noncariogenic, certain non–plaque-forming cariogenic streptococci (faecalis and liquefaciens) produce group 4 colonies (Table 15-2). Organisms in groups 1 and 2 generally produce dextran, ferment sorbitol and mannitol, and have been called *Streptococcus mutans* by a large number of dental scientists.

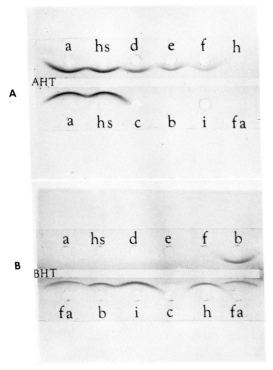

Fig. 15-9. Agar gel immunodiffusion reactions. Antisera to human strains of cariogenic streptococci are indicated in capital letters. Extracts of streptococcal strains are indicated in lower case letters; *a*, human streptococcal strain AHT; *b*, human streptococcal strain BHT; *c*, human streptococcal strain CHT; *d*, human streptococcal strain DHT; *e*, human streptococcal strain EHT; *f*, human streptococcal strain FHT; *h*, human streptococcal strain HHT; *i*, human streptococcal strain IHT; *hs*, hamster streptococcal strain HS, of Fitzgerald; *fa*, rat streptococcal strain FA, of Fitzgerald. **A,** Reactions to antisera of AHT. **B,** Reaction to antisera of BHT. (From Jablon, J. M., and Zinner, D. D.: J. Bact. **92:**1950, 1966.)

Those four groups may arbitrarily be separated into four antigenic groups. However, the four groups also are related immunologically. Agar gel immunodiffusion is one of several techniques used to demonstrate this relationship (Fig. 15-9). In this technique microscope slides, 3 inches by 1 inch, are coated with 1% melted agar to a depth of from 1 to 1.5 mm. After solidification a trough 2 mm. wide and 65 mm. long is cut in the agar along the length of the slide. Wells 2 mm. in diameter are cut above and below the trough. The antiserum is placed in the trough and the streptococcal extracts are placed in the wells. Diffusion of the antiserum and extracts toward each other is allowed to proceed for 48 hours at room temperature in a moist atmosphere. Positive reactions of antigen and corresponding antibody are indicated by precipitin bands. When there is an antigenic identity, the reaction bands are continuous; when the antigens are not identical, the reaction bands will cross or be present at different levels.

The reactions (Fig. 15-9, *A*) indicate that there is an antigenic relationship among the human streptococcal strains AHT, DHT, EHT, FHT, and the hamster cariogenic strain HS of Fitzgerald. The human strains react in a continuous band with the AHT antiserum. The extracts of streptococcal strains BHT, CHT, HHT, IHT, and the rat strain FA show no reactions.

There is also an antigenic relationship among the human BHT and IHT strains and the rat strain FA of Fitzgerald, as indicated by their reactions to the human BHT strain antiserum (Fig. 15-9, *B*). The CHT and HHT strains show cross-reactivity of some antigenic fractions to this antiserum, but these antigens are not identical because the antigen-antibody reaction bands cross the reaction bands of *fa* and *i*.

The CHT strain is noncariogenic and

the HHT strain is mildly cariogenic in hamsters. The latter organism is a strain of *Streptococcus salivarius,* which is commonly present in the human oral flora.

Further differentiation of cariogenic from noncariogenic streptococci is based on biochemical activities. Although many biochemical activities have been reported, differentiation is most widely accepted on the fermentation activities using two carbohydrates, sorbitol and mannitol. Most strains of cariogenic streptococci ferment sorbitol and mannitol, whereas most noncariogenic strains do not ferment these carbohydrates. Other studies have shown that cariogenic streptococci are less fastidious in their requirements for trace elements than noncariogenic strains. There is little or no difference between cariogenic and noncariogenic streptococci in amino acid composition of cell walls, vitamin requirements, or antibiotic spectrum.

The production of polysaccharide is another distinguishing characteristic of the cariogenic bacteria. In man the dental plaque of persons with caries contains a higher proportion of microorganisms capable of producing a strongly iodophilic polysaccharide than does plaque from persons without caries. This polysaccharide, which is produced from glucose, is intracellular and of the glycogen-amylopectin type. The storage of this intracellular polysaccharide may be significant as far as dental caries is concerned because streptococci during fasting periods are able to metabolize it with the formation of lactic acid.

Streptococci known to be cariogenic by gnotobiotic studies produce greater quantities of extracellular polysaccharides from sucrose than do certain noncariogenic streptococci. These polysaccharides are produced from sucrose but not from glucose, maltose, lactose, or fructose. The organisms that produce extracellular polysaccharide from sucrose usually produce intracellular polysaccharide from glucose.

The extracellular polysaccharide (capsular material) adheres to the side or bottom of culture vessels, forming a gelatinous mass. The capsular material can be responsible for the massive bacterial plaque accumulation observed on the teeth of animals inoculated with cariogenic streptococci. However, capsule formation is not always associated with dental caries in rats. The anatomic structure of the rat's molars with their narrow, deep fissures could allow for food accumulation that could undergo fermentation to produce acid and lead to the development of dental caries. It would be more likely to expect capsule formation on the teeth of rats to be associated with caries formation on the smoother buccal and lingual surfaces.

An extracellular polysaccharide produced by cariogenic bacteria (S. *mutans* or S. *sanguis*) has been characterized as dextran, a polymer of dextrose. Dextran is able to form with saliva an insoluble complex that adheres to the surface of the teeth. This complex cannot be readily dissolved. Furthermore, dextran is relatively resistant to hydrolysis by mixed bacterial population derived from samples of plaque and saliva. Dextran comprises about 2% of the total dried weight of plaque. Therefore, it is conceivable that the dextran-producing bacteria play a prominent role in plaque formation. It is possible that the plaque-forming bacteria enmesh non–plaque-forming cariogenic bacteria. This may explain why certain acidogenic bacteria are unable to produce caries in gnotobiotic test systems.

In contrast to dextran, a polymer of fructose, levan, an extracellular polysaccharide produced from sucrose by *Streptococcus salivarius*, is susceptible to hydrolysis by mixed bacterial populations. Nevertheless, organisms of this type have been shown to cause caries (Table 15-2). One organism (strain SS-2) resembling S. *salivarius* has induced caries in a gnotobiotic test system along with the formation of dental plaque. This organism formed levan but not dextran. In addition, strain ATCC 13419 of S. salivarius and a human isolate resembling S. salivarius have induced caries in gnotobiotic rats without the formation of plaque. Also, Streptococcus strain HHT is actually a strain of S. salivarius, and this particular strain induces caries in hamsters.

The causation of caries by S. salivarius, increases the complexity of the problem of understanding the origin of dental caries. It enhances the concept of multifactorial origin since it shows that certain levanas well as certain dextran-producing bacteria can cause caries.

The production of caries by specific bacteria has stimulated the search for a vaccine capable of inhibiting this disease. With conventional hamsters an attempt to produce an effective anticaries vaccine was not successful. With gnotobiotic rats success has been achieved with the organism Streptococcus faecalis. However, when the vaccine was tested in conventional rats, it was unsuccessful, probably because of the take-over of the cariogenic process by other bacteria. Just how an immune mechanism would operate in dental caries is still a matter of conjecture. With S. faecalis, agglutinins found in saliva in vaccinated gnotobiotic rats apparently are responsible for repressing the numbers of these bacteria in the oral cavity of these rats.

Another interesting approach in the development of a vaccine for dental caries has been to immunize animals with the enzyme dextransucrase (or glucosal transferase), the enzyme found in many cariogenic streptococci that catalyzes the conversion of sucrose to dextran. The rationale of this method is to block the organism's capacity to synthesize dextran without hindering its ability to exist in the oral environment. Reports on the success of this approach are in conflict.

Although the most recent information has been obtained with gnotobiotic rats, the bulk of research of dental caries has been with conventional animals.

Caries-test diets

Experiments investigating the factor of diet in the production of caries have been and still are considered important. Regardless of the oral flora and susceptibility of the host, caries will not develop unless an appropriate diet is fed to the subject. These diets have been termed "cariogenic diets"; recently the more appropriate term "caries-test diet" has been used.

The earlier caries-test diets consisted of coarse particles. In a classic study by Hoppert, Webber, and Canniff in 1932 it was shown that a diet consisting primarily of coarsely ground corn would produce caries in rats. When the corn was ground to the fineness of flour, caries was not produced. This diet was adequate for growth, bone development, and reproduction. Thus it was proven that nutritional inadequacy of a diet need not be a predisposing factor for caries. The composition of this diet was simple. In addition to the coarsely ground corn that comprised 60% of the diet, only whole-milk powder (30%), linseed meal (6%), alfalfa (3%), and salt (1%) constituted the entire composition of the diet. It is not known why rats developed caries on the coarse particle diet. A logical explanation is that the coarse particles caused the tooth to fracture, permitting easier penetration by microorganisms. However, evidence to the contrary does not allow us to accept this explanation. When penicillin is incorporated into the coarse particle diet, caries is inhibited and there is no evidence of fracture.

In order to simulate in experimentation the caries produced in human beings, diets containing 50% to 60% sucrose are used. The high sucrose diet under certain conditions is able to produce caries on the smoother surfaces of the teeth as well as in the fissures. With the coarse particle diet, caries develops largely in the fissures of the rat molars but not on the smooth surfaces.

In addition to sucrose, other sugars have been tested for their cariogenic potential. With the hamster the caries-producing capacity of the diet is much greater with sucrose than with glucose, lactose, or maltose. There is some evidence that sucrose produces greater caries activity than glucose in rats, although other studies have shown that glucose and sucrose are equally cariogenic. Caries-inducing streptococci are recovered in higher numbers from the oral cavities of hamsters when a diet containing sucrose is used, but with a diet containing glucose the same bacteria were recovered in low numbers. Animals fed sucrose in the form of confectioner's sugar have higher caries incidence than animals fed granulated sugar.

Certain studies have shown that dental caries in rats can be just as severe when diets contain glucose as when they contain sucrose. This has been demonstrated in both conventional and gnotobiotic studies. It has been reported that bacterial plaque and caries develop in rats whether they are fed diets containing glucose, maltose, or sucrose. Data are also available which show that with diets containing sucrose or glucose, caries can develop without the formation of a bacterial plaque. In these studies caries was not observed on the smooth surfaces of the teeth but in the sulci.

Neither the coarse particle nor the high sucrose diet is analogous to human diets. Furthermore, the carious lesions produced by these diets occurred to a great extent on occlusal surfaces and usually originated in the deep fissures of the teeth in rats. In order to simulate the development of caries on the buccal, lingual, and proximal tooth surfaces in animals, since these are tooth surfaces in human dentition that are susceptible to caries, diets containing processed cereal food with a low content of refined sugar and diets containing dry skim milk and dry whey powders were used. These diets caused a high incidence of smooth-surface caries, which occurs especially on lower buccal areas. The growth rate of the animals on these diets was poor, but growth was greatly improved by a supplement of lysine. The lysine supplement also inhibited the development of caries. Moreover, L-lysine and not D-lysine was biologically active. However, one diet that contained unautoclaved milk powder was not deficient in lysine but was distinctly cariogenic; addition of L-lysine to this diet gave variable results.

White bread and whole wheat flour have been identified as foods capable of producing caries on the smooth surfaces of the molar teeth of rats. Diets containing these substances are able to induce plaque formation on the smooth surfaces. Speculations as to why these substances induce plaque formation advance the explanation that these diets contain adhesive components or that they may support better growth and development of microorganisms capable of initiating and maintaining the bacterial plaque.

Rats that are pretreated with antibiotics and given a diet capable of inducing both sulcal and smooth-surface carious lesions develop only sulcal lesions. This indicates that a segment of the oral microflora that is essential for the induction of caries on smooth tooth surfaces has been selectively eliminated by the antibiotic treatment. Therefore in the rat, microorganisms exist that can induce only smooth-surface lesions, and there are other microorganisms that can induce sulcal lesions. However gnotobiotic studies have shown that certain specific microorganisms can induce both sulcal and smooth-surface carious lesions in rats.

Speculation as to which foods are cariogenic for human beings has usually implicated those containing high concentrations of sugar. It has been extremely difficult to conduct controlled experiments involving food consumption by human beings. In

Table 15-3. Comparison of caries scores produced by various foods*

Food material tested	Experiments with non-cariogenic supplement Mean of eight rats	Experiments with cariogenic supplement Mean of eight rats
Dog biscuits	0.0	0.0
Popcorn	0.0	1.8
Sorbitol	0.0	1.0
Peanuts	0.0	2.3
Whole milk†	0.0	4.2
Lemon‡	0.0	4.3
Corn chips	0.0	7.0
Cabbage	0.0	7.0
Lettuce	0.0	9.7
Control (basic diet only)	0.0	11.3
Dried apricots‡	0.0	11.3
Oranges‡	0.0	16.8
Soda crackers	0.3	11.6
Spinach	0.6	4.6
Cracked wheat bread	1.3	13.7
Potato chips	1.6	6.7
Whole wheat bread	2.0	17.7
Carrots†	2.1	21.1
Cornstarch†	3.3	10.2
White bread and butter	4.9	22.1
White bread and peanut butter	5.2	18.0
Graham crackers	8.7	22.7
Raisin bread	9.0	17.2
Melba toast	9.0	19.6
White bread	9.2	15.1
White bread and raspberry jam	10.2	33.0
Figs	10.3	29.0
Rye bread	12.7	29.0
Chewing gum	14.0	27.2
Caramels	16.0	50.4
Chocolate graham crackers	18.0	39.1
Baby cookies	18.5	22.0
Honey graham crackers	19.2	21.6
Apples‡	19.4	81.7
Vanilla wafers	19.7	30.2
Bananas	21.0	73.7
Chocolate sandwich cookies	23.8	92.2

*Adapted from Stephan, R. M.: J. Dent. Res. **45:** 1551, 1966.
†Produced a higher than average calculus score (greater than 1.5).
‡Produced dental erosion.

Table 15-3. Comparison of caries scores produced by various foods—cont'd

Food material tested	Experiments with non-cariogenic supplement Mean of eight rats	Experiments with cariogenic supplement Mean of eight rats
Grapes‡	24.1	42.4
Candy mints	24.7	42.1
Teething biscuits	29.0	29.2
Cola‡	29.6	40.2
Marshmallows	30.1	42.2
Dextrose	30.6	43.5
Raisins	30.9	61.6
10% sucrose water	32.3	20.6
Dates	32.7	38.5
Milk chocolate	34.1	41.2
White bread and jelly	36.7	36.2
Confectioner's sugar	38.4	60.2
10% dextrose water	41.3	45.5
Orange drink‡	43.5	26.1
Sucrose	62.1	51.9

order to evaluate which foods can lead to the development of caries in human beings, an experiment was conducted in rats in which fifty-three foods were added to a cariogenic and to a noncariogenic diet. The selection of most of these foods was based on the diets of persons with an extensively carious dentition. The cariogenic nature of these foods is given in Table 15-3. This table lists the mean caries score for experimental groups fed a noncariogenic basic diet and a cariogenic basic diet, respectively. The foods are listed in order of increasing caries scores for the experimental group fed the noncariogenic basic diet. The control group, listed tenth from the top, had a mean score of 11.3 when fed the cariogenic supplement. Therefore dog biscuits, popcorn, sorbitol, peanuts, and whole milk, which induce no caries with the noncariogenic supplement and significantly less caries than the control group with the cariogenic supplement, apparently contain anticariogenic substances.

The foods that are highly cariogenic have a high sugar content. The refined sugars, sucrose and dextrose, and certain fruits are able to induce high caries scores. Since fruits contain sugars such as sucrose, dextrose, fructose, or maltose, it is not too surprising that these foods are cariogenic. This finding furnishes evidence that fruits do not contain some unknown protective substance that renders them noncariogenic. Thus, there should be a reappraisal of current programs for preventing caries that advocate feeding fruits such as apples to children in schools. Instead, whole milk alone may serve as a beneficial noncariogenic between-meal snack. Whole milk as well as the noncariogenic supplement, which contains 50% lactose, are noncariogenic. This indicates that lactose or milk sugar is noncariogenic. Many oral microorganisms that ferment dextrose, fructose, and sucrose do not readily ferment lactose.

Saliva

Saliva has been adequately demonstrated to be a caries-inhibiting fluid in experimental animals. It has been found that if the salivary glands are extirpated from animals, there is a marked increase in susceptibility to dental caries. (The surgical removal of salivary glands has been termed desalivation, salivariadenectomy, or sialoadenectomy.) In rats that have undergone sialoadenectomy, there is an increase in the numbers of lactobacilli in the oral cavity. The removal of the salivary glands also removes the buffering capacity (Fig. 15-10), antibacterial activity, washing action, enzymatic activity, maturation potential, and so forth of saliva, all of which could influence the carious process.

The saliva of human beings has been studied extensively. Saliva from rodents has been studied to a lesser extent, partly be-

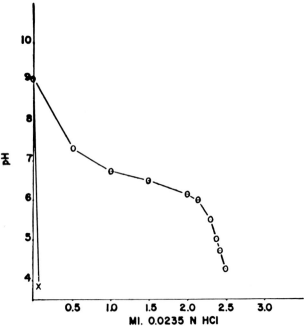

Fig. 15-10. Typical curve illustrating buffering capacity of diluted rat saliva compared with that of distilled water. O-O, 1 ml. rat saliva + 4 ml. distilled water; O = X, 4 ml. distilled water adjusted to pH 9.1 with sodium hydroxide. (From Sylvester, C. J., Rosen, S., Hoppert, C. A., and Hunt, H. R.: J. Dent. Res. **43**:528, 1964.)

cause the technique for collection was not developed until recently (Fig. 15-11). Basically, the technique of collecting rodent saliva consists of anesthetizing the animal and then administering a sialogogue such as pilocarpine hydrochloride or methyl choline. From 2 to 3 ml. of saliva can be collected from an adult rat in about 20 minutes.

As soon as saliva leaves the mouth, whether it be a rodent or a human mouth, changes occur in both its chemical and physical composition. Carbon dioxide is lost immediately, resulting in an increase in pH. Microbial activity can either raise or lower the pH. Changes in pH can cause precipitation of calcium phosphates or protein or both. Proper studies of saliva must take these rapid changes into consideration. Inserting a cannula into the salivary ducts and collecting saliva under oil is one method of obtaining it near its natural state. However, as soon as this saliva is used for a study, it will undergo certain rapid changes.

Both human and rodent salivas have a pronounced effect on the oral flora. Although there are reports indicating that saliva enhances the growth of certain bacteria, most reports indicate that it inhibits most species of microorganisms.

Fluoride

Animals have been used to study the effect of fluorides on dental caries. There is evidence that fluoride has an anticaries effect when administered systemically if given during the formation of the tooth. One of the findings that led to the suggestion of incorporating fluorides in the drinking water of human beings was that rat teeth formed with a submottling dosage of fluoride derived from placental and mammary transmission had increased

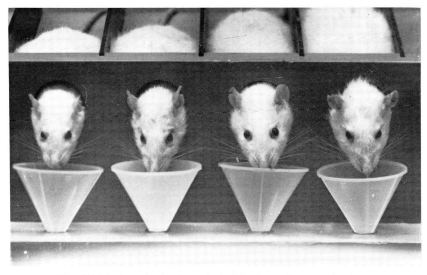

Fig. 15-11. Anesthetized rats in holder for collection of saliva.

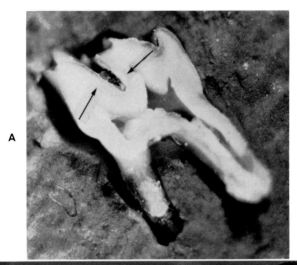

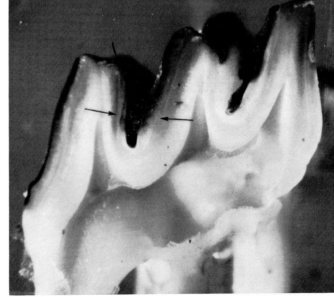

Fig. 15-12. Mineralization of rat molars revealed by staining with silver nitrate. Black areas indicate the penetration of silver nitrate into hypomineralized areas. **A,** A molar showing no hypomineralization. **B,** A molar showing a slight degree of hypomineralization. The blackened area in the enamel has not extended to the dentinoenamel junction. **C,** A molar showing a higher degree of hypomineralization. The blackened area extends up to the dentinoenamel junction. **D,** A molar showing hypomineralization extending beyond the dentinoenamel junction.

resistance to caries. Rats given fluoride by a tube inserted into the stomach, even those whose salivary glands had been removed, have shown greater resistance to dental caries. However, several reports indicate that fluoride exerts its anticariogenic effect through local rather than systemic action. Subcutaneous injection of fluoride into rats results in little or no protection from dental caries. The third molars of hamsters do not develop caries if treated with fluoride posteruptively, but preeruptive treatment does not retard the development of rampant caries.

The mechanism of caries inhibition by fluoride has not been established. Ex-

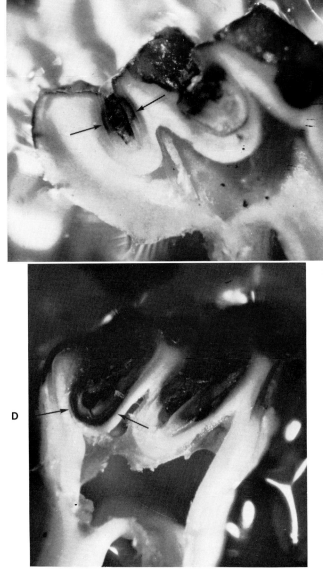

Fig. 15-12, cont'd. For legend see opposite page.

perimental evidence supports two main theories: that of the solubility depressing action on inorganic tooth structure and the enzyme inhibition theory.

It has been shown that fluoride interacts with enamel, resulting in a reduced solubility of enamel in acid. However, many other substances such as stannous chloride and certain cations (lead, silver, copper) reduce enamel solubility without increasing resistance to caries.

The enzyme inhibition theory is based on the fact that fluoride inhibits many enzymes, including those in the glycolytic cycle, that is, the breakdown of sugars to organic acids. The enzymes in the glycolytic cycle most sensitive to fluoride are phosphatase, enolase, and phosphoglyceromutase. It is known that very little fluoride (1 ppm.) is needed to inhibit acid production by oral bacteria and that the concentration of fluoride in human dental plaque is about 67 ppm. in low fluoride areas. The relatively high concentration of fluoride in plaque may not be present as free ions, but it is not known in what form this fluoride is present and what fraction of this fluoride is free to inhibit. There is evidence, however, that fluoride ions are released from enamel to an extent that is inhibitory to the production of lactate. This was shown in an experiment in which a pure culture of *Lactobacillus casei* was placed in a glass well containing nutrients held on the flattened surface of extracted incisor teeth of humans, some of which were pretreated with fluoride, some were from a natural fluoride area, and others were untreated, low fluoride controls. After 10 hours' incubation, there was significantly less lactate produced in the wells held on the naturally and artificially fluoridized teeth than in the wells held on the low fluoride controls.

Further evidence to support the enzyme inhibition theory has come from certain experiments with animals. Fluoride applied to the teeth of conventionally reared animals shows a maturation or enhanced mineralization effect (Fig. 15-12). There is no such effect in germ-free animals when fluoride- and nonfluoride-treated animals are compared. Penicillin, a known inhibitor of caries and gram-positive bacteria, also produces a maturation effect. These findings are best explained by reasoning that the oral microflora exerts a demineralization effect, whereas fluoride exerts a mineralizing effect by its antibacterial activity rather than its ability to reduce enamel solubility.

An interesting approach to the study of fluoride efficacy has been studied in animals. Applications of fluoride could be made with powders, solutions, or gels. Repeated daily applications were more effective than intermittent ones. Intensive applications also prevented copious deposit of plaque. Preeruptive benefits could not be demonstrated. As a follow-up study involving human beings, gels containing 0.5% fluoride ion were applied to children by means of custom-fitted vinyl applicators each day of the school year for almost two years. During this interval, children who were untreated developed an average of four grossly carious surfaces, whereas only one new surface broke down in the treated group. Unfortunately, there was no significant improvement in the oral hygiene status as a result of the treatment.

Anticariogenic agents other than fluoride

Animals have been used to test anticariogenic agents other than fluoride. Antibiotics have been tested extensively. The antibiotics that primarily inhibit the gram-positive flora, such as penicillin and bacitracin, are more effective as caries inhibitors than are broad-spectrum antibiotics such as chloramphenicol (Chloromycetin), streptomycin, chlortetracycline (Aureomycin), and oxytetracycline (Terramycin). Antibiotics are effective in reducing the numbers of oral streptococci and lactobacilli, and it is presumed that caries is inhibited by this mechanism.

Another inhibitor of caries that has proven effective in animal caries tests is sodium N-lauryl sarcosinate. This compound has the ability to inhibit glycolysis, to be retained in the plaque, and to inhibit caries in animals. It's efficacy in human beings, however, is unresolved.

In addition to the compounds just mentioned, an array of chemicals and antibiotics has been screened in animals for anticaries activity. The general nature of the effectiveness of these agents lies in their ability to be retained at the site of caries activity and to act by inhibiting the cariogenic flora or decreasing the solubility of enamel in acid or both.

The addition of phosphates to diets has inhibited the production of dental caries in animals. The mechanism of the activity of phosphates is not clearly defined. Various phosphates that are capable of inhibiting caries, such as orthophosphate, trimetaphosphate, hexametaphosphate, and pyrophosphate, may each have a different mode of action. Orthophosphate and pyrophosphate provide increased buffer action in the oral environment. In addition orthophosphate can counteract demineralization of the tooth by common ion effect, bring about replacements of carbonate and citrate with phosphate in the enamel surface, and promote formation of mineral in the enamel with a low solubility in acid.

The evidence for the effectiveness of phosphate in inhibiting caries is that it is a local rather than a systemic mechanism. Parenteral administration of phosphate is without effect in caries inhibition.

An understanding of the phosphate effect on caries could be of practical value since phosphates may be incorporated into human diets. Much of the phosphate content of certain foods is lost during refining; therefore one could justify the addition of phosphates to foods on this basis, just as vitamins are added to certain foods if it is known that during refining or processing some of the vitamin content has been lost. For example, in one study with rats the addition of 2% calcium monohydrogen phosphate to sugar-coated cereals resulted in significant reduction in dental caries.

Whether or not dietary phosphates affect the oral flora is still to be decided. There is positive correlation between enamel lesions and streptococci when animals receiving phosphate are killed after 47 days, but there is no correlation when they are killed after 68 days.

On the basis that dextran is an important constituent of the dental plaque, an experiment was conducted to determine if the enzyme dextranase, when incorporated into the diet or drinking water, could inhibit the formation of caries. This enzyme, obtained from the mold *Penicillum funiculosum,* was effective in inhibiting dental caries in hamsters that were infected with dextran-producing microorganisms.

Another plaque-inhibiting agent, chlorhexidine, has been found to inhibit plaque formation in the hamster when a 0.2% solution is swabbed onto the teeth. Chlorhexidine has an unusually strong affinity for enamel defects, dental caries, dental plaque, periodontal membranes, epithelium of the tongue, silicate cements, and some acrylates.

PERIODONTAL DISEASE
Experimental animals

Animals have been used in the study of periodontal disease. This disease is characterized by an inflammatory process affecting one or more of the supporting tissues of the teeth—the gingival tissue, the periodontal membrane, or the alveolar bone. Periodontal disease has been described in monkeys, dogs, albino rats, rice rats (Fig. 15-13), guinea pigs, Syrian hamsters, ferrets, mice, and marmosets (Fig. 15-14). The marmoset is a small primate possessing dentition similar to that

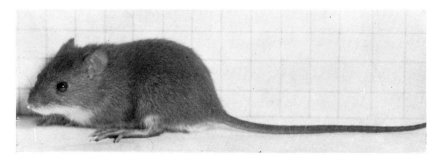

Fig. 15-13. Rice rat. (From Gupta, O. P., and Shaw, J. H.: Oral Surg. **9:**592, 1956.)

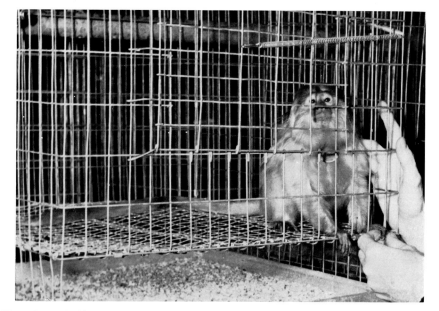

Fig. 15-14. Golden marmoset *(Leontocebus rosalia)*. (Courtesy B. Levy, Houston, Tex.)

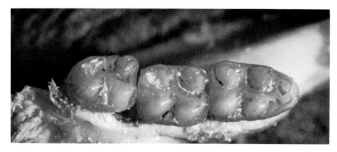

Fig. 15-15. Occlusal view of right mandibular molars of the rice rat. (From Gupta, O. P., and Shaw, J. H.: Oral Surg. **9:**592, 1956.)

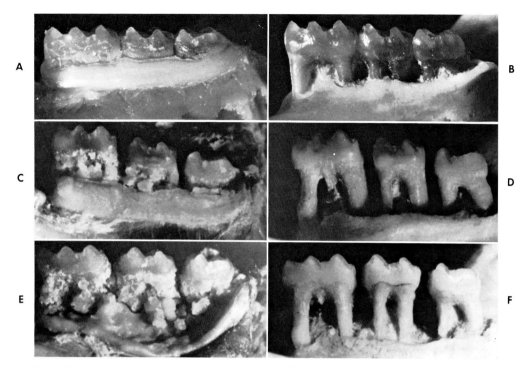

Fig. 15-16. Photographs of fixed preparations of jaws of rice rat that were selected to illustrate the extent of periodontal lesions. **A, C,** and **E,** Lingual aspects of mandibles with the soft tissue in situ. **B, D,** and **F,** Lingual aspects of the same mandibles after the soft tissues have been removed to reveal the amount of alveolar bone resorption. **A** and **B** show a moderate involvement of periodontal structures. **C** and **D** show more severe periodontal involvement. **E** and **F** illustrate extensive destruction of the periodontal structures. (From Gupta, O. P., and Shaw, J. H.: Oral Surg. **9:**727, 1956.)

of human beings. The rice rat has been made susceptible to periodontal disease by selective inbreeding. The dentition and effects of periodontal disease in this animal are presented in Figs. 15-15 to 15-20. Similar histologic effects are evident in the marmoset (Fig. 15-21).

Microbiology

Hairs in the gingival papillae of germ-free rats provoke a typical foreign-body reaction, accompanied in some cases by ulceration and profuse exudation. Germ-free mice lose alveolar bone at a rate comparable to conventional animals; however, the role of microorganisms in periodontal disease should not be minimized.

Although factors such as local irritants, nutrition, general health, and trauma from occlusion undoubtedly contribute toward the initiation and progression of periodontal disease, microorganisms are also an important etiologic factor.

The evidence from animal studies of the involvement of microorganisms in periodontal disease is as follows. Enterococci are recovered in greater numbers from rice rats with periodontal disease than from rice rats free of periodontal disease. However, periodontal disease of equal severity occurs in rice rats from which low numbers of enterococci are recovered. Penicillin, whether given *per os* or subcutaneously, successfully prevents the initiation and

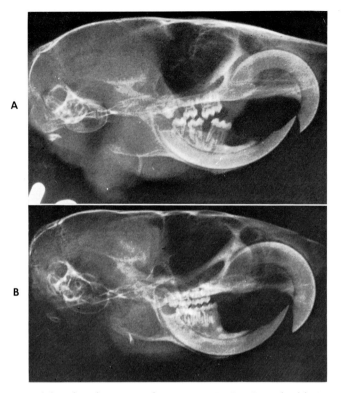

Fig. 15-17. Lateral head radiograms of rice rats. **A,** A 15-week-old rice rat susceptible to periodontal disease. Note the drifting of molar teeth resulting from loss of supporting bone. **B,** A 52-week-old rice rat resistant to periodontal disease. Note the properly aligned molar teeth. (From Mulvihill, J. E., Susi, F. R., Shaw, J. H., and Goldhaber, P.: Arch. Oral Biol. **12:**733, 1967.)

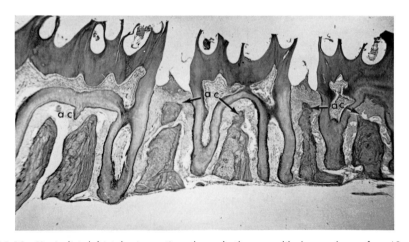

Fig. 15-18. Mesiodistal histologic section through the mandibular molars of a 48-week-old resistant rice rat. The interdental and interradicular bone height (alveolar crest, ac) and width are maximum. The papillae are pointed, and the interproximal space contains no debris. (From Mulvihill, J. E., Susi, F. R., Shaw, J. H., and Goldhaber, P.: Arch. Oral Biol. **12:**733, 1967.)

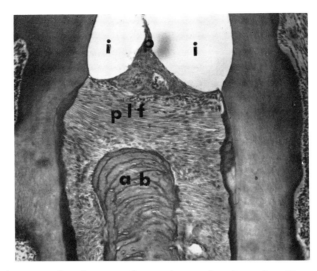

Fig. 15-19. High-power view between first and second molars of a 48-week-old resistant rice rat. Note the sharply pointed papilla, *p;* the high level of alveolar bone, *ab;* the continuity of the periodontal ligament fibers, *plf;* and the absence of interproximal accumulation of debris, *i.* (From Mulvihill, J. E., Susi, F. R., Shaw, J. H., and Goldhaber, P.: Arch. Oral Biol. **12:**733, 1967.)

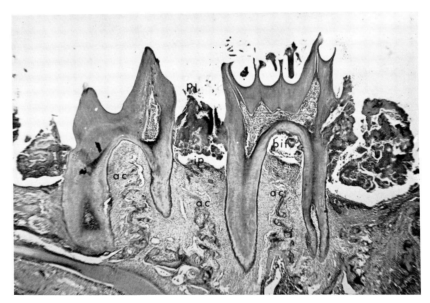

Fig. 15-20. Mesiodistal histologic section through first and second molars of a 15-week-old susceptible rice rat, showing the histopathologic picture of severe advanced periodontal disease. Note the marked recession of the interdental papilla, *ip,* and the overlying interproximal accumulation of basophilic-staining plaque material, *pl.* Also note the more apical position of the alveolar crest, *ac,* as well as the decreased width of aveolar bone due to bone resorption. There is bifurcation involvement of the first molar, *bif.* (From Mulvihill, J. E., Susi, F. R., Shaw, J. H., and Goldhaber, P.: Arch Oral Biol. **12:**733, 1967.)

progression of periodontal lesions, presumably by inhibiting the formation of plaque deposits. Rice rats resistant to periodontal disease and penicillin-pretreated, susceptible rice rats, when inoculated with microorganisms from rice rats with rapidly progressing periodontal lesions, demonstrate greatly increased rates of initiation and progression of periodontal lesions.

An active type of periodontal disease was observed in golden and cream hamsters fed a high carbohydrate diet, but not in the albino hamster. However, inoculat-

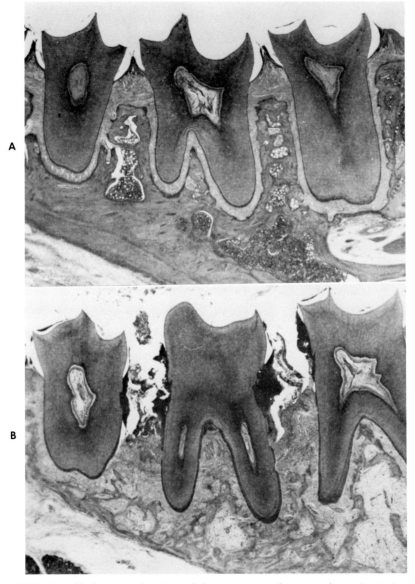

Fig. 15-21. Mandibular periodontium of the marmoset (hematoxylin-eosin stain; original magnification 10 x). **A,** Relatively normal periodontium. **B,** Periodontium with advanced chronic destructive periodontitis. (From Levy, B. M.: J. Dent. Res. **50:**246, 1971.)

ing the albino hamster with scrapings from the subgingival plaque of affected animals induced the disease. Once acquired, the disease may be transmitted from generation to generation.

An extension of thus study with hamsters has implicated aerobic gram-positive filamentous organisms as etiologic agents in periodontal disease in the albino hamster (Figs. 15-22 to 15-24). This origin was shown by inoculating albino hamsters with these organisms. Since the experiment was performed in a conventional environment, there could have been interactions with other bacteria that contributed to the disease.

When human gingival debris is inoculated into germ-free mice, there is an enhancement of bone loss without development of massive plaque accumulations typical of periodontal disease in other rodents.

As in studies in dental caries, it has been difficult to determine the cause of periodontal disease until gnotobiotic techniques have been applied. In gnotobiotic albino rats dextran- and levan-producing streptococci are able to cause alveolar bone loss (Figs. 15-25 to 15-27). In addition to streptococci, *Actinomyces naeslundii*, *Actinomyces viscosus*, and certain bacilli and diphtheroids produce marked subgingival plaque formation and alveolar bone loss in gnotobiotic albino rats or hamsters or both. In gnotobiotic rats a particular strain of *Actinomyces naeslundii* is capable of colonizing the cervical and root surfaces of teeth, and of forming destructive bacterial plaques that lead to pocket formation, destruction of alveolar bone, root caries, and exfoliation.

Microorganisms that induce alveolar bone loss in animals may also induce root caries. Certain dextran- and levan-forming streptococci (Figs. 15-27, 15-29) and *Acti-*

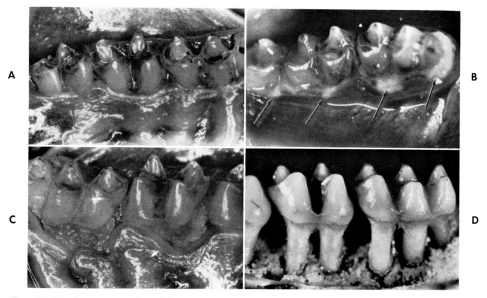

Fig. 15-22. Gross periodontal lesions induced in albino hamsters by aerobic gram-positive filamentous organism, strain T6A. **A,** Normal gingival tissue in a noninfected animal. **B,** Growth of subgingival plaque (arrows) on buccal surfaces of mandibular molars. **C,** Heavy accumulation of subgingival plaque and soft tissue displacement. **D,** Alveolar bone loss and root surface lesions in an inoculated hamster. (From Jordan, H. V., and Keyes, P. H.: Arch. Oral Biol. **9:**401, 1964.)

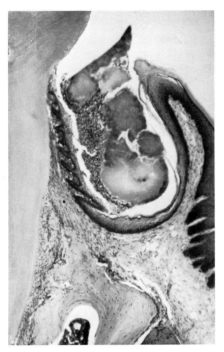 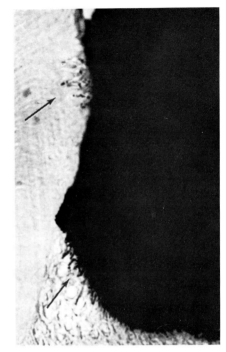

Fig. 15-23   **Fig. 15-24**

Fig. 15-23. Extensive plaque deposit associated with pocket formation, epithelial migration and invagination, inflammatory exudation, and alveolar crest resorption on the lingual surface of a maxillary molar in an albino hamster inoculated with filamentous strain T6. (From Jordan, H. V., and Keyes, P. H.: Arch. Oral Biol. **9:**401, 1964.)

Fig. 15-24. High-power photomicrograph of gram-stained section. Dense plaque accumulation (dark area) is evident in a gingival pocket of an albino hamster inoculated with a filamentous strain T6. Upper arrow indicates early penetration of dentin by the filamentous organism. Lower arrow shows filaments at periphery of plaque surrounded by an accumulation of inflammatory cells. (From Jordan, H. V., and Keyes, P. H.: Arch. Oral Biol. **9:**401, 1964.)

nomyces viscosus are known to cause root caries.

Material from human periodontal lesions, when inoculated intradermally into rabbits or guinea pigs, has produced infections. Sustained infection can also follow the injection of mixed microbial flora from an undiseased human mouth. It is now known that only certain combinations of oral bacteria can produce this infection. *Spirochaeta, Fusobacterium, Vibrio,* and anaerobic streptococci do not contribute to the experimental infection, but a com-

bination of four organisms—two *Bacteroides* (one of which is *B. melaninogenicus*), a motile gram-negative anaerobic rod, and a facultative diphtheroid—will produce the typical infection. *B. melaninogenicus* contains a glucolipid endotoxin and produces collagenase; the diphtheroid provides a vitamin K-like factor required by *B. melaninogenicus.*

That pathogenic microorganisms invade the soft tissues surrounding the teeth is debatable. Animal studies have not contributed any knowledge in this area.

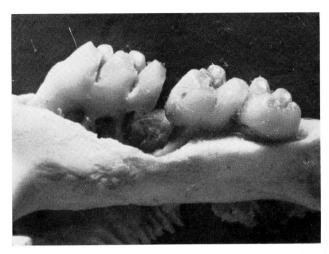

Fig. 15-25. Alveolar bone loss and root caries in a gnotobiotic rat inoculated with dextran-producing human streptococcus strain GS5. (From Gibbons, R. J., Berman, K. S., Knoellner, P., and Kapsimalis, B.: Arch. Oral Biol. **11:**549, 1966.)

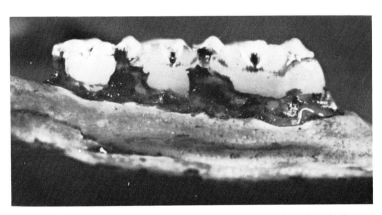

Fig. 15-26. Plaque accumulation in a gnotobiotic rat inoculated with levan-producing human streptococcus strain SS2. (Courtesy R. Gibbons, Boston, Mass.)

Animal studies have shown that massive plaque accumulation is associated with alveolar bone loss (Figs. 15-23, 15-26, 15-27). Such studies have not shown which disease-producing entities (for example, toxins, or enzymes such as hyaluronidase, collagenase, and beta-glucuronidase) are involved in periodontal disease.

Multifactorial origin

As in dental caries, there is multifactorial origin in periodontal disease; not only are different microorganisms in-

volved, but the interaction of local and systemic factors contributes to the initiation and progression of periodontal lesions. A strain of rice rat resistant to periodontal disease has been developed through selective inbreeding. Although the disease can be readily transmitted to the resistant rat, the rate and progression of the periodontal syndrome still does not equal that observed in susceptible rice rats.

The nature of the diet is another factor that should be considered in periodontal syndrome etiology. In studies with rice

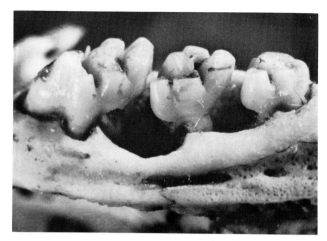

Fig. 15-27. Alveolar bone loss and root caries in a gnotobiotic rat inoculated with levan-producing human streptococcus strain SS2. (Courtesy R. Gibbons, Boston, Mass.)

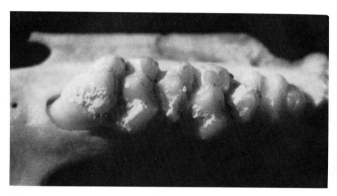

Fig. 15-28. Supragingival calculus on maxillary molars of a rat.

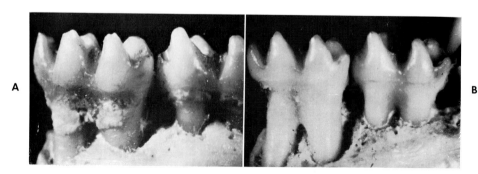

Fig. 15-29. A, Subgingival calculus on the lingual surface of the first mandibular molar of a hamster which was fed a high sucrose diet for 57 days and a laboratory stock diet for 40 days. **B,** Companion animal fed a high sucrose diet continuously for 97 days. Note typical root surface lesion and bone resorption but no calculus. (From Jordan, H. V., and Keyes, P. H.: Arch. Oral Biol. **9:**401, 1964.)

rats, when sucrose is replaced by maltose there is a significant reduction in the periodontal syndrome, and replacement by either whole wheat flour or white flour results in still greater reductions in the syndrome.

Parallels between human and animal periodontal disease

Periodontal disease in the rice rat exhibits many parallels to human periodontal disease, including an accumulation of debris around the teeth; gingival irritation leading to inflammation, ulceration, or atrophy of the gingival epithelium; resorption of alveolar bone and cementum; degeneration of the fibrous and cellular elements of the periodontal ligament; and gingival recession and pocket formation.

There are also certain differences between periodontal disease in rats and that in human beings. In the rice rat the disease is more generalized and progresses rapidly, presumably because of the rat's inability to cleanse the debris once initial lesions have occurred and because of predisposing systemic influences. Long-term antibiotic therapy is ineffective in preventing or arresting periodontal disease in human beings, whereas antibiotics are effective in preventing periodontal disease in animals.

CALCULUS

The production of calculus in experimental animals has been the subject of recent investigations. Calculus is a concretion that forms on the surfaces of teeth. It may occur supragingivally or subgingivally. It contains certain crystalline minerals—brushite, apatite (a carbonate-hydroxyl variety), whitlockite, and tetracalcium hydrogen triphosphate trihydrate (octacalcium phosphate)—as well as organic and inorganic matter. Its organic content ranges from 6% to 15%, water content from 6% to 20%, calcium from 30% to 40%, phosphorus from 6% to

20%, magnesium from 0.4% to 14%, and carbonate from 2% to 5%.

Mineralization of microorganisms

The initiation of calculus is dependent upon the formation of dental plaque. The conditions under which the plaque may calcify have not been determined. Apparently saliva with its supersaturated supply of calcium and phosphate and high carbon dioxide tension contributes substantially to the formation of calculus.

In vitro studies have shown that certain microorganisms become calcified when grown in a medium or placed in a solution containing mineral salts in concentrations found in saliva. Pieces of skin, tongue, lip, and mucous membrane do not calcify when placed in the same solution.

Animals have been employed in an unusual manner in the study of calculus formation. *Streptococcus salivarius,* an oral diphtheroid, *Actinomyces israelii, Actinomyces naeslundii, Bacterionema matruchotii,* and a preparation of collagen become mineralized with apatite when implanted in dialysis bags in the peritoneal cavities of rats for a period of 90 days. The first signs of mineralization are detected between 14 and 26 days. Apatite forms within from six to eight days in specimens containing acetone-treated or autoclaved cultures of *S. salivarius.* The mineralization of nonviable bacteria indicates that the metabolic process of bacteria is not essential for mineralization. Although a variety of organic material could serve as a nucleating site for calculus formation, it is apparent that one naturally occurring site is bacterial.

Calculus in animals

The formation of calculus has been observed on the teeth of certain experimental animals. A satisfactory diet for the reproducible, uniform production of calculus in rats has the following composition: 50% cornstarch, 32% nonfat dry milk powder,

3% liver powder, 5% celluflour, 1% cottonseed oil, 5% powdered sucrose, 1% $CaCl_2 \cdot 2H_2O$, 2.7% $NaH_2PO_4 \cdot H_2O$, and 0.3% $MgSO_4$. The powdered sucrose contained in the diet raises the calculus level probably because of increased bacterial plaque formation. The starch and milk powder contribute to calculus formation by providing the protein and physical texture to the diet that seem to encourage the formation of calculus. The inorganic salts are all necessary in the diet for optimum calculus formation. When fluoride was added to the diet, calculus increased probably because of the antisolubility property that fluoride imparts to apatite. The age of the animal does not appear to be important in experimental calculus, but the oral flora does have a slight affect on calculus accretion.

When the diet just described was used, supragingival calcareous deposits were observed on the molar teeth of albino rats (Fig. 15-28). These deposits were identified by x-ray diffraction as apatite. Neither chloramphenicol nor chlortetracycline, antibiotics capable of inhibiting a broad spectrum of microorganisms, exerts any inhibitory effects on the deposition of calculus.

Subgingival calculus has been observed on the lingual surface of hamster molars (Fig. 15-29). The formation of calculus in the hamster is enhanced by a laboratory stock diet.

Deposition of calculus has been reported in germ-free mice and rats. Hard, alizarin-staining deposits were found on the maxillary molars of germ-free mice. When a diet deficient in folic acid was used, brittle pellicular material collected from the first maxillary molar of germ-free rats was identified as apatite by x-ray diffraction.

The development of calculus in germ-free animals has been explained by the hydrolysis of fatty acid esters by esterase. The enzyme esterase is found in deposits on teeth and is thought to originate from epithelial cells, polymorphonuclear leukocytes, and macrophages. Fatty acids released by this enzymic action would then combine with calcium and magnesium to form soaps that, in turn, would be converted into less soluble forms of carbonate and phosphate.

Another explanation for the production of calculus in the germ-free animal is that salivary carbonic anhydrase catalyzes the formation of carbonate hydroxyapatite, using the inorganic constituents of the saliva and diet as a substrate. Using commercially available carbonic anhydrase, synthetic calculus was produced in vitro under circumstances that did not involve the presence of fatty acids.

Cornstarch has been identified as a calculus-inducing food substance in rats. Other available starches such as unmodified wheat, rice, arrowroot, tapioca, amioca, potato, and corn or pregelatinized potato, tapioca, amioca, and wheat do not form as much calculus as does cornstarch. Calculus has been induced by amylopectin, the insoluble fraction of starch, to a greater extent than by amylose, the soluble fraction.

REFERENCES AND ADDITIONAL READINGS

Baer, P. N., and White, C. L.: Studies on experimental calculus formation in the rat. X. The effect of various starches, J. Periodont. **38**:41, 1967.

Bagnall, J. S.: Bibliography on caries research, Ottawa, 1950, National Research Council of Canada.

Benarde, M. A., Fabian, F. W., Rosen, S., Hoppert, C. A., and Hunt, H. R.: A method for the collection of large quantities of rat saliva, J. Dent. Res. **35**:326, 1956.

Bowen, W. H.: A bacteriological study of experimental dental caries in monkeys, Int. Dent. J. **15**:12, 1965.

Briner, W. W., and Rosen S.: Effect of fluoride and penicillin on post-eruptive maturation of rat molars, Calc. Tiss. Res. **2**:60, 1968.

Briner, W. W., and Rosen, E.: Effect of fluoride on hypomineralized areas in the molars of rats fed a cariogenic diet, Arch. Oral Biol. **12**:1007, 1967.

Brislin, J. F., and Cox, G. J.: Survey of the literature of dental caries 1948-1960, Pittsburgh, Pa., 1964, University of Pittsburgh Press.

Brudevold, F., Amdur, B. H., Vogel, J. J., and Spinelli, M.: Effect of ingested supplementary phosphate on the tooth surface, J. Dent. Res. **43:**1168, 1964.

Burnett, G. W., and Scherp, H. W.: Oral microbiology and infectious disease, Baltimore, 1968, The Williams & Wilkins Co.

Englander, H. R., and Keyes, P. H.: Pre- and post-eruptive effect of sodium fluoride on dental caries in the syrian hamster, J. Dent. Res. **45:** 1149, 1966.

Fitzgerald, D. B., and Fitzgerald, R. J.: Induction of dental caries in gerbils, Arch. Oral Biol. **11:**139, 1966.

Fitzgerald, R. J., Jordan, H. V., and Archard, H. O.: Dental caries in gnotobiotic rats infected with a variety of *Lactobacillus acidophilus*, Arch. Oral Biol. **11:**473, 1966.

Fitzgerald, R. J., Jordan, H. V., and Stanley, H. R.: Experimental caries and gingival pathologic changes in the gnotobiotic rat, J. Dent. Res. **39:** 925, 1960.

Fitzgerald, R. J., and Keyes, P. H.: Demonstration of the etiologic role of streptococci in experimental caries in the hamster, J. Amer. Dent. Assoc. **61:**9, 1960.

Fitzgerald, R. J., and McDaniel, E. G.: Dental calculus in the germ-free rat, Arch. Oral Biol. **2:**239, 1960.

Francis, M. D., and Briner, W. W.: Animal calculus: Methods of evaluation and of dietary production and control, J. Dent. Res. **48:**1185, 1968.

Francis, M. D., and Briner, W. W.: The development and regression of hypomineralized areas of rat molars, Arch. Oral Biol. **11:**349, 1966.

Gibbons, R. J., and Banghart, S. B.: Synthesis of extracellular dextran by cariogenic bacteria and its presence in human dental plaque, Arch. Oral Biol. **12:**11, 1967.

Gibbons, R. J., Berman, K. S., Knoettner, P., and Kapsimalis, B.: Dental caries and alveolar bone loss in gnotobiotic rats infected with capsule forming streptococci of human origin, Arch. Oral Biol. **11:**549, 1966.

Gibbons, R. J., and Socransky, S. S.: Enhancement of alveolar bone loss in gnotobiotic mice harbouring human gingival bacteria, Arch. Oral Biol. **11:**847, 1966.

Grenby, T. H.: The effects of some carbohydrates on experimental dental caries in the rat, Arch. Oral Biol. **8:**27, 1963.

Gupta, O. P., Auskaps, A. M., and Shaw, J. H.: Periodontal disease in the rice rat. IV. The ef-

fects of antibiotics on the incidence of periodontal lesions, Oral Surg. **10:**1169, 1957.

Gupta, O. P., and Shaw, J. H.: Periodontal disease in the rice rat. I. Anatomic and histopathologic findings, Oral Surg. **9:**592, 1956.

Harris, R. S.: Art and science of dental caries research, (ed.) New York, 1968, Academic Press Inc.

Hoppert, C. A., Webber, P. A., and Canniff, T. L.: The production of dental caries in rats fed an adequate diet, J. Dent. Res. **12:**161, 1932.

Hunt, H. R., and Goodman, H. O.: The inheritance of resistance and susceptibility to dental caries, Int. Dent. J. **12:**306, 1962.

Jablon, J. M., and Zinner, D. D.: Differentiation of cariogenic streptococci by fluorescent antibody, J. Bact. **92:**1590, 1966.

Jordan, H. V., and Keyes, P. H.: Aerobic, gram-positive, filamentous bacteria as etiologic agents of experimental periodontal disease in hamsters, Arch. Oral Biol. **9:**401, 1964.

Keyes, P. H.: The infectious and transmissible nature of experimental dental caries: Findings and implications, Arch. Oral Biol. **1:**304, 1960.

Krasse, B.: Human streptococci and experimental caries in hamsters, Arch. Oral Biol. **11:**429, 1966.

Larson, R. H., Theilade, E., Fitzgerald, R. J.: The interaction of diet and microflora in experimental caries in the rat, Arch. Oral Biol. **12:**663, 1967.

Luckey, T. D.: Germfree life and gnotobiology, New York, 1963, Academic Press Inc.

McClure, F. J.: Dietary factors in experimental rat caries. In Sognnaes, R. F. (ed.) Advances in experimental caries research, Washington, D. C., 1955, American Association for the Advancement of Science.

MacDonald, J. B., Gibbons, R. J., and Socransky, S. S.: Bacterial mechanisms in periodontal disease, Ann. N. Y. Acad. Sci. **85:**467, 1960.

MacDonald, J. B., Socransky, S., and Sawyer, S.: A survey of the bacterial flora of the periodontium in the rice rat, Arch. Oral Biol. **1:**1, 1959.

Mulvihill, J. E., Susi, F. R., Shaw, J. H., and Goldhaber, P.: Histological studies of the periodontal syndrome in rice rats and the effects of penicillin, Arch. Oral Biol. **12:**733, 1967.

National Academy of Sciences, National Research Council: A survey of the literature of dental caries, Publication 225, Washington, D.C., 1952, The Academy.

Orland, F. J., Blayney, J. R., Harrison, R. W., Reyniers, J. A., Trexler, P. C., Ervin, R. F., Gordon, H. A., and Wagner, M.: Experimental caries in germ-free rats inoculated with enterococci, J. Amer. Dent. Assoc. **50:**259, 1955.

Rizzo, A. A., Martin, G. R., Scott, D. B., and Mergenhagen, S. E.: Mineralization of bacteria, Science **135**:439, 1962.

Rogosa, M., Johansen, E., and Disraely, M. N.: Relation of streptococci, lactobacilli, and the general oral and fecal flora to the progression of dental caries in the hamster, J. Dent. Res. **36**:695, 1957.

Rosen, S.: Comparison of sucrose and glucose in the causation of dental caries in gnotobiotic rats, Arch. Oral Biol. **14**:445, 1969.

Rosen, S., Hunt, H. R., and Hoppert, C. A.: A comparison of two methods of quantitative determinations of bacteria associated with teeth in rats, J. Dent. Res. **43**:717, 1964.

Rosen, S., Lenney, W. S., and O'Malley, J. E.: Dental caries in gnotobiotic rats inoculated with *Lactobacillus casei*, J. Dent. Res. **47**:358, 1968.

Rosen, S., Ragheb, H. S., Hunt, H. R., and Hoppert, C. A.: Effects of penicillin and Terramycin on dental caries and certain oral microflora in Hunt-Hoppert caries-susceptible rats, J. Dent. Res. **35**:399, 1956.

Shaw, J. H., Krumins, I., and Gibbons, R. J.: Comparison of sucrose, lactose, maltose and glucose in the causation of experimental oral diseases, Arch. Oral Biol. **12**:755, 1967.

Socransky, S. S., Hubersak, C., and Propas, D.: Induction of periodontal destruction in gnotobiotic rats by a human oral strain of *Actinomyces naeslundii*, Arch. Oral Biol. **15**:993, 1970.

Socransky, S. S., MacDonald, J. B., Sawyer, S. J., and Auskaps, A. M.: Quantitative studies of the bacterial flora of the periodontium in rice rats, Arch. Oral Biol. **2**:104, 1960.

Speirs, R. L.: Factors influencing "maturation" of developmental hypomineralized areas in the enamel of rat molars, Caries Res. **1**:15, 1967.

Sylvester, C. J., Rosen, S., Hoppert, C. A., and Hunt, H. R.: A comparison of certain properties from specific major salivary glands of caries-resistant and caries-susceptible rats, J. Dent. Res. **43**:528, 1964.

Wagner, M.: Specific immunization against *Streptococcus fecalis* induced dental caries in the gnotobiotic rat, American Society for Microbiology, Sixty-seventh Annual Meeting, New York, April-May, 1967.

Zinner, D. D., Jablon, J. M., Aran, A. P., and Saslaw, M. S.: Experimental caries induced in animals by streptococci of human origin, Proc. Soc. Exp. Biol. Med. **118**:766, 1965.

Zinner, D. D., Jablon, J. M., Aran, A. P., Saslaw, M. S., and Fitzgerald, R. J.: Comparative pathogenicity of streptococci of human origin in hamster caries, Arch. Oral Biol. **11**:1419, 1966.

Index